MOUNT SINAI
EXPERT GUIDES
Oncology

MOUNT SINAI EXPERT GUIDES

Oncology

EDITED BY

William K. Oh, MD
Chief, Division of Hematology and Medical Oncology
Deputy Director, The Tisch Cancer Institute
Professor of Medicine and Urology
Ezra M. Greenspan, MD Professor in Clinical Cancer Therapeutics
Icahn School of Medicine at Mount Sinai
New York, NY, USA

Ajai Chari, MD
Associate Professor of Medicine
Director Clinical Research, Multiple Myeloma Program
Associate Medical Director, Tisch Cancer Institute Clinical Trials Office
Icahn School of Medicine at Mount Sinai
New York, NY, USA

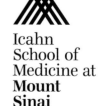

Icahn
School of
Medicine at
**Mount
Sinai**

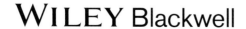

This edition first published 2019
© 2019 John Wiley & Sons Ltd

The right of William K. Oh and Ajai Chari to be identified as the editors of this work has been asserted in accordance with law.

Registered Office(s)
John Wiley & Sons, Inc., 111 River Street, Hoboken, NJ 07030, USA
John Wiley & Sons Ltd, The Atrium, Southern Gate, Chichester, West Sussex, PO19 8SQ, UK

Editorial Office
9600 Garsington Road, Oxford, OX4 2DQ, UK

For details of our global editorial offices, customer services, and more information about Wiley products visit us at www.wiley.com.

Wiley also publishes its books in a variety of electronic formats and by print-on-demand. Some content that appears in standard print versions of this book may not be available in other formats.

Library of Congress Cataloging-in-Publication Data

Names: Oh, William K., editor. | Chari, Ajai, editor.
Title: Mount Sinai expert guides. Oncology / [edited by] William K. Oh, Ajai Chari.
Other titles: Oncology
Description: Hoboken, NJ : Wiley, 2019. | Includes bibliographical references and index. |
Identifiers: LCCN 2019015625 (print) | LCCN 2019017014 (ebook) | ISBN 9781119189572 (Adobe PDF) | ISBN 9781119189589 (ePub) |
  ISBN 9781119189558 (pbk.)
Subjects: | MESH: Neoplasms | Medical Oncology–methods | Handbook
Classification: LCC RC263 (ebook) | LCC RC263 (print) | NLM QZ 39 | DDC 616.99/4–dc23
LC record available at https://lccn.loc.gov/2019015625

Cover image: © Raycat/Getty Images
Cover design by Wiley

Set in 8.5/12pt FrutigerLTStd by Aptara Inc., New Delhi, India
Printed and bound in Singapore by Markono Print Media Pte Ltd

10 9 8 7 6 5 4 3 2 1

Contents

Contributors, ix

Series Foreword, xvii

Preface, xviii

List of Abbreviations, xix

About the Companion Website, xxviii

Part 1: ONCOLOGY

1 Breast Cancer, 3
Jeanette Guziel and Charles L. Shapiro

2 Prostate Cancer, 23
Reza Mehrazin and William K. Oh

3 Bladder Cancer, 32
Matthew D. Galsky

4 Renal Cancer, 43
Bobby C. Liaw, Reza Mehrazin, and Che-Kai Tsao

5 Testicular Cancer, 56
Aditya V. Shreenivas and Seth M. Cohen

6 Lung Cancer, 66
Rajwanth Veluswamy and Jorge E. Gomez

7 Malignant Mesothelioma, 79
Nicholas C. Rohs and Zishuo I. Hu

8 Liver Cancer, 89
Augusto Villanueva, Myron E. Schwartz, and Josep M. Llovet

9 Gallbladder/Biliary Duct Cancers, 101
Rajwanth Veluswamy, Anuja Kriplani, and Celina Ang

10 Pancreas Cancer, 111
Max W. Sung

11 Colorectal Cancer, 118
Kenneth L. Angelino, Jason W. Steinberg, and Peter S. Kozuch

12 Gastric Cancer, 131
Sofya Pintova

13 Esophageal Cancer, 139
Madhuri Rao and Andrea S. Wolf

14 Anal Cancer, 153
Ashley J. D'Silva, Danielle S. Seiden, and Peter S. Kozuch

15 Invasive Epithelial Ovarian Cancer, 166
Brittney S. Zimmerman, Jeanette Guziel, and Amy Tiersten

16 Endometrial Cancer, 181
Jamal Rahaman and Carmel J. Cohen

17 Cervical Cancer, 194
Navya Nair, Ann Marie Beddoe, and Peter Dottino

18 Melanoma, 204
Philip Friedlander and Corazon B. Cajulis

19 Sarcomas, 214
Robert G. Maki

20 Thyroid Cancer, 221
Aaron M. Etra and Krzysztof Misiukiewicz

21 Head and Neck Cancer, 230
Le Min Lee and Bruce E. Culliney

22 Brain Tumors, 241
Rebecca M. Brown and Adília Hormigo

23 Neuroendocrine Tumors, 255
Richard R.P. Warner, Jacob A. Martin, and Michelle K. Kim

Part 2: MALIGNANT HEMATOLOGY

24 Myeloproliferative Neoplasms, 271
Sangeetha Venugopal, Daniel Aruch, and John Mascarenhas

25 Myelodysplastic Syndromes, 288
Thomas U. Marron and Lewis R. Silverman

26 Multiple Myeloma and Plasma Cell Disorders, 298
Siyang Leng and Ajai Chari

27 Acute Myeloid Leukemia, 308
Kevin Barley and Shyamala C. Navada

28 Acute Lymphoblastic Leukemia, 319
Jaclyn C. Davis and Birte Wistinghausen

29 Chronic Lymphocytic Leukemia, 332
Adam F. Binder and Janice L. Gabrilove

30 Non-Hodgkin Lymphoma, 342
Adam F. Binder and Joshua D. Brody

31 Hodgkin Lymphoma, 354
Jonah Shulman, Parth R. Rao and Akshay Sudhindra

32 Primary Central Nervous System Lymphoma, 364
Rebecca M. Brown and Adília Hormigo

Part 3: BONE MARROW TRANSPLANT

33 Autologous Stem Cell Transplantation for Plasma Cell Disorders, 379
Keren Osman

34 Allogeneic Stem Cell Transplantation Overview, 385
Parth R. Rao, Amir Steinberg, and Luis Isola

35 Allogeneic Stem Cell Transplantation for AML and MDS, 392
Alla Keyzner

36 Stem Cell Transplantation for Lymphoproliferative Disorders, 400
Doyun Park, Eileen Scigliano, and Amir Steinberg

37 Infectious Complications of Stem Cell Transplantation, 404
Meenakshi M. Rana and Amir Steinberg

38 Acute Graft Versus Host Disease, 412
Anne S. Renteria, James L.M. Ferrara, and John E. Levine

Part 4: MULTIDISCIPLINARY CARE OF CANCER PATIENTS

39 Oncologic Emergencies, 423
Scot A. Niglio and Adriana K. Malone

40 Thrombosis in Cancer Patients, 435
Doyun Park, Caroline Cromwell, Mala Varma, and Ilan Shapira

41 Imaging of Cancer Patients, 447
Idoia Corcuera-Solano, Mathilde Wagner, and Bachir Taouli

42 Overview of Radiation Oncology, 454
Ronald D. Ennis

43 Orthopedic Oncology, 463
Meredith K. Bartelstein and Ilya Iofin

44 Ophthalmologic Oncology, 473
Albert Y. Wu and Kalla A. Gervasio

45 Cardio-Oncology, 486
Gagan Sahni

46 Psychiatric and Psychologic Dimensions of Cancer Care, 501
Talia Wiesel

47 Geriatric Oncology, 514
Ali John Zarrabi, Ran Huo, and Cardinale B. Smith

48 Palliative Care, 519
Lori Spoozak and Bethann Scarborough

49 Nutrition and Symptom Management, 528
Paula Occiano, Melissa Nagelberg, and Raquela Adelsberg

50 Cancer Survivorship, 535
Lindsay Haines and Charles L. Shapiro

51 Pediatric Cancer: Solid Tumors and Lymphoma, 543
Surabhi Batra and Birte Wistinghausen

52 Pediatric Cancer: Brain Tumors, 556
Surabhi Batra and Birte Wistinghausen

Index, 566

Contributors

Raquela Adelsberg, MS, RD, CDN
Clinical Nutrition Coordinator
Icahn School of Medicine at Mount Sinai
New York, NY, USA

Celina Ang MD
Associate Professor
Icahn School of Medicine at Mount Sinai
New York, NY, USA

Kenneth L. Angelino MD
Icahn School of Medicine at Mount Sinai
New York, NY, USA

Daniel Aruch MD
Oncologist
Virginia Oncologist Associates
Virginia Beach, VA, USA

Kevin Barley MD
Hematologist
Hematology and Medical Oncology
Icahn School of Medicine at Mount Sinai
New York, NY, USA

Meredith K. Bartelstein MD
Fellow, Orthopedic Oncology
Memorial Sloan Kettering Cancer Center
New York, NY, USA

Surabhi Batra MD
Icahn School of Medicine at Mount Sinai
New York, NY, USA

Ann Marie Beddoe MD
Icahn School of Medicine at Mount Sinai
New York, NY, USA

Adam F. Binder MD
Icahn School of Medicine at Mount Sinai
New York, NY, USA

Joshua D. Brody
Icahn School of Medicine at Mount Sinai
New York, NY, USA

Rebecca M. Brown MD, PhD
Icahn School of Medicine at Mount Sinai
New York, NY, USA

Corazon B. Cajulis DNP, RN, ANP-BC
Icahn School of Medicine at Mount Sinai
New York, NY, USA

Ajai Chari MD
Associate Professor of Medicine
Director Clinical Research, Multiple Myeloma
    Program
Associate Medical Director, Tisch Cancer
    Institute Clinical Trials Office
Icahn School of Medicine at Mount Sinai
New York, NY, USA

Carmel J. Cohen MD
Professor Emeritus
Obstetrics, Gynecology and Reproductive
    Science
Icahn School of Medicine at Mount Sinai
New York, NY, USA

Seth M. Cohen MD
Icahn School of Medicine at Mount Sinai
New York, NY, USA

Idoia Corcuera-Solano MD
Translational and Molecular Imaging Institute
Department of Radiology
Icahn School of Medicine at Mount Sinai
New York, NY, USA

Caroline Cromwell MD
Assistant Professor
Medicine, Hematology, and Medical Oncology
Icahn School of Medicine at Mount Sinai
New York, NY, USA

Bruce E. Culliney MD
Assistant Professor
Medicine, Hematology, and Medical Oncology
Icahn School of Medicine at Mount Sinai
New York, NY, USA

Jaclyn C. Davis MD
Clinical Development Medical Director
Novartis Pharmaceuticals Corporation
East Hanover, NJ, USA

Peter Dottino MD
Icahn School of Medicine at Mount Sinai
New York, NY, USA

Ashley J. D'Silva MD
Icahn School of Medicine at Mount Sinai
New York, NY, USA

Ronald D. Ennis MD
Professor and Vice Chair of Network
   Integration and Quality
Department of Radiation Oncology
Cancer Institute of New Jersey
Robert Wood Johnson Medical School and
   New Jersey Medical School of Rutgers
   University
New Brunswick, NJ, USA

Aaron M. Etra MD
Assistant Professor
Medicine, Hematology, and Medical Oncology
Icahn School of Medicine at Mount Sinai
New York, NY, USA

James L.M. Ferrara MD
Professor, Medicine, Hematology and Medical
   Oncology
Professor, Pediatrics
Professor, Oncological Sciences
Icahn School of Medicine at Mount Sinai
New York, NY, USA

Philip Friedlander MD, PhD
Director of Melanoma Medical Oncology
   Program
Assistant Professor, Division of Hematology
   and Medical Oncology
Assistant Professor, Department of
   Dermatology
Icahn School of Medicine at Mount Sinai,
New York, NY, USA

Janice L. Gabrilove MD, PHD
Professor, Oncological Sciences
Professor, Medicine, Hematology, and Medical
   Oncology
Icahn School of Medicine at Mount Sinai
New York, NY, USA

Matthew D. Galsky MD
Professor of Medicine
Icahn School of Medicine at Mount Sinai
Director, Genitourinary Medical Oncology
Tisch Cancer Institute
New York, NY, USA

Kalla A. Gervasio MD
Ophthalmology Resident
Department of Ophthalmology
Wills Eye Hospital
Philadelphia, PA, USA

Jorge E. Gomez MD
Assistant Professor
Medicine, Hematology, and Medical Oncology
Icahn School of Medicine at Mount Sinai
New York, NY, USA

Jeanette Guziel MD
Hematology/Oncology
Kaiser Permanente
Southern California Permanente Medical
   Group
Woodland Hills, CA, USA

Lindsay Haines MD
Resident
Icahn School of Medicine at Mount Sinai
New York, NY, USA

Adília Hormigo MD, PhD
Director, Neuro-Oncology at Mount Sinai and
    Mount Sinai Health System
Professor of Neurology, Medicine, and
    Neurosurgery
Icahn School of Medicine at Mount Sinai
The Tisch Cancer Institute
New York, NY, USA

Zishuo I. Hu MD, PhD
Professor
Icahn School of Medine at Mount Sinai
New York, NY, USA

Ran Huo MD
Department of Hospital Medicine
The Everett Clinic
Providence Regional Medical Center
Everett, WA, USA

Ilya Iofin MD
Chief of Orthopaedic Oncology Service
Department of Orthopaedic Surgery
Icahn School of Medicine at Mount Sinai
New York, NY, USA

Luis Isola MD
Gerald J. Friedman Chair in Oncology
Professor of Medicine
Director, Cancer Clinical Programs, Mount
    Sinai Health System
Director, Bone Marrow and Stem Cell
    Transplantation Program, Tisch Cancer
    Institute
Director, Cancer Network, Mount Sinai Health
    Network
Icahn School of Medicine at Mount Sinai
New York, NY, USA

Alla Keyzner MD
Assistant Professor
Medicine, Hematology, and Medical Oncology
Icahn School of Medicine at Mount Sinai
New York, NY, USA

Michelle K. Kim MD
Professor
Center for Carcinoid and Neuroendocrine
    Tumors
Gastroenterology Division
Icahn School of Medicine at Mount Sinai
New York, NY, USA

Anuja Kriplani MD, MPH
Jack Martin Division of Pediatric
    Hematology-Oncology
Icahn School of Medicine at Mount Sinai
New York, NY, USA

Peter S. Kozuch MD
Icahn School of Medicine at Mount Sinai
New York, NY, USA

Le Min Lee MD
Icahn School of Medicine at Mount Sinai
New York, NY, USA

Siyang Leng MD
Instructor of Medicine
Division of Hematoloy/Oncology
Columbia University Irving Medical Center
New York, NY, USA

John E. Levine MD
Professor, Medicine, Hematology, and Medical
    Oncology
Professor, Pediatrics
Icahn School of Medicine at Mount Sinai
New York, NY, USA

Bobby C. Liaw MD
Assistant Professor
Medicine, Hematology, and Medical Oncology
Icahn School of Medicine at Mount Sinai
New York, NY, USA

Josep M. Llovet MD, PhD
Professor of Medicine
Division of Liver Diseases
Icahn School of Medicine at Mount Sinai
New York, NY, USA;
Liver Cancer Translational Research
    Laboratory, IDIBAPS, CIBEREHD
Hospital Clinic, Universitat de Barcelona;
Institució Catalana de Recerca i Estudis
    Avançats
Barcelona, Spain

Robert G. Maki MD, PhD, FACP
Northwell Cancer Institute and Cold Spring
    Harbor Laboratory
Long Island, NY, USA

Adriana K. Malone MD
Associate Professor
Tisch Cancer Institute Bone Marrow and Stem
    Cell Transplantation
Director, Hematology/Oncology and BMT
    Fellowship Programs
Icahn School of Medicine at Mount Sinai
New York, NY, USA

Thomas U. Marron MD, PhD
Assistant Professor
Medicine, Hematology, and Medical Oncology
Icahn School of Medicine at Mount Sinai
New York, NY, USA

Jacob A. Martin MD
Center for Carcinoid and Neuroendocrine
    Tumors
Gastroenterology Division
Icahn School of Medicine at Mount Sinai
New York, NY, USA

John Mascarenhas MD
Director, Adult Leukemia Program
Leader, Myeloproliferative Disorders Clinical
    Research Program
Associate Professor of Medicine
Tisch Cancer Institute, Division of
    Hematology/Oncology
Icahn School of Medicine at Mount Sinai
New York, NY, USA

Reza Mehrazin MD
Assistant Professor
Department of Urology
Icahn School of Medicine at Mount Sinai
New York, NY, USA

Krzysztof Misiukiewicz MD
Associate Professor, Medicine, Hematology,
    and Medical Oncology
Assistant Professor, Otolaryngology
Icahn School of Medicine at Mount Sinai
New York, NY, USA

Melissa Nagelberg MS, RD
Icahn School of Medicine at Mount Sinai
New York, NY, USA

Navya Nair MD
Icahn School of Medicine at Mount Sinai
New York, NY, USA

Shyamala C. Navada MD, MSCR
Assistant Professor
Tisch Cancer Institute
Icahn School of Medicine at Mount Sinai
New York, NY, USA

Scot A. Niglio MD
Fellow, Hematology and Medical Oncology
Icahn School of Medicine at Mount Sinai
New York, NY, USA

Paula Occiano RD, CDN, CSO
Clinical Nutrition Coordinator
Tisch Cancer Institute
Icahn School of Medicine at Mount Sinai
New York, NY, USA

William K. Oh MD
Chief, Division of Hematology and Medical
    Oncology
Deputy Director, Tisch Cancer Institute
Professor of Medicine and Urology
Ezra M. Greenspan, MD Professor in Clinical
    Cancer Therapeutics
Icahn School of Medicine at Mount Sinai
New York, NY, USA

Keren Osman MD
Bone Marrow Transplant Program
Mount Sinai Medical Center
New York, NY, USA

Doyun Park MD
Instructor, Department of Medicine
Blood and Bone Marrow Transplant Program
NYU School of Medicine
New York, NY, USA

Sofya Pintova MD
Division of Hematology and Medical Oncology
Icahn School of Medicine at Mount Sinai
New York, NY, USA

Jamal Rahaman MD
Associate Clinical Professor
Obstetrics, Gynecology and Reproductive
    Science
Icahn School of Medicine at Mount Sinai
New York, NY, USA

Meenakshi M. Rana MD
Icahn School of Medicine at Mount Sinai
New York, NY, USA

Madhuri Rao MD
Assistant Professor
Division of Thoracic and Foregut Surgery
University of Minnesota
Minneapolis, MN, USA

Parth R. Rao MD
Associate, Cancer Institute
Geisinger Medical Center
Danville, PA, USA

Anne S. Renteria MD
Leader, Acute Lymphoblastic Leukemia
Research and Clinical Service
Bone Marrow Transplant & Adult Leukemia
    Program
Assistant Professor of Medicine
Tisch Cancer Institute
Icahn School of Medicine at Mount Sinai
New York, NY, USA

Nicholas C. Rohs MD
Assistant Professor
Medicine, Hematology, and Medical
    Oncology
Icahn School of Medicine at Mount Sinai
New York, NY, USA

Gagan Sahni MD, FACC, FACP
Associate Professor of Medicine
Director of Cardio-Oncology
Director of Cardiology Consult Services
Mount Sinai Cardiovascular Institute
New York, NY, USA

Bethann Scarborough MD
Associate Director of Ambulatory
    Services
Assistant Professor of Palliative Medicine
Brookdale Department of Geriatrics and
    Palliative Medicine
Icahn School of Medicine at Mount Sinai
New York, NY, USA

Myron E. Schwartz MD
Professor of Surgery
Department of Surgery
Icahn School of Medicine at Mount Sinai
New York, NY, USA

Eileen Scigliano MD
Associate Professor of Medicine
Icahn School of Medicine at Mount Sinai
Physician Lead, World Trade Center Cancer
    Program
Department of Environmental Medicine and
    Public Health
New York, NY, USA

Danielle S. Seiden MD
Icahn Scool of Medicine at Mount Sinai
New York, NY, USA

Ilan Shapira MD
Assistant Professor
Medicine, Hematology, and Medical
    Oncology
Icahn School of Medicine at Mount Sinai
New York, NY, USA

Charles L. Shapiro MD, FASCO
Professor of Medicine, Division of Hematology
   and Oncology
Director of Translational Breast Cancer
   Research
Director of Cancer Survivorship
Icahn School of Medicine at Mount Sinai
Tisch Cancer Institute
New York, NY, USA

Aditya V. Shreenivas MD
Icahn Scool of Medicine at Mount Sinai
New York, NY, USA

Jonah Shulman MD
Assistant Professor
Division of Hematology and Oncology
Icahn School of Medicine at Mount Sinai
New York, NY, USA

Lewis R. Silverman MD
Tisch Cancer Institute
Icahn School of Medicine at Mount Sinai
New York, NY, USA

Cardinale B. Smith MD, PhD
Associate Professor of Medicine
Director of Quality for Cancer Services, Mount
   Sinai Health System
Division of Hematology/Medical Oncology and
   Brookdale Department of Geriatrics and
   Palliative Medicine
Icahn School of Medicine at Mount Sinai
New York, NY, USA

Lori Spoozak MD, MHS, FACOG
Clinical Assistant Professor
Division of Gynecologic Oncology
Department of Obstetrics and Gynecology
Clinical Assistant Professor
Palliative Medicine Division
Department of Internal Medicine
University of Kansas School of Medicine
Kansas City, KS, USA

Amir Steinberg MD, FACP
Associate Professor of Medicine
Unit Director, Quality Director, Bone Marrow
   Transplant Program
Icahn School of Medicine at Mount Sinai
New York, NY, USA

Jason W. Steinberg MD
Icahn School of Medicine at Mount Sinai
New York, NY, USA

Akshay Sudhindra MD
Icahn School of Medicine at Mount Sinai
New York, NY, USA

Max W. Sung MD
Associate Professor
Medicine, Hematology, and Medical Oncology
Icahn School of Medicine at Mount Sinai
New York, NY, USA

Bachir Taouli MD
Translational and Molecular Imaging Institute
Department of Radiology
Icahn School of Medicine at Mount Sinai
New York, NY, USA

Amy Tiersten MD
Professor of Medicine
Clinical Director, Breast Medical Oncology at
   Mount Sinai Hospital
Icahn School of Medicine at Mount Sinai
New York, NY, USA

Che-Kai Tsao MD
Associate Professor
Medicine, Hematology and Medical Oncology
Icahn School of Medicine at Mount Sinai
New York, NY, USA

Mala Varma MD
Assistant Clinical Professor
Medicine, Hematology and Medical Oncology
Icahn School of Medicine at Mount Sinai
New York, NY, USA

Rajwanth Veluswamy MD, MSCR
Assistant Professor
Medicine, Hematology and Medical Oncology
Icahn School of Medicine at Mount Sinai
New York, NY, USA

Sangeetha Venugopal MD
Fellow, Hematology and Medical Oncology
Tisch Cancer Institute
Icahn School of Medicine at Mount Sinai
New York, NY, USA

Augusto Villanueva MD, PhD
Assistant Professor of Medicine
Division of Liver Diseases
Division of Hematology and Medical Oncology
Icahn School of Medicine at Mount Sinai
New York, NY, USA

Mathilde Wagner MD
Translational and Molecular Imaging Institute
Department of Radiology
Icahn School of Medicine at Mount Sinai
New York, NY, USA

Richard R.P. Warner MD
Professor Emeritus
Center for Carcinoid and Neuroendocrine
  Tumors
Gastroenterology Division
Icahn School of Medicine at Mount Sinai
New York, NY, USA

Talia Wiesel PhD
Assistant Professor, Psychiatry
Icahn School of Medicine at Mount Sinai
New York, NY, USA

Birte Wistinghausen MD
Children's National Health System,
The George Washington University,
Washington, DC, USA

Andrea S. Wolf MD, MPH
Associate Professor
Department of Thoracic Surgery
Icahn School of Medicine at Mount Sinai
New York, NY, USA

Albert Y. Wu MD, PhD, FACS
Department of Ophthalmology
Stanford University School of Medicine
Palo Alto, CA, USA

Ali John Zarrabi MD
Assistant Professor of Medicine
Associate Director, Outpatient Supportive
  Care, Emory Healthcare
Division of Hospital Medicine
Emory University School of Medicine
Atlanta, GA, USA

Brittney S. Zimmerman MD
Fellow, Hematology and Medical Oncology
Icahn School of Medicine at Mount Sinai
New York, NY, USA

Series Foreword

Now more than ever, immediacy in obtaining accurate and practical information is the coin of the realm in providing high quality patient care. The Mount Sinai Expert Guides series addresses this vital need by providing accurate, up-to-date guidance, written by experts in formats that are accessible in the patient care setting: websites, smartphone apps, and portable books. The Icahn School of Medicine, which was chartered in 1963, embodies a deep tradition of preeminence in clinical care and scholarship that was first shaped by the founding of the Mount Sinai Hospital in 1855. Today, the Mount Sinai Health System, comprised of seven hospitals anchored by the Icahn School of Medicine, is one of the largest health care systems in the United States, and is revolutionizing medicine through its embracing of transformative technologies for clinical diagnosis and treatment. The Mount Sinai Expert Guides series builds upon both this historical renown and contemporary excellence. Leading experts across a range of disciplines provide practical yet sage advice in a digestible format that is ideal for trainees, mid-level providers, and practicing physicians. Few medical centers in the United States could offer this type of breadth while relying exclusively on its own physicians, yet here no compromises were required in offering a truly unique series that is sure to become embedded within the key resources of busy providers. In producing this series, the editors and authors are fortunate to have an equally dynamic and forward-viewing partner in Wiley Blackwell, which together ensures that health care professionals will benefit from a unique, first-class effort that will advance the care of their patients.

Scott Friedman MD
Series Editor
Dean for Therapeutic Discovery
Fishberg Professor and Chief, Division of Liver Diseases
Icahn School of Medicine at Mount Sinai
New York, NY, USA

Preface

In an era of innumerable sources of information yet ever increasing and competing demands on clinicians' time, it can be difficult to come up to speed quickly, yet reliably, on the rapidly evolving management of hematology and oncology patients. This is certainly true for those in training but also for busy practitioners treating a diversity of patients. In this Expert Guide we strive to provide concise summaries – using bullet points, tables, and figures in lieu of verbose texts, written by renowned disease experts at the Icahn School of Medicine at Mount Sinai, New York. The sections are divided into oncology, hematology, bone marrow transplant, and, importantly, an entire section on the multidisciplinary care of cancer patients. The content can be viewed in conventional print form or, for those preferring digital access, via the internet or a smartphone app. For those looking for more in-depth information, lists of further reading are also provided.

William K. Oh, MD
Chief, Division of Hematology and Medical Oncology
Deputy Director, The Tisch Cancer Institute
Professor of Medicine and Urology
Ezra M. Greenspan, MD Professor in Clinical Cancer Therapeutics
Icahn School of Medicine at Mount Sinai
New York, NY, USA

Ajai Chari, MD
Associate Professor of Medicine
Director Clinical Research, Multiple Myeloma Program
Associate Medical Director, Tisch Cancer Institute Clinical Trials Office
Icahn School of Medicine at Mount Sinai
New York, NY, USA

List of Abbreviations

AA	African American
AASLD	American Association for the Study of Liver Diseases
ABVD	Adriamycin-bleomycin-vinblastine-dacarbazine
ACE	angiotensin-converting enzyme
ACOG	American College of Obstetrics and Gynecology
ACS	American Cancer Society
ACTH	adenocorticotropic hormone
ADC	apparent diffusion coefficient
ADL	activities of daily living
ADT	androgen deprivation therapy
AFIP	Atlas of Tumor Pathology
AFP	alpha fetoprotein
aGVHD	acute graft versus host diesease
AI	aromatase inhibitor
AIHA	autoimmune hemolytic anemia
AIN	anal intraepithelial neoplasia
AJCC	American Joint Committee on Cancer
AKI	acute kidney insufficiency
AL	(primary) amyloidosis
ALCL	anaplastic large cell lymphoma
ALL	acute lymphoblastic leukemia
AlloSCT	allogeneic stem cell transplantation
ALP	alkaline phosphatase
ALT	alanine aminotransferase
AML	acute myeloid leukemia
ANC	absolute neutrophil count
APC	antigen-presenting cell
APL	acute promyelocytic leukemia
APR	abdominoperineal resection
aPTT	activated partial thromboplastin time
AR	androgen receptor
ARB	angiotensin receptor blocker
ASCO	American Society of Clinical Oncology
ASCT	autologous stem cell transplantation
AST	aspartate aminotransferase
ATA	American Thyroid Association
ATC	anaplastic thyroid cancer
ATRA	all-trans-retinoic acid
AUA	American Urological Association
AUC	area under the curve
AYA	adolescent and young adult

B-ALL	B-cell acute lymphoblastic leukemia
BCC	basal cell carcinoma
BCG	bacillus Calmette–Guérin
BCR	B-cell receptor
BCS	breast conserving therapy
BEP	bleomycin
bHCG	beta-human chorionic gonadotropin
BiTE	bi-specific T-cell engager
BMI	body mass index
BMP	basic metabolic panel
BMT	bone marrow transplantation
BPH	benign prostatic hyperplasia
BSO	bilateral salpingo-oophorectomy
BTC	biliary tract cancer
BUN	blood urea nitrogen
CA	cancer antigen
CABG	coronary artery bypass graft
CAD	coronary artery disease
CALGB	Cancer and Leukemia Group B
CAR	cancer-associated retinopathy
CARG	Cancer and Aging Research Group
CART	chimeric antigen receptor T-cell
CBC	complete blood count
CBCT	cone beam computed tomography
CCA	cholangiocarcinoma
CDC	Centers for Disease Control
CEA	carcinoembryonic antigen
CEL	chronic eosinophilic leukemia
CGA	Comprehensive Geriatric Assessment
cGVHD	chronic graft versus host disease
CHF	congestive heart failure
cHL	classic Hodgkin lymphoma
CHR	complete hematologic response
CHRPE	congenital hypertrophy of the retinal pigmented epithelium
CI	calcineurin inhibitor/confidence interval
CIBMTR	Center for International Blood and Marrow Transplant Research
CIS	carcinoma *in situ*
CLL	chronic lymphocytic leukemia
CML	chronic myelogenous leukemia
CMML	chronic myelomonocytic leukemia
CMP	comprehensive metabolic panel
CMR	complete molecular response
CMV	cytomegalovirus
CNL	chronic neutrophilic leukemia
CoC	Commission on Cancer
COPD	chronic obstructive pulmonary disease
CR	complete remission

CRABI	(syndrome of) hypercalcemia, renal failure, anemia, bone pain or lytic bone lesions, infection
CRASH	Chemotherapy Risk Assessment Scale for High age
CRC	colorectal cancer
CRP	C-reactive protein
CRPC	castrate-resistant prostate cancer
CRS	Cardiotoxicity Risk Score
CSF	cerebrospinal fluid
CT	computed tomography
CTLS	clinical tumor lysis syndrome
CTPA	computed tomographic pulmonary angiography
CTRCD	cancer therapeutics-related cardiac dysfunction
CyCR	cytogenetic response
D&C	dilatation and curettage
DAPT	dual antiplatelet therapy
DCIS	ductal carcinoma *in situ*
DFS	disease-free survival
3D C-XRT/3DCRT	three-dimensional conformal radiation therapy
D5W	dextrose 5% in water
DIC	disseminated intravascular coagulation
DIPSS	Dynamic International Prognostic Scoring System
DLBCL	diffuse large B-cell lymphoma
DLCO	diffusing capacity of the lungs for carbon monoxide
DPIG	diffuse intrinsic pontine glioma
DRE	digital rectal examination
DRESS	drug rash with eosinophilia and systemic symptoms
DRI	Disease Risk Index
DTC	differentiated thyroid cancer
DVT	deep venous thrombosis
DWI	diffusion weighted imaging
EASL	European Association for the Study of the Liver
EBCTCG	Early Breast Cancer Trialists' Collaborative Group
EBRT	external beam radiation therapy
EBUS	endobronchial ultrasound
EBV	Epstein–Barr virus
ECOG	Eastern Cooperative Oncology Group
EGD	esophagogastroduodenoscopy
EGFR	epidermal growth factor receptor
ELN	European LeukemiaNet
EOC	epithelial ovarian cancer
EP	etoposide
EPP	extrapleural pneumonectomy
ER	estrogen receptor
ERCP	endoscopic retrograde cholangiopancreatography
ESA	erythropoiesis stimulating agent
ESC	European Society of Cardiology
ESMO	European Society of Medical Oncology

ESR	erythrocyte sedimentation rate
ET	essential thrombocythemia
EUS	endoscopic ultrasound
EWS	Ewing sarcoma
FAB	French–American–British
FACT	Foundation for the Accreditation of Cellular Therapy
FAP	familial adenomatous polyposis
FDA	Food and Drug Administration
FDG	fluorodeoxyglucose
FFP	freedom from progression
FFPE	formalin fixed paraffin embedded
FIGO	International Federation of Gynecology and Obstetrics
FISH	fluorescence *in situ* hybridization
FLC	free light chain
FNA	fine needle aspiration
FOBT	fecal occult blood testing
5-FU	5-fluorouracil
GBC	gallbladder carcinoma
GBM	glioblastoma
GCB	germinal center B-cell
G-CSF	granulocyte colony-stimulating factor
GCT	giant/germ cell tumor
GEJ	gastroesophageal junction
GERD	gastroesophageal reflux disease
GGT	gamma-glutamyl transpeptidase
GIST	gastrointestinal stromal tumor
GLS	global longitudinal strain
GnRH	gonadotropin-releasing hormone
GVHD	graft versus host disease
HAART	highly active antiretroviral therapy
HB	hepatoblastoma
HBV	hepatitis B virus
HCC	hepatocellular carcinoma
HCG	human chorionic gonadotropin
HCV	hepatitis C virus
HD	Hodgkin disease
HD-MTX	high dose methotrexate
HDR	high dose rate
HEPA	high efficiency particulate air
HER2	human epidermal growth factor receptor 2
HGF	hepatocyte growth factor
5-HIAA	5-hydroxyindoleacetic acid
HIPEC	hyperthermic intraperitoneal chemotherapy
HIT	heparin-induced thrombocytopenia
HIV	human immunodeficiency virus
HL	Hodgkin lymphoma
HLA	human leukocyte antigen
HLRCC	hereditary leiomyomatosis and renal cell cancer

HMA	hypomethylating agent
HNC	head and neck cancer
HNPCC	hereditary nonpolyposis colorectal cancer
HPRC	hereditary papillary renal carcinoma
HPV	human papillomavirus
HR	hazard ratio
HRT	hormonal replacement therapy
HSCT	hematopoietic stem cell transplant
HSIL	high grade squamous intraepithelial lesion
HTLV	human T-cell lymphotropic virus
HVA	homovanillic acid
IBD	irritable bowel disease
IBMTR	International Bone Marrow Transplant Registry
IBS	irritable bowel syndrome
ICP	intracranial pressure
IDSA	Infectious Diseases Society of America
IFI	invasive fungal infection
IFRT	involved field radiation therapy
Ig	immunoglobulin
IG	image guidance
IHC	immunohistochemistry
IMDC	International Metastatic Database Consortium
IMiD	immunomodulatory imide drug
IMRT	intensity modulated radiation therapy
INR	International Normalized Ratio
IP	intraperitoneal
IPSS	International Prognostic Scoring System
ISH	*in situ* hybridization
ITP	idiopathic thrombocytopenic purpura
IUAC	International Union Against Cancer
IVC	inferior vena cava
IVFA	intravenous fluorescein angiography
IVP	intravenous pyelogram
IVT	incidental venous thrombosis
JIA	juvenile idiopathic arthritis
KPS	Karnofsky Performance Score
LCIS	lobular carcinoma *in situ*
LDH	lactate dehydrogenase
LDR	low dose rate
LFT	liver function test
LGL	large granular lymphocytic leukemia
LMWH	low molecular weight heparin
LTLS	laboratory tumor lysis syndrome
LVEF	left ventricular ejection fraction
LVI	lymphovascular invasion
MA	megestrol acetate
MAH	malignancy-associated hypercalcemia
MALT	mucosa-associated lymphoid tissue

MAPK	mitogen activated protein kinase
MAR	melanoma-associated retinopathy
MB	medulloblastoma
MBL	monoclonal B-lymphocytosis
MCL	mantle cell lymphoma
MCRPC	metastatic castration-resistant prostate cancer
MDS	myelodysplastic syndrome
MEN	multiple endocrine neoplasia
MF	mycosis fungoides
MIBG	methyl-iodine benzylguanine
MHC	major histocompatibility complex
MGUS	monoclonal gammopathy of undetermined significance
MM	malignant mesothelioma/multiple myeloma
MMR	major molecular response/measles, mumps, and rubella/mismatch repair
MPN	myeloproliferative neoplasm
MRCP	magnetic resonance cholangiopancreatography
MRI	magnetic resonance imaging
MRSA	methicillin-resistant *Staphylococcus aureus*
MS	multiple sclerosis
MSCC	malignant spinal cord compression
MSKCC	Memorial Sloan Kettering Cancer Center
MSM	men who have sex with men
MTC	medullary thyroid cancer
mTOR	mammalian target of rapamycin
MVAC	methotrexate, vinblastine, doxorubicin, plus cisplatin
NAFLD	nonalcoholic fatty liver disease
NCCN	National Comprehensive Cancer Network
NCI	National Cancer Institute
NET	neuroendocrine tumor
NHL	non-Hodgkin lymphoma
NICE	National Institute for Health and Clinical Excellence
NIH	National Institutes of Health
NK	natural killer/normal karyotype
NLPHL	nodular lymphocyte predominant Hodgkin lymphoma
NOAC	novel oral anticoagulant
NPVM	nonpulmonary visceral metastasis
NRM	nonrelapse mortality
NS	normal saline
NSAID	nonsteroidal anti-inflammatory drug
NSCLC	non-small cell lung cancer
NSGCT	nonseminomatous germ cell tumor
NT-proBP	N-terminal pro-brain natriuretic peptide
NYHA	New York Heart Association
OPT	optic pathway tumor
OR	odds ratio
OS	overall survival
PA	pilocytic astrocytoma
PARP	poly (ADP-ribose) polymerase

PAS	periodic acid–Schiff
PBRT	proton beam radiation therapy
PBSC	peripheral blood stem cell
PCD	plasma cell disorder
PCI	percutaneous coronary intervention
PCNSL	primary central nervous system lymphoma
PCP	*Pneumocystis jiroveci* pneumonia (formerly known as *Pneumocystis carinii* pneumonia)
PCR	polymerase chain reaction
PD	progression of disease
P/D	pleurectomy with decortication
PE	pulmonary embolism
PET	positron emission tomography
PFI	platinum-free interval
PFS	progression-free survival
PHI	Prostate Health Index
PI	proteasome inhibitor
PLCO	Prostate, Lung, Colorectal, and Ovarian Cancer Screening Trial
PMF	primary myelofibrosis
PNET	primitive neuroectodermal tumor
PNH	paroxysmal nocturnal hemoglobinuria
POEMS	(syndrome of) polyneuropathy, organomegaly, endocrinopathy, monoclonal gammopathy, and skin changes
PR	progesterone receptor
PSA	prostate-specific antigen
PSC	primary sclerosing cholangitis
PT	prothrombin time
PTLD	post-transplant lymphoproliferative disorder
PTT	partial thromboplastin time
PV	polycythemia vera
QOL	quality of life
RA	refractory anemia
RAEB	refractory anemia with excess blasts
RAI	radioactive iodine
RARS	refractory anemia with ringed sideroblasts
RBC	red blood cell
RCC	renal cell carcinoma
RCMD	refractory cytopenia with multilineage dysplasia
RCT	randomized controlled trial
RECIST	Response Evaluation Criteria In Solid Tumors
RFA	radiofrequency ablation
RMS	rhabdomyosarcoma
ROCA	risk of ovarian cancer algorithm
RP	radical pleurectomy
RPE	retinal pigmented epithelium
RPLND	retroperitoneal lymph node dissection
RR	relative rate/relative risk
RT	radiation therapy

RT-PCR	reverse transcription-polymerase chain reaction
RUQ	right upper quadrant
RVI	respiratory viral infection
SBRT	stereotactic body radiotherapy
SC	supportive care
SCC	squamous cell carcinoma
SCLC	small cell lung cancer
SCT	stem cell transplantation
SEER	Surveillance, Epidemiology, and End Results
SERD	selective estrogen receptor degrader
SERM	selective estrogen receptor modulator
SGO	Society of Gynecologic Oncology
SIFE	serum immunofixation
SLL	small lymphocytic lymphoma
SLN	sentinel lymph node
SMM	smoldering multiple myeloma
SNB	sentinel node biopsy
SNP	single-nucleotide polymorphism
SPECT	single proton emission computed tomography
SPEP	serum protein electrophoresis
SRE	skeletal-related event
SRS	stereotactic radiosurgery
SSPE	subsegmental pulmonary embolism
SSRI	selective serotonin reuptake inhibitor
SSRS	somatostatin receptor scintigraphy
SVC	superior vena cava
SVT	splanchnic venous thrombosis
TACE	transarterial chemoembolization
TAH	total abdominal hysterectomy
T-ALL	T-cell acute lymphoblastic leukemia
TBI	total body irradiation
TCC	transitional cell carcinoma
TCGA	The Cancer Genome Atlas
TEMPI	(syndrome of) telangiectasias, elevated erythropoietin and erythrocytosis, monoclonal gammopathy, perinephric fluid collection, and intrapulmonary shunting
TERT	telomerase reverse transcriptase
TIP	paclitaxel, ifosfamide, mesna, cisplatin
TKI	tyrosine kinase inhibitor
TLS	tumor lysis syndrome
TNBC	triple negative breast cancer
TNM	tumor, nodal, metastases
TORS	transoral robotic surgery
TPN	total parenteral nutrition
TSC	tuberous sclerosis complex
TSH	thyroid stimulating hormone
TTR	time to recurrence
TURBT	transurethral resection of bladder tumor
TURP	transurethral resection of the prostate

TVUS	transvaginal ultrasound
UIFE	24-hr urine collection for immunofixation
UPEP	24-hr urine collection for electrophoresis
UPSC	uterine papillary serous carcinoma
USPSTF	US Preventive Services Task Force
VEGF	vascular endothelial growth factor
VeIP	vinblastine, mesna, ifosfamide, cisplatin
VGPR	very good partial response
VHL	von Hippel–Lindau
VIP	mesna, ifosfamide, cisplatin, etoposide
VKA	vitamin K antagonist
VMA	vanillylmandelic acid
VOD	veno-occlusive disease
V/Q	ventilation–perfusion
VTE	venous thromboembolism
WBC	white blood cell
WBRT	whole brain radiation therapy
WHO	World Health Organization
WT	Wilms tumor

About the Companion Website

This series is accompanied by a companion website:

www.wiley.com/go/oh/mountsinaioncology

The website includes:
- Advice for patients
- Case studies with interactive MCQs
- ICD codes
- Color versions of images

PART 1

Oncology

CHAPTER 1

Breast Cancer

Jeanette Guziel[1] and Charles L. Shapiro[2]
[1] Southern California Permanente Medical Group, Woodland Hills, CA, USA
[2] Icahn School of Medicine at Mount Sinai, New York, NY, USA

OVERALL BOTTOM LINE

- Breast cancer is the second leading cause of cancer-related deaths among women aged <50 years.
- There has been an approximately 30% reduction in breast cancer mortality since 1990 as a result of screening and the increased detection of early stages of disease, and adjuvant therapy.
- Breast cancer is not a single disease. Based on molecular genetic profiling there are at least five major subtypes: luminal A, luminal B (high proliferation rate), luminal B human epidermal growth factor receptor 2 (HER2) overexpressing, HER2 overexpressing, and triple negative breast cancer (TNBC) is estrogen and progesterone receptor (ER, PR) and HER2 negative.
- Inherited germline mutations of *BRCA1* and *BRCA2* represent about 5–10% of all breast cancers. The lifetime risk of developing breast cancer increases by 80% and 60%, and ovarian cancer by 54% and 23% for *BRCA1* and *BRCA2* mutation carriers, respectively.
- The treatment of breast cancer is one of the earliest examples of using targeted treatments with the recognition of the ER and HER2 receptors serving as therapeutic targets and the development of effective drugs against these receptors.

Background
Definition of disease

- Breast cancers arise in the epithelial cells that line milk ducts or in breast alveolar lobules.
- Breast cancers consist of two major categories: invasive and noninvasive.
  - Invasive cancers include invasive ductal, lobular, mucinous, tubular, medullary, and papillary cancers.
  - Noninvasive cancers include ductal carcinoma *in situ* (DCIS) which is recognized as a pre-invasive lesion; and lobular carcinoma *in situ* (LCIS) that is recognized as a marker of increased risk of developing subsequent breast cancer in either breast.

Disease classification

Breast cancers can be phenotypically classified by their receptor status: ER and PR as measured by immunohistochemistry (IHC); by HER2/neu receptor status measured by IHC or *in situ* hybridization (ISH); or intrinsic molecular subtypes based on gene expression profiling (Table 1.1).

Mount Sinai Expert Guides: Oncology, First Edition. Edited by William K. Oh and Ajai Chari.
© 2019 John Wiley & Sons Ltd. Published 2019 by John Wiley & Sons Ltd.
Companion Website: www.wiley.com/go/oh/mountsinaioncology

Table 1.1 Subtypes of breast cancer.

	Luminal A	Luminal B	Luminal HER2	HER2 enriched	Triple negative/ basal like
Frequency	~55%	~15%		~20%	~10%
Receptors					
ER	+	+	+	−	−
PR	+/−	+/−	+/−	−	−
HER2	−	−	+	+	−
Grade	Low	Mod–high	Mod–high	High	High
Ki-67[a]	Low	High	High	High	High
Mutations[b]	PI3K (49%) PTEN[c] (13%) P53 (12%)	PI3K (32%) P53 (32%) PTEN[c] (24%)		P53 (75%) PI3K (42%) PTEN[c] (19%)	P53 (84%) PTEN[c] (35%) PI3K (7%)
Treatments					
Anti-estrogens[d]	+	+	+	−	−
Chemotherapy[e]	−	+/−	+/−	+	+
HER2 directed	−	−	+	+	−
Outcome	Favorable	Interm[f]	Interm[f]	Favorable	Poor

[a] Ki-67, proliferation marker; low <10–14%; high >14%.
[b] Most frequent mutations based on The Cancer Genome Atlas (TCGA).
[c] Loss or mutation.
[d] Tamoxifen and gonadotropin-releasing hormone (GnRH) agonists in premenopausal women; fulvestrant (selective estrogen receptor degrader, SERD), tamoxifen (selective estrogen receptor modulator, SERM), aromatase inhibitors (AI) in postmenopausal women.
[e] Anthracycline (cyclophosphamide, doxorubicin (AC) with or with paclitaxel (T) or non-anthracycline-containing regimens (docetaxel, cyclophosphamide (TC)). Trastuzumab (T), pertuzumab (P), lapatinib (L), and trastuzumab emtansine (T-DM1)
[f] Intermediate.

Incidence/prevalence
- Breast cancer is the most common cancer in females in the USA and the second most common cause of cancer death in women.
- There were approximately 225 000 new breast cancer cases and approximately 40 000 deaths in 2012, with an estimated 3 000 000 women living with breast cancer in the USA. There are about 5000 cases of male breast cancer annually.
- Black women have a lower incidence of breast cancer than white women, but a higher breast cancer-specific mortality rate. This is thought to be a result of more unfavorable biology (e.g. increase in triple negative subtype) and less access to care leading to a more advanced stage of disease at diagnosis.

Economic impact
- From 1970 to 2008, the number of breast cancer deaths in women aged 20–49 years was about 226 000 and accounted for 8 million years of potential life lost.
- The total productivity loss in 2008 was $5.5 billion and individual lifetime lost earnings was $1.1 million.

Etiology

- It is unclear what causes breast cancer; ~5–10% are linked to inherited germline mutations in *BRCA1, BRCA2, TP53, PTEN*, and the *ATM* genes.
- 15–20% of women will have a positive family history (with low penetrance genes).
- Environmental factors: endogenous and exogenous estrogen, radiation exposure (i.e. mantle field radiation in Hodgkin lymphoma), daily alcohol ≥2 drinks, and obesity (body mass index (BMI) >30) increase the risks of developing breast cancer.

Pathology/pathogenesis

- Figure 1.1 describes estrogen binding to ER in cytosol, translocation to the nucleus where the complex binds to DNA and initiates transcription. The *HER2* gene on chromosome 17q12 belongs to the epidermal growth factor receptor (EGFR) family. *HER2* overamplification occurs in 20% and is associated with an increased risk of distant recurrence, poorer response to chemotherapy, and increased mortality in the absence of *HER2*-directed therapy. A monoclonal antibody to an external domain of the *HER2* receptor, trastuzumab, has changed the natural history by improving OS in both the early and advanced stage setting.
- *BRCA1* on chromosome 17q21 and *BRCA2* on chromosome 13q12.3 proteins are involved in DNA repair. An inherited germline mutation from either the maternal or paternal line increases the lifetime risk of developing breast cancer by 80% (*BRCA1*) and 60% (*BRCA2*), and ovarian cancer by 54% (*BRCA1*) and 23% (*BRCA2*).

Predictive/risk factors

- Female gender.
- Aging.
- Elevated estrogen levels: early menarche, late menopause, late parity, nulliparity, and prolonged (>10–15 years) of hormone replacement therapy (HRT).
- Benign breast conditions: atypical ductal or lobular hyperplasia, or LCIS.
- Dense breast tissue.
- A personal history of breast cancer.
- A family history of breast cancer (strongly affected by the number of female first degree relatives).
- Inherited germline mutation in *BRCA1, BRCA2, p53, ATM,* and *PTEN*.
- Obesity: BMI ≥30 kg/m^2.
- Alcohol: dose–response relationship between alcohol and risk of breast cancer.
- Prior thoracic radiation.

However, 75–80% of newly diagnosed women with breast cancer do not have any of these risk factors.

Prevention

> **BOTTOM LINE/CLINICAL PEARLS**
> The key to prevention is:
> - Identification of germline genetic mutation carriers.
> - Age appropriate and high risk patient screening (i.e. magnetic resonance imaging (MRI) breast screening for mutation carriers of *BRCA* genes).
> - Modifiable lifestyle risk factors such as reducing daily alcohol consumption, weight management, and avoidance of obesity.

- Regular physical exercise may reduce the risk of breast cancer and reduces all cause mortality.
- Primary chemoprevention with tamoxifen in pre- and postmenopausal women, and raloxifene or aromatase inhibitors in postmenopausal women.
- Prophylactic salpingoopherectomy and mastectomy for *BRCA* germline mutation carriers.

Screening

- Mammographic screening is associated with a 15–30% decrease in breast cancer mortality, increased detection of earlier stage curable breast cancers, and an increase in breast conserving therapy (BCS). The role of ultrasound for whole breast screening is not established. Breast ultrasound is used to help clarify imaged mammographic abnormalities.
- Annual breast MRI for high risk women as defined by the following:
  - Known *BRCA* mutation carriers, start at age 25.
  - Untested and first degree relative of *BRCA* carrier, start at age 25.
  - Lifetime risk ≥20%.
  - Chest irradiation between ages 10 and 30 years.
  - Genetic syndromes (e.g. Cowden, Li–Fraumeni).
- Annual mammographic screening and clinical breast examination is indicated in women ≥50 years. The upper age limit of screening mammography has not been defined and decisions are based on functional age and comorbid conditions rather than chronologic age. There is controversy in women aged 40–49 with some policy-making organizations recommending decisions should be individualized with a thorough discussion of smaller absolute reductions in mortality and the potential harms of screening, whereas others recommend screening intervals every 1 or 2 years along with clinical breast examination. Promoting breast self-examination is controversial because overall mortality is not decreased. However, women can be empowered by performing breast self-examination but for other women it is a source of anxiety.

Primary prevention

- Breastfeeding for prolonged durations.
- Primary chemoprevention is indicated for women with a first degree relative with breast or ovarian cancer, history of thoracic irradiation, *BRCA* mutation carriers, LCIS, atypical hyperplasia or Gail Model risk assessment tool (https://bcrisktool.cancer.gov/) predicting a 5-year breast cancer risk ≥1.7%. Five years of tamoxifen, raloxifene, or the aromatase inhibitors exemestane or anastrozole reduces the risk of developing breast cancer by 50–75%.
- Prophylactic bilateral mastectomy: reduces the risk of breast cancer by 99% in *BRCA* germline mutation carriers.
- Prophylactic bilateral salpingoopherectomy: decreases risk of ovarian cancer by 99% in *BRCA* mutation carriers.

Secondary prevention

- Weight maintenance and avoid obesity.
- Reduce alcohol to ≤1 serving/day.
- There is emerging evidence that physical activity lessens the risks of developing breast cancer.

Diagnosis

BOTTOM LINE/CLINICAL PEARLS
- Most women present with a nonpalpable mammographic abnormality. Only about 20% of these biopsied mammographic abnormalities will be breast cancer. Up to 30–40% of the cancers diagnosed based on mammographic abnormality will be DCIS.
- 15% of women have a breast mass that is not detected on mammogram.
- Women without access or who do not choose not to have mammograms typically present with a palpable breast or axillary mass with or without skin changes and advanced stage at diagnosis.
- Women with a palpable breast lesion should undergo biopsy of the lesion regardless of whether the imaging is positive or negative.

Differential diagnosis

Differential diagnosis	Features
Proliferative benign breast changes	Ductal hyperplasia, papilloma, radial scar, sclerosing adenosis, cysts, and fibroadenoma
Atypia	Atypical ductal or lobular hyperplasia
DCIS	A precursor lesion to invasive breast cancer characterized by the size of the lesion, nuclear grade, presence and extent of comedo necrosis, architectural pattern, and ER status
LCIS	Typically, found incidentally when a breast biopsy is performed Serves as marker of increased risk of developing breast cancer in either breast
Other cancers	Sarcoma and lymphoma

DCIS, ductal carcinoma *in situ*; LCIS, lobular carcinoma *in situ*.

History
- Family history of breast and ovarian cancer in the maternal and paternal lineage and the age of diagnosis of these cancers.
- Age of menarche.
- Age of menopause.
- Number of years of HRT.
- Prior exposure to mediastinal radiation.
- Establish any symptoms related to the breast (e.g. bloody nipple discharge, erythema of the skin, palpable masses in the breast or axillae) or suggestive of metastatic disease including any new or persistent symptoms in any part of the body.

Physical examination
Breast imaging and a clinical breast examination are always indicated. Clinical breast examination includes upright and supine inspection of the breasts, palpation of all the four quadrants of the breast and of the lymph-bearing areas including the cervical, supraclavicular, and axillae. A complete physical examination is also indicated.

Disease severity classification

Staging is based on the TNM system of the American Joint Committee on Cancer (AJCC 8th edition; website: https://cancerstaging.org).

List of diagnostic tests

- Pathology review of a breast biopsy requires histologic type, grade, and receptor classification.
- Tumor markers: CA 27-29, CA 15-3, and carcinoembryonic antigen (CEA) are sometimes useful to monitor treatment response in the metastatic setting. They should not be used to "screen" for metastatic disease in asymptomatic women.
- If metastatic lesion is suspected, biopsy is essential to document the histology and confirm ER/PR/HER2 status. For example, in women treated for early stage breast cancer the appearance of solitary lung nodule is a primary lung cancer in up to 50–60%. Discordance between receptor status of the primary breast cancer and metastatic site occurs in up to 10–15%.
- Oncotype DX® is a 21-gene reverse transcription-polymerase chain reaction (RT-PCR) assay commercially available since 2004, used in women with HER2 negative, ER positive, node-negative, or 1–3 node-positive breast cancers. The results are a recurrence score from 1 to 100. The recurrence score predicts the 10-year risk of distant metastases in node-negative women, and may predict the 5-year risk of distant recurrence in 1–3 node-positive disease. More importantly, only the high risk recurrence score group (≥25) derives benefit from adjuvant chemotherapy in addition to anti-estrogen treatments, whereas the low risk group (0–11) derives no benefit from the additional chemotherapy. Recently, the low risk recurrence score was prospectively validated (Sparano et al. 2015). The intermediate recurrence score group (11–25) has been reported (Sparano et al. 2018). For women over the age of 50 years, recurrence scores of <25 are associated with no chemotherapy benefit whereas recurrence scores ≥25 are associated with benefit. For women ≤50 years, recurrence scores of 16–20 are associated with a 1.6% absolute benefit of chemotherapy and scores of 21–25 are associated with 6.5% absolute benefit.
- A prospective validation of Oncotype DX was recently completed in axillary node 1–3 positive but has not been reported.
- Mammoprint is based on the 70-gene risk predictor and classifies into low risk (favorable) or high risk (unfavorable) prognosis. It is indicated for both ER positive and negative breast cancers. Prospective validation of its use as a prognostic test and a predictive test (i.e. which patients respond to chemotherapy) is available.
- PAM50 is a multigene RT-PCR test, which measures 50 classifier genes and five control genes. It can be used to categorize patients into five intrinsic breast cancer subtypes that confers prognostic information: luminal A, luminal B, HER2-enriched, basal-like, and normal-like. It is in commercial use.
- Breast Cancer Index is a five-classifier of late (after 5 years) recurrences in ER positive women. Prospective validation of this test is not available.

Lists of imaging techniques

- Bilateral digital diagnostic mammography and breast ultrasound. Breast MRI as clinically indicated (see section on Screening).
- Any new or persistent symptoms require imaging as clinically indicated. If the review of systems is negative, the likelihood of finding occult asymptomatic metastases is very low in clinical stages I–IIIA and no imaging or blood tests are recommended.
- In asymptomatic stage IIIB or higher, the likelihood of finding occult metastatic disease is higher and either a computed tomography (CT) scan of chest, abdomen, pelvis, and bone scan or positron emission tomography (PET)/CT is indicated.

- If, based on symptoms, central nervous system disease is suspected a brain MRI scan with contrast is indicated and is superior to a head CT with contrast.

Treatment
Treatment rationale

The primary goal of treatment for stages I–III is personal cure (i.e. dying of a cause other than breast cancer).

- Anti-estrogen treatments tamoxifen (for pre- and postmenopausal women) and aromatase inhibitors (only for postmenopausal women) are given in all cases of ER and PR positive breast cancers.
- Chemotherapy is routinely given to women with breast cancers that are HER2 positive, TNBC, ER/PR positive with high risk Oncotype DX recurrence score or Mammoprint in histologically proven multiple axillary node-positive disease.
- The primary goal of treatment for stage IV disease is to palliate symptoms, increase quality of life, and, in some cases, increase OS.

Table of treatment

Local treatment	Comments
Breast surgery	Multiple randomized controlled trials (RCTs) show that BCS (also called lumpectomy or partial mastectomy) with whole breast radiation/boost and modified radical mastectomy show the same OS. There is slightly higher overall local recurrence with BCS; however, the individual RCT varied with respect to adequacy of surgical margins and the use of boost. Standard treatment option in stage I and II breast cancers is BCS. However, both BCS and mastectomy options should be discussed. Absolute contraindications to BCS include: • Two or more primary tumors in different quadrants of the breast or diffuse malignant appearing calcifications throughout the breast on presurgical breast imaging • Breast cancer during pregnancy • Prior history of breast radiation • History of scleroderma • Persistently positive surgical margins after attempted surgical re-excisions of the lumpectomy bed Relative contraindications include: • Centrally placed tumor with removal of the nipple–areolar complex • Relatively large tumor in a smaller breast in which asymmetry would be the result of BCS (relative to the contralateral breast) Stage IIIA (T3 or >5 cm tumors with N0 or N1) breast cancers often receive neoadjuvant chemotherapy Absolute contradictions to breast surgery include: • Direct extension to skin or chest wall, ulceration, or skin nodules (T4, any N) • Fixed or matted axillary nodes (any T, with N2–N3) • Internal mammary and supraclavicular nodal positivity For noninvasive DCIS either lumpectomy with (or without) radiation, or mastectomy are standard options
Sentinel node biopsy (SNB)	Standard practice for stage I–III (operable) breast cancers is sentinel node mapping and biopsy. SNB reduces the risk of lymphedema vs. full level I and II axillary dissection without comprising OS

(Continued)

(Continued)

Local treatment	Comments
Breast radiation	For invasive cancers: after BCS follows whole breast radiation/boost. After mastectomy, decisions about chest wall radiation are based on increasing the number of positive axillary nodes, initial tumor size, extranodal extension, or subtype of breast cancer For noninvasive DCIS: after lumpectomy whole breast radiation/boost is the standard practice. Obviating radiation is a consideration in women over the age of 70 years with stage I breast cancer who receive anti-estrogen treatments or women who have small, low grade, ER positive DCIS
Systemic treatments	Early stage I–III breast cancers: • RCTs of postoperative adjuvant chemotherapy vs. preoperative neoadjuvant chemotherapy show comparable clinical results. The advantages of neoadjuvant therapy are downstaging to allow BCS • The benefits of chemotherapy are greater in pre- than in postmenopausal women, in ER negative or low vs. high ER expression and high vs. low grade breast cancers • The use of anthracyclines (doxorubicin) in chemotherapy regimens for stage I–III breast cancer is controversial. This is because of the small risk of developing cardiomyopathy, about $\leq 1\%$ with doxorubicin-based regimens and about 3% with trastuzumab/taxane-based regimens following doxorubicin-based regimens. It is important to distinguish doxorubicin-related cardiomyopathy (causes myocardial cell death and is related to total cumulative dose) from trastuzumab-related myocardial dysfunction (does not cause myocardial cell death, is not dose-related, and 50% of patients can be retreated with trastuzumab when their left ventricular fraction improves). Several randomized trials show that outcomes are similar or better (results of one randomized trial) with non-anthracycline than with anthracycline-based regimens. Women with pre-existing cardiac problems should receive non-anthracycline-based regimens Systemic treatment decisions are based on the expression of three receptors: ER, PR, and HER2 ER and/or PR positive, HER2 negative (luminal A: see Table 1.1): • ER and/or PR positivity is defined as $\geq 1\%$ positive cells. Treated with anti-estrogen treatments such as tamoxifen (pre- and postmenopausal women) or one of the aromatase inhibitors (e.g. anastrozole, exemestane, or letrozole). RCTs of 10 vs. 5 years of tamoxifen show benefits favoring treatment for 10 years. RCTs of 10 vs. 5 years of aromatase inhibitor have been completed and the results show treatment durations of more than 5 years show no differences for the low risk patients, but the high risk multiple nodal positive patients may benefit. The MA-17 trial showed a benefit for 10 years of letrozole over 5 years but the patients in that trial had all completed 4–5 years of prior tamoxifen. The majority of benefit was in contralateral risk reduction • Oncotype DX assay is a predictive test (high recurrence score predicts [25 or greater] benefit from chemotherapy) ER and/or PR positive, HER2 positive (luminal B): • These breast cancers typically receive trastuzumab-based chemotherapy regimens and then anti-estrogens. • Luminal B is also defined by ER and/or PR positive and high proliferation rate as measured by Ki-67. However, the Ki-67 assays are problematic in varying methods and interpretation of cut-points that separate high and low proliferating tumors. Therefore, Ki-67 is not considered as a standard marker. The majority of non-HER2 positive luminal B cancers, but not all, are high grade. The Oncotype DX assay is also used in this group. Many will receive chemotherapy and then anti-estrogen treatments. Identification of luminal B, non-HER positive breast cancers will be easier when PAM 50 is routinely used to subtype breast cancers

(Continued)

Local treatment	Comments
	HER2 positive: • For less than 3 cm, node-negative, adjuvant paclitaxel in combination with trastuzumab results in a 3-year invasive disease-free survival of over 97% • Trastuzumab and pertuzumab with concurrent chemotherapy (either docetaxel or paclitaxel alone for six cycles every 21 days alone, docetaxel and carboplatin for six cycles every 21 days, or cyclophosphamide and doxorubicin for four cycles every 2 weeks followed by 12 weeks of weekly paclitaxel) is standard practice as neoadjuvant therapy or postoperative adjuvant therapy (Table 1.2) • Trastuzumab given for 2 years has not been shown to be superior to 1 year • The Katherine Trial is for patients with residual disease after neoadjuvant HER2 targeted containing chemotherapy. The randomization was to 1 year of trastzumab emtansine (TDM-1) or trastuzmab. TDM-1 was statistically and clinically significant and is the new standard of care • Concurrent administration of anthracycline and trastuzumab results in an unacceptably high risk of cardiomyopathy and is contraindicated TNBC: • Postoperative adjuvant or neoadjuvant chemotherapy is the only option. TNBC responding to DNA-damaging drugs such as carboplatin or cisplatin are more frequent in *BRCA1* germline mutation carriers • The hallmark of TNBC is early distant recurrences (i.e. the first 1–2 years after completing treatment). Distant recurrences after 5–6 years are rare and most women who remain disease-free will experience personal cures. This is in contrast to ER positive, luminal A cancers in which $\geq$50% of metastatic recurrences occur after 5 years • Carboplatin added to paclitaxel increases the pathologic complete response rate in neoadjuvant chemotherapy. A trial of carboplatin added to paclitaxel in the postoperative adjuvant setting is ongoing • Poly (ADP-ribose) polymerase (PARP) inhibitors, inhibiting homologous recombination DNA repair, are still being evaluated in TNBC Treatment of stage IV metastatic breast cancer: • OS has improved for women with metastatic breast cancer • The first site of metastatic disease is bone only in 40% • Treatment continues until progression of disease or dose-limiting side effects in most cases • For women with ER positive metastatic disease, there is no advantage in OS to starting initial treatment with chemotherapy over anti-estrogen treatments • Besides ER expression, prediction of response to a subsequent anti-estrogen treatment is based on the prior response to current anti-estrogen treatment. Progression of disease $\leq$6–12 months usually predicts for no or minimal response to subsequent anti-estrogen treatment • RCTs demonstrate the mammalian target of rapamycin (mTOR) inhibitor, everolimus, when combined with exemestane (Bolero-2 trial) provides superior PFS but not OS relative to exemestane alone in postmenopausal women with ER positive, HER2 negative metastatic disease who progressed on an aromatase inhibitor as the first line treatment for metastatic disease. The main side effects of everolimus include mouth sores, myelosuppression, diarrhea, and pneumonitis (rare)

(Continued)

(Continued)

Local treatment	Comments
	• In RCTs the cyclin-dependent kinase inhibitor 4 and 6, palbociclib, in combination with letrozole as first line treatment (Paloma III trial) and in combination with fulvestrant as second line treatment (Paloma III trial) for postmenopausal, ER positive, HER2 negative, metastatic disease improves PFS. The main side effect of palbociclib is neutropenia. The OS results of palbociclib trials are not yet available. In the second line treatment of ER positive metastatic disease, in planned subset analysis in those patients with prior endocrine sensitivity, fulvestrant plus palbociclib showed an OS advantage over fulvestrant plus placebo. During the past 2 years the Monarch (ambeciclib) and Monalessa (ribociclib) trials have been published showing essentially comparable benefits in PFS in the first line (with letrozole) and second line (with fulvestrant). There are no OS results as yet • Chemotherapy remains the standard of care for metastatic triple-negative breast cancer (TNBC), however TNBC is more immunogenic than other breast cancer subtypes. The FDA approved the combination of Atezolizumab and nab-paclitaxel in November 2018 for TNBC based on the Impassion130 trial. This demonstrated an improved PFS compared to nab-paclitaxel alone and the benefit was more pronounced (25 vs. 15.5 months) for those with PDL1 expressing tumors Chemotherapy: • Clinical trials, if available and the woman is eligible, should always be considered when discussing therapeutic options • The goals of treatment are to palliate symptoms, improve quality of life, and in some cases extend OS (in particular, OS in metastatic breast cancer has improved for women with HER2 positive tumors) • There are a number of single drugs and chemotherapy combination regimens that are Food and Drug Administration (FDA) approved or commonly used for metastatic breast cancer, neoadjuvant or postoperative adjuvant (Table 1.2) • For non-HER2 positive metastatic disease, sequential use of single drugs is preferred over combinations because of fewer side effects and generally no differences in OS. The use of combination chemotherapy results in higher response rates but at the expense of more side effects

Table 1.2 FDA-approved chemotherapy drugs and regimens in breast cancer.

Drug (metastatic)[¶]		Dose (mg/m²)	Schedule (week/cycle[a])	Major side effects
Paclitaxel (T)	IV	80	Every week	Pain, alopecia, neuropathy
Nab[a]-T	IV	260	Every 3 weeks	Neuropathy
Docetaxel (D)	IV	100 or 75	Every 3 weeks	Myelosuppression; mucositis, alopecia, hand-foot; fluid accumulation[c]
Capecitabine	oral	2000	Days 1–14 every 3 weeks	Hand-foot; diarrhea
Vinorelbine	IV	15–20	Days 1, 8 every 3 weeks Days 1, 8, 15 every 4 weeks	Constipation/ileus; neuropathy
Gemcitabine	IV	1250	Days 1, 8 every 3 weeks Days 1, 8, 15 every 4 weeks	Myelosuppression

Table 1.2   (*Continued*)

Drug (metastatic)[¶]		Dose (mg/m²)	Schedule (week/cycle[a])	Major side effects
Eribulin[d]	IV	1.4	Days 1, 8 every 3 weeks	Myelosuppression, alopecia, peripheral neuropathy
Ixabepilone	IV	40	Every 3 weeks	Myelosuppression, hand-foot, alopecia, peripheral neuropathy
Pegylated liposomal doxorubicin[d]	IV	40	Every 4 weeks	Hand-foot
HER2 (metastatic)[¶]				
D Trastuzumab (H) Pertuzumab (P)	IV	75 6 mg/kg[e] 420 mg[f]	Every 3 weeks[b] Every 3 weeks (HP)	Myelosuppression; mucositis, hand-foot, fluid accumulation[c], and diarrhea
THP	IV	80 6 mg/kg 420 mg	Every week[b] Every 3 weeks (HP)	Myelosuppression, alopecia, peripheral neuropathy, diarrhea
TH	IV	80 6 mg/kg	Every week[b] Every 3 weeks (H)	Myelosuppression, alopecia, peripheral neuropathy
Capecitabine and lapatinib	oral	2000 125 mg	Days 1–14 every 3 weeks Daily	Myelosuppression; hand-foot; diarrhea
TDM-1	IV	3.6	Every 3 weeks	Thrombocytopenia; neuropathy
HER2 (neoadjuvant) and adjuvant				
D CarboHP	IV	75 AUC = 6 6 mg/kg 420 mg	Every 3 weeks × 6 Every 3 weeks × 17 Every 3 weeks × 6	Myelosuppression, mucositis, alopecia, hand-foot, fluid accumulation[c], and diarrhea
Doxorbicin Cyclophosphamide (C)-THP	IV	60 600 80 2 mg/kg 6 mg/kg 420 mg	Every 2 weeks × 4 (AC) Weekly × 12 (T) Weekly × 12 (H) Every 3 weeks × 14 (H) Every 3 weeks × 4 (P)	Myelosuppression, mucositis, alopecia, hand-foot, diarrhea, cardiac (~3%), leukemia (≤0.1%)
THP	IV	80 2 mg/kg 6 mg/kg 420 mg	Every week × 12 (T) Every week × 12 (H) Every 3 weeks × 14 (H) Every 3 weeks × 4 (P)	Myelosuppression, alopecia, diarrhea
THP-Fluorouracil (F) Epirubicin (E) C	V	80 2 mg/kg 6 mg/kg 420 mg 500 75 500	Every week × 12 (T) Weekly × 12 (H) Every 3 weeks × 14 (H) Every 3 weeks × 4 (P) Every 3 weeks × 4	Myelosuppression, alopecia, diarrhea Myelosuppression, alopecia, cardiac (~3%), leukemia (≤0.1%)
TH	IV	80 2 mg/kg 6 mg/kg	Every week × 12 (T) Every week × 12 (H) Every 3 weeks × 14 (H)	Myelosuppression, alopecia, cardiac (~3%), leukemia (≤0.1%)

(Continued)

Table 1.2 (*Continued*)

Drug (metastatic)[¶]		Dose (mg/m²)	Schedule (week/cycle[a])	Major side effects
TNBC (neoadjuvant)				
PCarbo-AC	IV	80 AUC 6 60 600	Every week × 12 (T) Every 3 weeks × 4 (Carbo) Every 2 weeks × 4 (AC)	Myelosuppression, alopecia, mucositis, cardiac (≤1%); leukemia (≤0.1%)
AC-T	IV	60 600 80	Every 2 weeks × 4 (AC) Every week × 12 (T)	Myelosuppression; alopecia, mucositis, cardiac (≤1%); pain, peripheral neuropathy, leukemia (≤0.1%)
Adjuvant				
AC-T	IV	60 600 80	Every 2 weeks × 4 (AC) Every week × 12 (T)	Myelosuppression; alopecia, mucositis, cardiac (≤1%); pain, peripheral neuropathy, leukemia (≤0.1%)
DC	IV	75 600	Every 3 weeks × 4	Myelosuppression; alopecia, mucositis, hand-foot, fluid accumulation
CAF	IV	600 60 600	Every 3 weeks × 6	Myelosuppression; alopecia, mucositis, cardiac (≤1%), leukemia (≤0.1%)
CEF	IV	500 75 500	Every 3 weeks × 6	Myelosuppression; alopecia, mucositis, cardiac (≤1%), leukemia (≤0.1%)
C Methotrexate (M)F	IV	600 50 600	Every 3 weeks × 6	Myelosuppression; alopecia[g], mucositis, diarrhea

[¶] Treatment until disease progression or dose-limiting side effects.
[a] Nanoparticle albumin bound (Nab).
[b] Chemotherapy until maximal benefits or dose-limiting side effects, then H continues.
[c] Taking dexamethasone before, during, and after treatment mitigates fluid accumulation.
[d] Three-month median OS advantage vs. physician's choice for women with ≥2 lines of chemotherapy for metastatic disease (Embrace RCT).
[e] First loading dose is 8 mg/kg then 2 or 6 mg/kg.
[f] First loading dose is 840 then 480 mg.
[g] Partial alopecia is common, but most women do not have to wear a wig.

Prevention/management of complications

Bone metastases

- Cause pain and skeletal-related events (SRE) including spinal cord compression, pathologic fracture, necessity of radiation to provide pain relief, and hypercalcemia.
- As adjunctive treatment to women with bone metastases, either every 1 or 3 month intravenous zoledronic acid, an osteoclast inhibitor, or monthly subcutaneous denosumab, a monoclonal antibody to the RANK ligand, for a 2-year duration are standard options. In an RCT comparing monthly zoledronic acid with denosumab the only endpoint that was statistically significant in favor of denosumab was the time to multiple SRE events. For OS and, for most individuals, SRE there were no significant differences between the two drugs. In cost-effectiveness analyses,

denosumab is about 20 times the cost of zoledronic acid. The main side effects of zoledronic acid are temporally associated fevers, myalgia, arthralgia, renal and osteonecrosis (very rare). The main side effects of denosumab are asymptomatic hypocalcemia and osteonecrosis (very rare).

- Orthopedic fixation of an impending pathologic fracture is always preferred to an operative procedure after fracture. Retrospective criteria for an impending pathologic fracture in a weight-bearing bone include pain, ≥50% cortical involvement, or metastasis ≥2.5 cm. After orthopedic fixation, a course of radiation therapy is usually indicated.
- Radiation is an effective means of providing pain relief if the pain is localized to one area or region of bone and systemic treatments and pain medications do not control the pain. Repeated radiation to large areas of the bone marrow can comprise systemic chemotherapy so if at all possible should be avoided.

Brain metastases

- Increased incidence of metastatic disease to brain in HER2 positive and TNBC subtypes.
- For solitary lesions in an area of the brain that is not critical for neurologic function resection of lesion followed by whole brain radiation, or stereotactic radiation, is used for smaller (up to ≤3 cm) and up to 1–3 lesions. For ≥4 brain metastases and for multiple lesions >3 cm whole brain radiation is generally indicated.

Cardiotoxicity

Trastuzumab is associated with reversible New York Heart Association (NYHA) class III–IV cardiomyopathy in 2–4%. In contrast to anthracycline-induced cardiomyopathy (occurs in ≤1% in women who receive a total cumulative dose of 240 mg/m^2), it is not dose-dependent, does not cause myocardial cell death, the ejection improves in most cases with cardiac medications, and retreatment is possible once the ejection fraction improves.

CLINICAL PEARLS
- When there is an opportunity to try anti-estrogen treatment first, then try it. There are fewer side effects and no advantages to chemotherapy first in the initial treatment of metastatic breast cancer.
- Most women with newly diagnosed invasive cancers will experience personal cures and die of something else.
- There has been enormous progress made in drugs that target the HER2 receptor. In the absence of HER2 targeted drugs ≤20 years ago, HER2 overexpression was an independent adverse prognostic factor. However, the multitude of drugs to target the HER2 receptor and pathways has changed the natural history of this subtype by improving OS.

Special populations
Pregnancy

The treatment of breast cancer during pregnancy can be modified in such a way that the mother can receive optimal breast cancer treatment without the risk of harming the fetus/baby. The basic principles are the following: (i) This is considered as a "high risk" pregnancy by most obstetricians and close communication between the oncologist and obstetrician is essential. (ii) Routine staging studies such as CT, bone, and PET scans are contraindicated. With appropriate shielding mammograms, chest radiographs and liver ultrasounds can be performed. (iii) Chemotherapy should be avoided in the first trimester, but can be given during the second and third trimesters without harm to the fetus in terms of increased congenital abnormalities. The babies that are delivered are normal in terms of APGAR scores and developmental milestones. (iv) If breast surgery has to be performed during pregnancy the only option is mastectomy because radiation after BCS is contraindicated. (v) There is no evidence that a pregnancy subsequent to breast cancer treatment increases the risks of recurrence or decreases OS.

Elderly

- Risk of developing breast cancer increases with aging such that the lifetime risk of "1 in 9 women" will develop it in the sixth to ninth decades of life. Consequently, over the next 25 years and beyond most breast cancers will be in elderly women. Unfortunately, there is a relative lack of knowledge about this group because most RCTs over the past 40+ years either excluded women over 65–70 years or recruited only a minority of women in this age group.
- Women of this age often have comorbid conditions, the primary one being heart disease. For example, a woman who has coronary artery disease and a myocardial infarction has a greater risk of mortality from heart disease than from a stage I or II breast cancer. This has to be taken into consideration when discussing treatment options.
- It is functional age and comorbid disease rather then chronologic age that determines OS and treatment options. Matched for performance status and end organ function, the side effects and toleration of chemotherapy are similar in younger and elderly women.
- A comprehensive geriatric assessment should be performed in women aged 65 years and older to establish functional assessment. These can be CRASH score (https://www.moffitt.org/eforms/crashscoreform) or Cancer and Aging Research Group (CARG) Chemotoxicity calculator (www.mycarg.org).
- Several RCTs performed specifically in elderly women (65+ years) have established the following: (i) radiation can be omitted from BCS in selected stage IA, ER positive women treated with anti-estrogens. (ii) standard combination chemotherapy with either anthracycline or non-anthracycline-based adjuvant chemotherapy has better clinical outcomes than single-agent capecitabine.

Prognosis

> **BOTTOM LINE/CLINICAL PEARLS**
> - Women with early stage breast cancer have a better OS than those diagnosed with later stages of disease. Hence, the emphasis is on screening mammography and early detection of breast cancer.
> - African American (AA) women have worse OS than Caucasians. In part, this is because of access to care, with AA women presenting at more advanced stages. However, even controlling for stage of disease at initial presentation, AA women have higher mortality rates.
> - Low BMI ≤18 or obesity with BMI ≥30 is associated with poorer prognoses.
> - The 21-gene Oncotype DX assay recurrence score is prognostic is for 10-year risk of distant (metastatic) recurrence in women with ER positive, node-negative breast cancers and a prospective randomized trial in ER positive, axillary node 1–3 positive disease has been completed.

Follow-up tests and monitoring

Routine surveillance for asymptomatic women after stage I–III breast cancer treatment:

- History and physical examination every 3–4 months for the first 3 years, then every 6 months for years 4 and 5, then annually thereafter. Unless they receive anti-estrogen treatment for up to 10 years, in which case every 6 months until they finish treatment.
- Mammogram 6 months after radiation for BCS and then annually.

- Periodic review of family history of cancer and referral to a genetic counselor as clinically indicated.
- Bone density every 2 years for women on aromatase inhibitors, with recommended amounts for daily calcium intake (ideally from food sources) and vitamin D3.
- All the routine preventative health care that women without a history of breast cancer receive including immunizations and periodic nonbreast cancer screening examinations.

References and reading list

Cortazar P, Zhang L, Untch M, et al. Pathological complete response and long-term clinical benefit in breast cancer: the CTNeoBC pooled analysis. Lancet 2014;384:164–172.

Davies C, Pan H, Godwin J, et al. Long-term effects of continuing adjuvant tamoxifen to 10 years versus stopping at 5 years after diagnosis of oestrogen receptor-positive breast cancer: ATLAS, a randomised trial. Lancet 2013;381:805–816.

Early Breast Cancer Trialists' Collaborative Group, Peto R, Davies C, Godwin J, et al. Comparisons between different polychemotherapy regimens for early breast cancer: meta-analyses of long-term outcome among 100,000 women in 123 randomised trials. Lancet 2012;379:432–444.

Early Breast Cancer Trialists' Collaborative Group, Darby S, McGale P, Correa C, et al. Effect of radiotherapy after breast-conserving surgery on 10-year recurrence and 15-year breast cancer death: meta-analysis of individual patient data for 10,801 women in 17 randomised trials. Lancet 2011;378:1707–1716.

Gnant M, Mlineritsch B, Luschin-Ebengreuth G, et al. Adjuvant endocrine therapy plus zoledronic acid in premenopausal women with early-stage breast cancer: 5-year follow-up of the ABCSG-12 bone-mineral density substudy. Lancet Oncol 2008;9:840–849.

Krop I, Kim SB, Martin A, et al. Trastuzumab emtansine versus treatment of physician's choice in patients with previously treated HER2-postive metastatic breast cancer (TH3RESA): final overall survival results from a randomised open-label phase 3 trial. Lancet Oncol 2017;18:743–754.

Perez EA, Romond EH, Suman VJ, et al. Trastuzumab plus adjuvant chemotherapy for human epidermal growth factor receptor 2-positive breast cancer: planned joint analysis of overall survival from NSABP B-31 and NCCTG N9831. J Clin Oncol 2014;32:3744–3752.

Perez EA, Barrios, C, Eiermann W, et al. Trastuzumab emtansine with or without pertuzumab versus trastuzumab plus taxane for human epidermal growth factor 2-positive advanced breast cancer: primary results from the phase MARIANNE study. J Clin Oncol 2017;35:141–148.

Rugo HS, Finn RS, Diéras V, et al. Palbociclib plus letrozole as first line therapy in estrogen receptor positive/human epidermal growth factor 2-negative advanced breast cancer with extended follow-up. Breast Cancer Res Treat 2019. doi: 10.1007/s10549-018-05125-4.

Schmid P, Adams S, Rugo HS, et al. Atezolizuman and nab-paclitaxel in adavanced triple negative breast cancer. N Engl J Med 2018;379:2108–2121.

Slamon DJ, Leyland-Jones B, Shak S, et al. Use of chemotherapy plus a monoclonal antibody against HER2 for metastatic breast cancer that overexpresses HER2. N Engl J Med 2001;344:783–792.

Sparano JA, Gray RJ, Makover DF, et al. Prospective validation of a 21-gene expression assay in breast cancer. N Engl J Med 2015;373:2005–2014.

Sparanoi JA, Gray, RJ, Markover DF, et al. Adjuvant chemotherapy guided by a 21-gene assay in breast cancer. N Engl J Med 2018;379:111–121.

Swain SM, Baselga J, Kim SB, et al. Pertuzumab, trastuzumab, and docetaxel in HER2-positive metastatic breast cancer. N Engl J Med 2015;372:724–734.

Turner N, Slamon D, Ro I, et al. Overall survival with palbociclib and fulvestrant in advanced breast cancer. N Engl J Med 2018;379:1926–1936.

Verma S, Miles D, Gianni L, et al. Trastuzumab emtansine for HER2-postive advanced breast cancer. N Engl J Med 2012;367:1783–1791.

Suggested websites

American Society of Clinical Oncology (ASCO). http://www.asco.org

National Comprehensive Cancer Network (NCCN). https://www.nccn.org/professionals/physician_gls/f_guidelines.asp

National Cancer Institute (NCI). http://www.cancer.gov/

Clinical Trials. http://www.cancer.gov/about-cancer/treatment/clinical-trial

Guidelines
National society guidelines

Title	Source	Date and weblink
National Comprehensive Cancer Network (NCCN) Clinical Practice Guidelines in Oncology: Breast Cancer	Consensus Committee made up of surgical, radiation, and medical oncologists from NCCN member institutions	Version 1.2016 http://www.nccn.org/professionals/physician_gls/f_guidelines_nojava.asp
American Cancer Society (ACS)/American Society of Clinical Oncology (ASCO) Breast Cancer Survivorship Care Guideline	Systematic literature review performed by Expert Panel	2015 http://www.instituteforquality.org/american-cancer-societyamerican-society-clinical-oncology-breast-cancer-survivorship-care-guideline
ASCO Clinical Practice Guideline: Chemo- and Targeted Therapy for Women with HER2 Negative (or unknown) Advanced Breast Cancer	Systematic literature review performed by an Expert Panel	2014 http://www.instituteforquality.org/chemo-and-targeted-therapy-women-her2-negative-or-unknown-advanced-breast-cancer-american-society
ASCO Clinical Practice Guideline Focused Update: Adjuvant Endocrine Therapy for Women With Hormone Receptor-Positive Breast Cancer	Systematic literature review performed by an Expert Panel	2014 http://www.instituteforquality.org/adjuvant-endocrine-therapy-women-hormone-receptor positive-breast-cancer-american-society-clinical
ASCO Clinical Practice Guideline: Systemic Therapy for Patients With Advanced Human Epidermal Growth Factor Receptor 2-Positive Breast Cancer	Systemic literature review performed by an Expert Panel	2014 http://www.instituteforquality.org/systemic-therapy-patients-advanced-human-epidermal-growth-factor-receptor-2-positive-breast-cancer
ASCO Clinical Practice Guideline Update: Sentinel Lymph Node Biopsy for Patients with Early-Stage Breast Cancer	Systematic literature review performed by an Expert Panel	2014 http://www.instituteforquality.org/sentinel-lymph-node-biopsy-patients-early-stage-breast-cancer-american-society-clinical-oncology
ASCO Clinical Practice Guideline Update: Use of Pharmacologic Interventions for Breast Cancer Risk Reduction	Systematic literature review performed by an Expert Panel	2013 http://www.instituteforquality.org/use-pharmacologic-interventions-breast-cancer-risk-reduction-american-society-clinical-oncology

(Continued)

Title	Source	Date and weblink
ASCO Clinical Practice Guideline Update: Breast Cancer Follow-Up and Management After Primary Treatment	Systematic literature review performed by an Expert Panel	2013 http://www.instituteforquality.org/breast-cancer-follow-and-management-after-primary-treatment-american-society-clinical-oncology
ASCO Clinical Practice Guideline Update: Role of Bone-Modifying Agents in Metastatic Breast Cancer	Literature search using Medline and Cochrane Collaboration Library performed by an Expert Panel	2011 http://www.instituteforquality.org/asco-clinical-practice-guideline-update-role-bone-modifying-agents-metastatic-breast-cancer

Evidence

Type of evidence	Title and comment	Date and weblink
Genomic study	Molecular portraits of human breast cancer **Comment:** Paradigm shifting first evidence that breast cancer can be divided into subtypes (Table 1.1) based on molecular genetic profiling	2000 http://www.ncbi.nlm.nih.gov/pubmed/10963602
RCT	Use of chemotherapy plus a monoclonal antibody against HER2 for metastatic breast cancer that overexpresses HER2 **Comment:** Pivotal trial that first demonstrated that trastuzumab improved the OS for women with HER2 positive metastatic disease	2001 http://www.ncbi.nlm.nih.gov/pubmed/11248153
Early Breast Cancer Trialists' Collaborative Group (EBCTCG) Meta-analysis	Effects of chemotherapy and hormonal therapy for early breast cancer on recurrence and 15-year survival: an overview of the randomized trials **Comment:** Largely of historic interest establishes multidrug adjuvant chemotherapy with an anthracycline-based chemotherapy (compared with no chemotherapy) reduces breast cancer mortality by 30% (absolute reduction in mortality in about 12% of women < 50 years) and 20% (absolute mortality reduction of about 6% in women aged 50–69). Five years of adjuvant tamoxifen irrespective of age and use of adjuvant chemotherapy (compared to with no treatment) reduces breast cancer mortality by 30% (absolute reduction in mortality of 9%)	2005 http://www.ncbi.nlm.nih.gov/pubmed/15894097
EBCTCG Meta-analysis	Effect of radiotherapy after breast-conserving surgery on 10-year recurrence and 15-year breast cancer death: meta-analysis of individual patient data for 10,801 women in 17 randomized trials **Comment:** Radiation after BCS confers a small, statistically significant OS benefit in addition to improved local control	2011 http://www.ncbi.nlm.nih.gov/pubmed/22019144

(Continued)

(*Continued*)

Type of evidence	Title and comment	Date and weblink
RCT	Lumpectomy plus tamoxifen with or without irradiation in women age 70 years or older with early breast cancer: long-term follow-up of CALGB 9343 **Comment:** No OS benefit to radiation, but local/regional breast recurrences were 2% and 10% with and without radiation. Omitting radiation is a viable option	2013 http://www.ncbi.nlm.nih.gov/pubmed/23690420
RCT	Adjuvant chemotherapy in older women with early-stage breast cancer **Comment:** Standard multidrug adjuvant chemotherapy was superior to single-drug oral capecitabine. Provides justification for not undertreating women aged ≥65	2009 http://www.ncbi.nlm.nih.gov/pubmed/19439741
RCT	Improved outcomes from adding sequential paclitaxel but not from escalating doxorubicin dose in an adjuvant chemotherapy regimen for patients with node-positive primary breast cancer **Comment:** First trial to show paclitaxel after standard doses of doxorubicin and cyclophosphamide improves disease-free and OS	2003 http://www.ncbi.nlm.nih.gov/pubmed/12637460
RCT	Trastuzumab plus adjuvant chemotherapy for human epidermal growth factor receptor 2-positive breast cancer: planned joint analysis of OS from NSABP B-31 and NCCTG N9831 **Comment:** The addition of trastuzumab to adjuvant chemotherapy results in 10% absolute improvement in OS. These results are consistent with two other RCTs	2014 http://www.ncbi.nlm.nih.gov/pubmed/25332249
RCT	Effect of anastrozole and tamoxifen as adjuvant treatment for early-stage breast cancer: 10-year analysis of the ATAC trial **Comment:** Largest trial with longest follow-up that shows anastrozole was superior to tamoxifen in time to recurrence (TTR) by about 21% (absolute difference of 4.3%) but there was no difference in OS. Consistent with the results of two other RCTs of other aromatase inhibitors (exemestane or letrozole) vs. tamoxifen	2010 http://www.ncbi.nlm.nih.gov/pubmed/21087898
RCT	Effect of preoperative chemotherapy on the outcome of women with operable breast cancer **Comment:** Established that neoadjuvant and postoperative result in similar OS	1998 http://www.ncbi.nlm.nih.gov/pubmed/9704717
RCT	Lumpectomy and radiation therapy for the treatment of intraductal breast cancer: findings from National Surgical Adjuvant Breast and Bowel Project B-17 Tamoxifen in treatment of intraductal breast cancer: National Surgical Adjuvant Breast and Bowel Project B-24 randomized controlled trial **Comment:** These two RCTs established modern treatment of DCIS with BCS, radiation, and tamoxifen for ER-positive DCIS	1998 http://www.ncbi.nlm.nih.gov/pubmed/9469327 1999 http://www.ncbi.nlm.nih.gov/pubmed/10376613

(Continued)

Type of evidence	Title and comment	Date and weblink
RCT	Everolimus in postmenopausal hormone-receptor-positive advanced breast cancer **Comment:** Established the use exemestane and everolimus for treatment of postmenopausal women who progressed on aromatase inhibitor	2012 http://www.ncbi.nlm.nih.gov/pubmed/22149876
RCT	The cyclin-dependent kinase 4/6 inhibitor palbociclib in combination with letrozole versus letrozole alone as first line treatment of estrogen receptor-positive, HER2-negative, advanced breast cancer (PALOMA-III): a randomized phase 3 trial **Comment:** With median follow-up of 38 months, 27.6 vs. 14.5 months ($p < 0.0001$) in median PFS with letrozole + palbociclib vs. letrozole, respectively in postmenopausal women with ER-positive metastatic disease, first line treatment for metastases	2019 https://doi.org/10.1007/s/10549-018 05125-4
RCT	OS with palbociclib and fulvestrant in advanced breast cancer **Comment:** With a median follow-up of 45 months, OS for fulvestrant + palbociclib vs. fulvestrant + placebo in postmenopausal women with ER-positive metastatic disease was 35 versus 28 months ($p = 0.09$), as second line treatment for metastases. However, in a preplanned subset analysis in patients that had previouly responded to endocrine therapy (79% of overall population), the median OS was 40 months for combination versus 30 months (hazard ratio 0.72; 95% CI 0.55–0.94)	2018 https://www.ncbi.nlm.nih.gov/pubmed/30345905
RCT	Trastuzumab emtansine (TDM-1) in previously treated HER/2 overexpressing breast cancer **Comment:** The EMILA trial (versus lapatinib and capecitabine) and the TH3rRESA (versus physicians choice of standard chemotherapy) led to 6–7 month median OS favoring TDM-1. The MARIANNE trial was first line chemotherapy for metastatic HER2 overexpressing breast cancer patients randomizing to paclitaxel and trastuzumab, TMD-1, or TDM-1 and pertuzumab. These treatments were comparable	2012 https://www.ncbi.nlm.nih.gov/pubmed/23020162 2017 https://www.ncbi.nlm.nih.gov/pubmed/28526538 2017 https://www.ncbi.nlm.nih.gov/pubmed/28056202
RCT	PDL-1 inhibitor in triple negative breast cancer (TNBC) **Comment:** Metastatic TNBC were randomized to nab-paclitaxel +/– atezolizumab. The median trial follow-up was 12.9 months. Overall, there was a 1.7 month statistically significant improvement ($p = 0.0025$) for combination. In a preplanned interim subgoup analysis, in the TNBC group who had PDL-1 expression of $\geq 1\%$ in tumor-infiltrating lymphocytes (41% of the total trial population), the overall median survial was 25 months for combination vs. 15.5 months for nab-paclitaxel alone (stratified hazard ratio for death was 0.62 (95% CI 0.45–0.86)	2018 https://www.ncbi.nlm.nih.gov/pubmed/30345906

Image

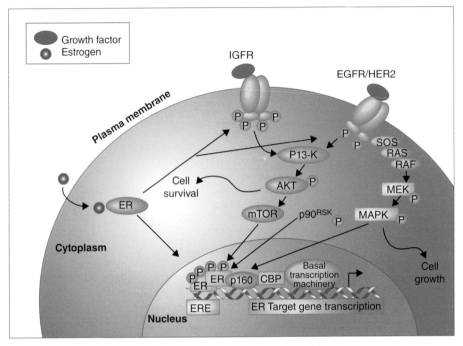

Figure 1.1 ER and HER2 pathways in breast cancer (used with permission).

Additional material for this chapter can be found online at:
www.wiley.com/go/oh/mountsinaioncology

This includes advice for patients, a case study, and multiple choice
questions.

CHAPTER 2

Prostate Cancer

Reza Mehrazin and William K. Oh
Icahn School of Medicine at Mount Sinai, New York, NY, USA

OVERALL BOTTOM LINE

- Prostate cancer has been the most common internal malignancy in US men over the last three decades. Approximately 1 out of 7 men are diagnosed with prostate cancer and roughly 1 out of 35 men die of prostate cancer, making it the second leading cause of cancer death in US men.
- Both physician and patient should discuss the benefits and risks of prostate cancer screening prior to initiating testing.
- Radical prostatectomy and radiation therapy have been standard treatments for localized prostate cancer in a healthy man with a life expectancy of at least 10 years.
- Active surveillance is a consideration for older men and those with less aggressive disease.
- Men with advanced prostate cancer often require more than one treatment (e.g. radiation, androgen deprivation therapy, or chemotherapy).
- Multidisciplinary treatment by Urology, Medical Oncology, and Radiation Oncology departments improves cancer treatment outcome and quality of life for the patient, while keeping treatment-related side effects as low as possible.

Background
Definition of disease

Prostate cancer is the development of malignancy within the prostate gland. Although it is mostly slow growing and confined within the prostate, it can be aggressive in nature and invade the seminal vesicles and metastasize to pelvic lymph nodes, bone, lung, or liver.

Incidence/prevalence

- Prostate cancer is the most common noncutaneous malignancy in US men with an estimated annual incidence of 220 500 new cases and ~27 500 cancer-specific mortality in 2015.
- Although it can occur at any age, patients often present at age ≥65.
- The use of prostate-specific antigen (PSA) testing for screening has greatly impacted the incidence, and arguably the mortality, of prostate cancer worldwide.

Economic impact

- Population-based studies have ranked prostate cancer as the fifth most expensive cancer to treat in the USA, projecting estimated total cost of care at around $16 billion by 2020.

Mount Sinai Expert Guides: Oncology, First Edition. Edited by William K. Oh and Ajai Chari.
© 2019 John Wiley & Sons Ltd. Published 2019 by John Wiley & Sons Ltd.
Companion Website: www.wiley.com/go/oh/mountsinaioncology

Etiology

- The exact etiologic factors leading to carcinoma of the prostate are not well defined. However, substantial evidence suggest genetics and environmental risk factors predispose certain patients to prostate cancer.
- Common risk factors: family history (first degree relative > second degree), race (African Americans experience >55% higher incidence rates than whites), and age (older than 65 years).
- Environmental risk factors: chronic inflammation, obesity (associated with higher treatment failure and cancer mortality), smoking (increases disease recurrence and death from cancer).
- Molecular genetic risk factors: BRCA and HOXB13 genes increase an individual's risk. Epigenetic regulation of gene expression (e.g. methylation or chromatin remodeling) has a key role in development and progression of prostate cancer. Alteration in androgen receptors is important in progression of castrate-resistant prostate cancer (CRPC).

Pathology/pathogenesis

- Prostate cancer (most commonly adenocarcinoma) arises from the epithelial cell layer. Other less common types (<5%): transitional cell, small cell, sarcoma.
- The development and progression of prostate cancer widely depends on the androgen receptor (AR) signaling pathway. AR is a protein made up of 919 amino acids and encoded by a single copy gene, located on the X-chromosome (Xq11.2-q12). The activity of AR is largely regulated by two ligands: testosterone and dihydrotestosterone. Mutation or amplification in AR genes are recognized in locally advanced prostate tumors and in men with hormone refractory prostate cancer.
- DNA hypermethylation, causing gene silencing, is the most well-known epigenetic alteration in prostate cancer. Chromatin remodeling is an epigenetic mechanism that also affects gene regulation.
- Gene fusion between TMPRSS2 and ERG has been identified in 50–60% of localized prostate cancers.
- Chronic inflammation causing cellular hyperproliferation can also contribute to development of prostate cancer

Predictive/risk factors

Risk factor	Odds ratio
Age >65	2.1
African Americans	2.4
Family history:	
• First degree	2.6–4.2
• Second degree	1.1–2.6

Prevention

No interventions have been proven to prevent the development of the disease. Smoking cessation is the only known preventive measure. Although not clear if smoking cessation reduces the risk of developing cancer, it may reduce the risk of having aggressive prostate cancer. No vitamin supplement or medication is known to be effective in prevention.

Screening
- Even though the pattern of annual screening is controversial, PSA and digital rectal examination (DRE) are often performed.
- The American Urological Association (AUA) does not recommend routine screening in men younger than 55 years, older than 70, or those with less than 10-year lifes expectancy. Shared decision making is recommended in men aged 55–69 years.
- The decision to perform screening should be individualized and based on the patient's values and preferences.
- Prostate biopsy is used to confirm the presence of cancer within the gland.

Primary prevention
- No dietary supplements or medication are known to be effective in prevention.
- Smoking cessation appears to reduce the risk of developing aggressive cancer.

Secondary prevention
- Adjuvant radiation reduces the chance of recurrence in men with positive surgical margins.
- Salvage radical prostatectomy or cryotherapy are sometimes used for treatment of non-metastatic cancer recurrence after radiotherapy.
- Use of androgen deprivation therapy, prior to initiation of radiotherapy, in high risk men, achieves a higher disease-free and OS.

Diagnosis (Algorithm 2.1)

Algorithm 2.1 Diagnosis of prostate cancer

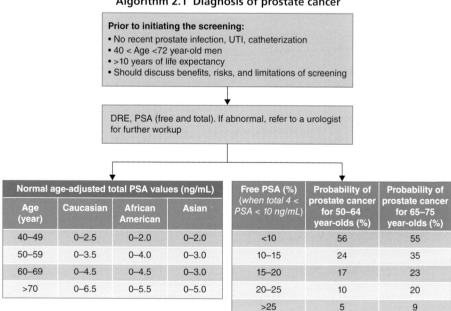

Prior to initiating the screening:
- No recent prostate infection, UTI, catheterization
- 40 < Age <72 year-old men
- >10 years of life expectancy
- Should discuss benefits, risks, and limitations of screening

DRE, PSA (free and total). If abnormal, refer to a urologist for further workup

Normal age-adjusted total PSA values (ng/mL)				Free PSA (%) (when total 4 < PSA < 10 ng/mL)	Probability of prostate cancer for 50–64 year-olds (%)	Probability of prostate cancer for 65–75 year-olds (%)
Age (year)	Caucasian	African American	Asian			
40–49	0–2.5	0–2.0	0–2.0	<10	56	55
50–59	0–3.5	0–4.0	0–3.0	10–15	24	35
60–69	0–4.5	0–4.5	0–3.0	15–20	17	23
>70	0–6.5	0–5.5	0–5.0	20–25	10	20
				>25	5	9

> **BOTTOM LINE/CLINICAL PEARLS**
> - Prostate cancer screening should be strongly considered in men older than 50 years (with + 10 years life expectancy), family history of prostate cancer, and/or African Americans.
> - Abnormal DRE (e.g. nodular or hard prostate) and/or elevated age-adjusted PSA should be further evaluated by a urologist.
> - Percentage free PSA, PSA density, prostate cancer gene 3 (*PCA3*), Prostate Health Index (PHI), multiparametric MRI, transrectal ultrasound and prostate biopsy are common tests that are used by urologists to predict the presence of neoplasm within the prostate.
> - A single abnormal test should not prompt immediate prostate biopsy.

Differential diagnosis

Differential diagnosis	Features
Prostatitis	Also causes rise in total PSA level
Benign prostatic hypertrophy	Also causes rise in total PSA level
Prostatic trauma (e.g. catheterization)	Also causes rise in total PSA level
Long rides (e.g. airplane, cycling, car rides)	Also causes rise in total PSA level

Typical presentation
Most patients with localized prostate cancer are asymptomatic on presentation. Those with advanced cancers can present with urinary retention, hematuria, irritative voiding complaints, hydronephrosis, or bone pain.

Clinical diagnosis
History
A complete personal and family history significant for prostate cancer should be obtained. It is important to note if a family member died with disease or because of it. Although not specific for cancer, the presence of lower urinary tract symptoms such as irritative voiding complaints, dysuria, hematuria, frequency, or hesitancy should be documented.

Physical examination
DRE should be performed to estimate the size of the gland and to determine if a palpable nodule is present. An abnormal DRE is often associated with increased risk of detecting high grade cancer.

Useful clinical decision rules and calculators
There are several individualized risk assessment calculators which can be found on the Internet (e.g. riskcalc.org or myprostatecancerrisk.org). They are often used to aid clinicians in determining whether biopsy is needed and the likelihood of cancer-specific mortality.

Disease severity classification
The Gleason score grading system is commonly used to report on severity of the cancer. It is based on the pathologic architectural pattern of prostatic glands. The two common patterns are graded 1–5, and then added to obtain the Gleason score. The higher the score, the worse the prognosis; Gleason scores of 8–10 are considered high risk cancers.

Laboratory diagnosis
List of diagnostic tests
- **PSA:** secreted in high concentrations into seminal fluid. It circulates in free (unbound) or complex (bound) forms. The levels vary with age, prostate size, race, amount of androgens present, and presence of prostate disease (e.g. cancer, benign prostatic hyperplasia [BPH], infection).
- **Free PSA:** A lower percentage of PSA circulating in an unbound or free form is often associated with prostate cancer. It has been shown to improve the ability to distinguish men with cancer when used in conjunction with total PSA.
- **Prostate cancer gene 3 (*PCA3*):** a noncoding mRNA urine test to detect *PCA3* which is overexpressed in prostate cancer tissue (i.e. a higher *PCA3* score indicates a higher risk of detecting cancer on biopsy).
- **PHI:** a combination test of total and free PSA and [-2]proPSA.

Lists of imaging techniques
- **Ultrasound:** often used at the time of prostate biopsy. Although not sensitive, at times hypoechoic lesions seen on ultrasound could represent prostate cancer.
- **MRI:** functional sequences such as diffusion-weighted images and dynamic contrast-enhanced images are being commonly used to localize and evaluate the extent of cancer.
- **Pelvic CT:** used when nomogram indicates >10% chance of lymph node involvement (PSA >20, Gleason score >8, clinical stage T3–T4).
- **Bone scan:** obtained if symptoms suggestive of metastatic cancer (elevated alkaline phosphatase [ALP], bone pain) or when PSA >20, Gleason score >8, or clinical stage T3–T4.

Potential pitfalls/common errors made regarding diagnosis of disease
- Prostate cancer screening is associated with potential harms of psychologic and physical stress of overtreatment of an indolent cancer.
- Prostate biopsy has risks of hematuria (14–50%), hematochezia, hematospermia (10–70%), dysuria, sepsis (4%), and pain.

Treatment (Algorithm 2.2)
Treatment rationale
- Treatment of prostate cancer is dependent on Gleason score, PSA, stage, and extent of disease.
- Standard treatments for localized disease: radical prostatectomy, external beam radiation, brachytherapy, cryotherapy, and surveillance.
- For high risk cancer, brachytherapy or cryotherapy alone have lower cure rates and are not recommended.
- Androgen deprivation therapy (ADT) is often used as a neoadjuvant or adjuvant treatment in men with high risk prostate cancer. It is the treatment of choice in men with metastatic prostate cancer but has no role as a solitary treatment for cT1-T2N0M0.
- Docetaxel chemotherapy added to ADT improves survival in men with newly diagnosed metastatic disease.
- Abiraterone, enzalutamide, sipuleucel T, and cabazitaxel radium-223 are therapeutic options for men with castration-resistant metastatic disease. All have been shown to improve OS in randomized clinical trials.

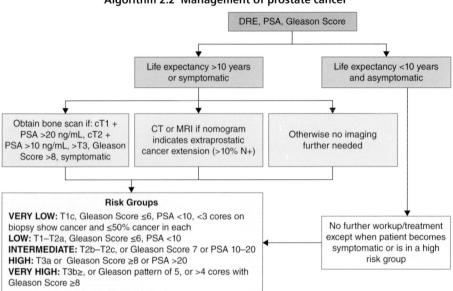

Algorithm 2.2 Management of prostate cancer

When to hospitalize

- **Ureteral obstruction:** pelvic adenopathy from metastatic cancer can cause ureteral obstruction leading to renal failure. In these situations, either ureteral stent or percutaneous nephrostomy tubes are used to relieve the obstruction.
- **Bladder outlet obstruction:** managed by urethral catheter, suprapubic tube, or transurethral resection of the prostate (TURP).
- **Persistent prostatic bleeding:** managed by TURP, ADT, or embolization.
- **Acute spinal cord compression from metastasis:** treated with IV bolus of dexamethasone 100 mg, followed by oral dose for 3 days. Then, the patient should be immediately castrated by ketoconazole, bilateral orchiectomy, or GnRH antagonists. Surgical decompression can sometimes be necessary.

Table of treatment

Treatment	Comments
Conservative	
Active surveillance	An option for men either with low risk disease and/or life expectancy <10 years
Surgical	
Radical prostatectomy	Either performed in a conventional open approach, robotic assisted laparoscopically, or standard laparoscopic approach. It is a standard treatment approach in men with nonmetastatic prostate cancer
Cryotherapy	By intracellular ice formation, the prostate cancer cells are killed at −40°C. It is typically recommended for treatment of low risk cancer or as a salvage treatment after failed radiotherapy

(Continued)

Treatment	Comments
Radiotherapy	
Intensity modulated radiation therapy (IMRT)	Delivers less radiation to surrounding tissues than three-dimensional conformal radiation therapy (3D C-XRT) and associated with fewer short- and long-term side effects. External beam radiation is fractionated over several weeks
Brachytherapy ("seeds")	Permanent radioactive seed implants: iodine 125 (half-life 60 days), palladium 103 (half-life 17 days), or cesium 131 (half-life 9.5 days). Seed monotherapy has a higher failure rate in men with intermediate disease
Proton beam therapy	Similar to IMRT but its benefits over IMRT are not clear
Medical	
Docetaxel	Considered first line chemotherapy, docetaxel is a taxane and functions by disrupting normal microtubule function. It is administered IV every 3 weeks × 10 cycles
Cabazitaxel	Also a taxane. It is administered IV every 3 weeks × 10 cycles
Mitoxantrone	Disrupts DNA synthesis and then intercalates into DNA. Also inhibits topoisomerase II. Used to treat pain arising from advanced cancer
Sipuleucel-T (Provenge)	An autologous cellular immunotherapy. Used in asymptomatic or minimally symptomatic metastatic castration-resistant prostate cancer (MCRPC). Exact mechanism of action is unknown but likely it programs the T-cells to destroy cells that express prostatic acid phosphatase
Abiraterone (Zytiga)	Inhibits CYP17 which is needed for androgen synthesis. Dose: 1 g/day PO on an empty stomach. Can cause hyperaldosteronism so prednisone 5 mg twice daily is given
Enzalutamide (Xtandi)	A nonsteroidal antiandrogen that competitively inhibits androgen binding. Dose: 160 mg/day PO
Zoledronic acid (Zometa)	Inhibits osteoclast activity and prevents bone resorption. Used in patients with CRPC and bone metastasis. Dose: 4 mg IV every 4 weeks
Denosumab (Xgeva)	A monoclonal antibody that binds to RANK ligand and prevents bone resorption in patients with CRPC and bone metastasis. Dose: 120 mg subcutaneously every 4 weeks
Radium-223 (Xofigo)	Has a similar behavior to calcium and is taken up with increased bone metabolism. Used in men with CRPC and symptomatic bone metastasis
Lifestyle modification	
Smoking cessation	Can reduce cancer progression in some studies
Diet	Low fat, high fiber, lycopene, green tea, vitamin D, E, and selenium can inhibit the growth of cancer

Prevention/management of complications

- Stress urinary incontinence and erectile dysfunction are the two common side effects of radical prostatectomy. Pelvic floor muscle exercises and medical therapies are the first line treatment. Infertility and aspermia are always seen after surgery.
- Urinary and bowel incontinence, erectile dysfunction, urethral stricture, infertility, hemorrhagic cystitis, bladder and rectal irritation are side effects of radiotherapy.

> **CLINICAL PEARLS**
> - The optimal treatment of prostate cancer depends on assessment of the patient's life expectancy and the disease risk.
> - Active surveillance means actively monitoring the course of the disease in patients with very low risk disease with the expectation to intervene if the cancer progresses. This prevents the side effects of an unnecessary definitive therapy.
> - Radical prostatectomy or radiation is appropriate for any men with life expectancy >10 years, whose tumor is clinically confined to the prostate.
> - In patients with metastatic prostate cancer, castrate levels of serum testosterone (<50) should be maintained.

Special populations

Elderly

Prostate cancer screening in men older than 70 years or those with less than 10 years' life expectancy is not recommended by most guidelines. The decision on screening and treatment of cancer should be individualized and based on the patient's values and preferences.

Prognosis

> **BOTTOM LINE/CLINICAL PEARLS**
> - Appropriate risk group stratification provides a better basis for appropriate treatment recommendation than just clinical stage.
> - Preoperative high PSA at diagnosis, Gleason score ≥8, PSA velocity >2.0 ng/mL per year, and positive DRE all increase the risk of death from prostate cancer.
> - Positive surgical margin correlates with a higher risk of death from cancer.
> - After radiotherapy, if PSA rises and doubles in less than 3 months, the chance of death from cancer is high.
> - Relapse of cancer rarely occurs without a rise in PSA.

Natural history of untreated disease

The natural history of untreated disease depends on the stage, Gleason score, and PSA. For instance, the 10-year prostate cancer mortality in men >65 years with Gleason score 6 not receiving treatment is about 9%, while it is estimated at 25% for Gleason score 8.

Follow-up tests and monitoring

- PSA is used after a definitive treatment for surveillance. A rise in PSA is associated with cancer recurrence.
- CT and/or bone scans are used for initial evaluation and surveillance of skeletal or distant metastases.

Reading list

Carter HB, Albertsen PC, Barry MJ, et al. American Urological Association (AUA) Guideline on Early Detection of Prostate Cancer. American Urological Association, 2013.

European Association of Urology Guidelines on Prostate Cancer. EAU/ESTRO/SIOG, 2017.

McDougal WS, Wein AJ, Kavoussi LR, et al. (eds.) Campbell-Walsh Urology, 11th edition. Part XIV The Prostate. Elsevier, 2016, pp. 408–475.

National Comprehensive Cancer Network (NCCN) Guidelines for Prostate Cancer, 2016.

Guidelines
National society guidelines

Title	Source	Date and weblink
Early detection of prostate cancer	NCCN	2016 http://www.nccn.org/professionals/physician_gls/pdf/prostate.pdf
	AUA	2013, updated 2018 https://www.auanet.org/guidelines/prostate-cancer-early-detection-(2013-reviewed-for-currency-2018)

International society guidelines

Title	Source	Date and weblink
Guidelines on prostate cancer	EAU	2014 http://uroweb.org/wp-content/uploads/1607-Prostate-Cancer_LRV3.pdf

Evidence

Type of evidence	Title and comment	Date and weblink
RCT	PLCO and ERSPC Trials **Comment:** Although highly questioned by urologic societies, these trials showed screening did not reduce risk of mortality	2012 https://www.ncbi.nlm.nih.gov/pubmed/22228146 2014 https://www.ncbi.nlm.nih.gov/pubmed/25108889
RCT	Göteborg Trial **Comment:** With median follow-up of 14 years, the relative reduction in cancer mortality with screening is 40%	2010 https://www.ncbi.nlm.nih.gov/pubmed/20598634
Systematic review and meta-analysis of the published literature	Statement released by AUA on prostate cancer detection and screening	2013, reviewed 2018 https://www.auanet.org/guidelines/prostate-cancer-early-detection-(2013-reviewed-for-currency-2018)

Additional material for this chapter can be found online at:
www.wiley.com/go/oh/mountsinaioncology

This includes advice for patients, a case study, multiple choice questions, and ICD codes.

CHAPTER 3

Bladder Cancer

Matthew D. Galsky
Icahn School of Medicine at Mount Sinai, New York, NY, USA

OVERALL BOTTOM LINE
- Bladder cancer is the second most commonly diagnosed genitourinary cancer.
- Cigarette smoking accounts for at least half of bladder cancer diagnoses.
- Gross hematuria is the most common presenting sign of bladder cancer.
- The majority of patients with bladder cancer present with cancer that does not invade the muscularis propria (i.e. non-muscle-invasive bladder cancer). Non-muscle-invasive bladder cancer is frequently curable with transurethral resection of tumor with or without the application of intravesical chemotherapy or immunotherapy.
- Bladder cancer invading the muscularis propria (i.e. muscle-invasive bladder cancer), in the absence of radiographic evidence of metastatic disease, is managed with definitive local therapy. This most commonly involves surgical removal of the bladder (radical cystectomy) although radiation therapy represents a potential bladder-sparing treatment option for a subset of patients. Outcomes are suboptimal with single-modality treatment approaches and the integration of systemic chemotherapy should be considered for all patients without contraindications to such treatment.

Background
Definition of disease
Bladder cancer is a malignancy of the urinary bladder that most commonly arises from the urothelium, which is the cell lining of the bladder.

Disease classification
- The vast majority of bladder cancers are urothelial cancers although mixed histologies and less common variant histologies (e.g. squamous carcinoma) can occur.
- Because the urothelium extends from the urethra to the renal pelvis, urothelial cancers can arise from anywhere along this urothelial tract although cancers arising in the bladder are the most common.

Incidence/prevalence
- Approximately 70 000 patients are diagnosed with bladder cancer each year in the USA and approximately 16 000 patients each year succumb to the disease.
- The majority of patients present with non-muscle-invasive disease.

Mount Sinai Expert Guides: Oncology, First Edition. Edited by William K. Oh and Ajai Chari.

Economic impact

The need for frequent cystoscopic surveillance for non-muscle-invasive disease means that bladder cancer is considered among the most expensive malignancies to treat on a per patient basis.

Etiology

- Although the precise etiology of bladder cancer is not known, several risk factors have been identified.
- Tobacco smoking is the most important risk factor for bladder cancer and accounts for approximately half of all diagnoses.
- Environmental exposures have been associated with bladder cancer including aluminum, dye, paint, petroleum, and rubber.
- Occupations involving exposure to combustion gases have been associated with bladder cancer.
- An endemic form of bladder cancer caused by the trematode *Schistosoma haematobium* occurs in the Middle East and other parts of the world and is most commonly squamous cell cancer rather than urothelial cancer.

Pathology/pathogenesis

- Hematuria is the most common presenting sign of bladder cancer.
- Urothelial cancer, formerly known as transitional cell carcinoma, is the most common histologic subtype, and accounts for approximately 90–95% of bladder cancers in the USA.
- Less common histologic subtypes include squamous cell carcinoma, adenocarcinoma, and small cell carcinoma.
- Gene expression profiling has identified subtypes of bladder cancer that resemble molecular subtypes of breast cancer and are associated with distinct therapeutic targets and clinical outcomes.

Predictive/risk factors

Risk factor	Comment
Tobacco smoking	Responsible for approximately 50% of bladder cancer
Occupational exposure	Responsible for approximately for 20% of bladder cancer

Prevention

> **BOTTOM LINE/CLINICAL PEARL**
> - Smoking cessation is the most important intervention to decrease the risk of bladder cancer.

Screening

- There are currently no reliable screening tests for bladder cancer.
- While bladder cancer is commonly associated with hematuria, asymptomatic microscopic hematuria is very rarely caused by bladder cancer, highlighting the limitation of urinalysis as a general screening tool. Genitourinary cancers account for approximately 5% of microscopic hematuria. Therefore, routine urinalyses have not been shown to be an effective screening strategy for the general population.

Primary prevention

- Smoking cessation.

Secondary prevention
- Intravesical treatment with bacillus Calmette–Guérin (BCG) or chemotherapy for non-muscle-invasive disease has been shown to reduce recurrence and/or progression.
- Perioperative systemic chemotherapy for muscle-invasive bladder cancer, particularly neoadjuvant cisplatin-based combination chemotherapy, has been shown to decrease the risk of metastatic recurrence.

Diagnosis

> **BOTTOM LINE/CLINICAL PEARLS**
> - A medical history should ascertain the presence of gross hematuria and other urinary tract symptoms, as well as constitutional symptoms (e.g. fatigue, weight loss). The latter can be an indication of metastatic disease.
> - Physical examination should assess for the presence of any palpable masses or lymphadenopathy which may indicate the presence of metastatic disease.
> - Urine cytology can be helpful for diagnosing bladder cancer but has the greatest sensitivity for the diagnosis of carcinoma *in situ*.
> - Cystoscopy, which allows direct visualization of the inner lining of the bladder, is critical in diagnosing bladder cancer. Cystoscopy, particularly rigid cystoscopy performed in the operating room, allows endoscopic resection of a visualized bladder tumor. This procedure, known as a transurethral resection of bladder tumor (TURBT), is generally a diagnostic procedure but in some cases can also serve as a definitive therapeutic procedure.
> - Cross-sectional imaging (e.g. computed tomography scan of the chest, abdomen, and pelvis) should be performed in all patients with muscle-invasive bladder cancer to rule out regional or distant metastases.

Differential diagnosis

Differential diagnosis	Features
Cancer arising elsewhere in the genitourinary tract	Gross hematuria in the setting of a normal cystoscopy should prompt an evaluation of the upper urinary tract with a computed tomography scan, retrograde pyelography, or direct visualization with ureteroscopy
Glomerular disease of the kidney	Urinalysis should be performed in patients with gross hematuria to rule out findings that could suggest glomerular bleeding (e.g. casts)

Typical presentation
- Gross hematuria in a patient >40 years old requires evaluation of the entire genitourinary tract to rule out cancer.
- Gross painless hematuria is the most common presentation of bladder cancer.
- Patients can have irritative voiding symptoms such as urinary urgency, frequency, or dysuria. The presence of pain, fatigue, anorexia, and/or weight loss could indicate the presence of locally advanced or metastatic disease and should prompt an evaluation to rule out the same.

Clinical diagnosis
History
The clinical history should ascertain the presence of hematuria or lower urinary tract symptoms. In addition, constitutional symptoms and/or pain, which could indicate the presence of metastatic

disease, should be excluded. A prior history of bladder cancer should be documented as patients initially presenting with non-muscle-invasive disease are generally at high risk for recurrence and/or progression. Prior radiation to the pelvis can increase the risk of bladder cancer and can impact treatment selection and so should be ascertained.

Physical examination

- The physical examination should rule out the presence of any masses or adenopathy that could indicate the presence of metastatic disease.
- A referral to a urologist is indicated if there is a suspicion of bladder cancer (e.g. gross hematuria in a patient >40 years old). A urologist will generally perform a flexible cystoscopy in the office which allows direct visualization of the lining of the bladder and any tumors; the ability to obtain biopsies with flexible cystoscopy is limited. If there is a tumor or other suspicious findings, the urologist will perform a rigid cystoscopy in the operating room facilitating endoscopic TURBT. The TURBT is generally considered a "biopsy" implying that it is commonly a diagnostic rather than a therapeutic procedure; however, in certain cases, TURBT can also be a definitive surgical procedure. The TURBT specimen is submitted to the pathologist for evaluation. The diagnosis of bladder cancer can only be made by pathologic inspection of tumor tissue.

Disease severity classification

- While standard TNM (tumor, nodal, metastases) staging applies to bladder cancer, there are distinct clinical disease states that are directly linked to treatment and prognosis.
- Clinical staging refers to information derived from the examination, imaging, and the pathologic review of the TURBT specimen. Pathologic staging refers to the extent of disease as determined by pathologic review of the bladder and regional lymph nodes after surgical removal (i.e. cystectomy and lymphadenectomy specimen).
- Bladder cancer can broadly be categorized as non-muscle-invasive, muscle-invasive, or metastatic. The distinction between non-muscle-invasive disease and muscle-invasive disease is made by the pathologist upon review of the TURBT specimen. Hence, muscle (muscularis propria) must be present in the specimen to rule out muscle invasion adequately and the absence of muscle in the specimen is an indication for a repeat TURBT.
- Non-muscle-invasive bladder cancer includes:
  - Ta: papillary tumors that are most often low grade and present as "polyps" in the bladder. These tumors are located above the basement membrane. They frequently recur but uncommonly progress to more invasive disease.
  - Carcinoma *in situ* (CIS): CIS is flat and often has a velvety appearance. CIS is typically high grade and has a high propensity for progression to more invasive disease.
  - T1: these tumors invade the lamina propria. They are most commonly high grade and associated with the worst prognosis among the non-muscle-invasive tumors. Approximately 50% of patients with T1 tumors will develop muscle-invasive bladder cancer within 10 years.
- Muscle-invasive bladder cancer involves tumor invasion into or through the muscularis propria. Approximately 50% of patients undergoing cystectomy for muscle-invasive bladder cancer will experience metastatic recurrence.
- Metastatic bladder cancer is most commonly suspected based on abnormal findings on cross-sectional imaging which is then verified by obtaining a biopsy. Bladder cancer most commonly metastasizes to the lymph nodes, lungs, liver, and bone.

Laboratory diagnosis
List of diagnostic tests
- Urine cytology.

- Complete blood count particularly to evaluate for the presence of anemia as a consequence of hematuria.
- Comprehensive metabolic profile particularly to evaluate for renal dysfunction as a consequence of potential ureteral obstruction from tumor, elevated alkaline phosphatase as a potential indicator of bone metastases, and liver function test abnormalities as a potential indicator of liver metastases.
- Cystoscopy and TURBT.

Lists of imaging techniques
- Cross-sectional imaging to evaluate for the presence of a bladder tumor, hydronephrosis as a consequence of potential ureteral obstruction, and any metastatic disease. Imaging can include a computed tomography (CT) scan of the abdomen and pelvis (Figure 3.1) or magnetic resonance imaging (MRI) of the abdomen and pelvis.
- For patients with muscle-invasive disease, chest imaging to rule out metastases with a chest X-ray or preferably a CT of the chest should be performed.
- A bone scan should be performed in the setting of an elevated alkaline phosphatase level or signs or symptoms worrisome for bone metastases.

Potential pitfalls/common errors made regarding diagnosis of disease
Adults with gross hematuria and a normal cystoscopy require evaluation of the upper urinary tract to rule out the presence of tumors of the ureter, renal pelvis, or kidneys. This can be accomplished with cross-sectional imaging of the abdomen and pelvis but may also require visualization of the upper urinary tracts with retrograde pyelograms or ureteroscopy.

Treatment (Algorithm 3.1)

Algorithm 3.1 Management of bladder cancer

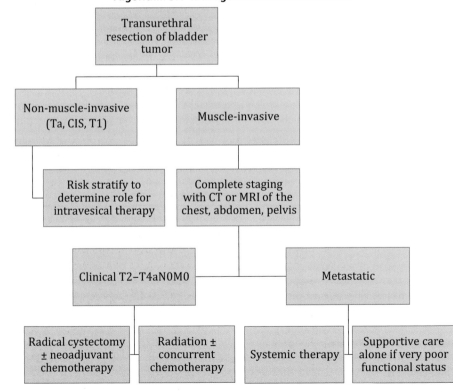

Treatment rationale

Non-muscle-invasive bladder cancer

- All patients should undergo a complete TURBT which is diagnostic and can be therapeutic depending on the depth of invasion of the cancer into the bladder wall.
- For patients at low risk of recurrence (i.e. low grade solitary Ta tumors <3 cm), a single instal-lation of intravesical chemotherapy (e.g. mitomycin) post-TURBT is recommended to decrease the risk of recurrence.
- For patients at intermediate risk of recurrence/progression (i.e. multiple tumors, recurrent Ta tumors, or grade 1–2 T1 tumors), a single instillation of chemotherapy (e.g. mitomycin) post-TURBT should be administered in addition to treatment with intravesical BCG. BCG is a live attenuated strain of *Mycobacterium bovis*. While the precise mechanism of action of BCG for non-muscle-invasive bladder cancer is not completely known, BCG has been shown to induce both an innate and adaptive anticancer immune response. BCG immunotherapy is given for six weekly doses (referred to as induction) followed by maintenance. Maintenance BCG should be continued for at least 1 year for intermediate risk patients.
- For patients at high risk for recurrence/progression (i.e. CIS or grade 3 Ta or T1 tumors), follow-ing TURBT, patients should be treated with intravesical BCG induction and maintenance should be continued for 3 years.
- Radical cystectomy is an alternative for patients with high grade T1 tumors and early cystec-tomy should be considered for patients with recurrent high grade T1 disease despite prior treatment.

Muscle-invasive bladder cancer

- Surgical removal of the bladder (radical cystectomy) and pelvic lymph node dissection is the mainstay of treatment for muscle-invasive bladder cancer though bladder-sparing treatments (e.g. radiation therapy ± concurrent chemotherapy) can be also be considered.
- Radical cystectomy involves removal of the bladder and prostate in men and removal of the bladder and reproductive organs in women.
- With removal of the bladder, the urine can be diverted into a segment of intestine which is connected to the abdominal wall and drains to an external collection bag (ileal conduit urinary diversion), can be diverted into a segment of bowel which is connected to the abdominal wall and can be intermittently catheterized so an external collection bag is not needed, or a small segment of bowel can be fashioned into a "neobladder" which is anastomosed to the urethra so patients can void in a fashion that approximates normal voiding.
- Approximately 50% of patients with muscle-invasive bladder cancer develop metastatic recur-rence after surgery prompting the evaluation of perioperative systemic chemotherapy in an attempt to increase cure rates.
- Two randomized trials and a meta-analysis support the use of neoadjuvant (i.e. systemic chemotherapy given prior to surgery in an attempt to eradicate micrometastatic disease) cisplatin-based combination chemotherapy prior to cystectomy for muscle-invasive bladder can-cer based on a significant improvement in survival.
- The data supporting adjuvant chemotherapy (i.e. systemic chemotherapy given after surgery in an attempt to eradicate micrometastatic disease) are somewhat less compelling based on small and underpowered clinical trials. However, most guidelines support consideration of cisplatin-based combination chemotherapy in the adjuvant setting for patients with pathologic ≥T3 disease and/or patients with pathologic lymph node involvement based on review of the cys-tectomy/lymphadenectomy specimen.
- Radiation therapy administered with concurrent chemotherapy can be potentially curative in patients with muscle-invasive bladder cancer and represents a "bladder-sparing" option. While

predictors of patients optimally suited for this approach remain elusive, patients with a solitary T2 tumor that can be completely resected upon TURBT, not involving the ureteral orifice, and without concomitant CIS, are likely the best candidates. Two randomized trials have demonstrated an improvement in local regional control with the addition of concurrent chemotherapy to radiation. However, no trials have been adequately powered to demonstrate a survival benefit with the addition of concurrent chemotherapy and there have been no prospective randomized trials comparing cystectomy with chemoradiation.

Metastatic bladder cancer

- Cisplatin-based combination chemotherapy is standard first line treatment for patients with metastatic bladder cancer. The most commonly administered regimens are gemcitabine plus cisplatin or MVAC (methotrexate, vinblastine, doxorubicin, plus cisplatin).
- The median survival of patients with metastatic bladder cancer is approximately 14 months. However, patients experience heterogeneous outcomes and the most important prognostic factors are a patient's functional status and the presence of metastatic disease involving non-lymph node sites.
- A large subset of patients with metastatic bladder cancer are ineligible for cisplatin chemotherapy due to renal impairment or poor functional status. In such cases, carboplatin is commonly substituted.
- In 2016–2017, five immune checkpoint inhibitors (PD-1 or PD-L1 inhibitors) were approved by the US Food and Drug Administration (FDA) for the treatment of patients with metastatic bladder cancer progressing despite prior treatment with platinum-based chemotherapy: atezolizumab, pembrolizumab, nivolumab, durvalumab, and avelumab. Most of these approvals were based on single-arm trials demonstrating durable responses in approximately 15–25% of patients. A randomized phase 3 trial has demonstrated an improvement in survival in patients with metastatic bladder cancer progressing despite platinum-based chemotherapy treated with pembrolizumab versus standard chemotherapy.
- Two immune checkpoint inhibitors, atezolizumab and pembrolizumab, have also been approved by the US FDA for first line treatment of patients with metastatic bladder cancer who are considered "cisplatin-ineligible"; that is patients for whom the risks of cisplatin-based chemotherapy are felt to outweigh the potential benefits based on poor renal function or other comorbidities. While these drugs were initially approved for all chemotherapy-naïve cisplatin-ineligible patients, the label was subsequently restricted to patients with tumors expressing a high level of PD-L1 by immunohistochemistry based on emerging data.

Table of treatment
Non-muscle-invasive bladder cancer

Treatment	Comments
Surgical	TURBT is standard management and can be both diagnostic and therapeutic
Medical	Intravesical administration of chemotherapy (e.g. mitomycin) post-TURBT is indicated for patients with low or intermediate risk of disease recurrence. A meta-analysis of seven RCTs has demonstrated a significant decrease in the risk of recurrence with single dose intravesical chemotherapy in the immediate postoperative period
	Intravesical administration of BGC is indicated for patients with intermediate or high risk disease. BCG intravesical immunotherapy has been shown in RCTs to decrease the risk of recurrence and progression as well as improve disease-specific survival

Muscle-invasive bladder cancer

Treatment	Comments
Surgery	Radical cystectomy and pelvic lymph node dissection is a standard treatment for patients with muscle-invasive bladder cancer. Outcomes after radical cystectomy are associated with pathologic disease stage. In a large series, recurrence-free survival at 5 years was 89% for pT2 tumors, 62–78% for pT3 tumors, and 35% for patients with pathologic evidence of lymph node involvement
Medical	Neoadjuvant (prior to surgery) cisplatin-based combination chemotherapy has been shown to improve surgical results when administered prior to radical cystectomy in patients with muscle-invasive bladder cancer. A meta-analysis of RCTs has demonstrated an absolute survival benefit of 5% with neoadjuvant cisplatin-based combination chemotherapy
	Adjuvant (after surgery) cisplatin-based combination chemotherapy can improve survival in patients with ≥pT3 or node-positive disease
	The MVAC regimen is best supported by Level I evidence though the combination of gemcitabine plus cisplatin is often substituted based on potentially better tolerability
Radiation	Radiation is a "bladder-sparing" option for treatment of muscle-invasive bladder cancer
	Radiation should be administered with concurrent chemotherapy in patients without contraindications to systemic chemotherapy. An RCT of concurrent 5-FU plus mitomycin given concurrently with radiation demonstrated a 13% absolute improvement in locoregional disease-free survival at 2 years compared with radiation alone. Other studies have most commonly explored concurrent cisplatin

Metastatic bladder cancer

Treatment	Comment
Medical	Cisplatin-based combination chemotherapy is standard first line treatment for metastatic bladder cancer. The two most commonly utilized regimens are MVAC (methotrexate, vinblastine, doxorubicin, plus cisplatin) and gemcitabine plus cisplatin. An RCT demonstrated similar efficacy between these regimens but less toxicity with gemcitabine plus cisplatin
	Carboplatin is substituted for cisplatin in patients with renal impairment or poor functional status. The most commonly prescribed regimen is the combination of gemcitabine plus carboplatin
	The immune checkpoint inhibitors atezolizumab or pembrolizumab are treatment options for chemotherapy-naïve patients with metastatic bladder cancer who are considered "cisplatin-ineligible" and with tumors expressing high levels of PD-L1 by immunohistochemistry
Surgical	Surgical resection of metastatic disease should be considered in patients with solitary sites of metastatic disease particularly after achieving a response to chemotherapy
Radiation	Radiation therapy should be considered for solitary sites of metastatic disease that are causing complications such as pain

Prevention/management of complications
- Ureteral obstruction from bladder cancer can result in hydronephrosis and renal impairment and can often be managed, at least temporarily, with placement of a ureteral stent or nephrostomy tube.
- Hematuria from bladder cancer can often be managed with transurethral resection of the tumor. For patients with refractory hematuria and contraindications to cystectomy, palliative radiation therapy can be considered.

> **CLINICAL PEARLS**
> - Gross hematuria in a patient >40 years old should be considered indicative of a genitourinary malignancy until proven otherwise.
> - Muscularis propria must be present in the TURBT specimen to evaluate accurately for the presence of muscle-invasive bladder cancer. Absence of muscularis propria in the TURBT specimen is an indication for a repeat TURBT.
> - Multimodality therapy is generally required to optimize the likelihood of cure for patients with muscle-invasive bladder cancer without radiographic evidence of metastatic disease.
> - A subset of patients with radiographic metastatic disease involving only lymph nodes are curable with chemotherapy with or without post-chemotherapy surgical consolidation.

Special populations
Elderly
- Bladder cancer is a disease of the elderly, with a median age of diagnosis in the seventh decade.
- Radical cystectomy is a major operation and requires careful preoperative risk assessment particularly in elderly patients often with smoking-related comorbidities. However, untreated, muscle-invasive bladder cancer often progresses to metastatic disease within months to years of diagnosis and this must be balanced with the potential for morbidity and/or mortality with definitive therapy and viewed in the context of the estimated life expectancy of the patient.
- A Comprehensive Geriatric Assessment, or more abbreviated assessment tool, should be considered in all elderly patients to assess the potential risks and benefits of bladder cancer therapies (www.mycarg.org).
- Prediction tools have been developed and validated by the Cancer and Aging Research Group to determine the likelihood of chemotherapy-related toxicity in elderly patients (www.mycarg.org/Chemo_Toxicity_Calculator).

Others
- Pure variant histologies of bladder cancer (e.g. squamous cell carcinoma, adenocarcinoma, small cell carcinoma) are uncommon in the USA and account for <10% of bladder cancers.
- Adenocarcinoma and squamous cell carcinoma of the bladder are generally less chemosensitive than urothelial cancer and muscle-invasive disease is best managed with cystectomy alone.
- Adenocarcinoma of the dome of the bladder commonly represents a tumor originating in the urachus (a remnant of a channel between the bladder and the umbilicus). Such tumors can be managed surgically with partial cystectomy and en bloc resection of the urachus.
- Small cell carcinoma of the bladder is very chemotherapy sensitive but rapidly develops resistance to treatment. The optimal treatment for patients with disease localized to the bladder is not clear but retrospective series support initial treatment with cisplatin-based chemotherapy followed by cystectomy in patients without evidence of disease progression.

Prognosis

> **BOTTOM LINE/CLINICAL PEARLS**
> - Non-muscle-invasive bladder cancer is curable in the majority of patients.
> - Approximately 50% of patients with muscle-invasive bladder cancer will develop metastatic recurrence despite undergoing curative-intent therapy (e.g. radical cystectomy).
> - The median survival of patients with metastatic bladder cancer is approximately 14 months.

Follow-up tests and monitoring

- Patients with non-muscle-invasive disease require frequent cystoscopic surveillance and urine cytology to monitor for recurrent disease.
- Patients treated with definitive therapy for muscle-invasive bladder cancer are typically monitored with periodic cross-sectional imaging studies (e.g. CT scans of chest, abdomen, and pelvis). While the optimal schedule has not been established, a common approach is to perform scans every 3 months for the first 1.5 years after definitive treatment, every 6 months for the next 1.5 years, and then yearly for up to 5 years post-definitive treatment. Ongoing cystoscopic surveillance is also required for patients treated with bladder-sparing approaches.

Reading list

Suggested websites

National Cancer Institute bladder cancer treatment summary. http://www.cancer.gov/types/bladder/hp/bladder-treatment-pdq

Bladder Cancer Advocacy Network. http://www.bcan.org

American Cancer Society. http://www.cancer.org/cancer/bladdercancer/

Guidelines

National society guidelines

Title	Source	Date and weblink
National Comprehensive Cancer Network Bladder Cancer Guidelines	NCCN	2018 https://www.nccn.org/professionals/physician_gls/default.aspx
Guideline for the Management of Nonmuscle Invasive Bladder Cancer	American Urological Association (AUA)	2016 https://www.auanet.org/guidelines/bladder-cancer-non-muscle-invasive

International society guidelines

Title	Source	Date and weblink
Guidelines on Non-muscle-invasive Bladder Cancer (Ta, T1 and CIS)	European Association of Urology (EAU)	2015 http://uroweb.org/wp-content/uploads/EAU-Guidelines-Non-muscle-invasive-Bladder-Cancer-2015-v1.pdf
Guidelines on Muscle-invasive and Metastatic Bladder Cancer	European Association of Urology (EAU)	2015 http://uroweb.org/wp-content/uploads/EAU-Guidelines-Muscle-invasive-and-Metastatic-Bladder-Cancer-2015-v1.pdf

Evidence

Type of evidence	Title and comment	Date and weblink
RCT	Maintenance bacillus Calmette–Guérin immunotherapy for recurrent TA, T1 and carcinoma in situ transitional cell carcinoma of the bladder: a randomized Southwest Oncology Group Study **Comment:** Established the benefit of maintenance BCG in non-muscle-invasive bladder cancer	2000 http://www.jurology.com/article/S0022-5347(05)67707-5/abstract

(Continued)

(*Continued*)

Type of evidence	Title and comment	Date and weblink
RCT	Neoadjuvant chemotherapy plus cystectomy compared with cystectomy alone for locally advanced bladder cancer **Comment:** Demonstrated a survival benefit with the use of neoadjuvant chemotherapy followed by cystectomy vs. cystectomy alone for muscle-invasive bladder cancer	2003 http://www.nejm.org/doi/full/10.1056/NEJMoa022148
RCT	Radiotherapy with or without chemotherapy in muscle-invasive bladder cancer **Comment:** Demonstrated a significant improvement in locoregional disease-free survival with concurrent chemoradiation vs. radiation alone for muscle-invasive bladder cancer	2012 http://www.nejm.org/doi/full/10.1056/NEJMoa1106106
RCT	Gemcitabine and cisplatin versus methotrexate, vinblastine, doxorubicin, and cisplatin in advanced or metastatic bladder cancer: results of a large, randomized, multinational, multicenter, phase III study **Comment:** Demonstrated similar survival in patients treated with metastatic bladder cancer treated with gemcitabine plus cisplatin vs. MVAC albeit with much less toxicity with gemcitabine plus cisplatin	2000 http://jco.ascopubs.org/content/18/17/3068.full
RCT	Pembrolizumab as second-line therapy for advanced urothelial carcinoma **Comment:** Demonstrated improvement in survival with pembrolizumab compared with standard chemotherapy in patients with metastatic bladder cancer progressing despite prior platinum-based chemotherapy	2017 https://www.nejm.org/doi/full/10.1056/NEJMoa1613683

Image

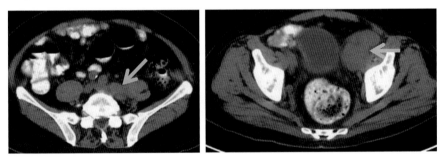

Figure 3.1 Computed tomography scan demonstrated metastatic bladder cancer to the pelvic (right panel) and retroperitoneal lymph nodes (left panel).

Additional material for this chapter can be found online at: www.wiley.com/go/oh/mountsinaioncology

This includes advice for patients, a case study, and ICD codes.

CHAPTER 4

Renal Cancer

Bobby C. Liaw, Reza Mehrazin, and Che-Kai Tsao
Icahn School of Medicine at Mount Sinai, New York, NY, USA

OVERALL BOTTOM LINE
- Renal cancer encompasses a collection of different disease entities, the most common of which are renal cell carcinoma (RCC) and transitional cell carcinoma (TCC).
- Diagnosis is often made incidentally, although some patients still present with the classic triad of hematuria, flank pain, and palpable abdominal mass.
- A subset of RCC is associated with hereditary syndromes for which genetic mutations have been identified.
- Management of localized RCC is surgical, whereas management of metastatic RCC is comprised of immunotherapeutic and molecularly targeted agents.
- TCC of the renal pelvis is managed in a similar way to transitional cell bladder cancer.

Background
Definition of disease
- RCCs originate within the renal cortex and comprise the majority (80–85%) of all adult primary kidney cancers.
- TCCs arise from the renal pelvis and are the second most common subtype (8%).
- Rare tumor types make up the remainder of renal cancers.

Disease classification
- The World Health Organization (WHO) classifies renal cancer based on pathologic and genetic characteristics.
- An inherited familial syndrome is present in fewer than 4% of renal cancers.

Incidence/prevalence
- Renal cancer incidence rates vary by geographic region. Rates in Europe and North America are generally higher than those in Asia and South America.
- In 2015, there were an estimated 61 560 new diagnoses and 14 080 deaths from kidney and renal pelvis cancers in the USA.
- RCC comprises 3.7% of all new cancer diagnoses, and 2.4% of all cancer deaths.

Economic impact
- The National Institute for Health and Clinical Excellence (NICE) in the UK initially declined to reimburse targeted therapies, citing cost ineffectiveness despite having clinical benefits. This

---

Mount Sinai Expert Guides: Oncology, First Edition. Edited by William K. Oh and Ajai Chari.
© 2019 John Wiley & Sons Ltd. Published 2019 by John Wiley & Sons Ltd.
Companion Website: www.wiley.com/go/oh/mountsinaioncology

decision sparked intense debate and was later reversed, but drew considerable attention to the economic impact of RCC on healthcare spending.
- With newly approved targeted therapies such as nivolumab, the economic burden of RCC treatment will continue to grow.

Etiology
- Development of RCC is a result of interactions between medical comorbidities, environmental exposures, and some degree of inherent genetic susceptibility. Risk factors include the following.
  - **Cigarette smoking:** peripheral blood lymphocyte DNA damage and presence of chromosomal 3p deletion are more commonly observed in active smokers and those chronically exposed to passive smoking. These changes are thought to result from tobacco-specific *N*-nitrosamine compounds and chronic tissue hypoxia.
  - **Acquired cystic disease of the kidney:** renal hypertrophy by proto-oncogene activation and growth factor stimulation.
  - **Occupational exposure:** associated with genetic damage or mutations in tumor suppressors such as von Hippel–Lindau (VHL), or activation of oncogenes.
  - **Obesity:** proposed mechanisms including chronic tissue hypoxia, compensatory hyperinsulinemia from relative insulin resistance, and reactive oxygen species formation from lipid peroxidation.
  - Other risk factors include hypertension, diuretic use, analgesic use, and nephrolithiasis.

Pathology/pathogenesis
- RCC has multiple histologic subtypes including clear cell (75–85%), papillary (10–15%), chromophobe (5–10%), oncocytoma (3–7%), and collecting duct (Bellini) (<1%).
- RCC is associated with several hereditary syndromes, but they only account for 1–4% of RCC.
  - **VHL:** autosomal dominant mutation of the VHL gene (3p25). A second-hit loss of the remaining VHL gene leads to loss of the functional VHL product that is involved in the ubiquitination of hypoxia-inducible factor 1 alpha and 2 alpha (HIF1α, HIF2α). Unregulated activity of HIF1α/2α promotes transcription of hypoxia response factors (VEGF, PDFG-β, TGF-α, EPO, EGFR), increasing angiogenesis and survival in anaerobic environments.
  - **Hereditary papillary renal carcinoma (HPRC):** autosomal dominant mutation of the *MET* oncogene codes for a hepatocyte growth factor (HGF) binding tyrosine kinase receptor that activates intracellular pathways (RAS, ERK, PI3K, cSRC) which promote cell proliferation and inhibit apoptosis.
  - **Tuberous sclerosis complex (TSC):** autosomal dominant mutation of hamartin (TSC1, 9q34) or tuberin (TSC2, 16p13), which function as tumor suppressors, predisposing to development of benign tumors of the brain, heart, kidneys, lungs, and skin (hamartomas), but also increased frequency of renal cancers.
  - **Hereditary leiomyomatosis and renal cell cancer (HLRCC):** autosomal dominant fumarate hydratase (FH) mutation, has a role in the mitochondrial tricarboxylic acid cycle and acts as a tumor suppressor.
  - **Birt–Hogg–Dubé syndrome:** autosomal dominant folliculin (FLCN) mutation, which regulates the cellular energy and nutrient sensing system. Affected individuals are at risk of bilateral, multifocal kidney cancer in addition to cutaneous (fibrofolliculomas) and pulmonary lesions.
  - **Hereditary paraganglioma/pheochromocytoma:** autosomal dominant mutation in one of the four subunits that comprise succinate dehydrogenase (SDH) leading to development of paragangliomas and pheochromocytomas, but can also be associated with early onset RCC.

- Sporadic RCC comprises the majority of RCC diagnoses.
  - Loss of the short arm of chromosome 3 (3p), contains VHL and BAP1, two members of the ubiquitin-mediated proteolysis pathway (UMPP), is commonly observed (94%) in clear cell RCC. PBRM1, a tumor suppressor, also maps to 3p. Overexpression of p53 and p53 mutations are also implicated in the development of clear cell RCC.
  - Somatic mutations of *MET* are uncommon, but associated with papillary RCC.
  - Chromophobe RCC is associated with up-regulation of the *KIT* oncogene and elevation of telomerase reverse transcription (TERT) expression.
  - Oncocytomas arise from the intercalated cells of the collecting duct, but have higher association with cyclin D1 (CCND1) rearrangements.
  - Even in the absence of a definable hereditary genetic mutation, a meta-analysis finds a 2.2-fold increase in risk for RCC in individuals with a first degree relative with an RCC diagnosis. The risk is even higher among siblings (RR 3.91–4.02), suggesting germline mutations with low penetrance.

Predictive/risk factors

Risk factor	Relative risk
Obesity	1.0–1.9, increases progressively with higher baseline BMI
Hypertension	1.0–2.2, increases progressively with higher baseline diastolic and systolic blood pressures
Occupational exposure	1.5–2.3, depending on type and level of exposure
NSAIDs/analgesics	0.81–2.92, depending on dose and duration of use
Acquired cystic disease of the kidney	Varied reports, but significantly elevated
Chronic hepatitis C	1.77
Cigarette smoking	1.30
• Current smoker	1.33
• Former smoker	1.17
• Passive smoking	1.43
Nephrolithiasis	
• RCC	1.76
• TCC	2.14
Family history of RCC	
• First degree relative	2.2
• Sibling	3.91–4.02

Prevention

No interventions have been demonstrated to prevent the development of renal cancer.

Screening

Given the relatively low prevalence of RCC in the general population, screening in the asymptomatic patient is not recommended. However, for persons at higher risk for development of RCC, periodic imaging (ultrasound, CT, or MRI) to evaluate for disease can be considered:
- Diagnosis of a hereditary syndrome associated with RCC

- Strong family history of RCC
- End-stage renal disease on long-term dialysis
- History of radiation to kidney.

Primary prevention
- For most renal cancers, the underlying etiology is not known.
- Modification of risk factors may be helpful:
  - Smoking cessation
  - Maintain healthy/ideal weight
  - Healthy diet
  - Decrease alcohol consumption
  - Maintain good blood pressure control
  - Avoid occupational exposures.

Secondary prevention
- Following complete surgical resection, median time to RCC recurrence is 15–18 months, with 85% of relapses occurring within 3 years.
- In the phase III ASSURE trial, patients with RCC at high risk for recurrence were randomized 1 : 1 : 1 to receive adjuvant sunitinib, sorafenib, or placebo. Neither drug improved disease-free survival compared with placebo.
- Adjuvant treatment is not recommended for RCC, although trials are ongoing to evaluate pazopanib, axitinib, and everolimus.

Diagnosis (Algorithm 4.1)

> **BOTTOM LINE/CLINICAL PEARLS**
> - The majority of patients are free of symptoms or signs at presentation. Physical examination can yield a palpable abdominal mass.
> - Initial investigation should include complete blood count (CBC), comprehensive metabolic panel (CMP), urine studies, and abdominal imaging.
> - A diagnostic biopsy is not always required, as specific radiographic signs can often be pathognomonic, leading to planning of nephrectomy.

Differential diagnosis of renal mass

Differential diagnosis	Features
Renal cyst	Simple thin-walled appearance on ultrasound
Renal abscess	Enhancing abscess wall with low density fluid-filled mass
Benign neoplasm (adenoma)	Similar to RCC on imaging
Renal infarction	Hypodense and cortically located on CT
Sarcoma	Similar to RCC on imaging
Angiomyolipoma	Presence of fat on contrast enhanced CT
Metastasis from a distant primary lesion	Lymphoma > lung > breast > colon > melanoma

Algorithm 4.1 Diagnosis of renal cancer

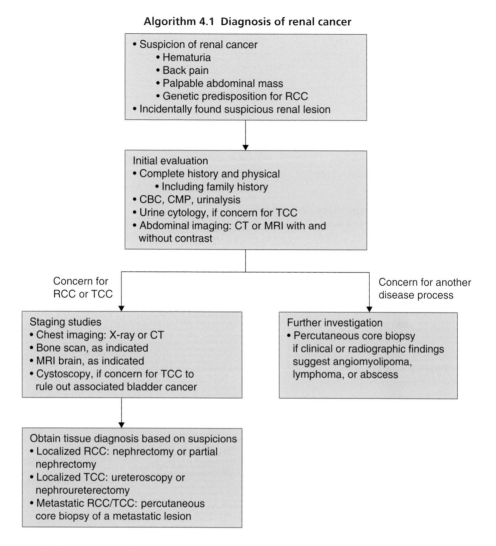

- Suspicion of renal cancer
  - Hematuria
  - Back pain
  - Palpable abdominal mass
  - Genetic predisposition for RCC
- Incidentally found suspicious renal lesion

Initial evaluation
- Complete history and physical
  - Including family history
- CBC, CMP, urinalysis
- Urine cytology, if concern for TCC
- Abdominal imaging: CT or MRI with and without contrast

Concern for RCC or TCC

Concern for another disease process

Staging studies
- Chest imaging: X-ray or CT
- Bone scan, as indicated
- MRI brain, as indicated
- Cystoscopy, if concern for TCC to rule out associated bladder cancer

Further investigation
- Percutaneous core biopsy if clinical or radiographic findings suggest angiomyolipoma, lymphoma, or abscess

Obtain tissue diagnosis based on suspicions
- Localized RCC: nephrectomy or partial nephrectomy
- Localized TCC: ureteroscopy or nephroureterectomy
- Metastatic RCC/TCC: percutaneous core biopsy of a metastatic lesion

Typical presentation
- Often asymptomatic in early stages, with symptoms presenting as it progresses in size and stage. The majority (>50%) of disease is now incidentally discovered.
- Classic triad of hematuria, back/flank pain, and palpable mass now only observed in <10% of newly diagnosed cases.
- Other presenting symptoms: anemia, fatigue, decreased appetite, weight loss, hypercalcemia, erythrocytosis, thrombocytosis, scrotal varicoceles, lower extremity edema, venous thromboembolism, and unexplained fevers.

Clinical diagnosis
History
A complete medical history to evaluate for risk factors and disease-related symptoms is necessary if RCC is suspected:
- Personal or family history of RCC or hereditable cancer syndrome.
- Hematuria, back/flank pain, palpable mass.

- Passage of blood clots in the urine suggests heavier bleeding from a nonglomerular source, more concerning for a urinary tract malignancy.
- Fatigue, decreased appetite, weight loss, unexplained fevers, and lower extremity edema are less specific.

Physical examination
The classic examination finding is an abdominal mass, typically smooth, firm, and nontender. It may not be palpable depending on size, or if it is located away from the lower pole of the kidney. Lower extremity edema, ascites, and scrotal varicoceles (in men), may be present if there is disease invasion into adjacent renal vein and inferior vena cava (IVC).

Useful clinical decision rules and calculators
See Algorithm 4.1.

Disease severity classification
RCC is commonly graded on the Fuhrman histologic scale based on appearance and characteristics of cancer cell nuclei. Grade 1 most resembles normal kidney cell nuclei (size, shape, number of nucleoli, chromatin clumping) and carries the best prognosis, whereas grade 4 carries the worst prognosis.

Laboratory diagnosis
List of diagnostic tests
- **CBC:** patients with renal cancers often present with anemia. Patients with RCC can also uncommonly present with polycythemia caused by excessive erythropoietin production.
- **CMP:** electrolyte abnormalities such as hypercalcemia are sometimes seen in RCC. Liver function test (LFT) abnormalities can indicate liver metastases.
- **Urinalysis:** approximately half of renal cancer patients will have some amount of blood in their urine.
- **Urine cytology:** may detect presence of TCC.

Lists of imaging techniques
- **CT:** CT with and without IV contrast is considered the standard modality of imaging for disease staging in RCC and TCC.
- **Ultrasound:** not as sensitive as CT, but can be used to confirm presence of a renal mass. Ultrasound can distinguish between simple cysts, complex cystic lesions, and solid masses.
- **MRI:** an alternative to CT if there are contraindications for IV contrast. MRI with gadolinium is superior to CT for the evaluation of vascular invasion, CNS involvement, and spinal cord involvement. In patients with renal insufficiency, diffusion weighted imaging (DWI) can be used.
- **Bone scan:** indicated when concern for osseous metastasis is high (bone pain, hypercalcemia, elevated alkaline phosphatase).
- **Intravenous pyelogram (IVP):** used in the investigation of TCC, evaluates abnormalities of the renal pelvis and ureter.
- **Ureteroscopy:** allows direct visualization of the upper urinary tract, including the ureter and renal pelvis collecting system. Brush biopsy can be performed on suspected TCC to confirm pathologic diagnosis. In addition, ureteral stents can be deployed to alleviate urinary obstruction.

Potential pitfalls/common errors made regarding diagnosis of disease
- The wide variety of renal cancer histologic subtypes means that pathologic interpretation is challenging when the tumor sample is limited or has an unusual appearance.
- CT imaging demonstrates high specificity (98%), but poor specificity (46%), in the evaluation of perinephric invasion, affecting confidence in differentiating between stage T2 and T3a disease.

Treatment (Algorithm 4.2)

Algorithm 4.2 Management of renal cancer

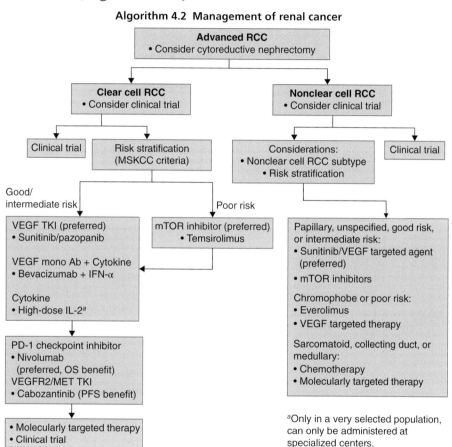

Treatment rationale
Treatment of renal cancer is dependent on stage and extent of disease.
- **Localized RCC (stages I–III):** intent of therapy prioritizes cure.
  - Definitive surgical options include partial and radical nephrectomy. Radical nephrectomy is favored for stage II–III disease, centrally located tumors, suspected lymph node involvement, renal vein or IVC thrombosis, or disease extension into adjacent structures. Similar long-term outcomes observed whether approach is open or laparoscopic/robotic.
  - For surgery ineligible patients, nephron-sparing or localized therapy such as surgical enucleation, radiofrequency ablation, cryotherapy, radiotherapy, or arterial embolization can be considered, but are not considered curative.

- For select cases of early stage RCC, active surveillance is a suitable alternative, especially in patients with medical comorbidities or limited life expectancy.
- Adjuvant therapy is not recommended as studies have not demonstrated any clinical benefit.
- **Metastatic RCC (stage IV):** intent of therapy emphasizes disease control, as well as maintaining quality of life.
  - Cytoreductive nephrectomy – considered to be standard of care prior to systemic therapy based on two randomized trials demonstrating definitive survival benefit in conjunction with cytokine therapy.
  - Clear cell RCC: first line
    - VEGF pathway inhibitors – sunitinib, pazopanib (considered standard of care for first line therapy, less toxicities and better tolerability than cytokine therapy)
    - cytokine therapy: bevacizumab + IFN-α, high-dose IL-2 (significant treatment-related toxicities, long-term durable remission in 10%)
    - mTOR inhibitor: temsirolimus – first line for poor-risk RCC (see section on Prognosis).
  - Clear cell RCC: second line
    - Following first line cytokine therapy, consider VEGF TKI.
    - Following VEGF-targeted therapy:
      - PD-L1 inhibitor: nivolumab (preferred, OS benefit in phase III study compared with everolimus after first line VEGF TKI)
      - VEGFR2 and MET TKI: cabozantinib (PFS benefit in phase III study compared with everolimus after at least one VEGF TKI).
  - Clear cell RCC: third line and beyond
    - Optimal management not established; mTOR inhibitors, bevacizumab, cytokine therapies and other VEGF TKIs can be considered.
    - Clinical trial is encouraged.
  - Nonclear cell RCC
    - Optimal management not established in any line of therapy, consider clinical trial.
  - Phase III ASPEN trial suggests that first line sunitinib is associated with a longer radiographic PFS than everolimus. Although hypothesis generating, in subgroup analysis, both chromophobe histology and poor-risk RCC subgroups had better suggested outcomes with everolimus.
  - For those with collecting duct histology or clear cell with predominant sarcomatoid differentiation, chemotherapy alone (e.g. doxorubicin, gemcitabine) or in combination with targeted therapy can be considered (e.g. gemcitabine + sunitinib).
- Localized TCC (stage I–III)
  - Neoadjuvant cisplatin-based chemotherapy can be considered; improves disease-free survival when compared with historic controls.
  - Surgical resection
    - Nephrourectomy +/− lymph node dissection
    - Distal/segmental ureterectomy.
  - Adjuvant radiation therapy can decrease chances of local recurrence but does not influence distal recurrences or OS.
  - Adjuvant chemotherapy does not have a well-defined role, but can be considered for select high risk patients.
  - Postoperative surveillance cystoscopies are necessary as 20–50% of TCC will develop bladder cancer.

- Metastatic TCC (stage IV)
  - Treatment is extrapolated from data on advanced urothelial bladder cancer.
  - First line treatment includes several platinum-based chemotherapy regimens (cisplatin is preferred if patient is eligible).
  - Outcomes of second line treatments remain extremely poor. Clinical trial participation is encouraged.

Table of treatment

Treatment	Comment
Conservative	
Active surveillance	Option in patients with small asymptomatic lesions, significant medical comorbidities, or limited life expectancy
Surgical: RCC	
Partial nephrectomy	Preferred for stage I RCC
Radical nephrectomy	Preferred for stage II and III RCC
Cytoreductive nephrectomy	Consider prior to initiation of systemic therapy in metastatic RCC if can safely debulk ≥75% of tumor volume
Medical: RCC	
High dose IL-2	Cytokine therapy, associated with significant treatment toxicity
Sunitinib 50 mg/day PO (4 weeks on/2 weeks off)	First line VEGF TKI
Pazopanib 800 mg/day PO	First line VEGF TKI, equivalent clinical benefits to sunitinib but with more favorable toxicity profile
Bevacizumab 10 mg/kg IV every 2 weeks + IFN-α SQ 9 MIU TIW	VEGF monoclonal antibody + cytokine therapy Bevacizumab can be used as monotherapy in later lines of therapy
Axitinib 5 mg/day PO	VEGF TKI, approved for second line therapy
Sorafenib 400 mg PO twice daily	VEGF TKI, generally used in later lines of therapy
Cabozantinib 60 mg/day PO	VEGFR2 and MET inhibitor, improved PFS and ORR compared with everolimus in patients previously treated with a VEGF TKI
Everolimus 10 mg/day PO	mTOR inhibitor, inferior to sunitinib in the first line, and nivolumab and cabozantinib in the second line
Temsirolimus 25 mg IV weekly	mTOR inhibitor, first line indication for poor-risk RCC
Nivolumab 3 mg/kg IV every 2 weeks	PD-1 inhibitor, improved OS and better tolerated than everolimus after first line VEGF TKI
Surgical: TCC	
Nephroureterectomy	Gold standard for localized tumors of the renal pelvis or ureter

(Continued)

(Continued)

Treatment	Comment
Distal/segmental ureterectomy	Option in select patients with localized, low grade, early stage disease
Medical: TCC	
Platinum-based regimens (MVAC, GC)	Carboplatin is a reasonable substitute for those ineligible for cisplatin treatment, but considered inferior in efficacy

Prevention/management of key treatment complications
VEGF TKIs (sunitinib, pazopanib, sorafenib, axitinib, cabozantinib)
- Palmar-plantar erythrodysesthesia
  - Avoid hot water, constrictive footwear, excessive friction to hands/feet
  - Trim calluses, keep palms and soles dry but moisturized
  - Mild to moderate symptoms: dose reduction, topical emollients, topical urea or salicylic acid, topical corticosteroid
  - Severe symptoms: withhold treatment until improved, restart at 50% dose reduction and slow titration if tolerating.
- Hypertension
  - Optimize blood pressure control and have patients keep a blood pressure journal prior to initiation of VEGF TKI
  - Mild to moderate symptoms: aggressive pharmacologic management. No one class of anti-hypertensives has been shown to be more effective than others
  - Severe symptoms: reduce dosage or withhold treatment
  - Cytopenias can affect one or multiple cell lines. Reduce dosage or withhold treatment.

VEGF monoclonal antibodies (bevacizumab)
- Proteinuria
  - Monitor with dipstick urine analysis, if 2+ or greater, further assess with 24-hour urine collection. Withhold treatment if ≥2 g proteinuria/24 hours, resume when proteinuria is <2 g/24 hours.
- Hypertension
  - Optimize blood pressure control and have patients keep a blood pressure journal prior to initiation of VEGF TKI
  - Mild to moderate symptoms: aggressive pharmacologic management. No one class of anti-hypertensives has been shown to be more effective than others
  - Severe symptoms: reduce dosage or withhold treatment.
- Hemorrhage
  - Do not administer in patients with recent history of hemorrhage
  - Discontinue if hemorrhage occurs in the setting of treatment.
- Arterial/venous thrombotic events
  - Discontinue if thrombotic event occurs in the setting of treatment. Safety of restarting treatment after resolution of thrombotic event has not been studied.

mTOR inhibitors (everolimus, temsirolimus)
- Non-infectious pneumonitis: class effect of rapamycin derivatives
  - Rule out infection

- Mild to moderate symptoms: withhold drug until improved, consider corticosteroids, restart at 50% dose reduction and slow titration if tolerating
  - Severe symptoms: discontinue therapy, start corticosteroids.
- Infection risk: immunosuppressive properties predispose to bacterial, fungal, viral, and parasitic infections
  - Definitively treat any pre-existing infections prior to initiation of therapy
  - Appropriate antibiotic or antifungal therapy
  - Withhold and/or discontinue drug treatment.
- Oral ulcers
  - Promote good oral hygiene, brushing, flossing, and frequent rinsing
  - Mild to moderate symptoms: nonalcoholic, salt water, or topical anesthetic mouthwash. Topical corticosteroids can be added
  - Severe: withhold and restart at lower dose, or discontinue therapy.

PD-1 checkpoint inhibitors (nivolumab)
- Immune-related adverse effects: immunologic augmentation can lead to autoimmune phenomena including colitis, hepatitis, pneumonitis, dermatitis, and endocrinopathies.
  - Mild to moderate symptoms: withhold treatment until symptoms improve, then restart. Corticosteroids (prednisone 0.5 mg/kg/day or equivalent) should be initiated if symptoms do not resolve within a week.
  - Severe symptoms: permanently discontinue, and start high dose corticosteroids (prednisone 1–2 mg/kg/day or equivalent) until symptoms improve. Taper steroids slowly over at least a month.

CLINICAL PEARLS
- Surgical resection offers the best chance of cure in localized renal cancer.
- Neoadjuvant and adjuvant therapy are not recommended for RCC.
- There is not a clearly defined role for neoadjuvant or adjuvant therapy in TCC, but it can be considered in high risk patients.
- Multiple immunotherapeutic and molecularly targeted therapies are approved for the treatment of metastatic RCC, although the optimal sequence is debated.
- The mainstay of treatment of metastatic TCC is platinum-based chemotherapy. Carboplatin is a reasonable but inferior option for those who are cisplatin-ineligible.

Special populations
Pregnancy
- For localized disease, timing of surgical resection is dependent on clinical behavior of the tumor and the neonatal survival rates for the stage of gestation in question.
- For metastatic disease, none of the systemic agents are well-studied in the pregnant patient and cannot be recommended.

Children
- Wilms tumor is the most common childhood kidney cancer. Treatment involves primary surgical resection and adjuvant chemotherapy, with the addition of radiation therapy in stage III and IV disease.

Elderly
- Approach to RCC and TCC management in elderly patients is the same as in the adult patient, although active surveillance is an alternative to consider.

Sickle cell disease
- Renal medullary carcinoma is almost entirely found in patients with sickle cell trait or sickle cell disease, typically presenting before the age of 20.

Prognosis

BOTTOM LINE/CLINICAL PEARLS
- Multiple prognostic models exist for metastatic RCC, although the most commonly used are the Memorial Sloan Kettering Cancer Center (MSKCC) and International Metastatic Database Consortium (IMDC) models.
- The IMDC model more accurately captures outcomes incorporating modern use of targeted therapies.

Natural history of untreated disease
- Early institutional series report that small renal lesions generally grow slowly, with intermediate term follow-up metastasis being rare (2%).
- RCC spreads by direct extension and by invasion of lymphatics and renal veins.
- Tumor thrombus is often observed in intrarenal veins, renal veins, and IVC.
- Approximately 25% of newly diagnosed renal cancers present as locally advanced or metastatic disease.
- Common sites of metastases: lungs, lymph node, liver, and bone.

Prognosis for treated patients
- The IMDC reevaluated the MSKCC prognostic model in the modern era of VEGF-targeted therapies and found six baseline clinical parameters to be prognostic: KPS <80%, hgb <LLN, corrected Ca >ULN, neutrophils >ULN, platelets >ULN, and time from diagnosis to treatment of <1 year:
  - 0 risk factors: low risk – mOS not reached; 2 year OS 75%
  - 1–2 risk factors: intermediate risk – mOS 27 months; 2 year OS 53%
  - ≥3 risk factors: poor risk – mOS 8.8 months; 2 year OS 7%.

Follow-up tests and monitoring
- History and physical examination every 6–16 weeks while receiving systemic therapy.
- Laboratory tests depending on type of therapeutic agent being used.
- CT or MRI of abdomen every 6–16 weeks per physician discretion.
- Imaging of head, MRI spine, and bone scan as clinically indicated.

Reading list
Bellmunt J, Negrier S, Escudier B, et al. Taskforce S. The medical treatment of metastatic renal cell cancer in the elderly: position paper of a SIOG Taskforce. Crit Rev Oncol Hematol 2009;69:64–72.

Beroukhim R, Brunet JP, Di Napoli A, et al. Patterns of gene expression and copy-number alterations in Von-Hippel Lindau disease-associated and sporadic clear cell carcinoma of the kidney. Cancer Res 2009;69:4674–4681.

Choueiri TK, Escudier B, Powles T, et al. Cabozantinib versus everolimus in advanced renal-cell carcinoma. N Engl J Med 2015;373:1814–1823.

Chow WH, Dong LM, Devesa SS. Epidemiology and risk factors for kidney cancer. Nat Rev Urol 2010;7:245–257.

Clague J, Lin J, Cassidy A, et al. Family history and risk of renal cell carcinoma: results from a case–control study and systematic meta-analysis. Cancer Epidemiol Biomarkers Prev 2009;18:801–807.

Escudier B, Porta C, Bono P, et al. Randomized, controlled, double-blind, cross-over trial assessing treatment preference for pazopanib versus sunitinib in patients with metastatic renal cell carcinoma: PISCES Study. J Clin Oncol 2014;32:1412–1418.

Heng DY, Xie W, Regan MM, et al. Prognostic factors for overall survival in patients with metastatic renal cell carcinoma treated with vascular endothelial growth factor-targeted agents: results from a large, multicenter study. J Clin Oncol 2009;27:5794–5799.

Linehan WM, Spellman PT, Ricketts CJ, et al. Comprehensive molecular characterization of papillary renal-cell carcinoma. N Engl J Med 2016;374:135–145.

Motzer RJ, Escudier B, McDermott DF, et al. Nivolumab versus everolimus in advanced renal-cell carcinoma. N Engl J Med 2015;373:1803–1813.

Motzer RJ, Hutson TE, Cella D, et al. Pazopanib versus sunitinib in metastatic renal-cell carcinoma. N Engl J Med 2013;369:722–731.

Guidelines
National society guidelines

Title	Source	Date and weblink
NCCN	National Comprehensive Cancer Network	2015 http://www.nccn.org/professionals/physician_gls/pdf/kidney.pdf
AUA	American Urological Association	2017 https://www.auanet.org/guidelines/renal-mass-and-localized-renal-cancer-new-(2017)

International society guidelines

Title	Source	Date and weblink
EAU	European Association of Urology	2014 http://uroweb.org/wp-content/uploads/10-Renal-Cell-Carcinoma_LR.pdf
ESMO	European Society for Medical Oncology	2016 http://www.esmo.org/Guidelines/Genitourinary-Cancers/Renal-Cell-Carcinoma

Evidence

Type of evidence	Title	Weblink
RCT	NCCN Guidelines for Kidney Cancer	http://www.nccn.org/professionals/physician_gls/pdf/kidney.pdf

Additional material for this chapter can be found online at:
www.wiley.com/go/oh/mountsinaioncology

This includes a case study, ICD codes, and multiple choice questions.

CHAPTER 5

Testicular Cancer

Aditya V. Shreenivas and Seth M. Cohen
Icahn School of Medicine at Mount Sinai, New York, NY, USA

OVERALL BOTTOM LINE
- Seminoma and nonseminoma, the main histologic categories of testicular cancers, are managed with different approaches.
- Active surveillance is an increasingly important management option for patients with early stage disease.
- Management of advanced disease is guided by a risk adapted classification system.
- Combined modality treatment strategies are employed to achieve a high likelihood of cure, with a focus on reducing long-term morbidity.
- In light of the high likelihood of cure, survivorship issues have an important role in the long-term management of patients with testicular cancer.

Background
Definition of disease
- Malignancy of the testicle.
- Most common cancer in males aged 15–35 years.

Disease classification
- Germ cell tumor
  - Seminoma: seminoma with or without syncytiotrophoblastic cells
  - Nonseminomatous germ cell tumor: embryonal carcinoma, teratoma, choriocarcinoma, yolk sac tumor.
- Sex cord stromal tumor: Sertoli cell tumor, Leydig cell tumor, granulosa cell tumor.
- Other: paratesticular rhabdomyosarcoma, adenocarcinoma of the rete testis.

Incidence/prevalence
- One percent of all cancers in males.
- Four times more common in white people than in black people.
- Approximately 8400 cases of testicular cancer were diagnosed in 2016.
- Approximately 380 men died of testicular cancer in 2016.

Etiology
- Cryptorchidism is associated with an increased risk of testicular cancer.
- *In utero* exposure to diethylstilbestrol is associated with an increased risk of cryptorchidism and testicular cancer.
- Agent Orange exposure is associated with an increased risk of testicular cancer.

Mount Sinai Expert Guides: Oncology, First Edition. Edited by William K. Oh and Ajai Chari.
© 2019 John Wiley & Sons Ltd. Published 2019 by John Wiley & Sons Ltd.
Companion Website: www.wiley.com/go/oh/mountsinaioncology

Pathology/pathogenesis

Pathogenesis

The exact pathogenesis of testicular cancer is not known. However, testicular cancer is often associated with chromosomal abnormalities. Eighty percent of all histologic subtypes have an isochromosome of the short arm of chromosome 12 (i12p), while 20% have excess 12p genetic material, suggesting that one or more genes at this location are involved in the development of germ cell tumors. Target genes include cyclin D2 gene (CCDN2), present at 12p13, or SOX1, JAW1, and KRAS, which map to 12p11.2-12.1.8. CCDN2 activates cdk4/6, which makes the cancerous cell cross the G1-S checkpoint and proliferate.

Pathology

Histologically, seminomas are composed of a diffuse sheet-like pattern of polygonal cells which replace the testicular parenchyma. Seminoma cells have clear to eosinophilic cytoplasm, central nuclei, and 1–2 nucleoli. They are periodic acid–Schiff (PAS) positive. Embryonal carcinoma exhibits poorly differentiated pleomorphic cells in cords, and yolk sac tumors comprise poorly differentiated endothelial-like or cuboidal cells.

Immunohistochemistry

- Seminomas express placental alkaline phosphatase (PLAP), CD117 (CKIT), OCT4, and SALL4, and are negative for cytokeratins and CD30.
- Embryonal carcinoma expresses cytokeratin, epithelial membrane antigen, CD30, OCT4, and SALL4, with ~50% expressing PLAP.
- Yolk sac tumors express cytokeratin, AFP, and SALL4 and are negative for CD117 and CD30.
- Choriocarcinoma uniformly expresses human chorionic gonadotropin (HCG).

Risk factors

Risk factor	Relative risk ratio
Cryptorchidism	8–10
Hypospadias	2.13
Testicular microlithiasis	8.5
Contralateral testicular cancer	1.9% 15-year cumulative risk
Family history	8–10
HIV	0.7–1.8

Prevention

> **BOTTOM LINE/CLINICAL PEARLS**
> - Surgical correction cryptorchidism with orchiopexy reduces the risk of development of testicular cancer.

Screening

There is no proven method of screening. Some providers recommend testicular self examination (Lin and Sharangpani 2010).

Primary prevention
- Orchiopexy in young adults with cryptorchidism reduces the risk of subsequent testicular cancer (Pettersson et al. 2007).

Secondary prevention
- Adjuvant carboplatin in clinical stage 1 seminoma reduces the risk of having contralateral testicular cancer.

Diagnosis

> **CLINICAL PEARLS**
> - Painless swelling or nodule in testicle. About one-third of patients complain of heaviness or dull ache in lower abdomen, scrotum, or perineum.
> - Firm, nontender nodule or mass in testicle is found on examination.
> - Ultrasound of testis, and tumor markers including alpha fetoprotein (AFP), HCG, and lactate dehydrogenase (LDH).

Differential diagnosis

Differential diagnosis	Features
Epididymitis	Associated with testicular discomfort, dysuria. Ultrasound of testis for confirmation
Hydrocele and spermatocele	Soft painless swelling, rapidly changes size as fluid enters or leaves. Ultrasound of testis needed to confirm
Inguinal hernia	Soft swelling, enlarges on cough or straining
Varicocele	Scrotal swelling prominent on standing. Diagnosed with ultrasound of testis

Typical presentation
- A young male presents with painless, hard testicular swelling or mass associated with heavy sensation in lower abdominal area. Sometimes advanced stage germ cell tumors are diagnosed incidentally on biopsy of retroperitoneal, mediastinal lymph node or neck mass, or patients will present with cough, dyspnea, anorexia, weight loss, back pain, or bone pain.

Clinical diagnosis
History
- Painless swelling associated with dull ache or heavy sensation in the lower abdomen.
- Palpable mass and/or nodule in testicle.
- Gynecomastia is found in nearly 5% of testicular germ cell tumors that produce HCG.
- Patients with metastatic testicular cancer present with neck mass or other palpable lymphadenopathy, anorexia, weight loss, cough, chest pain, shortness of breath, hemoptysis, or neurologic symptoms.

Physical examination
- Painless solid mass within testis.
- Unilateral or bilateral leg swelling caused by iliac vein obstruction/thrombosis is often associated with testicular cancer.

- Gynecomastia and supraclavicular lymphadenopathy are some of the other pertinent physical findings.

Useful clinical decision rules and calculators
Germ cell tumor staging:
- Special TNM staging developed by AJCC which incorporates serum tumor markers AFP, HCG, and LDH.

Disease severity classification
Risk stratification according to International Germ Cell Consensus Classification.

Seminoma
- **Good risk:** any primary or markers without pulmonary or visceral metastasis.
- **Intermediate risk:** any primary or markers with nonpulmonary visceral metastasis.

Nonseminoma
- **Good risk:** testis or retroperitoneal primary with good risk markers and no nonpulmonary visceral metastasis.
- **Intermediate risk:** testis or retroperitoneal primary with intermediate risk markers and no nonpulmonary visceral metastasis.
- **Poor risk:** mediastinal primary, or testis or retroperitoneal primary, with either poor risk markers or nonpulmonary visceral metastasis.

Laboratory diagnosis
List of diagnostic tests (Algorithm 5.1)

Algorithm 5.1 Diagnosis of testicular mass

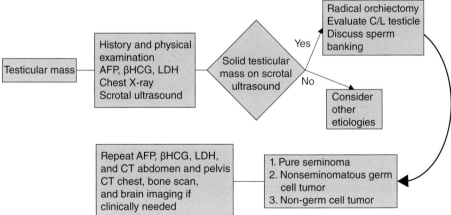

- Tumor markers including AFP, HCG, and LDH are measured as part of staging, to assess for treatment response, and to assess for residual disease.
- Increased AFP is pathognomonic of nonseminoma and is not seen in seminoma. HCG and LDH can be elevated in both.
- AFP can also be elevated in liver cancer, cirrhosis, and even colorectal or gastric cancer.
- HCG level may be elevated as a result of hypogonadism or marijuana use.

Lists of imaging techniques

- Ultrasound of testis is performed to diagnose a testicular mass.
- Staging performed with chest X-ray, with CT of the chest if the chest X-ray is abnormal, and either CT or MRI of the abdomen and pelvis.
- Bone scan if skeletal symptoms are present or there is increased alkaline phosphatase.
- MRI of brain if neurologic symptoms are present.

Potential pitfalls/common errors made regarding diagnosis of disease

- False positive tumor markers: LDH can be elevated secondary to other medical problems including hemolysis, recent myocardial infarction, or lymphoma. AFP can be elevated in hepatocellular carcinoma or other liver disorders. HCG can be falsely elevated in hypogonadism or with marijuana use.

Treatment (Algorithm 5.2)
Treatment rationale

Orchiectomy is performed for diagnosis.

Algorithm 5.2 Management of testicular mass: (A) treatment of stage I seminoma; (B) treatment of stage II, III seminoma; (C) treatment of stage I nonseminoma; (D) treatment of stage II, III nonseminoma

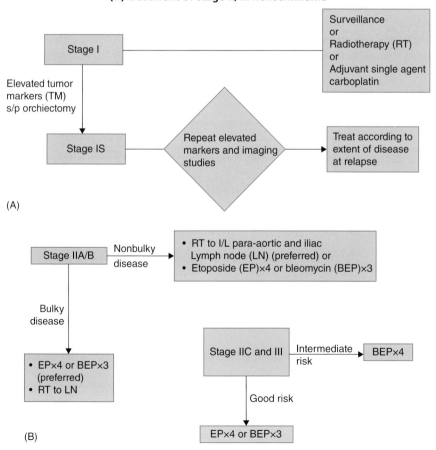

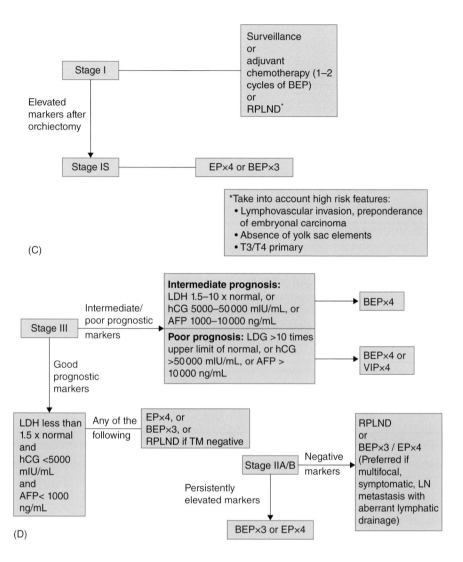

(C)

(D)

Seminoma

- **Stage IA, IB:** can be surveilled (preferred) or treated with adjuvant carboplatin AUC7 for one cycle or radiation (RT) (20 Gy in 10 fractions). Stage IS: repeat elevated markers and restaging with imaging studies. Treat according to extent of disease.
- **Stage IIA/nonbulky stage IIB:** typically treated with RT 30 Gy to para-aortic and ipsilateral iliac lymph nodes, followed by a small optional boost to the involved nodal areas, although chemotherapy is an option for nonbulky stage IIB disease, with cisplatin and etoposide (EP)×4 or with the addition of bleomycin (BEP)×3. Bulky stage IIB disease is typically treated with chemotherapy comprising EP×4 or BEP×3.
- **Stage IIC, III:** good risk disease is treated with EP×4 or BEP×3; intermediate risk disease is treated with BEP×4. Following chemotherapy, if there is no residual mass, or mass <3 cm, and normal markers, then follow patient. If residual mass >3 cm and normal markers, then PET scan at least 6 weeks after chemotherapy with surgery reserved for those with hypermetabolism if feasible.

Nonseminoma

- **Stage IA:** surveillance or nerve sparing retroperitoneal lymph node dissection (RPLND) although surveillance is preferred. In case of lymphovascular invasion (LVI) or predominant embryonal carcinoma histology, one might favor intervention over surveillance. Stage IB: RPLND or BEP×1 or 2, or surveillance for T2 lesions. Stage IS: EP×4 or BEP×3.
- **Stage IIA with markers negative:** EP×4 or BEP×3 or RPLND in selected cases.
- **Stage IIB with markers negative:** EP×4 or BEP×3, but could consider RPLND if lymph node in expected sites.
- More advanced disease or stage IIA–IIB with persistent marker elevation, treat according to risk stratification: good risk stage IIAS1, IIBS1, IIC, IIIA treated with EP×4 or BEP×3; immediate risk stage IIIA/B treated with BEP×4; poor risk stage IIIC treated with BEP×4 or VIP×4 (mesna, ifosfamide, cisplatin, etoposide).

Post chemotherapy

If there is complete response, then surveillance based on original staging is preferred. If there is a partial response or residual mass with negative markers, then follow-up surgical resection of residual mass should be performed. Further management is based on histologic features of residual mass. Residual teratomas are usually followed with surveillance, whereas residual embryonal, yolk sac, choriocarcinoma, and seminoma elements are treated with an additional two cycles of EP/TIP (paclitaxel, ifosfamide, mesna, cisplatin) or VIP. Incomplete responses are treated with second line chemotherapy.

Patients with brain metastases

Primary chemotherapy with RT and/or neurosurgical resection as indicated.

Second line therapy

Clinical trial, VeIP (vinblastine, mesna, ifosfamide, cisplatin) or TIP or high dose chemotherapy with carboplatin, etoposide followed by autologous stem cell transplantation. Surgical resection of residual masses always need to be considered. Palliative chemotherapy options for cisplatin refractory disease include gemcitabine/oxaliplatin, gemcitabine/paclitaxel, and gemcitabine/oxaliplatin/paclitaxel.

Table of treatment

Treatment	Comments
Conservative	Clinical stage I seminoma/nonseminoma
Medical	Cisplatin and etoposide are the main chemotherapeutic agents
Surgical	Retroperitoneal lymph node dissection in stage I nonseminoma and for residual masses
Radiation	Radiation for stage I and II seminoma
Psychologic	Testicular cancer survivors are at risk for anxiety disorder but not for depression and may benefit from behavioral therapy
Complementary	1. Sperm banking should be discussed with all patients 2. Baseline pulmonary function testing in patients treated with bleomycin 3. Consider baseline audiometry testing for patients treated with cisplatin

Prevention/management of complications

- Patients with respiratory compromise and smoking history should avoid bleomycin-based regimens as it can lead to pneumonitis and pulmonary fibrosis.

- Cisplatin is associated with neurotoxicity, ototoxicity, and nephrotoxicity.
- Myelosuppression is common but rarely associated with infectious complications.
- Chemotherapy, radiation, and surgery can all adversely affect reproductive capability.
- Treated patients are at increased risk for metabolic syndrome, cardiovascular disorders, and secondary malignancies.

CLINICAL PEARLS
- PET/CT is useful in triaging patients with seminoma who have residual masses, but not in patients with nonseminoma.
- One must avoid overtreatment due to low levels of markers which not infrequently represent false positives.
- Surveillance for clinical stage I germ cell tumors is an increasingly important and preferred management option.

Special populations
Others
Avoid bleomycin in patients with underlying lung disorders and in some patients with primary mediastinal nonseminoma in whom future significant intrathoracic surgery is felt to be likely.

Prognosis

BOTTOM LINE/CLINICAL PEARLS
- International Germ Cell Consensus Classification is used as a prognostic classification.
- High risk features of clinical stage I nonseminoma include lymph vascular invasion, preponderance of embryonal carcinoma, absence of yolk sac elements, and/or T3/T4 primary.
- For advanced nonseminoma, adverse factors include mediastinal primary site, presence of nonpulmonary visceral metastasis (NPVM), and markedly elevated tumor markers.
- For advanced seminoma, the predominant adverse risk factor is NPVM.
- The overall 5-year survival rate is over 95%.

Follow-up tests and monitoring
Follow-up includes taking a periodic history and physical examination, markers in the context of nonseminoma, and imaging, with frequency depending on histology, risk factors, initial stage, and response to treatment.

References and reading list
Edge SB, Byrd DR, Compton CC, et al. AJCC Cancer Staging Handbook, 7th edn. Springer, 2011.

International Germ Cell Cancer Collaborative Group. International Germ Cell Consensus Classification: a prognostic factor-based staging system for metastatic germ cell cancers. J Clin Oncol 1997;15:594–603.

Jameson JL, Kasper D, Hauser S, et al. Harrison's Principles of Internal Medicine, 20th edn. McGraw-Hill Education, 2018.

Lin K, Sharangpani R. Screening for testicular cancer: an evidence review for the US Preventive Services Task Force. Ann Intern Med 2010;153:396–399.

Pettersson A, Richiardi L, Nordenskjold A, et al. Age at surgery for undescended testis and risk of testicular cancer. N Engl J Med 2007;356:1835–1841.

Vogelzang N, et al. Comprehensive Textbook of Genitourinary Oncology. Lippincott Williams and Wilkins, 2011.

Suggested websites
www.nccn.org
www.cancer.gov
www.uptodate.com

Guidelines
National society guidelines

Title	Source	Date and weblink
Testicular cancer version 1.2016	NCCN	2015 www.nccn.org

Evidence

Type of evidence	Title and comment	Date and weblink
RCT	Long-term follow-up of a phase III study of three versus four cycles of bleomycin, etoposide, and cisplatin in favorable-prognosis germ-cell tumors: the Indian University experience **Comment:** There is no statistically significant difference in survival between three or four cycles of BEP chemotherapy in patients with favorable prognosis germ cell carcinoma	1998 https://www.ncbi.nlm.nih.gov/pubmed/?term=saxman,+finch
RCT	Randomized phase III trial comparing retroperitoneal lymph node dissection with one course of bleomycin and etoposide plus cisplatin chemotherapy in the adjuvant treatment of clinical stage I nonseminomatous testicular germ cell tumors: AUO trial AH 01/94 by the German Testicular Cancer Study Group **Comment:** Showed superiority of one course of adjuvant BEP over RPLND to prevent recurrence in clinical stage I nonseminomatous germ cell tumor (NSGCT)	2008 https://www.ncbi.nlm.nih.gov/pubmed/?term=18458040
Randomized noninferiority trial	Randomized trial of carboplatin versus radiotherapy for stage I seminoma: mature results on relapse and contralateral testis cancer rates in MRC TE19/EORTC 30982 study (ISRCTN27163214) **Comment:** Carboplatin had a noninferior relapse-free rate compared with radiation and had reduced contralateral germ cell tumor for clinical stage I seminoma	2011 https://www.ncbi.nlm.nih.gov/pubmed/?term=21282539
RCT	Randomized comparison of cisplatin and etoposide and either bleomycin or ifosfamide in treatment of advanced disseminated germ cell tumors: an Eastern Cooperative Oncology Group, Southwest Oncology Group, and Cancer and Leukemia Group B Study **Comment:** BEP and VIP produce comparable favorable response rates and survival in patients with poor-risk germ cell tumors	1998 https://www.ncbi.nlm.nih.gov/pubmed/?term=9552027
Nonrandomized prospective study	One course of adjuvant BEP in clinical stage I nonseminoma: mature and expanded results from the SWENOTECA group **Comment:** Suggested that BEP×1 cycle should be standard therapy for +LVI, stage I NSGCT, where surveillance or BEP×1 are options for –LVI NSGCT	2014 https://www.ncbi.nlm.nih.gov/pubmed/25114021

Additional material for this chapter can be found online at:
www.wiley.com/go/oh/mountsinaioncology

This includes advice for patients, a case study, ICD codes, and
multiple choice questions.

CHAPTER 6

Lung Cancer

Rajwanth Veluswamy and Jorge E. Gomez
Icahn School of Medicine at Mount Sinai, New York, NY, USA

OVERALL BOTTOM LINE
- Accurate staging of early stage disease minimizes over- and undertreatment, providing the best outcomes for all stages.
- Early lung cancer is curable, and should be managed by multidisciplinary teams that include surgery, radiation oncology, and medical oncology.
- All nonsquamous tumors should undergo genomic sequencing to identify driver mutations that can be treated with targeted therapies. Targeted therapies provide better PFS than chemotherapy in the first line setting.
- Chemotherapy improves survival over best supportive care in advanced non-small cell lung cancer (NSCLC).
- Immunotherapy provides better survival than docetaxel in the second line setting in NSCLC.

Background
Definition of disease
Lung cancer is a neoplastic disease of the lower respiratory tract, including multiple histologic subtypes and biologically diverse genotypes, which is associated with a high mortality despite treatment.

Disease classification
Lung cancers are classified according to their histologic subtype into several broad categories.
- Adenocarcinoma, with identifiable patterns such as acinar, papillary, solid, micropapillary, lepidic mucinous, and lepidic nonmucinous.
- Squamous cell carcinoma.
- NSCLC-NOS, a non-small cell carcinoma without clear adenocarcinoma, squamous, or neuroendocrine morphology or staining.
- Non-small cell carcinoma with neuroendocrine markers and morphology.
- Non-small cell carcinoma with neuroendocrine morphology and no neuroendocrine markers.
- Small cell carcinoma.
- Sarcomatoid carcinoma.
- Pleomorphic carcinoma.

Mount Sinai Expert Guides: Oncology, First Edition. Edited by William K. Oh and Ajai Chari.
© 2019 John Wiley & Sons Ltd. Published 2019 by John Wiley & Sons Ltd.
Companion Website: www.wiley.com/go/oh/mountsinaioncology

Incidence/prevalence
- Lung cancer is the second most common cancer in both men and women and accounts for approximately 14% of all cancers.
- The yearly incidence of lung cancer in the USA is approximately 225 000 cases.
- The yearly incidence of lung cancer in the world is approximately 1.8 million cases.

Economic impact
The National Institutes of Health (NIH) has estimated that the cost of care for lung cancer in 2010 was $12.1 billion. The estimated cost in 2020 will be $17 billion.

Etiology and risk factors
Tobacco smoking is the most important risk factor in the development of lung cancer, accounting for approximately 80% of lung cancer deaths in the USA. Tobacco cessation programs in the USA have produced a decrease in the incidence of lung cancer in both men and women. Exposure to passive smoking also increases the risk of lung cancer.
- Exposure to radon, asbestos, ionizing radiation, industrial chemicals, and air pollution are less common risk factors.
- Multiple cohort studies have suggested that first degree relatives of patients with lung cancer have an increased risk of developing lung cancer.
- The role of genetic susceptibility in the development of lung cancer is under investigation. Genome-wide association studies have identified multiple genetic polymorphisms that are associated with lung cancer risk.
- Several single-nucleotide polymorphisms (SNPs) at 15q25.1 in genes that encode nicotinic-acetylcholine receptors have been associated with nicotine dependence.
- An SNP in 5p15.33, which contains the gene encoding for TERT has been associated with increased lung cancer risk.

Pathology/pathogenesis
- The pathogenesis of tobacco-related lung cancer (squamous carcinoma, small cell carcinoma, and the majority of adenocarcinomas) may be different from that of lung cancer in never smokers (predominantly adenocarcinoma).
- The pathogenesis of squamous carcinoma of the lung follows a pattern of progressive molecular abnormalities that start in the normal epithelium. Squamous dysplasia is the preneoplastic lesion for squamous carcinoma and progresses to carcinoma *in situ* and squamous cell carcinoma. The chain of molecular events begins with loss of heterozygosity at chromosomes 3p and 9p. Subsequent changes include abnormalities of *TP53* and *RB1*, followed by loss of heterozygosity at 8p and 5q. Amplification of *SOX2* has also been identified in squamous carcinomas and precursor lesions.
- Adenocarcinomas are believed to arise from Clara cells and type II pneumocytes. Although the exact pathogenesis of adenocarcinoma is unknown, adenomatous hyperplasia has been identified as a precursor lesion. *KRAS* mutations are predominant among tobacco-related adenocarcinomas and *EGFR, HER2*, and *BRAF* mutations, *ALK* rearrangements, and *ROS1* rearrangements are common among never-smoker adenocarcinomas.
- Loss of function of *TP53* and *RB1* has been found in animal models to drive small cell lung cancer (SCLC) development, and is commonly found in this disease.

Prevention

> **BOTTOM LINE/CLINICAL PEARLS**
> - Smoking cessation can significantly decrease the risk of developing or dying from lung cancer.

Screening
- A low dose CT scan performed in high risk subjects can decrease lung cancer mortality by 20%. High risk subjects are 55–80 years of age, with a 30 pack/year or greater smoking history, and are currently smoking, or have quit within the past 15 years (National Lung Screening Trial Research Team 2011).

Primary prevention
- Smoking cessation can significantly decrease the risk of developing or dying from lung cancer compared with people who continue to smoke. The magnitude of the benefit can vary according to length of tobacco exposure and age at cessation.
- Multiple clinical trials studying vitamins, NSAIDs, and other substances have yielded no positive results.

Secondary prevention
- Smoking cessation after treatment for early stage lung cancer can significantly decrease the risk of developing or dying from lung cancer compared with people who continue to smoke.

Diagnosis (Algorithm 6.1)

> **BOTTOM LINE/CLINICAL PEARLS**
> - Accurate smoking history can guide the diagnostic pathway. Never smokers will predominantly have adenocarcinoma, and have a high probability of harboring activating mutations.
> - Bronchoscopy with endobronchial ultrasound and CT-guided lung biopsy are the standard methods for obtaining diagnostic tissue, and can be important in staging.
> - Accurate histologic diagnosis is critical before deciding treatment. Treatments for small cell carcinoma, adenocarcinoma, and squamous carcinoma can differ significantly.
> - All non-squamous NSCLC should undergo genomic sequencing to test for activating mutations before making treatment decisions.

Typical presentation
- Early stage lung cancer is frequently asymptomatic and is often found as an incidental finding during the investigation of other medical problems or through lung cancer screening.
- Advanced lung cancer typically presents with a clinical picture of respiratory symptoms from both the upper and lower respiratory tract. Pneumonia, increasing unexplained dyspnea, and hemoptysis are frequent presenting signs.
- Symptoms arising from distant metastatic disease such as bone pain from bone metastases or neurologic complaints from brain metastases are also common forms of presentation.
- Paraneoplastic syndromes such as hypercalcemia, syndrome of inappropriate antidiuretic hormone secretion (SIADH), or hyponatremia, while uncommon, can sometimes be the presenting clinical scenario for lung cancer.

Algorithm 6.1 Diagnosis of lung cancer

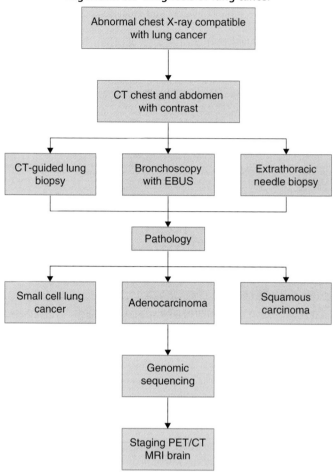

Clinical diagnosis/history
- Respiratory findings such as cough, hemoptysis, dyspnea, chest pain, or pneumonia are the most common presenting events.
- Smoking history is a marker of lung cancer risk.
- Weight loss and cachexia are common in patients with advanced lung cancer, and can impact prognosis.
- Hoarseness can suggest recurrent laryngeal nerve involvement.
- Pain can indicate bone or soft tissue involvement.
- Recent changes in mental status or behavior can point to hyponatremia, hypercalcemia, or brain metastasis.

Physical examination
- **Head and neck:** ptosis, miosis, and anhidrolysis suggest the presence of a superior sulcus tumor. The presence of enlarged supraclavicular lymph nodes indicate stage IIIB disease while cervical lymph nodes indicate stage IV disease. Dilated neck veins with facial edema can indicate superior vena cava obstruction.

- **Cardiac:** distant cardiac sounds and pulsus paradoxus can imply the presence of pericardial effusion. Arrhythmias such as atrial fibrillation and atrial flutter are common in patients with lung cancer.
- **Respiratory:** decreased breath sounds, wheezing, rales, and rhonchi may be present in patients with lung lesions. Dullness to percussion suggests pleural effusion.
- **Gastrointestinal:** hepatomegaly can be present with liver metastases.
- **Musculoskeletal:** tenderness, swelling, or decreased range of motion can indicate bone metastases.
- **Neurologic:** changes in mental status and sensorimotor deficits can be signs of metastases or paraneoplastic syndromes.
- **Extremities:** nail clubbing and bone/joint pain can be a sign of hypertrophic osteoarthropathy. Lower extremity edema, especially unilateral, can be present with deep venous thrombosis.

Useful clinical decision rules and calculators
- The Eastern Cooperative Oncology Group (ECOG) performance status is a scale used to measure a patient's daily living abilities. It has significant research utility and is useful when evaluating patients for eligibility for anticancer treatment (Table 6.1).

Disease severity classification
The American Joint Commission on Cancer staging system, seventh edition, provides an excellent prognostic and treatment framework in lung cancer (Table 6.2).

Laboratory diagnosis
List of diagnostic tests
- Genomic sequencing of formalin fixed paraffin embedded (FFPE) tissue specimens can identify activating mutations that have important implications in the treatment of lung cancer (*EGFR, HER2, BRAF, KRAS*).
- Fluorescence *in situ* hybridization (FISH) performed on FFPE can identify rearrangements in *ALK* and *ROS1* that have important implications in the treatment of lung cancer.
- Genomic sequencing of circulating tumor DNA can identify driver mutations in lung cancer. However, this testing has significant limitations, primarily the scarcity of cell free circulating DNA.
- CBC and a basic or CMP that includes calcium are important in monitoring treatment toxicity.

Table 6.1 Eastern Cooperative Oncology Group (ECOG) performance status scale.

Grade	ECOG performance status
0	Fully active, able to carry out all predisease performance without restriction
1	Restricted in physically strenuous activity but ambulatory and able to carry out work of a light or sedentary nature (e.g. light house work, office work)
2	Ambulatory and capable of all self-care but unable to carry out any work activities; up and about more than 50% of waking hours
3	Capable of only limited self-care; confined to bed or chair more than 50% of waking hours
4	Completely disabled; cannot carry out any self-care; totally confined to bed or chair
5	Dead

Table 6.2 American Joint Commission on Cancer staging system.

T/M descriptor	T/M	N0	N1	N2	N3
T1 (≤2 cm)	T1a	IA	IIA	IIIA	IIIB
T1 (>2–3 cm)	T1b	IA	IIA	IIIA	IIIB
T2 (≤5 cm)	T2a	IB	IIA	IIIA	IIIB
T2 (>5–7 cm)	T2b	IIA	IIB	IIIA	IIIB
T2 (>7 cm)	T3	IIB	IIIA	IIIA	IIIB
T3 invasion		IIB	IIIA	IIIA	IIIB
T4 (same lobe nodules)		IIB	IIIA	IIIA	IIIB
T4 (extension)	T4	IIIA	IIIA	IIIB	IIIB
M1 (ipsilateral lung)		IIIA	IIIA	IIIB	IIIB
T4 (pleural effusion)	M1a	IV	IV	IV	IV
M1 (contralateral lung)		IV	IV	IV	IV
M1 (distant)	M1b	IV	IV	IV	IV

Lists of imaging techniques
- A CT scan of chest and abdomen with contrast will identify disease in the lung, liver, adrenal system, and bone. In the thorax, the addition of IV contrast aids in the clinical staging of the mediastinum.
- PET is a standard staging tool that can identify areas of metastatic disease in bone or soft tissue. In addition, high fluorodeoxyglucose (FDG) uptake values have been found to correlate with worse outcomes.
- MRI of the brain, although not necessary in every case, can recognize early brain metastases before they become symptomatic.
- A Bone scan can identify areas of bone metastasis.

Potential pitfalls/common errors made regarding diagnosis of disease
- While fine needle aspiration biopsy may be sufficient for an adequate diagnosis of lung cancer, it is not uncommon for there to be insufficient tissue for genomic analysis. It is important to communicate with the pathologist that the minimum amount of tissue should be used to establish the lung cancer subtype in order to have tissue for genomic testing.

Treatment (Algorithm 6.2)
Treatment rationale
Limited SCLC (LSCLC)
- While surgery does not have a significant role in SCLC, resection may be appropriate for patients with small tumors without nodal involvement. This should be followed by adjuvant chemotherapy.
- The optimal treatment of SCLC includes chemotherapy with a platinum regimen and radiation, usually given concurrently. Concurrent treatment improves median survival compared with sequential treatment (27 vs. 19 months).
- Twice daily radiation improves survival by 4 months over once daily radiation, but, because of toxicity, should be performed only in selected, fit patients.
- Prophylactic cranial irradiation improves 3-year survival by 5.4% (20.7 vs. 15.3 months).

Algorithm 6.2 Management of non-small cell lung cancer

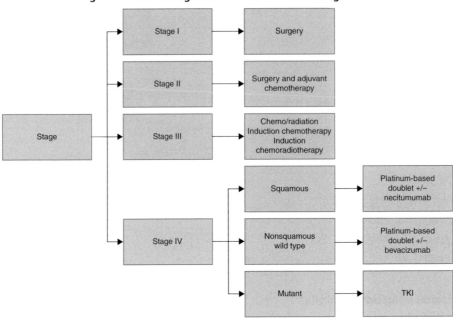

Extensive SCLC (ESCLC)

- Chemotherapy with a platinum-based regimen is the standard treatment for extensive SCLC.
- Etoposide/cisplatin provides equivalent efficacy to doxorubicin-based regimens, but is better tolerated.
- Etoposide/cisplatin seems to be equivalent to irinotecan/cisplatin in the western population. Response rates are in the range of 60–80%.
- Second line chemotherapy with topotecan provides equivalent efficacy as a doxorubicin regimen with less toxicity.
- Prophylactic cranial irradiation after chemotherapy improves survival by 1.3 months in ESCLC.
- Consolidation radiotherapy to the chest increases 2-year survival from 3% to 13% and increases 6-month PFS from 7% to 23%.
- The addition of atezolizumab to carboplatin and etoposide in extensive stage small cell lung cancer improves OS from 10.3–12.3 months in the 1st line setting.

Early stage NSCLC

- Approximately one-third of NSCLC patients present with early stage disease amenable to surgical resection (stage I–IIIA). Based on the Lung Cancer Study Group Trial, the standard surgical approach for stage I–II NSCLC is lobectomy with systematic lymph node sampling. The most common surgical approach is open thoracotomy, although minimally invasive techniques such as video-assisted thorascopic surgery are being increasingly adopted.
- For patients who are unable to tolerate lobectomy or have good prognostic tumors (i.e. <2 cm) potentially not requiring lobectomy, limited resection (segmentectomy vs. wedge resection) may be an acceptable alternative. Stereotactic radiation treatment also appears to be a promising option for patients who cannot tolerate surgery.
- Many NSCLC patients who undergo potentially curative surgery experience local and distant relapse of disease causing significant morbidity and mortality. Postoperative radiotherapy has

demonstrated improved local control, but has not been shown to improve OS rates. Platinum-based chemotherapy, on the other hand, significantly improved long-term survival following surgical resection of stage II or III tumors (i.e. positive lymph node involvement) in randomized controlled trials (ANITA trial, LACE meta-analysis).

Locally advanced NSCLC

- The management of locally advanced NSCLC remains controversial, and treatment decisions are made with curative intent. For potentially resectable disease ("non-bulky," stage IIIA), induction cisplatin-based chemotherapy alone or with radiation treatment prior to surgery is usually considered to allow for early treatment of micrometastatic disease and possibly decrease tumor size to improve surgical outcomes. Surgical resection following chemoradiotherapy was associated with a significantly longer PFS and a trend towards improved OS rates in the phase III intergroup 0139 trial. For patients unable to tolerate surgery, definitive radiotherapy remains an option. Adjuvant chemotherapy and/or radiation treatment is often used to attenuate the high risk of local and distant failure following surgery.
- Adjuvant chemotherapy with a cisplatin-based regimen provides a 5% survival benefit in patients with stage II and III NSCLC after resection.
- The treatment of choice for unresectable stage IIIA (N2) or stage IIIB disease is a combination of chemotherapy and definitive radiation treatment. The results of two RCTs (RTOG and a Japanese phase III trial) demonstrated a clear survival benefit with the use of concurrent chemoradiation, albeit at the expense of increased toxicity. The patient's functional status, age, and comorbidities must be carefully considered. Chemotherapy regimens appropriate for chemoradiation are:
  - Platinum/etoposide
  - Platinum/vinca alkaloid
  - Platinum/pemetrexed
  - Caroplatin/paclitaxel.

Metastatic NSCLC

- Stage IV NSCLC is not curable. The goal of treatment is to prolong survival and improve quality of life. Cytotoxic chemotherapy has been the mainstay of treatment for several decades associated with modest improvements in survival. As our understanding of molecular mechanisms of tumorogenesis and tumor interactions with the immune system improves, novel treatments including targeted inhibitors and immunotherapies are showing promising therapeutic efficacy with fewer toxicities.
- All lung cancers with adenocarcinoma histology should undergo molecular testing for driver mutations in *EGFR, ALK,* and *ROS* genes. In patients with these actionable mutations, targeted treatment is recommended in the first line setting. Several RCTs have shown superior response and disease-free survival outcomes with TKIs (i.e. erlotinib, gefitinib, afatinib for *EGFR*; crizotinib for *ALK/ROS1*) compared with chemotherapy in patients whose tumors are driven by these mutations.
- In patients without driver mutations, first line therapy with a platinum-based doublet with or without bevacizumab is recommended after being shown to have a clear survival advantage over monotherapy. However, no particular two-drug combination has been shown to be superior. Cisplatin appears to be more efficacious than carboplatin, but also carries a more significant side effect profile and is more difficult to tolerate. More recently, a phase III trial demonstrated pemetrexed (thymidylate synthase inhibitor; antifolate) with platinum to have improved OS and better toxicity profile than another platinum-based doublet in a prespecified analysis of nonsquamous cell cancers.

- The addition of bevacizumab to chemotherapy was shown to have a significant 2-month survival benefit (12.3 vs. 10.3 months) in the ECOG 4599 phase III trial. However, because of the risk of bleeding, only patients with nonsquamous call cancers and without other significant bleeding risks should receive bevacizumab.
- The initial chemotherapy regimen is usually given for four to six cycles. If the patient responds to first line chemotherapy, maintenance chemotherapy aims to prolong the survival benefit while limiting toxicity from continued treatment. Maintenance pemetrexed after standard chemotherapy produces better survival than best supportive care (13.4 vs. 10.6 months). Bevacizumab improves OS by 2 months when added to paclitaxel and carboplatin (12.3 vs. 10.3 months). Bevacizumab, pemetrexed, and erlotinib are currently approved in the maintenance setting.
- Necitumumab, an EGFR monoclonal antibody, improves survival when added to gemcitabine and cisplatin when compared with chemotherapy alone (median survival 11.5 vs. 9.9 months) in advanced, chemotherapy naïve squamous carcinoma.
- Unfortunately, all patients will eventually have disease progression following initial treatment and subsequent lines of treatment should be considered in accordance with the patient's performance status. For patients who had a durable response to initial chemotherapy, they can be rechallenged with the same regimen. If they did not have a satistfactory reponse to first line treatment, patients can be offered immunotherapy, another combination regimen, monotherapy, or an EGFR inhibitor.
- Immune checkpoint inhibitors such as PD-1 antibodies are the latest class of drugs that have received accelerated approval for the management of NSCLC patients who progressed on or following treatment with platinum-based chemotherapy. Nivolumab (does not require PD-L1 expression testing) is now approved for both squamous cell (CHECKMATE-017 trial) and non-squamous (CHECKMATE-057) NSCLC after demonstrating improved OS rates over docetaxel in the second line setting (CHECKMATE 017, 9.2 vs. 6 months; CHECKMATE 057, 12.2 vs. 9.4 months). Pembrolizumab (requires PD-L1 expression testing) is a PD-1 inhibitor that showed impressive response rates, PFS, and OS in the KEYNOTE 010 trial (outcomes correlated with PD-L1 expression). The KEYNOTE 010 trial pembrolizumab showed improved survival compared to docetaxel in second line treatment of PD-L1 positive NSCLC (12.7 vs. 8.5 months).
- Ramucirumab, a VEGFR2 monoclonal antibody, improves survival when added to docetaxel when compared with chemotherapy alone (median survival 10.5 vs. 9.1 months) in advanced NSCLC in the second line setting.
- Ceritinib produces a 40% response rate vs. 6% for chemotherapy after failure of first line TKI in *ALK* mutant NSCLC.
- Alectinib produces a 40–50% response rate after failure of first line TKI in *ALK* mutant NSCLC.
- Osimertinib produces a response rate of approximately 60% in patients with a *T790M* mutation who have failed a first line TKI.

Immunotherapy
- In the second-line setting, atezolizumab improves OS from 9.6 months to 13.8 months when compared to docetaxel in non-small cell lung cancer.
- The combination of pembrolizumab and platinum-based chemotherapy improves median survival from 12.1 months to 16.7 months compared to chemotherapy alone in the first line treatment of non squamous non-small-cell lung cancer.
- The combination of atezolizumab and chemotherapy with carboplatin and Nab paclitaxel improves PFS from 5.6–6.3 months compared to chemotherapy alone in squamous non-small cell lung cancer in the first line setting.

- The addition of atezolizumab to platinum and pemetrexed in the first line setting improves OSl from 13.6 months to 18.1 months in nonsquamous non-small cell lung cancer.
- The addition of atezolizumab to bevacizumab plus chemotherapy improves OS from 14.7 months to 19.2 months in nonsquamous non-small cell lung cancer in first line setting.
- The addition of pembrolizumab to platinum/taxane in the first line setting improves OS from 11.3 months to 15.9 months in squamous non-small cell lung cancer.
- Twelve months of consolidation durvalumab after concurrent chemotherapy and radiation for stage III non-small cell lung cancer improves PFS from 5.6 months to 16.8 months.
- The addition of atezolizumab.

Targeted therapy
- Brigatinib improves PFS, objective response rate, and intracranial response rate in ALK mutant patients in the first line setting when compared to crizotinib.
- Ceritinib improves PFS from 8.1 months to 16.6 months when compared to standard chemotherapy in the first line setting in ALK mutant patients.
- Lorlatinib, and ALK and ROS1 inhibitor produces response rates of 90% in TKI naive ALK positive patients, 69% in patients treated with crizotinib, and 38.7% in patients with 2 or more previous ALK TKI.
- Dacomitinib improves OS from 26.8 months to 34.1 months over gefitinib in the first line setting in patients with EGFR mutations.

Table of treatment

Treatment	Comments
Conservative	
Best supportive care	Best supportive care should be offered to patients who are more likely to experience more harm than benefit from treatment (i.e. ECOG performance status 3–4; poor pulmonary function). Localized palliative treatment (i.e. radiation) should still be considered to alleviate symptoms
Medical	
Chemotherapy agents • Cisplatin (60–100 mg/m^2 IV every 21 days) • Paclitaxel (175–225 mg/m^2 IV every 3 weeks) • Carboplatin (AUC 6 IV every 21 days) • Pemetrexed (500 mg/m^2 IV every 21 days) • Gemcitabine (1250 mg/m^2 IV on day 1 and 8 of 21-day cycle) • Docetaxel (75 mg/m^2 IV every 21 days) • Nab-Paclitaxel (100 mg/m^2 IV on days 1, 8, and 15 of 21-day cycle) • Etoposide (100 mg/m^2 IV days 1–3 every 28 days)	• Nephrotoxicity, ototoxicity, peripheral neuropathy, cytopenias • Cytopenias, peripheral neuropathy, fatigue, hair loss • Cytopenias, nausea, hair loss, fatigue, nephrotoxicity (less common than cisplatin) • Cytopenias, nausea, fatigue, rash. Patients must take vitamin B12 and folic acid throughout treatment • Cytopenias, hair loss, nausea, dehydration, fatigue, liver injury • Cytopenias, hair loss, fatigue, nausea, myalgias, diarrhea • Cytopenias, peripheral neuropathy, hair loss, nausea, fatigue • Cytopenias, nausea, anorexia, diarrhea or constipation, fatigue, hair loss, mouth sores • Cytopenias, fatigue, nausea, constipation or diarrhea, peripheral neuropathy, hepatic impairment, hair loss

(Continued)

(*Continued*)

Treatment	Comments

• Vinorelbine (25 mg/m² IV every week)
 	
• Irinotecan (60 mg/m² IV days 1, 8, 15 of 28-day cycle)
 	
Molecular targeted therapy
• *EGFR* inhibitors (PO)
  • Erlotinib (150 mg/day)
  • Gefitinib (250 mg/day)
  • Afatinib (40 mg/day)
  • Osimertinib (80 mg/day)
• *ALK/ROS1* inhibitors (PO)
  • Crizotinib (250 mg twice daily)
  • Ceritinib (400 mg/day)
  • Alectinib (600 mg twice daily)
  • Brigatinib 180 mg daily
  • Lorlatinib 100 mg daily
  • Dacomitinib 45 mg daily
• Bevacizumab (15 mg/kg IV every 3 weeks)
 	
Immunotherapy (PD-1)
• Nivolumab (240 mg IV every 2 weeks)
• Pembrolizumab (2 mg/kg IV every 3 weeks)
• Atezolizumab 1200 mg IV every 3 weeks
• Durvalumab 10 mg/kg IV every 2 weeks
	• Diarrhea, nausea/vomiting, cytopenias, fatigue, anorexia, hair loss, mouth sores, interstitial lung disease
	
	• Diarrhea, fatigue, rash, cough, dyspnea, anorexia, pneumonitis, hepatic impairment, stomatitis, paronychia, dry skin
	
	• Diarrhea, nausea/vomiting, blurry vision, rash, hepatotoxicity, pneumonitis, fatigue
	
	• Bleeding, hypertension, gastrointestinal perforation, delayed wound healing, proteinuria, rash, headache
	Colitis (diarrhea), pneumonitis (SOB, cough), hepatic impairment, pancreatitis, rash, thyroid and adrenal insufficiency

Surgical	
• Pneumonectomy • Lobectomy • Segmentectomy • Wedge resection	Comprehensive assessment based on factors such as tumor characteristics, performance status, age, comorbidities and preoperative pulmonary function tests (e.g. FEV$_1$, DLCO) to calculate predicted postoperative pulmonary function
Radiologic	
External beam radiation therapy (EBRT) • 3D conformal radiation therapy • Intensity modulated radiation therapy • Stereotactic body radiation therapy Brachytherapy (internal radiation therapy)	Depending on the stage of lung cancer, radiation treatment can be the definitive treatment (with or without chemotherapy) for localized cancers that are not resectable or in patients who cannot tolerate surgical resection. Radiation treatment is also often used to treat a single area of cancer metastasis (e.g. brain). Additionally, radiation treatment is used to palliate symptoms caused by tumors (e.g. airway obstruction)

Prevention/management of complications

• Esophagitis from concurrent chemoradiation can be treated with topical viscous lidocaine and narcotic analgesics, in addition to nutritional support. More severe cases can require gastrostomy tube placement.
• Nivolumab and pembrolizumab can produce severe pneumonitis. This can be treated with systemic steroids.

CLINICAL PEARLS
- Targeted therapies should be used in the first line setting for patients with advanced NSCLC.
- All patients with stage IIIA NSCLC should be considered for resection by a multidisciplinary group.
- Adjuvant chemotherapy with a cisplatin-based regimen must be considered for patients with stage II and III NSCLC after resection.
- Pembrolizumab and nivolumab produce a 3-month survival benefit after standard docetaxel in the second line setting for patients with advanced NSCLC.

Special populations
Elderly
- Older patients with few comorbidities and excellent performance status may derive the same survival benefit from standard treatments as younger patients, and should not be denied treatment based solely on age.
- The accumulation of comorbidities and age-related decline in renal, cardiac, pulmonary, and hematologic function increases the likelihood of higher grade toxicities.
- A thorough evaluation of comorbid issues, social support, nutrition, and cognitive function is key in predicting toxicities and outcomes.

Prognosis

BOTTOM LINE/CLINICAL PEARLS
- The 5-year OS for all patients diagnosed with lung cancer in the USA is 17% (Table 6.3).
- In patients with advanced disease, where the median survival is approximately 12 months, quality of life is an extremely important goal of care.

Table 6.3 Stage of disease and survival rates for patients with non-small cell lung cancer.

NSCLC stage	7th edition of TNM stage subdivision	5-year survival
I	IA	50%
	IB	43%
II	IIA	36%
	IIB	25%
III	IIIA	19%
	IIIB	7%
IV	IV	2%

Reference
National Lung Screening Trial Research Team, Aberle DR, Adama AM, Berg CD, et al. Reduced lung-cancer mortality with low-dose computed tomographic screening. N Engl J Med 2011;365:395–409.

Guidelines
National society guidelines

Title	Source	Weblink
Lung Cancer Guidelines	NCCN	www.nccn.org
Lung Cancer Guidelines	ASCO	www.asco.org
Lung Cancer Guidelines	ACCP	http://journal.publications.chestnet.org

Evidence

Type of evidence	Title	Date and weblink
Systematic review	Lung adjuvant cisplatin evaluation: a pooled analysis by the LACE Collaborative Group	2008 https://www.ncbi.nlm.nih.gov/pubmed/18506026
Systematic review	Meta-analysis of concomitant versus sequential radiochemotherapy in locally advanced non-small cell lung cancer	2010 https://www.ncbi.nlm.nih.gov/pubmed/20351327
RCT	Comparison of four chemotherapy regimens for advanced non-small cell lung cancer	2002 https://www.ncbi.nlm.nih.gov/pubmed/11784875
RCT	Paclitaxel-carboplatin alone or with bevacizumab for non-small cell lung cancer	2006 https://www.ncbi.nlm.nih.gov/pubmed/17167137
RCT	Maintenance pemetrexed plus best supportive care versus placebo plus best supportive care for non-small cell lung cancer: a randomised, double-blind, phase 3 study	2009 https://www.ncbi.nlm.nih.gov/pubmed/19767093
RCT	Phase III study comparing cisplatin plus gemcitabine with cisplatin plus pemetrexed in chemotherapy-naive patients with advanced-stage non-small cell lung cancer	2008 https://www.ncbi.nlm.nih.gov/pubmed/18506025
RCT	Gefitinib or carboplatin–paclitaxel in pulmonary adenocarcinoma	2009 https://www.ncbi.nlm.nih.gov/pubmed/19692680
RCT	Crizotinib versus chemotherapy in advanced ALK-positive lung cancer	2013 https://www.ncbi.nlm.nih.gov/pubmed/23724913
RCT	Pembrolizumab versus docetaxel for previously treated, PD-L1-positive, advanced non-small cell lung cancer (KEYNOTE 010): a randomised controlled trial	2016 https://www.ncbi.nlm.nih.gov/pubmed/26712084
RCT	Nivolumab versus docetaxel in advanced nonsquamous non-small-cell lung cancer	2015 https://www.ncbi.nlm.nih.gov/pubmed/26412456

Additional material for this chapter can be found online at:
www.wiley.com/go/oh/mountsinaioncology

This includes a case study, ICD code, and multiple choice questions.

CHAPTER 7

Malignant Mesothelioma

Nicholas C. Rohs and Zishuo I. Hu
Icahn School of Medicine at Mount Sinai, New York, NY, USA

OVERALL BOTTOM LINE
- Malignant mesothelioma (MM) is a rare malignant tumor of the lung pleura, peritoneum, pericardium, or tunica vaginalis testis primarily found in males between 50 and 80 years of age.
- Approximately 70–80% of pleural mesotheliomas are associated with direct or indirect asbestos exposure.
- Epithelial histology confirms better prognosis than either sarcomatoid or biphasic/mixed histology.
- Patients should be managed by high volume centers where they can be evaluated for trimodality therapy including surgery, radiation, chemotherapy, and immunotherapy.
- Most patients are diagnosed with advanced disease with median OS of approximately 1 year. First line chemotherapy includes cisplatin and pemetrexed +/– bevacizumab. Despite aggressive management, overall outcomes remain poor.

Section 1: Background
Definition of disease

A neoplasm arising from the mesothelial cells that form the serosal lining of the pleural, pericardial, and peritoneal cavities. The majority are malignant with an aggressive clinical course.

Incidence/prevalence

- A rare disease with approximately 2500 new cases in the USA annually. The majority are pleural in origin.
- 5 : 1 male to female ratio with median age at diagnosis of 72 and higher prevalence in Caucasian and Hispanic than in African or Asian populations.
- Incidence in the USA is leveling off whereas it is increasing in Australia, Russia, China, India, and Western Europe (likely because of reduced occupational exposure caused by earlier asbestos regulation and abatement efforts instituted in the USA).

Economic impact

- An estimated 17 potential years of life are lost in patients with MM.
- Estimated spending on asbestos litigation through 2002 was about $70 billion, with gross compensation around $49 billion.

Mount Sinai Expert Guides: Oncology, First Edition. Edited by William K. Oh and Ajai Chari.
© 2019 John Wiley & Sons Ltd. Published 2019 by John Wiley & Sons Ltd.
Companion Website: www.wiley.com/go/oh/mountsinaioncology

Etiology
- Asbestos (70–80% of cases) – chrysotile and amphibole are the two main types with crocidolite, an amphibole subtype, being the most oncogenic.
- Thorotrast (radiocontrast agent containing thorium dioxide).
- Ionizing radiation (i.e. previous mantle radiation for Hodgkin lymphoma).
- Erionite (mineral found in gravel roads).
- Possible increased familial risk resulting from germline mutations in the *BAP1* gene.
- Smoking is *not* a risk factor.

Pathology/pathogenesis
- Direct physical effect of asbestos on chromosomes; production of hydroxyl radicals and super-oxide anions leading to DNA strand breaks and deletions; stimulation of EGFR phosphorylation, activation, and signal transduction; increased production of inflammatory cytokines.
- Simian virus 40 large-tumor antigen can also contribute as its expression is elevated in 85% of MM cells.

Odds ratios for select risk factors

Risk factor	Odds ratio
Any asbestos	3.7 : 1
Amphibole asbestos	7 : 1
Male sex	5 : 1

Prevention
Prevention
- Avoidance of asbestos and radiation exposure.

Screening
- Screening is not recommended as there are no data to support that screening improves survival.

Primary prevention
- Ensure appropriate protective equipment use when exposed to asbestos and avoid bringing asbestos dust home on clothing.

Secondary prevention
- Primary treatment is the only intervention to prevent recurrence.

Diagnosis (Algorithm 7.1)

> **BOTTOM LINE/CLINICAL PEARLS**
> - Mesothelioma development is largely attributed to previous asbestos exposure.
> - Patients commonly present with dyspnea, cough, chest pain, fatigue, or unilateral pleural effusion.
> - Pleural aspiration and biopsy, thoracosopy, immunohistochemistry, and radiologic imaging are used to confirm diagnosis. Fine needle aspiration is *not* recommended for diagnosis.

Algorithm 7.1 Diagnosis of malignant mesothelioma

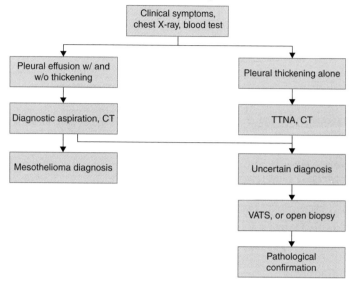

TTNA, trans-thoracic needle aspiration; VATS, video-assisted thoracoscopic surgery.

Differential diagnosis

Differential diagnosis	Features
Metastatic adenocarcinoma	Similar radiographic appearance, but with unique immunohistochemical profile
Chronic, organizing empyema	Empyema typically do not involve entire pleural wall and are loculated
Lymphoma	Lymphoma often has mediastinal and retrocrural lymphadenopathy, fevers, and night sweats
Thymoma	Thymomas can occasionally metastasize into pleura, but usually have a primary anterior mediastinal mass which is rare for MM

Typical presentation
- Long latency period of 30–40 years with usual presentation from 50 to 70 years old. Median time from symptom onset to diagnosis is 2–3 months. Most common presenting symptoms are nonpleuritic posterolateral chest pain and dyspnea. Chest X-ray will typically reveal a unilateral pleural effusion, with 60% being right-sided. Only 5% have bilateral disease at presentation.
- Less common symptoms include fatigue, insomnia, fever, cough, and chills. Patients with advanced disease present with anorexia/cachexia, asymmetric chest wall expansion, or palpable chest wall masses.

History
- It is crucial to ask about previous occupational and household exposure to asbestos. High risk occupations include shipyard workers, building insulators, asbestos miners, brake mechanics, railroad workers, and electricians. Household members can also be at risk through exposure from family members' contaminated clothing. Less common historic exposures include radiation, intrapleural thorium dioxide, and erionite.

Physical examination
- Decreased breath sounds, crackles, or dullness to percussion. Local spread of the disease can also develop with signs of chest wall invasion, superior vena cava syndrome, spinal cord compression, and pericardial involvement.

Useful clinical decision rules and calculators
- CALGB Prognostic Index (see website Addendum 7.1: Summary table of prognostic scores for MM).
- EORTC Prognostic Index (see website Addendum 7.1: Summary table of prognostic scores for MM).

Disease severity classification
- **TNM staging** (stage I–IV): (Figure 7.1) (see website Addendum 7.2: Visual representation of TNM staging for MM).
- **Histology:** epithelial histology (approximately 50% of cases) confers better prognosis. Biphasic/mixed histology (34%) includes both subtypes and prognosis is dependent on the percent composition. Sarcomatoid (16%) confers the worst prognosis.

Laboratory diagnosis
- **CBC:** 60–90% of patients with MM have thrombocytosis.
- **Blood-based diagnostics:** several blood-based tests have been evaluated to aid in diagnosis and include homocysteine, soluble mesothelin-related peptide (commercially available), osteopontin, and fibulin 3 (see website Addendum 7.3: Laboratory diagnosis).
- **Tissue biopsy with histologic evaluation:** microscopic evaluation by a pathologist to determine epithelial, sarcomatoid, or biphasic/mixed histology. Fine needle aspirate is *not* recommended. Immunohistochemical staining in MM is usually positive for calretinin, cytokeratin 5/7, WT1, and D2-40 and negative for CEA, CD15, Ber-EP4, Moc-31, TTF-1, and B72.3.

Lists of imaging techniques
- **Chest X-ray:** good initial test which may show a pleural effusion or pleural thickening.
- **Chest CT:** useful for detecting invasion into mediastinal structures, chest wall, and ribs (Figure 7.2).
- **MRI:** used for detecting diaphragmatic, endothoracic fascial, or spinal cord invasion.
- **PET CT:** useful in differentiating benign from malignant disease and ruling out metastatic disease, particularly in surgical candidates. Also used to assess treatment response.
- **Echocardiography:** to rule out cardiac involvement.

Potential pitfalls/common errors made regarding diagnosis of disease
- Commonly mistaken for pulmonary infection or other malignancies.

Treatment (Algorithm 7.2)
- Given the rarity of MM there is no standard of care and treatment should be individualized as determined by a multidisciplinary team including surgeons, radiation oncologists, and medical oncologists at a high volume center. The optimal sequencing of these modalities is undefined.
- Age, comorbidities, pulmonary and cardiac function, disease histology, and disease extent all have a major role in treatment decision.
- There are currently no approved targeted or biological therapies although research in this area is ongoing.
- Standard treatment for all but localized mesothelioma is generally not curative.

Algorithm 7.2 Treatment of malignant mesothelioma

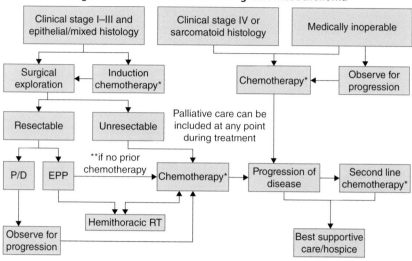

P/D, pleurectomy/decortication; EPP, extrapleural pneumonectomy.   *Consider clinical trial

When to hospitalize
- Uncontrollable disease-related symptoms including pain, shortness of breath, and anorexia/cachexia.
- Uncontrollable treatment-related symptoms including nausea, vomiting, diarrhea, or severe infections such as febrile neutropenia.

Managing the hospitalized patient
- Aggressive pain control including evaluation for palliative radiation.
- Pulmonary support including supplemental oxygen and consideration of thoracentesis or talc pleurodesis for management of pleural effusion.

Table of treatment

Treatment	Comments
Conservative	
• Pain control (NSAIDs, opioids) • Thoracentesis/talc pleurodesis	• Advanced stage patients with multiple comorbidities or patients who decline treatment • Talc pleurodesis should be performed after PET CT staging as it can affect results
Medical	
• Clinical trials • Cisplatin 75 mg/m², pemetrexed 500 mg/m² (FDA approved) • Cisplatin 75 mg/m², pemetrexed 500 mg/m², bevacizumab 15 mg/kg • Carboplatin AUC5, pemetrexed 500 mg/m² • Cisplatin 80–100 mg/m², gemcitabine 1000–1250 mg/m²	• Due to rarity of MM always consider a clinical trial • Common side effects of chemotherapy include fatigue, anorexia, nausea, vomiting, dyspnea, and cytopenias • Pemetrexed should be taken with folate and vitamin B12 supplements • Bevacizumab can cause bleeding, gastrointestinal perforation, hypertension, or wound healing issues • HIPEC (hyperthermic intraperitoneal chemotherapy) is only for peritoneal mesothelioma

(*Continued*)

Treatment	Comments
• Single agent pemetrexed 500 mg/m², liposomal doxorubicin 30 mg/m², or vinorelbine 25–30 mg/m² • Second line – rechallenge with pemetrexed 500 mg/m² or single agent vinorelbine 25–30 mg/m² or gemcitabine 1000–1250 mg/m² • Second line immunotherapy: nivolumab 3 mg/kg IV +/– ipilimumab 1 mg/kg IV; pembrolizumab 10 mg/kg IV • HIPEC with cisplatin or doxorubicin	• Immune therapy can cause a wide array of immune-related side effects and patient should be monitored closely • Immune-related side effects should be treated with steriods and supportive care

Surgical

• Pleurectomy with decortication (P/D): complete removal of the pleura and all gross tumor. Perioperative mortality of <2% • Radical pleurectomy (RP): complete lung-sparing resection of the visceral and parietal pleura +/– diaphragmatic, pericardial, or wedge resection. Perioperative mortality of 2.9% • Extrapleural pneumonectomy (EPP): en bloc resection of pleural, lung, ipsilateral diaphragm, and, often, pericardium. Perioperative mortality of 6–30%	• Surgeon should have experience with MM resection • Can be employed for curative (rare) or palliative intent • Goal of complete gross cytoreduction. If not possible surgery should be aborted • Generally not recommended for sarcomatoid histology • Mediastinal lymph node sampling of at least three nodal stations is recommended • P/D can also be used to prevent recurrent pleural effusions. • RP, also called an "extended P/D," is a newer technique to improve gross resection but limit morbidity • EPP results in lower recurrence rate although no survival benefit has been proven. Because of its involved nature it should be reserved for patients who are <65 years and with good performance status

Radiologic

• Curative intent adjuvant radiation (45–60 Gy) • Palliative radiation for pain relief (20–40 Gy) • Local/residual tumors (60 Gy or more) • Prophylactic radiation to surgical sites (21 Gy)	• A dose of 54 Gy to the entire hemithorax, thoracotomy incision, and chest drains is generally well tolerated. • Palliative intent doses are 4 Gy daily, but ideal total dosage is still unclear. While pain relief is significant, duration may be brief • Dose may be limited by adjacent structures • Some experienced practitioners use brachytherapy and intraoperative external beam radiation • Extensive nodal irradiation is not recommended

Psychologic

• Encourage family/friend involvement • Social work support • Mental health provider as indicated	• Poor prognosis disease with significant symptomatology • Consider early involvement of palliative care team

Complementary

• Management of nausea/vomiting • Complementary/alternative interventions: acupuncture, Reiki therapy, massage therapy, etc.	• Antiemetics are given as part of chemotherapy treatment • Alternative treatments have not shown any proven effect on disease outcome, but can improve patient's quality of life

Other

• Intraoperative treatment with heated chemotherapy (cisplatin, mitomycin, and cytarabine) or photodynamic therapy	• These modalities are still under investigation, but in small studies have shown to reduce tumor size and control effusions. They can be considered for locally aggressive disease

Prevention/management of complications
- Ensuring proper antiemetic treatment is important.
- Supplementation with vitamin B12 and folate before initiating pemetrexed is important to prevent toxicity.
- Fatal radiation pneumonitis: radiation oncologists will attempt to limit the dose of radiation as significantly as possible.
- Close perioperative observation for complications of surgery.

CLINICAL PEARLS
- Encourage interdisciplinary discussion of cases to assess appropriateness of trimodality therapy.
- Aggressive symptom management during treatment is important.
- Even with treatment prognosis is poor and early involvement of palliative care is reasonable and encouraged.

Special populations
Pregnancy
- Extremely rare in this population. Limited literature exists regarding MM in pregnancy.

Children
- Childhood MM is a very rare disease and has a poor prognosis. Unlike malignant mesothelioma in adults, there is no clear causal association between asbestos exposure and MM in children.

Elderly
- With a median age at diagnosis of 72 most patients with MM are elderly. Overall functional status and comorbidities must be actively integrated into treatment planning. Carboplatin may be better tolerated in the elderly population than cisplatin.

Prognosis
- There are multiple prognostic scoring systems (CALGB, EORTC, IALSC) which include different prognostic variables. No unified system has been established (see website Addendum 7.1 Summary table of prognostic scores for MM).
- While multiple studies are investigating the role of genetic alterations and gene expression profiling in MM, there are no currently approved tests.

Natural history of untreated disease
- Patients with untreated mesothelioma die from respiratory compromise or pneumonia. As the disease progresses, arrhythmias, heart failure, and stroke can develop as a consequence of myocardial involvement. Dysphagia results from the tumor mass compressing against the esophagus.

Prognosis for treated patients
- Treatment with cisplatin and pemetrexed increases survival by 3–4 months compared with cisplatin alone.
- In patients under 76 years old with unresectable MM the addition of bevacizumab to pemetrexed and cisplatin had a survival advantage of 2.7 months.
- Overall prognosis remains poor even with treatment.

Follow-up tests and monitoring

- A modified Response Evaluation Criteria in Solid Tumors (RECIST) for mesothelioma is used with CT scanning to determine response rate. PET scans are also used to assess chemotherapy response.

Reading list

Cao C, Tian D, Manganas C, et al. Systematic review of trimodality therapy for patient with malignant pleural mesothelioma. Ann Cardiothorac Surg 2012;1:428–437.

Curran D, Sahmoud T, Therasse P, et al. Prognostic factors in patients with pleural mesothelioma: the European Organization for Research and Treatment of Cancer Experience. J Clin Oncol 1998;16:145–152.

Flores RM, Pass HI, Seshan VE, et al. Extrapleural pneumonectomy versus pleurectomy/decortication in the surgical management of malignant pleural mesothelioma: results in 663 patients. J Thorac Cardiovasc Surg 2008;135:620–626.

Herndon JE, Green MR, Chahinian AP, et al. Factors predictive of survival among 337 patients with mesothelioma treated between 1984 and 1994 by the Cancer and Leukemia Group B. Chest 1998;113:723–731.

Lin RT, Takahashi K, Karjalainen A, et al. Ecological association between asbestos-related diseases and historical asbestos consumption: an international analysis. Lancet 2007;369:844–849.

Mossman BT, Shukla A, Heintz NH, et al. New insights into understanding the mechanisms, pathogenesis, and management of malignant mesothelioma. Am J Pathol 2013;182:1065–1073.

Norbet C, Joseph A, Rossi SS, et al. Asbestos-related lung disease: a pictorial review. Curr Probl Diagn Radiol 2015;44:371–382.

Remon J, Reguart N, Corral J, et al. Malignant pleura mesothelioma: new hope on the horizon with novel therapeutic strategies. Cancer Treat Rev 2014;41:27–34.

Wong RM, Ianculescu I, Sharma S, et al. Immunotherapy for malignant pleural mesothelioma: current state and future prospects. Am J Respir Cell Molec Biol 2014;50:870–874.

Suggested websites

American Cancer Society: www.cancer.org/malignant-mesothelioma

Diagnosis and treatment algorithms based on clinical trials and expert opinion: www.nccn.org

National Institutes of Health/National Cancer Institute: www.cancer.gov/types/mesothelioma

Registry of all clinical trials in the USA: www.clinicaltrials.gov

Guidelines
National society guidelines

Title	Source	Date and weblink
NCCN Guidelines	NCCN	2019 http://www.nccn.org/professionals/physician_gls/pdf/mpm.pdf
ATC Guidelines	ASTRO/ACR IMRT	2006 http://rrp.cancer.gov/content/docs/imrt.doc
JTD Guidelines	Journal of Thoracic Disease	2013 http://jtd.amegroups.com/article/view/1903

International society guidelines

Title	Source	Date and weblink
Malignant pleural mesothelioma: ESMO Clinical Practice Guidelines for diagnosis, treatment and follow-up	European Society for Medical Oncology (ESMO)	2015 http://www.esmo.org/Guidelines/Lung-and-Chest-Tumours/Malignant-Pleural-Mesothelioma

Evidence

Type of evidence	Title	Date and weblink
Phase III RCT	Bevacizumab for newly diagnosed pleural mesothelioma in the Mesothelioma Avastin Cisplatin Pemetrexed Study (MAPS): a randomised, controlled, open-label, phase 3 trial	2016 https://www.ncbi.nlm.nih.gov/pubmed/26719230
Phase III RCT	Phase III study of pemetrexed in combination with cisplatin versus cisplatin alone in patients with malignant pleural mesothelioma	2003 https://www.ncbi.nlm.nih.gov/pubmed/12860938
Randomized feasibility study	Extra-pleural pneumonectomy versus no extra-pleural pneumonectomy for patients with malignant pleural mesothelioma	2011 https://www.ncbi.nlm.nih.gov/pubmed/21723781

Images

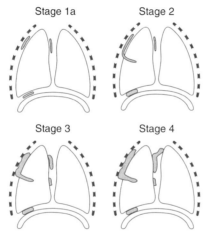

Figure 7.1 Simplified pictorial representation of pleural mesothelioma staging. (Source: http://mesothelioma.com/stages/)

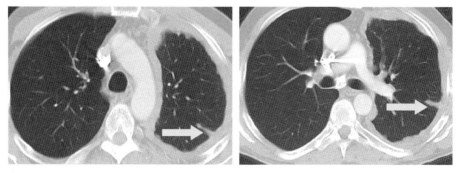

Figure 7.2 CT imaging of pleural mesothelioma involving both the mediastinal and parietal pleura. The arrows show fissural involvement of disease. (Source: Norbet et al. 2015. Reproduced with permission from Elsevier.)

Additional material for this chapter can be found online at:
www.wiley.com/go/oh/mountsinaioncology

This includes Addenda 7.1–7.3, advice for patients, a case study,
multiple choice questions, and ICD codes.

CHAPTER 8

Liver Cancer

Augusto Villanueva, Myron E. Schwartz, and Josep M. Llovet

Icahn School of Medicine at Mount Sinai, New York, NY, USA

OVERALL BOTTOM LINE
- Liver cancer is the forth leading cause of cancer-related death worldwide, with a mortality rate that has increased by more than 50% in the last 20 years.
- Liver cancer develops mainly in patients with chronic liver disease; the leading risk factors being viral hepatitis (B or C), alcohol abuse, and nonalcoholic fatty liver disease.
- Around 30% of patients are diagnosed at early stages, where curative treatment options (e.g. resection, ablation, or transplantation) provide 5-year survival of 70%.
- Chemoembolization is the accepted treatment for intermediate stages with liver only disease.
- Sorafenib and lenvatinib (first line) and regorafenib, cabozantinib, and ramucirumab (if AFP >400 ng/mL) (second line) are the systemic agents able to increase survival at advanced stages. Nivolumab and pembrolizumab have received accelerated FDA approval in second line treatment, based on phase 2 clinical trials.

Background
Definition of disease
Liver cancer is a primary hepatic malignant tumor resulting from an uncontrolled and unrestricted proliferation of hepatic cells.

Disease classification
- Primary liver cancer can be classified according to its histologic type. The most frequent form is hepatocellular carcinoma (HCC), which accounts for 90% of all cases, followed by intrahepatic cholangiocarcinoma. Other less frequent subtypes include fibrolamellar carcinoma, angiosarcoma, and hemangioendothelioma.

Incidence/prevalence
- Liver cancer is a major public health problem with an annual worldwide incidence of 850 000 cases.
- Liver cancer is the fourth highest cause of cancer-related mortality worldwide.
- In the USA, recent data estimate that in 2014 there were 33 190 new liver cancer cases.
- Mortality from liver cancer has risen more than any other cancer in the USA in the last 20 years.

Economic impact
The overall per-patient cost of HCC is $32 907 (as per estimates from 2009). Considering that the USA HCC incidence is around 33 000 cases annually, it is estimated that HCC-related annual costs are around $1 billion.

Mount Sinai Expert Guides: Oncology, First Edition. Edited by William K. Oh and Ajai Chari.
Companion Website: www.wiley.com/go/oh/mountsinaioncology

Etiology
- Almost 90% of all liver cancer develops on the background of chronic liver disease.
- Cirrhosis of any etiology is the main risk factor for liver cancer development.
- Viral hepatitis (B and/or C) and alcohol abuse are the main causes of liver cancer worldwide. Exposure to aflatoxin B1 further increases liver cancer risk in the background of chronic hepatitis B virus (HBV) infection.
- Nonalcoholic fatty liver disease in the context of type 2 diabetes and metabolic syndrome is becoming a major cause of liver cancer in Western countries.

Pathology/pathogenesis
- During the preneoplastic stage, there is an up-regulation of mitogenic pathways leading to the selection of certain clones of dysplastic cells. These clones, organized as dysplastic nodules and surrounded by fibrous septae of connective tissue, acquire a malignant phenotype after exposure to additional genomic alterations.
- Analysis of close to 1000 HCC samples using next-generation sequencing technologies identified mutations in TERT promoter (60%), TP53 (30%), CTNNB1 (25%), ARID2 (7%), AXIN1 (5%), ARID1A (5%), and NFE2L2 (4%).
- High-level DNA amplifications affect chromosome 11q13 (CCND1, FGF19) and chromosome 6p21 (VEGFA) in around 5–7% of cases.
- Environmental factors such as hepatitis B or exposure to aflatoxin B1 can directly damage the DNA through direct mutagenesis or viral insertion.

Predictive/risk factors

Risk factor	Adjusted odds ratio
Male gender	1 : 2–3
HCV infection	13.3
HBV infection	9.1
Obese (BMI >30 kg/m^2)	2.1
High ethanol intake	1.7

Prevention

> **BOTTOM LINE/CLINICAL PEARLS**
> - No interventions have been prospectively shown to decrease liver cancer incidence other than those designed to eliminate known risk factors (see section on Primary prevention for details).
> - Surveillance programs for early liver cancer detection in at-risk populations increase the applicability of curative therapies and are highly recommended.

Screening for HCC
- **Screening method:** abdominal ultrasound every 6 months, with or without measurement of serum alpha-fetoprotein levels, according to guidelines from the American Association for the Study of Liver Diseases (AASLD) and the European Association for the Study of the Liver (EASL).

- **Target population:** patients at high risk of liver cancer development as defined by an estimated annual risk higher than 1.5%. Specifically:
  - Cirrhotic patients of any etiology, Child–Pugh A and B
  - Cirrhotic patients of any etiology, Child–Pugh C awaiting liver transplantation
  - Noncirrhotic hepatitis C virus (HCV) patients with advanced fibrosis defined as F3
  - Noncirrhotic HBV carriers with active hepatitis or family history of HCC
  - Noncirrhotic HBV carriers older than 40 (males) or 50 (females) years; or African Americans older than 20 years (AASLD guidelines).

Primary prevention
- Hepatitis B vaccination.
- Adequate HBV suppression. Treatment objective: undetectable HBV-DNA levels in blood.
- Sustained virologic response in HCV (evidence derived from IFN-based treatment regimes, but likely to be reproduced with new direct-acting antiviral agents).

Secondary prevention
- Prevention of recurrence has not been demonstrated in 15 randomized studies, and thus there is no formal recommendation according to guidelines.

Diagnosis (Algorithm 8.1)

BOTTOM LINE/CLINICAL PEARLS
- Diagnosis is based upon noninvasive criteria (radiology) or tissue biopsy.
- Most patients with liver cancer have some form of underlying liver disease, either chronic hepatitis or established cirrhosis.
- Noninvasive diagnosis: patients with cirrhosis and a liver nodule larger than 1 cm that fulfills the radiologic hallmark of HCC (contrast uptake in the arterial phase and washout in the venous/late phase on 4-phase CT or dynamic contrasted enhanced MRI).
- Tissue biopsy and biomarkers: histologic confirmation is required for those patients not fulfilling noninvasive diagnostic criteria. Tissue markers are useful in small nodules (1–2 cm). The combination of at least two positive markers among HSP70, GPC2, and GS was adopted by the International Consensus Group of Hepatocelluar Neoplasia to diagnose HCC. High AFP levels are frequent in patients with HCC, but this is not required for a definitive HCC diagnosis.

Differential diagnosis

Differential diagnosis	Features
Intrahepatic cholangiocarcinoma	Specific radiologic features with frequent capsule retraction High CA19.9 levels Histologic confirmation is required
Hepatic adenoma	Usually occurs in young women taking oral contraceptives Absence of chronic liver disease Specific radiologic features Normal AFP levels
Focal nodular hyperplasia	Absence of chronic liver disease Specific radiologic features Normal AFP levels

(Continued)

(*Continued*)

Differential diagnosis	Features
Nodular regenerative hyperplasia	Associated with other diseases causing portal hypertension without cirrhosis (e.g. portal vein thrombosis, primary portal hypertension) Specific radiologic features
Atypical hemangioma	Absence of chronic liver disease Specific radiologic features Normal AFP levels
Liver metastasis	Absence of chronic liver disease Specific radiologic features Known primary malignancy
Hepatic angiomyolipoma	Absence of chronic liver disease Specific radiologic features Immunohistochemical staining for HMB-45

Algorithm 8.1 Diagnosis of hepatocellular carcinoma

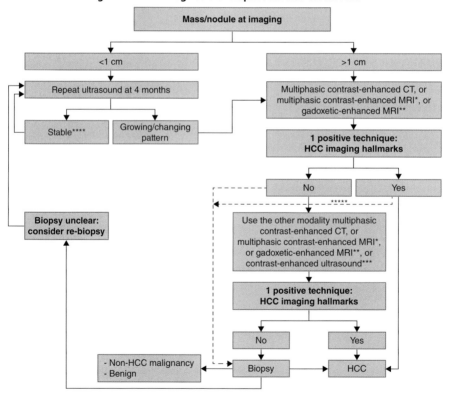

*Using extracellular MR contrast agents or gadobenate dimeglumine. **Diagnostic criteria: arterial phase hyperenhancement (APHE) and washout on the portal venous phase. ***Diagnostic criteria: APHE and mild washout after 60 seconds. ****Patients with a lesion <1 cm stable for 12 months (three controls after 4 months) can return to regular surveillance. *****Optional for center-based programmes. (Source: 2018 EASL Practice Guidelines: Management of Hepatocellular Carcinoma. Reproduced with permission from Elsevier.)

Typical presentation
- **Patients enrolled in a surveillance program:** includes identification of a new liver nodule on abdominal ultrasound, and diagnostic confirmation using either noninvasive criteria or biopsy. These patients are generally asymptomatic and have early stage HCC.
- **Patients diagnosed outside surveillance:** usually present at advanced stages with large tumors, portal vein invasion, and extrahepatic disease (lymph nodes, lungs, or bone). Symptoms include malaise, weight loss, anorexia, abdominal discomfort, or signs related to advanced liver dysfunction (see section on Physical examination).

Clinical diagnosis
History
- All patients with established cirrhosis should be considered at risk for HCC development.
- Past medical history should include active assessment for known risk factors for chronic liver disease such as HCV or HBV infection (e.g. blood transfusions, intravenous drug use, tattoos, unprotected sex with multiple partners), alcohol abuse (e.g. CAGE questionnaire), nonalcoholic fatty liver disease (NAFLD; e.g. high BMI, diabetes) and hemochromatosis (e.g. joint pain, fatigue, diabetes).

Physical examination
- Look for signs of chronic liver disease:
  - Spider nevi
  - Palmar erythema
  - Splenomegaly
  - Ascites
  - Jaundice
  - Peripheral edema
  - Flapping tremor.

Disease severity classification
- The currently accepted staging system by the AASLD and EASL is the Barcelona Clinic Liver Cancer (BCLC). It classifies HCC in five stages based on tumor burden, patient symptoms (ECOG performance status), and degree of underlying liver disease (Algorithm 8.2).

Laboratory diagnosis
List of diagnostic tests
- Complete liver screen to identify potential causes of chronic liver disease:
  - Hepatitis B and C serology
  - Alpha-1 antitrypsin
  - Ceruloplasmin
  - Ferritin, transferrin, serum Fe
  - Immunoglobins and protein electrophoresis
  - Autoantibody screen (ANA, SMA, LKM, AMA).
- Laboratory data of liver dysfunction and/or portal hypertension:
  - Low white cell count
  - Low platelet count (<100 000 is an indicator of significant portal hypertension)
  - Elevated bilirubin
  - Decreased albumin
  - Decreased INR
  - Mild elevation of ALT, AST, ALP.

- Elevated AFP (tumor marker, not always present). Also useful as a prognostic biomarker, particularly AFP >400 ng/mL indicates poor outcome).
- Histologic findings:
  - Discriminate between HCC, cholangiocarcinoma, and mixed tumors
  - Tumor hepatocytes are polygonal, with eosinophilic granular cytoplasm, rounded nuclei, and prominent nucleoli. Different degrees of cell pleomorphism
  - Histologic variants include clear cell, scirrhous, sarcomatoid, and sclerosing
  - Stromal invasion is key to differentiate high grade dysplastic nodule from early HCC.

Algorithm 8.2 Management of HCC (adopted from EASL Guidelines)

"Preserved liver function" refers to Child–Pugh A without any ascites, considered optimal to maximize treatment benefit. [2]PS 1 refers to tumor induced modification of performance capacity as quantified by the ECOG Performance Status Test. [3]Optimal surgical candidacy is based on a multiparametric evaluation including compensated Child–Pugh class A liver function with MELD score <10, to be matched with grade of portal hypertension, acceptable amount of remaining parenchyma and possibility to adopt a laparoscopic/minimally invasive approach. [4]The stage migration strategy is a therapeutic choice by which a treatment theoretically recommended for a different stage is selected as best 1st line treatment option. [5]Systemic therapies shown to be effective in phase 3 clinical trials include: sorafenib and lenvatinib (first line); and regorafenib, ramucirumab, cabozantinib (second line). (Source: J Hepatol 2012;56:908–943. Reproduced with permission from Elsevier.)

Lists of imaging techniques

- **Abdominal ultrasound:** gold standard for HCC surveillance. It should be performed every 6 months in at-risk patients.
- **Dynamic contrast-enhanced CT scan or MRI:** gold standard for HCC noninvasive diagnosis. Should be performed when a focal liver lesion >1 cm is identified on ultrasound. They can also help identify radiologic features of chronic liver disease or portal hypertension (e.g. irregular hepatic surface, ascites, splenomegaly, collateral shunts).
- **Thoracic CT scan:** used for staging purposes (presence of lung metastasis).
- **Bone scan:** used for staging purposes (presence of bone metastasis).

Potential pitfalls/common errors made regarding diagnosis of disease
- Any patient with established cirrhosis and a focal liver lesion on ultrasound should be evaluated for a potential HCC.
- Noninvasive radiologic criteria for HCC diagnosis are only applicable in patients with cirrhosis. The Liver Imaging Reporting and Data System (LI-RADS) is used to classify hepatic nodules based on their likelihood of being HCC. In noncirrhotic livers, HCC diagnosis should be established with tumor biopsy.
- A negative biopsy does not rule out the diagnosis of HCC, and inconclusive results should follow Algorithm 8.1.
- Patients with chronic hepatitis C can have fluctuating serum levels of AFP. Diagnosis is based on imaging or biopsy, not AFP levels.

Treatment
Treatment rationale
- The primary goal for treatment is to increase survival. Treatment decision should consider three parameters encapsulated in the BCLC algorithm (Algorithm 8.2):
  - Tumor burden: as determined by imaging techniques
  - Patient's symptoms: medical history and ECOG-PS (performance status)
  - Degree of underlying liver dysfunction: Child–Pugh Score, MELD score.
- In addition to the primary treatment of the tumor, patients should also be considered for treatments to improve the underlying liver dysfunction such as antiviral therapies or alcohol abstinence.

When to hospitalize
- Signs of ruptured HCC:
  - Abdominal distension and pain or fever
  - Signs of hypovolemic shock (e.g. hypotension, cyanosis, drop in hemoglobin levels, tachycardia).
- Admission because of complications related to liver dysfunction: evidence of altered mental status indicating hepatic encephalopathy, gastrointestinal bleeding, suspicious of infection (e.g. spontaneous bacterial peritonitis, pneumonia).

Table of treatment
See Algorithms 8.2 and 8.3.

Treatment	Comments
Surgical	
Surgical resection, liver transplantation	Patients at **early stage** (BCLC-A): • Liver resection in patients with single nodules, without clinically significant portal hypertension (Level 2A) • Liver transplantation for patients with 2–3 nodules (all <3 cm) or with one nodule less than 5 cm not suitable for resection (Level 2A)
Locoregional (TACE, RFA)	Patients at **early stage** (BCLC-A): • RFA in patients with single nodules (<5 cm) or three nodules <3 cm (Level 1) not candidates for surgical therapies Patients at **intermediate stage** (BCLC-B): • TACE with drug eluting beads in patients with multinodular HCC, compensated liver disease, and ECOG-PS 0 (Level 1A)

(Continued)

(Continued)

Treatment	Comments
Medical	
Sorafenib (400 mg twice daily PO)	Patients at **advanced stage** (BCLC-C), Child–Pugh A class. Level 1A
Lenvatinib [12 mg daily (for bodyweight ≥60 kg) or 8 mg daily (for bodyweight <60 kg)]	Patients with less than 50% occupation of the liver with tumors without invasion of the bile duct or main portal vein. Child–Pugh A class. Level 1A.
Regorafenib (160 mg twice daily PO)	Patients who **progressed to sorafenib**, Child–Pugh A class. Level 1A
Cabozantinib (60 mg daily PO)	Child–Pugh A class. Level 1A
Ramucirumab (8 mg/kg for 1 hour every 14 days)	Patients with AFP levels ≥400 ng/mL. Child–Pugh A class. Level 1A

Prevention/management of complications

- **Surgical resection:** perioperative mortality <2%.
- **Liver transplantation:** perioperative mortality: 3–4%.
- **Radiofrequency ablation (RFA):** local infection, seeding <1%.
- **Transarterial chemoembolization (TACE):** treatment-related mortality <2%. Liver abscess 1%. In patients with limited hepatic functional reserve there is a risk of hepatic decompensation following TACE. Patients may develop ascites, but it is generally reversible. In some cases, it can be life-threatening. TACE should not be considered in patients with decompensated liver disease.
- **Sorafenib:** Grade 3–4 hand-foot skin reaction leading to discontinuation: 10–15%
- **Lenvatinib:** Grade 3–4 hypertension: 23%
- **Regorafenib:** Grade 3–4 hand-foot skin reaction: 13%
- **Cabozantinib:** Grade 3–4 hand-foot skin reaction: 17%
- **Ramucirumab:** Grade 3–4 hypertension: 13%

Algorithm 8.3 Systemic drugs for patients with advanced HCC

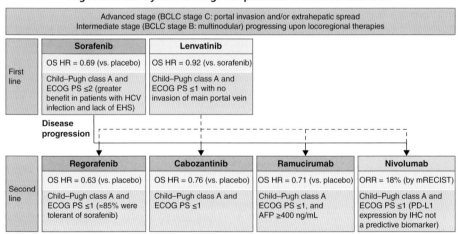

(Source: Llovet et al. Nat Rev Clin Oncol 2018, https://www.ncbi.nlm.nih.gov/pubmed/?term=30061739.)

CLINICAL PEARLS
- HCC arise mostly in cirrhotic patients or those with chronic HBV infection.
- Resection has no size limit, as long as the patient has a single nodule, good performance status, and lacks clinically significant portal hypertension.
- Stage migration: patients who progress to a given therapy or who do not fulfill all the criteria for the treatment allocation for their stage should be offered the next most suitable option within the same stage or the next prognostic stage. For instance BCLC-B failing to TACE are offered sorafenib.
- Treatment response should be evaluated using the modified RECIST criteria.
- Conventional chemotherapy has not been shown to improve survival in patients with HCC and has potentially life-threatening complications in patients with cirrhosis.

Special populations
Children
- The most common liver tumor in children is hepatoblastoma, which is treated by resection and systemic chemotherapy.

Others
- Patients with NAFLD frequently have cardiovascular comorbidities that limit the applicability of surgical therapies.

Prognosis

BOTTOM LINE/CLINICAL PEARLS
- The BCLC algorithm outperforms other prognostic staging systems when compared head-to-head.
- In advanced cases, presence of ECOG:1–2, and portal vein invasion are poor prognostic factors.
- High AFP blood levels (>400 ng/mL) correlate with poor outcome.
- Staging systems that disregard the degree of underlying liver dysfunction do not adequately capture HCC prognosis.

Natural history of untreated disease
- Patients with advanced liver dysfunction (Child–Pugh score C) who are not candidates for liver transplantation have poor survival (<1 year) regardless of tumor characteristics.
- Median survival for patients: natural history without treatment at early (BCLC-A), intermediate (BCLC-B), and advanced (BCLC-C) stages are 36, 16, and 8 months, respectively.

Prognosis for treated patients
- Median survival for patients at early stage (BCLC-A) treated with resection transplantation or local ablation is 60 months, at intermediate stage (BCLC-B) treated with TACE is 25–30 months, and at advanced stage (BCLC-C) treated with sorafenib or lenvatinib (first line) and regorafenib or cabozantinib (second line) are 12–13 and 10–11 months, respectively.

Follow-up tests and monitoring
- Monitoring of treated patients to discard recurrence/progression should include CT scan or MRI every 3 months during the first 2 years and every 6 months thereafter.

Reading list

Bruix J, Qin S, Merle P, et al. Regorafenib for patients with hepatocellular carcinoma who progressed on sorafenib treatment: a randomized, double-blind, placebo-controlled, phase 3 trial. Lancet 2017;389:56–66.

Cheng AL, Kang YK, Chen Z, et al. Efficacy and safety of sorafenib in patients in the Asia-Pacific region with advanced hepatocellular carcinoma: a phase III randomised, double-blind, placebo-controlled trial. Lancet Oncol 2009;10:25–34.

EASL Clinical Practice Guidelines: Management of hepatocellular carcinoma. J Hepatol 2018;69:182–236.

Heimbach JK, Kulik LM, Finn RS, et al. AASLD guidelines for the treatment of hepatocellular carcinoma. Hepatology 2018;67:358–380.

Lang K, Danchenko N, Gondek K, et al. The burden of illness associated with hepatocellular carcinoma in the United States. J Hepatol 2009;50:89–99.

Llovet JM, Montal R, Sia D, et al. Molecular therapies and precision medicine for hepatocellular carcinoma. Nat Rev Clin Oncol 2018;15:599–616.

Llovet JM, Ricci S, Mazzaferro V, et al. Sorafenib in advanced hepatocellular carcinoma. N Engl J Med 2008;359:378–390.

Llovet JM, Zucman-Rossi J, Pikarsky E, et al. Hepatocellular carcinoma. Nat Rev Dis Primers 2016;2:16018.

Villanueva A, Hernandez-Gea V, Llovet JM. Medical therapies for hepatocellular carcinoma: a critical view of the evidence. Nat Rev Gastroenterol Hepatol 2013;10:34–42.

Villanueva A. Hepatocellular carcinoma. N Engl J Med 2019; 380:1450–1462.

Zucman-Rossi J, Villanueva A, Nault JC, et al. Genetic landscape and biomarkers of hepatocellular carcinoma. Gastroenterology 2015;149:1226–1239.

Guidelines
National society guidelines

Title	Source	Date and weblink
Management of hepatocellular carcinoma: an update	American Association for the Study of Liver Diseases (AASLD)	2018 https://www.ncbi.nlm.nih.gov/pubmed/?term=29624699

International society guidelines

Title	Source	Date and weblink
EASL Clinical Practice Guidelines: Management of hepatocellular carcinoma	European Association for the Study of the Liver (EASL)	2018 https://www.journal-of-hepatology.eu/article/S0168-8278(18)30215-0/fulltext

Evidence

Type of evidence	Title and comment	Date and weblink
RCT	Sorafenib in advanced hepatocellular carcinoma **Comment:** First clinical trial to demonstrate survival improvement using a systemic agent (i.e. sorafenib) in patients with HCC	2008 https://www.ncbi.nlm.nih.gov/pubmed/?term=18650514

(*Continued*)

Type of evidence	Title and comment	Date and weblink
RCT	Regorafenib for patients with hepatocellular carcinoma who progressed on sorafenib treatment (RESORCE): a randomised, double-blind, placebo-controlled, phase 3 trial **Comment:** First clinical trial to demonstrate survival benefit in second line (i.e. regorafenib) in advanced HCC	2017 https://www.ncbi.nlm.nih.gov/pubmed/?term=27932229
RCT	Lenvatinib versus sorafenib in first line treatment of patients with unresectable hepatocellular carcinoma: a randomised phase 3 non-inferiority trial **Comment:** Lenvatinib noninferior to sorafenib for OS in first line for HCC patients at advanced stages	2018 https://www.ncbi.nlm.nih.gov/pubmed/?term=29433850
RCT	Cabozantinib (C) versus placebo (P) in patients (pts) with advanced hepatocellular carcinoma (HCC) who have received prior sorafenib: results from the randomized phase III CELESTIAL trial **Comment:** Cabozantinib superior to placebo in advanced HCC – second line	2018 https://www.ncbi.nlm.nih.gov/pubmed/?term=29972759
RCT	Ramucirumab after sorafenib in patients with advanced hepatocellular carcinoma and increased α-fetoprotein concentrations (REACH-2): a randomised, double-blind, placebo-controlled, phase 3 trial **Comment:** First biomarker-based positive clinical trial in patients with advanced HCC	2019 https://www.ncbi.nlm.nih.gov/pubmed/?term=30665869
RCT	Arterial embolisation or chemoembolisation versus symptomatic treatment in patients with unresectable hepatocellular carcinoma: a randomised controlled trial Randomized controlled trial of transarterial lipiodol chemoembolization for unresectable hepatocellular carcinoma **Comment:** These trials conducted in different geographic areas showed survival improvement in patients receiving TACE	2002 https://www.ncbi.nlm.nih.gov/pubmed/?term=12049862 https://www.ncbi.nlm.nih.gov/pubmed/?term=11981766
Systematic review	Systematic review of randomized trials for unresectable hepatocellular carcinoma: chemoembolization improves survival **Comment:** Systemic review and meta-analysis that provided the evidence to recommend TACE in patients at intermediate stages (BCLC-B)	2003 https://www.ncbi.nlm.nih.gov/pubmed/?term=12540794
Cohort study	Liver transplantation for the treatment of small hepatocellular carcinomas in patients with cirrhosis **Comment:** Landmark study to define the criteria that provide good survival results in HCC patients treated with transplantation	1996 https://www.ncbi.nlm.nih.gov/pubmed/?term=8594428

Additional material for this chapter can be found online at:
www.wiley.com/go/oh/mountsinaioncology

This includes a case study, ICD codes, and multiple choice
questions.

CHAPTER 9

Gallbladder/Biliary Duct Cancers

Rajwanth Veluswamy, Anuja Kriplani, and Celina Ang

Icahn School of Medicine at Mount Sinai, New York, NY, USA

OVERALL BOTTOM LINE
- Biliary tract cancers comprise of a diverse disease group characterized by different etiologies, risk factors, molecular characteristics, and clinical features.
- Despite known biologic differences, the treatment of these cancers overlaps significantly and they are often grouped together in clinical trials because of their rarity. Collectively, these cancers tend to be diagnosed at an advanced stage and carry a poor prognosis.
- Patients with biliary tract cancers require a multidisciplinary and multimodality approach in order to optimize outcomes and address potential complications.

Background
Definition of disease
- Biliary tract cancers (BTCs) arise from the epithelial lining of the gallbladder and bile ducts and are associated with late diagnosis and poor outcomes.
- There are several histologic subtypes of BTCs, 90% of which are adenocarcinomas. The remaining cases comprise of squamous cell carcinomas and other rarer types such as adenosquamous carcinoma, carcinoid tumor, lymphoma, sarcoma, oat cell carcinoma, and metastatic tumors.

Disease classification
- BTCs are anatomically classified as cholangiocarcinomas (CCAs) arising from intrahepatic, perihilar, or distal biliary tree, or gallbladder carcinomas (GBCs) (Figure 9.1):
  - Perihilar CCAs (Klatskin tumors) involving the hepatic duct bifurcation are further classified according to the Bismuth–Corlette system (Figure 9.1)
  - Mixed hepatocellular CCA is a distinct subtype of primary liver cancer consisting of cells of both hepatocyte and biliary differentiation.
- BTCs are graded as well, moderately, or poorly differentiated (majority are well and moderately differentiated).
- Adenocarcinomas can be further classified as:
  - **GBCs:** infiltrative (diffuse thickening/induration of wall; possible fistula formation), exophytic (irregular, cauliflower mass growing into lumen and walls), and papillary (can fill entire gallbladder; most favorable prognosis) subtypes
  - **CCAs:** nodular (constricting annular lesions of the bile duct), sclerosing (intense desmoplastic reaction), and papillary (rare; bulky masses causing biliary obstruction) subtypes.

Mount Sinai Expert Guides: Oncology, First Edition. Edited by William K. Oh and Ajai Chari.

© 2019 John Wiley & Sons Ltd. Published 2019 by John Wiley & Sons Ltd.

Companion Website: www.wiley.com/go/oh/mountsinaioncology

Incidence/prevalence
- Biliary tract tumors are uncommon and account for approximately 3% of all gastrointestinal malignancies with 10 310 extrahepatic tumors (two-thirds of which are GBCs; the remainder are extrahepatic CCAs) and approximately 5000 intrahepatic CCAs diagnosed annually:
  - Approximately two-thirds of all CCAs are perihilar, about 25% are distal tumors, and the remainder are intrahepatic
  - GBCs are most often an incidental pathologic finding in 0.2–3% of patients undergoing cholecystectomy for cholelithiasis.

Etiology and risk factors
Gallbladder carcinoma
- There is a close association with gallstones which are present in 65–90% of patients with GBC, though only 1–3% of patients with gallstones develop cancer.
- Women are affected 2–6 times more often than men and the incidence steadily increases with age. There are wide geographic, ethnic, and cultural variations in the incidence of GBCs suggesting major genetic and environmental influences (i.e. diet, lifestyle).
  - The highest incidences worldwide are seen in the indigenous population of the Andes mountains, northern Europeans, and Israelis. In the USA, GBCs occur more often in Mexican Americans and Native Americans.
- Other known risk factors include calcified or porcelain gallbladder, gallbladder polyps, anomalous pancreaticobiliary duct junction, and carcinogens (e.g. methylcholanthrene, O-aminoazotulene, nitrosamines).

Cholangiocarcinoma
- Primary sclerosing cholangitis (PSC) is the most common predisposing condition for CCA in developed countries, with the lifetime incidence ranging 5–10%. Approximately 50% of patients who develop CCA are diagnosed within 2 years of PSC diagnosis.
- There is a very high incidence (113 per 100 000) of CCA in Southeast Asia because of the high prevalence of hepatobiliary flukes (i.e. *Opisthorchis viverrini* and *Clonorchis sinensis*).
- Hepatitis B and C, obesity, alcohol, metabolic syndrome, and other conditions associated with cirrhosis have been recognized as risk factors for CCAs, especially intrahepatic tumors. Hepatolithiasis and biliary enteric drainage, which predisposes to bile duct infections, are also known risk factors.

Pathology/pathogenesis
- Chronic inflammation is an inciting factor in the progression of BTC from dysplasia to carcinoma *in situ* and eventually becoming invasive malignancy.
- Oncogenic transformation is mediated by genomic alterations and signaling pathway aberrations that may become targets of emerging therapies.
  - Mutational spectrum of oncogenes:
    - *KRAS* and *BRAF* are mutually exclusive driver mutations in the pathogenesis of BTCs. Based on their respective frequencies, activation of the RAF/MAPK pathway is a major event in the majority of BTCs.
    - EGFR and HER2/NEU tyrosine kinases are overexpressed or amplified in a subset of BTCs. Of note, *HER2/NEU* mutations are generally not found in intrahepatic CCAs.
    - Although *PIK3CA* mutations are rarely found in BTCs, there is evidence of indirect activation of this pathway in BTC oncogenesis.
    - Expression of IGF1-R and other AKT/mTOR signaling components have been implicated in the majority of GBCs and may be an effective target for therapy.
    - FGFR2 fusions and gain of function mutations in IDH1/2 are present in approximately 15% and 20% of intrahepatic CCAs, respectively, and represent novel therapeutic targets.

- Mutational spectrum of tumor suppressor genes
  - The loss of function of tumor suppressor genes is similar to that seen in other gastrointestinal malignancies. The most common genes involved are *TP53, CDKN2A/P16INK4A*, and *SMAD4*.

Prevention

- There are no established primary or secondary preventions for BTCs. Adherence to treatment and subsequent surveillance for viral hepatitis, avoidance of alcohol, maintaining a healthy weight, and other lifestyle modifications may reduce risk of developing BTCs, although these interventions have not been directly studied.

Screening

- No screening program has shown clinical or cost effectiveness because of the low incidence of biliary tract tumors in the general population.
- In patients with PSC, annual ultrasounds are recommended to detect mass lesions in the gallbladder (AASLD/EASL Practice Guidelines, Level 1C).
- Inadequate information exists regarding the utility of screening (biochemical or imaging) for CCA in PSC (AASLD/EASL Practice Guidelines).

Diagnosis (Algorithm 9.1)

Algorithm 9.1 Diagnosis of gallbladder/biliary duct cancers

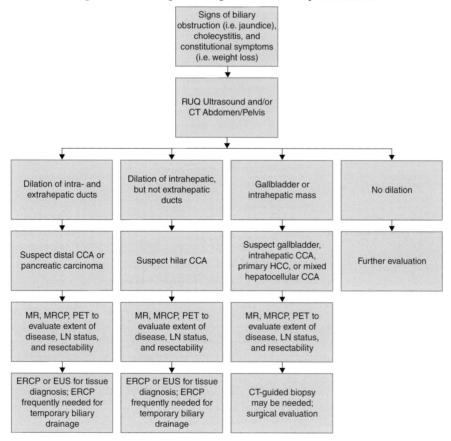

> **BOTTOM LINE/CLINICAL PEARLS**
> - BTCs can develop with symptoms of biliary tract obstruction, acute/chronic cholecystitis, and constitutional symptoms such as weight loss.
> - Signs of biliary tract obstruction and systemic signs signifying more advanced disease may be observed on physical examination.
> - The diagnosis is made using a combination of laboratory imaging and tissue evaluation. GBCs are often associated with gallstones and intraoperative and postoperative evaluation for GBC should be part of all cholecystectomies.

Differential diagnosis

Differential diagnosis	Features
Cholelithiasis	Sporadic/unpredictable episodes. Pain of biliary colic begins postprandially, lasts 1–5 hours and may radiate to right scapula (Collins sign). Imaging (i.e. right upper quadrant (RUQ) ultrasound) confirms diagnosis but ultrasound is less sensitive (15–40%) for choledocholithaisis – may need magnetic resonance cholangiopancreatography (MRCP)
Bile duct strictures	Benign strictures; usually iatrogenic (e.g. operative trauma)
Cholangitis	Fever, RUQ pain, and jaundice (Charcot triad). Signs of infection (e.g. leukocytosis; positive blood cultures). Can lead to bacteremia and sepsis. Caused by biliary obstruction
Cholecystitis	Peritoneal irritation, fever, nausea, and vomiting. Palpable gallbladder or RUQ fullness (30–40% of patients). Signs of infection
Choledochal cysts	Congenital bile duct anomaly
Primary hepatocellular carcinoma	Normally arises in setting of cirrhosis. Strong association with prior history of hepatitis B/C and alcoholic liver disease. Characterized by arterial hyperenhancement followed by venous washout on contrast-enhanced, multiphasic imaging
PSC	Chronic liver disease with progressive cholestasis with inflammation and fibrosis of bile ducts. Strongly associated with inflammatory bowel disease. High risk of CCA and colorectal cancer. Autoimmune disease: marked increase in ANCA, ANA, anticardiolipin antibodies
Pancreatic head tumor	Many similar symptoms and signs. Imaging and tissue diagnosis to differentiate

Typical presentation
- Patients with GBCs often present with nonspecific symptoms that can be grouped into the following clinical syndromes: (i) acute or chronic cholecystitis; (ii) biliary tract disease with symptoms of jaundice and RUQ pain (usually indicating extensive disease); (iii) systemic signs/symptoms such as anorexia, weight loss, weakness, and symptoms of local tumor invasion (extensive, metastatic disease); and (iv) gastrointestinal bleeding or obstruction. GBC can be diagnosed preoperatively during symptom evaluation, during surgical exploration, or postoperatively on pathology following cholecystectomy for cholelithiasis.
- The clinical presentation of CCAs depends on tumor location. Patients with extrahepatic tumors classically present with signs of biliary obstruction (i.e. painless jaundice, pale stools, dark urine, pruritus). Those with intrahepatic tumors often present with nonspecific symptoms such as weakness, weight loss, and abdominal pain.

Clinical diagnosis
History
- Clinicians should explore symptoms of biliary tract obstruction and constitutional symptoms.
- Enquire about risk factors for biliary tract pathology and conditions associated with chronic inflammation of the biliary epithelium: biliary stones, PSC, exposure to carcinogens (i.e. nitrosamines, dioxins, alcohol, tobacco), travel (endemic areas of liver fluke infestation such as Thailand), viral hepatitis.
- In patients with a long history of chronic cholecystitis with gallstones, a change in symptom quality (e.g. pain) may be reported.
- Family history to assess for an inherited predisposition to developing BTCs such as Lynch syndrome.

Physical examination
- Jaundice, scratch marks of pruritus, hepatomegaly, and RUQ tenderness might be observed.
- Patients with advanced disease may present with a palpable gallbladder mass (Courvoisier law), hard nodular liver, and malignant ascites from carcinomatosis.
- Stigmata of cirrhosis such as ascites, gynecomastia, caput medusa, and spider angiomata.

Laboratory diagnosis
List of diagnostic tests
- Biochemical tests including markers of cholestasis, liver injury, and synthetic function (transaminases, alkaline phosphatase, bilirubin, albumin, INR/PTT). Hematologic and renal function laboratory tests.
- Serum tumor markers: carcinoembryonic antigen (not sensitive or specific alone) and cancer antigen (CA) 19-9 (sensitivity: 67–89%; specificity: 86–98%).
- HIV and hepatitis B and C serologies in patients at risk for exposure.
- Tissue diagnosis.

Lists of imaging techniques
- Abdominal ultrasound or CT are usually the first imaging studies performed to evaluate for symptoms/signs concerning for BTCs.
- When a biliary tract tumor is suspected, further imaging such as MRI and MRCP can evaluate tumor extension and nodal status in greater detail.
- If there is concern for obstructive jaundice, ERCP can locate and alleviate the obstruction. Bile duct cytology may also help to make the diagnosis.
- Endoscopic ultrasound (EUS) can help with the diagnosis and staging of distal CCAs.

Disease severity classification
Table 9.1 shows the American Joint Commission on Cancer Staging System for gallbladder cancer and cholangiocarcinoma.

Potential pitfalls/common errors made regarding diagnosis of disease
- While tumor markers help support the diagnosis of biliary tract tumors, they are neither sensitive nor specific enough to be diagnostic on their own.
  - CA 19-9 can be elevated because of nonmalignant causes of hyperbilirubinemia.
  - Alternatively, CA 19-9 may be normal in the presence of malignancy in individuals who are Lewis antigen negative.
- Endosopic or percutaneous biopsies have high specificity; however, because of desmoplastic components of the lesion, they have low sensitivity and may be nondiagnostic.

Table 9.1 American Joint Commission on Cancer Staging System.

Gallbladder cancer				Cholangiocarcinoma			
Stage 0	T_{is}	N_0	M_0	Stage 0	T_{is}	N_0	M_0
Stage I	T_1	N_0	M_0	Stage I	T_1	N_0	M_0
Stage II	T_2	N_0	M_0	Stage II	T_2	N_0	M_0
Stage IIIA	T_3	N_0	M_0	Stage III	T_1 or T_2	N_1 or N_2	M_0
Stage IIIB	T_{1-3}	N_1	M_0	Stage IVA	T_3	Any N	M_0
Stage IVA	T_4	N_2	M_0	Stage IVB	Any T	Any N	M_1
Stage IVB	Any T	N_2 Any N	M_0 M_1				

T_{is}, carcinoma *in situ*; T_1, tumor invades lamina propria or muscular layer; T_2, tumor invades perimuscular connective tissue; T_3, tumor perforates serosa and/or directly invades adjacent organs/structures; T_4, tumor invades main portal vein or hepatic artery or invades ≥ 2 extrahepatic organs/structures	T_{is}, carcinoma *in situ*; T_1, tumor invades the subepithelial connective tissue; T_2, tumor invades perifibromuscular connective tissue; T_3, tumor invades adjacent organs
N_0, no regional lymph node metastases; N_1, metastasis to nodes along cystic duct, common bile duct, hepatic artery, and/or portal vein; N_2, metastasis to periaortic, percaval, superior mesenteric artery, and/or celiac artery lymph nodes	N_0, no regional lymph node metastases; N_1, metastasis to hepatoduodenal ligament lymph nodes; N_2, metastasis to peripancreatic, periduodenal, periportal, celiac, and/or superior mesenteric artery lymph nodes
M_0, no distant metastasis; M_1, distant metastasis	M_0, no distant metastasis; M_1, distant metastasis

Treatment (Algorithms 9.2 and 9.3)

Algorithm 9.2 Management of gallbladder cancer

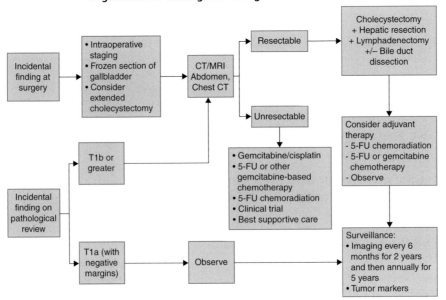

Algorithm 9.3 Management of cholangiocarcinoma

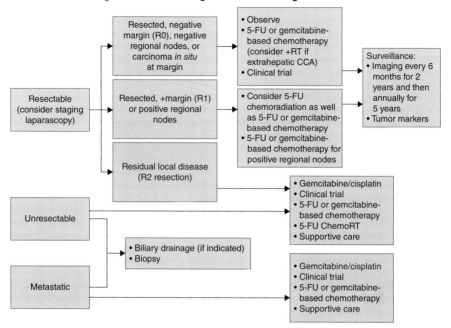

Treatment rationale

- Resection represents the only meaningful chance for cure or long-term survival in patients with BTCs. However, only a small proportion of patients can be considered for surgery on presentation (criteria for resectability varies).
  - Contraindications include: multiple liver, peritoneal or other distant metastases, ascites, extensive involvement of hepatoduodenal ligament, encasement or occlusion of major vessels, poor performance status.
- Adjuvant therapy is often recommended given the high incidence of locoregional spread and recurrence. Most oncologists use gemcitabine or 5-FU based chemotherapy with/without radiotherapy. Evidence supporting this practice comes from three randomized phase 3 studies and a large meta-analysis.
  - The European Study Group for Pancreatic Cancer (ESPAC-3) periampullary trial randomized 428 patients (297 with ampullary, 96 with bile duct and 35 with other cancer) to observation or chemotherapy with 5-FU or gemcitabine. The difference in median survival in the chemotherapy cohorts vs. the observation group was not significant (43.1 months vs. 35.2 months, respectively; $p = 0.25$). However, multivariate analysis adjusting for age, type of cancer, tumor differentiation, and lymph node status found a significant difference favoring chemotherapy (hazard ratio for chemotherapy vs. observation was 0.75; $p = 0.03$).
  - A study assessed adjuvant mitomycin and 5-FU chemotherapy in resected stage II–IV pancreaticobiliary carcinomas. Of the 508 patients investigated, 335 patients had BTCs. Patients with noncuratively resected GBCs had significantly better 5-year survival (26% vs. 14.4%; $p = 0.0367$) and 5-year disease-free survival (20.3% vs. 11.6%; $p = 0.021$) with chemotherapy than with observation. These outcomes were not found in other BTCs.
  - A meta-analysis of 6712 (Horgan et al. 2012) demonstrated a nonsignificant survival benefit with adjuvant therapy for resected BTCs (pooled odds ratio [OR] 0.74; $p = 0.06$). Benefit was

greatest in patients with lymph node-positive disease (OR 0.49; $p = 0.004$) or positive margins (OR 0.36; $p = 0.002$).

- Most recently, the phase III BILCAP study (Primrose et al., 2019) which randomized patients with curatively resected CCA or muscle invasive GBC to observation vs. surgery followed by 6 months of adjuvant capecitabine.

- Systemic therapy is recommended for patients with unresectable or metastatic BTCs and an adequate performance status to forestall disease progression, palliate symptoms, and prolong survival.

  - Combination chemotherapy instead of monotherapy is preferred in patients with a good performance status. A randomized phase 3 trial reported significant improvements in disease control rates, PFS and OS (11.7 vs. 8.1 months, HR 0.64; $p < 0.001$) with gemcitabine plus cisplatin vs. gemcitabine alone (Valle et al. 2010).

  - Fluoropyrimidines, oxaliplatin, irinotecan, and taxanes are also active in BTCs and may be used as first line or in subsequent lines of therapy.

- Molecular alterations in BTCs provide a rationale for the use of targeted therapies. Inhibitors of angiogenesis (bevacizumab), EGFR (erlotinib, cetuximab), and MAP kinase signaling (sorafenib, selumetinib) have been evaluated alone or combined with chemotherapy in mostly single-arm phase 2 studies.

  - In a randomized phase 3 study, the addition of erlotinib to gemcitabine and oxaliplatin (GEMOX) significantly increased objective responses but did not improve PFS or OS compared with GEMOX alone.

  - Studies of agents targeting *IDH 1/2, FGFR2, ALK, and BRAF* (and others) in molecularly enriched patient subpopulations are underway, and preliminary results appear promising. Clinical trial enrollment is encouraged where available.

- Liver directed therapies (chemoembolization, radioembolization, external beam radiotherapy, hepatic arterial infusion) demonstrate promising results in patients with unresectable liver-dominant disease but are considered investigational. These do not replace chemotherapy but may be used to "consolidate" a favorable response to chemotherapy.

Prevention/management of complications

- Patients with BTCs can develop biliary obstruction which causes significant morbidity and limits treatment options. Patients require multimodal evaluation (CT, MRCP, ERCP) and multispecialty management (e.g. gastroenterology for ERCP stenting or interventional radiology for percutaneous drainage).

Follow-up tests and monitoring

- Following definitive treatment, surveillance imaging is recommended every 6 months for the first 2 years and then annually for the next 5 years.
- There are no established guidelines for monitoring tumor markers, though they can be used in conjunction with imaging surveillance to evaluate for recurrence.

Prognosis

- The overall prognosis of BTCs is poor, related to the often advanced stage at diagnosis. Fewer than 10% of symptomatic patients and approximately 20% of incidentally diagnosed gallbladder cancer patients have early stage disease. Most CCAs are found only after they have grown enough to cause symptoms, and are also unlikely to be operable. As such, jaundice is an indicator of poor prognosis – it is associated with unresectable disease in about 44% of patients.

- According to survival data provided by NCI's SEER database, intrahepatic CCAs have 5-year relative survival rates of 15%, 6%, and 2% for localized, regional, and distant disease, respectively. Extrahepatic CCAs have 5-year relative survival rates of 30%, 24%, and 2% for localized, regional, and distant disease, respectively.
- Gallbladder cancer 5-year survival rates range from 50% for stage I tumors to 28% for stage II cancer, below 10% for stage III–IV cancer, and 4–2% for stage IV cancer.

CLINICAL PEARLS

- Surgery offers the best chance for cure and long-term survival but recurrences are frequent. Adjuvant chemotherapy with or without radiation should be considered for patients with lymph node-positive disease or positive resection margins.
- Systemic chemotherapy improves disease control and survival in patients with advanced BTCs. Gemcitabine and cisplatin is a common first line regimen but there are other active chemotherapies. Clinical trial enrollment should be encouraged.
- Emerging options include the study of targeted therapies in molecularly enriched patient subgroups, and the use of liver-directed therapies.

References and reading list

Bridgewater J, Galle PR, Khan SA, et al. Guidelines for the diagnosis and management of intrahepatic cholangiocarcinoma. J Hepatol 2014;60:1268–1289.

Hezel AF, Zhu Ax. Systemic therapy for biliary tract cancers. Oncologist 2008;13:415–423.

Horgan AM, Amir E, Walter T, et al. Adjuvant therapy in the treatment of biliary tract cancer: a systemic review and meta-analysis. J Clin Oncol 2012;30:1934–1940.

Primrose JN, Fox RP, Palmer DH, et al. Capecitabine compared with observation in resected biliary tract cancer (BILCAP): a randomised, controlled, multicentre, phase 3 study. Lancet Oncol 2019;29:663–673.

Valle JW, Wasan HS, Palmer DD, et al. Cisplatin plus gemcitabine versus gemcitabine for biliary tract cancer. N Engl J Med 2010;362:1273–1281.

Wang SJ, Lemieux A, Kalpathy-Cramer J, et al. Nomogram for predicting the benefit of adjuvant chemoradiotherapy for resected gallbladder cancer. J Clin Oncol 2011;29:4627–4632.

Suggested website

www.nccn.org/professionals/physician_gls/f_guidelines.asp

Guidelines
National society guidelines

Title	Source	Date
National Comprehensive Cancer Network Guidelines	NCCN	2016 Version I

Image

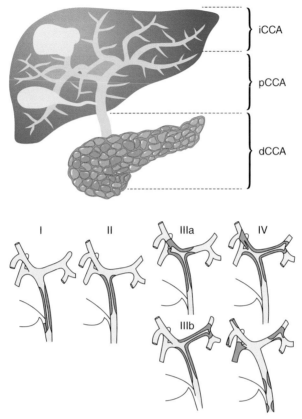

Figure 9.1 Classification of cholangiocarcinoma (CCA). Top panel: overall classification of CCA. Intrahepatic CCAs (iCCA) originate from intrahepatic ductules/ducts proximal to the bifurcation of the right and left hepatic ducts. Extrahepatic tumors are divided into perihilar (pCCA) and distal (dCCA) cholangiocarcinomas – the transition occurring where the common bile duct lies posterior to the duodenum and distal to the insertion of the cystic duct into the common bile duct. Bottom panel: Bismuth classification of perihilar cholangiocarcinomas. Classified according to the patterns of involvement of the hepatic ducts. (Reproduced with permission of Elsevier.)

Additional material for this chapter can be found online at: www.wiley.com/go/oh/mountsinaioncology

This includes a case study, ICD codes, and multiple choice questions.

CHAPTER 10

Pancreas Cancer

Max W. Sung

Icahn School of Medicine at Mount Sinai, New York, NY, USA

OVERALL BOTTOM LINE

- Advances in combination chemotherapy have improved survival of patients with advanced pancreas cancer over single agent gemcitabine, the first drug approved by the FDA for pancreas cancer in 1996.
- Combination chemotherapy as well as radiation therapy used in the neoadjuvant and adjuvant settings following curative resection has improved survival in patients with early stage pancreas cancer.
- Supportive care including interventions for obstructive jaundice has improved the quality of life for patients with pancreas cancer.
- Identification of environmental and genetic risk factors is paving the way towards earlier detection of pancreas cancer.
- Adenocarcinomas and neuroendocrine cancers of the pancreas have significant differences in prognosis. Response to intervention needs to be made through histologic and serologic evaluation.

Background
Definition of disease

Cancers arising from the ductal and acinar cells of the exocrine pancreas are commonly referred to as pancreas cancers (95%), while those arising from the neuroendocrine cells are termed pancreatic neuroendocrine tumors (5%).

Disease classification

- TNM classification of exocrine pancreatic tumors is based on primary tumor size and extent of invasion, nodal involvement, and distant metastases.
- WHO and Atlas of Tumor Pathology (AFIP) histologic classification of exocrine pancreas tumors is based on histologic assessment of low, moderate, and high grade dysplasia corresponding to benign, borderline, and noninvasive carcinoma.

Incidence/prevalence

- Estimated incidence, mortality, and 5-year prevalence of pancreas cancers worldwide in 2012 was 337 872 (2.4%), 330 391 (4.0%), and 211 544 (0.6%), respectively.
- For the USA, estimated incidence and mortality in 2016 was 53 070 (3%) and 41 780 (7%), respectively, while estimated prevalence in 2012 was 45 702.

Mount Sinai Expert Guides: Oncology, First Edition. Edited by William K. Oh and Ajai Chari.

© 2019 John Wiley & Sons Ltd. Published 2019 by John Wiley & Sons Ltd.

Companion Website: www.wiley.com/go/oh/mountsinaioncology

- Pancreas cancer ranks as the fourth leading cause of cancer-related deaths in the USA and seventh in the world.

Economic impact
- In the USA, the direct medical care costs (84% related to hospitalization) were estimated to be $881 million annually, while total costs (direct and indirect costs) were estimated at $4.9 billion annually.

Etiology
- Hereditary factors, including hereditary pancreatitis, germline mutations in *BRCA1/2, PALB2, STK11* (Peutz–Jeghers), *CDKN2A* (FAMM), p16 Leiden (FAMM-pancreatic carcinoma), and *ORSS1* (hereditary pancreatitis).
- Familial pancreatic cancer syndromes (germline mutations not yet identified).
- Nonhereditary pancreatitis and pancreatic cysts are associated with pancreas cancer.
- Cigarette smoking, obesity, and nonphysical activity increase risk.
- Diabetes mellitus has been linked to pancreas cancer.

Pathology/pathogenesis
- Pancreas cancer, by its growth within the pancreas, can cause ductal obstruction resulting in pancreatic insufficiency and pancreatic atrophy distal to the obstruction, and obstruction of the common bile duct as it courses through the head of the pancreas with resulting obstructive jaundice. By its growth beyond the pancreas, it can cause duodenal obstruction, gastric ulceration, and peritoneal carcinomatosis.
- Recent studies on the sequencing of protein-coding exons from pancreas cancer samples have provided early information in the genetic pathogenesis of pancreas cancers, including activation of oncogene mutations (*KRAS*), inactivation of tumor suppressor genes (*ITP53, p16/CDKN2A, SMAD4*), and inactivation of DNA mismatch repair genes (*hMLH1, MSH2*). Germline mutations also provide hereditary mechanisms for the pathogenesis of pancreas cancers.

Predictive/risk factors

Risk factor	Odds ratio (95% CI)
Cigarette smoking	2.2 (1.7–2.8)
Obesity	1.47 (1.23–1.75)
Chronic pancreatitis	2.62 (1.88–3.66)
Diabetes	2.1 (1.6–2.8)
Familial pancreatic cancer	3.2 (1.8–5.6)

Prevention

BOTTOM LINE/CLINICAL PEARL
- No interventions have been shown to prevent the development of the disease.

Screening
- There are no guidelines for the screening of high risk patients for pancreatic cancer from the American Gastroenterological Association or the National Comprehensive Cancer Network.

- The use of imaging modalities (CT, MRI, EUS) for the screening of pancreatic cancer in asymptomatic high risk individuals is considered investigational, although it has been recommended by some groups such as the Consensus Committees of the European Registry of Hereditary Pancreatic Diseases, the Midwest Multicenter Pancreatic Study Group, and the International Association of Pancreatology.

Primary prevention
- Cessation of cigarette smoking can reduce pancreatic cancer related deaths in the USA by 25% annually.
- A "healthy" diet of higher intake of fruits and vegetables and lower intake of saturated fats.
- Physical activity, particularly for overweight individuals.

Secondary prevention
- Adjuvant chemotherapy (gemcitabine) following curative resection: the CONKO-001 trial showed significant improvement in OS compared with observation only control group (hazard ratio [HR] 0.76; 95% confidence interval [CI] 0.61–0.95). Five-year OS was 20.7% in the treated group vs. 10.4% for the control group.
- Adjuvant chemotherapy (gemcitabine + capecitabine): the ESPAC-4 trial (gemcitabine-capecitabine vs. gemcitabine) showed significant survival benefit for the combination (median OS 28 vs. 25.5 months; HR for death 0.82; 95% CI 0.68–0.98). Five-year OS was 19% for the combination group compared with 9% for gemcitabine alone.
- Adjuvant chemoradiotherapy following curative resection has not been definitely shown to confer survival benefit in randomized clinical trials.

Diagnosis (Algorithm 10.1)

> **BOTTOM LINE/CLINICAL PEARLS**
> - **History:** weight loss, abdominal pains, recent onset diabetes, steatorrhea.
> - **Examination findings:** jaundice, epigastric tenderness, ascites.
> - **Investigations:** CT of the abdomen with and without contrast, ERCP, EUS and biopsy, and MRCP.

Differential diagnosis

Differential diagnosis	Features
Pancreatic cystic neoplasms	Cystic lesions on CT, MRCP
Pancreatic neuroendocrine cancers	Pathology differences in morphology, immunostains from pancreatic adenocarcinomas

Typical presentation
The patient typically presents with jaundice, darkening of urine, light-colored stools, postprandial diarrhea and abdominal cramps, and epigastric pain penetrating through to the mid back which is exacerbated on lying supine. Tumors in the pancreatic body or tail can present as left upper quadrant discomfort in the absence of obstructive jaundice.

Algorithm 10.1 Diagnosis of pancreas cancer

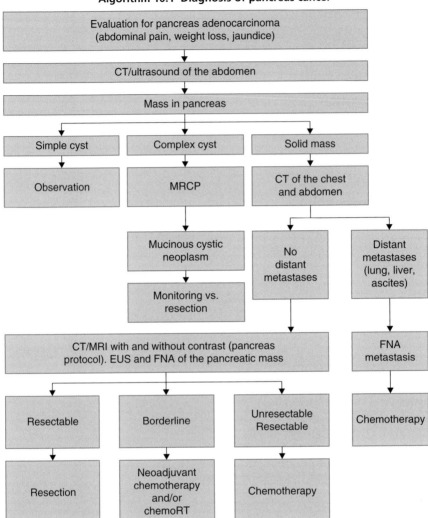

Clinical diagnosis

History
- Recent weight loss, upper abdominal discomfort, loose stools, recent onset diabetes, recent depressive symptoms. Family history for pancreatic cancer.

Physical examination
- Assess scleral jaundice in white light, assess for epigastric tenderness on deep palpation, and for abdominal distention caused by ascites. Assess for metastases to left supraclavicular node.

Useful clinical decision rules and calculators
- Elevated serum tumor markers such as CA19-9 for pancreatic adenocarcinomas and elevated serum chromogranin A for pancreatic neuroendocrine tumors is not diagnostic but may be useful for diagnosis and management.

Disease severity classification
- Assessment for borderline resectable disease: no distant metastases; venous involvement of superior mesenteric vein/portal vein demonstrating tumor abutment with or without impingement and narrowing of the lumen, encasement of the superior mesenteric vein/portal vein but without encasement of the nearby arteries, or short segment venous occlusion resulting from either tumor thrombus or encasement, but with suitable vessel proximal and distal to the area of vessel involvement, allowing for safe resection and reconstruction; gastroduodenal artery encasement up to the hepatic artery with either short segment encasement or direct tumor abutment of the hepatic artery, but without extension to the celiac axis; tumor abutment of the superior mesenteric artery not to exceed >180 degrees of the circumference of the vessel wall.

Laboratory diagnosis
List of diagnostic tests
- **Serum liver function tests:** total bilirubin, direct bilirubin, alanine transferase, aspartate transferase, albumin.
- **CBC:** white blood cell count, red blood cell count, hemoglobin, hematocrit, differential, platelet count, prothrombin time, partial thromboplastin time.
- **Biopsy of pancreatic mass:** percutaneous CT/ultrasound guided or endoscopic ultrasound guided.

List of imaging techniques
- Abdominal ultrasound to assess pancreatic mass, biliary obstruction.
- CT of the chest, abdomen, and pelvis to complete staging, evaluation for metastatic disease, and ascites.
- MRI/MRA/MRCP to assess for biliary tract and vascular involvement.
- EUS to assess for resectability and fine needle cytology/biopsy to confirm malignant pancreatic tumor.

Potential pitfalls/common errors made regarding diagnosis of disease
- Benign pancreatic serous cyst.
- Pancreatic benign cystadenoma.
- Pancreatic neuroendocrine tumor.

Treatment
Treatment rationale
- **Resectable disease:** surgical resection with curative intent.
- **Borderline resectable disease:** neoadjuvant treatment to include chemotherapy (FOLFIRINOX or gemcitabine-nab-paclitaxel) and/or chemoradiation therapy (EBRT concurrent with capecitabine or gemcitabine).
- **Unresectable and metastatic disease:** systemic chemotherapy (FOLFIRINOX or gemcitabine-nab-paclitaxel) or participation in clinical trials.
- Biliary stent placement for obstructive jaundice.

When to hospitalize
- Ascending cholangitis because of biliary tract obstruction for intravenous antibiotics.
- Intestinal obstruction from pancreatic tumor.
- Intractable pain from pancreatic tumor.
- Neutropenic sepsis from chemotherapy.

Managing the hospitalized patient

- Ascending cholangitis to be treated with intravenous antibiotics and biliary stent placement if there is biliary tract obstruction.
- Consideration of laparoscopic or open gastrojejunostomy for intestinal bypass.
- Intravenous antibiotics for neutropenic sepsis secondary to chemotherapy.

Table of treatment

Treatment	Comments
Conservative	
	Palliative care with aims to pain control and comfort care for patients with tumor progression and who are not candidates for further chemotherapy radiation therapy or surgical treatments
Medical	
FOLFIRINOX Gemcitabine-nab-paclitaxel Gemcitabine Gemcitabine-capecitabine MM398-leucovorin-fluorouracil	Neoadjuvant treatment for borderline resectable disease and for unresectable and metastatic disease
Surgical	
Pancreaticoduodenectomy Distal pancreatectomy	Resectable patients and patients rendered resectable with neoadjuvant treatment
Radiologic	
EBRT concurrent with capecitabine or gemcitabine	Neoadjuvant treatment for borderline resectable disease
Psychologic	
	Antidepressants
Complementary	
	Pain control and appetite stimulants Pancreatic enzyme replacement

Prevention/management of complications

- Disabling peripheral neuropathy from oxaliplatin or nab-paclitaxel; omit these chemotherapy drugs on development of symptoms.
- Neutropenic sepsis: use of granulocyte colony stimulating factors and outpatient antibiotics with neutropenia.
- Diarrhea and dehydration from pancreatic insufficiency or chemotherapy related (irinotecan): vigorous rehydration, use of antidiarrheals.

CLINICAL PEARLS
- Borderline resectable patients to be treated with neoadjuvant treatment: chemotherapy such as FOLFIRINOX, gemcitabine-nab-paclitaxel, and/or radiation therapy concurrent with capecitabine or gemcitabine to render patients resectable for curative resection.
- Use of sequential chemotherapy regimens to extend survival.

Special populations
Elderly
- Elderly patients with comorbidities may be at high risk for pancreaticoduodenectomy resections and should be considered for noninvasive treatments. Elderly patients may also not tolerate multiagent chemotherapy regimens such as FOLFIRINOX which should be avoided.

Prognosis

BOTTOM LINE/CLINICAL PEARLS
- High rates of tumor recurrence and metastases occur despite curative resection: 5-year survival 10–25% and median survival 10–20 months.
- Increased survival with newer chemotherapy regimens such as FOLFIRINOX and gemcitabine-nab-paclitaxel up to 11 months.
- Ampullary cancer has twice the expected survival compared with pancreatic adenocarcinoma.

Reading list
Burris HA, Moore MJ, Andersen J, et al. Improvements in survival and clinical benefit with gemcitabine as first-line therapy for patients with advanced pancreas cancer: a randomized trial. J Clin Oncol 1977;15:2403–2413.

Conroy T, Desseigne F, Ychou M, et al. FOLFIRINOX versus gemcitabine for metastatic pancreatic cancer. N Engl J Med 2011;364:1817–1825.

Krushman M, Dempsey N, Maldonaldo JC, et al. Full dose neoadjuvant FOLFIRINOX is associated with prolonged survival in patients with locally advanced pancreatic adenocarcinoma. Pancreatology 2015;15:667–673.

Neoptolemos JP, Palmer JP, Ghaneh P, et al. Comparison of adjuvant gemcitabine and capecitabine with gemcitabine monotherapy in patients with resected pancreatic cancer (ESPAC-4): a multicentre, open-label, randomised, phase 3 trial. Lancet 2017;389:1011–1024.

Von Hoff DD, Ervin T, Arena FP, et al. Increased survival in pancreatic cancer with nab-paclitaxel plus gemcitabine. N Engl J Med 2013;369:1691–1703.

Guidelines
International society guidelines

Title	Comment	Date and weblink
NCCN	Unresectability	2009 https://www.nccn.org/professionals/physician_gls/pdf/pancreatic.pdf
Consensus	Borderline resectable	2017 https://www.ncbi.nlm.nih.gov/pubmed/29191513
NCCN	All stages	2019 https://www.nccn.org/professionals/physician_gls/pdf/pancreatic.pdf

---

Additional material for this chapter can be found online at:
www.wiley.com/go/oh/mountsinaioncology

This includes advice to patients, a case study, ICD codes, and multiple choice questions.

CHAPTER 11

Colorectal Cancer

Kenneth L. Angelino, Jason W. Steinberg, and Peter S. Kozuch
Icahn School of Medicine at Mount Sinai, New York, NY, USA

OVERALL BOTTOM LINE
- Most colorectal cancers (CRCs) grow slowly over 10–15 years and often do not produce symptoms until they reach >1 cm.
- CRC is the third leading cause of cancer death in the USA, resulting in approximately 50 000 deaths yearly, and 8% of all cancer mortality.
- If detected early, CRC can be prevented or cured.
- Systemic therapy is the cornerstone of unresectable disease.
- Stage at time of diagnosis is the most important prognostic indicator, although genetic features such as microsatellite instability, *BRAF* and *KRAS* mutational status are prognostic and predictive, respectively.

Background
Definition of disease
- Malignant cells form in the inner lining (mucosa) of the colon or rectum as an adenomatous polyp, then grow slowly through the layers of the large bowel.

Disease classification
- Adenocarcinoma is the most prevalent type (95%) of CRC and is further subdivided into cribriform comedo-type, medullary, micropapillary, mucinous, serrated, and signet-ring cell. Other types include adenosquamous, spindle cell, squamous cell (epidermoid), and undifferentiated.

Incidence/prevalence
- In the USA, CRC is the third most common cancer in both men and women, with more than 130 000 new cases per year. Nearly 50 000 deaths are attributed to this disease, making it the third leading cause of cancer-related mortality (Figure 11.1).
- CRC rarely occurs in individuals under 49 years (1.7–3.5%).
- Over the last several decades, overall CRC incidence and mortality rates have decreased because of increased screening and improved treatments.
- However, incidence rates are increasing among men and women under age 50 years by about 1.5% per year per 100 000 individuals.

Economic impact
- In 2010, the medical cost of colorectal care was $14 billion in the USA, which is projected to increase to as much as $20 billion by 2020.

Mount Sinai Expert Guides: Oncology, First Edition. Edited by William K. Oh and Ajai Chari.
© 2019 John Wiley & Sons Ltd. Published 2019 by John Wiley & Sons Ltd.
Companion Website: www.wiley.com/go/oh/mountsinaioncology

Etiology

- Although 20–30% have a familial component, only 5% of CRCs are caused by well-defined genetic syndromes. About 70% of CRCs are caused by sporadic mutations leading to genetic instability. Amplifications, rearrangements, and deletions result in the accumulation of hundreds to thousands of genetic aberrations as a premalignant adenoma progresses to invasive colon cancer.

Pathology/pathogenesis

- Colorectal tumors are divided into non-neoplastic polyps, neoplastic polyps, and cancers. Hamartomatous, hyperplastic, inflammatory, juvenile, and lymphoid polyps have low malignant potential. Neoplastic polyps such as adenomas are the primary precursor to CRC, although of these only 5% or less progress to invasive malignancy over 10–15 years. Adenomas demonstrating a villous component, high grade dysplasia, or which are larger than 1 cm are considered advanced and at higher risk for malignant transformation (Figure 11.2).
- The progression from adenoma to carcinoma occurs through the accumulation of changes in gene expression patterns and mutations. Along with measurement of chromosomal and microsatellite instability status (CIN and MSI, respectively) and clinical and pathologic findings, a worldwide consensus defines four consensus molecular subtypes (CMS1–4) for *future* clinical stratification and subtype-based targeted interventions (Table 11.1).

Table 11.1 Consensus molecular subtypes.

Consensus subtype	Prevalence (%)	Characteristics	5-year OS (all stages) (%)	Median survival after relapse (months)
CMS1	14	*BRAF* mutations, MSI, hypermutated, immune activation, right-sided tumors, older, female	74	9
CMS2	37	Highly proliferative, high CIN, TP53 mutations, EGFR up-regulated, WNT/MYC activated, left-sided and rectal tumors	77	35
CMS3	13	Low CIN, *KRAS* and *PIK3CA* mutations, WNT/MYC activated	75	20
CMS4	23	Mesenchymal/TGF-beta activation, NOTCH3/VEGFR2 overexpression, younger	62	24
No consensus assignment	13			

Predictive/risk factors

Risk factor	Relative risk (RR)
Alcohol (5 drinks per week)	1.06
BMI >30	1.10
Cigarette smoking (5 pack-years)*	1.06
Inflammatory bowel disease	2.93
Red meat (5 servings per week)	1.13

- Lifetime risk for CRC developing in individuals with inherited disorders such as familial adenomatous polyposis (FAP), Turcot syndrome, and hereditary nonpolyposis colorectal cancer (HNPCC) approach 80–100%.
- Compared with those with no family history, a single first degree relative with CRC diagnosed before age 45 increases risk two- to fourfold.
- A personal history of adenomas (RR 2.1) or inflammatory bowel disease (RR up to 5) can contribute to an increased lifetime risk of up to 18%.
- The risk of CRC increases with age from 65; 140/100 000 to 260/100 000 person-years in the sixth, seventh, and eighth decades of life, respectively.
- Some environmental factors linked with risk include: high caloric diet, diabetes mellitus, metabolic syndrome, and radiation exposure.
- In metastatic disease compared with left-sided tumors, right-sided tumors have a worse prognosis and an inferior response to EGFR antibodies.

Prevention

BOTTOM LINE/CLINICAL PEARLS

Modality	Surveillance interval (years)
Colonoscopy	10
CT colonography	5
Double-contrast barium enema	5
Flexible sigmoidoscopy	5
Fecal immunochemical test	1
Guaiac-based fecal occult blood test	1

- Removal of polyps during colonoscopy can prevent or delay onset of CRC.
- The only effective preventative intervention for patients with FAP is colectomy.
- Aspirin and other NSAID use continuously for over 5 years can prevent CRC.
- Increased physical activity and diets high in fruits and/or vegetables are associated with lower risk.

Screening
Screening choices for average risk adults aged 50 and older

- In the USA, colonoscopy is the most commonly used screening test and the gold standard for detection and prevention. Stool-based chemical tests, while noninvasive and inexpensive, may detect early cancer but cannot prevent it. Flexible sigmoidoscopy requires less extensive bowel preparation and patient sedation than colonoscopy, but only visualizes the distal 40–60 cm of bowel. Radiologic examinations such as CT colonography or double-contrast barium enema visualize the entire colon but, like other tests, abnormal findings require follow-up optical colonoscopy.

Follow-up after index colonoscopy

Recommended surveillance interval	Findings on baseline colonoscopy
10 years	- No polyps, or - Small hyperplastic polyps
5–10 years	- 1–2 small tubular adenomas

(*Continued*)

Recommended surveillance interval	Findings on baseline colonoscopy
3 years	• 3–10 tubular adenomas, *or* • Tubular adenoma ≥1 cm, *or* • Villous adenoma, *or* • Adenoma with high grade dysplasia
<3 years	• >10 adenomas

- Higher risk populations require more intensive screening. In patients with inflammatory bowel disease, colonoscopy should be performed 8–12 years after onset of disease and annually thereafter. Patients with HNPCC should be screened starting at age 20–25 every 1–2 years. Some expert guidelines recommend to begin screening African Americans at age 45 given higher CRC incidence, mortality rates, and frequency under age 50 in this population.
- In all populations, when to stop screening depends on each patient's life expectancy and risks for the procedure.

Primary prevention

- Regular physical activity (RR 0.76) and diets high in fruits and vegetables are associated with protection from developing CRC.
- Very high risk patients with FAP and polyps that cannot be managed endoscopically undergo prophylactic colectomy.
- Aspirin and other NSAIDs, after a latent period of 5 years, reduce the incidence of CRC (HR 0.74). The US Preventative Services Task Force recommends daily low-dose aspirin for at least 10 years for the primary prevention of cardiovascular disease and CRC in adults aged 50–59 years who are not at increased risk for bleeding.

Secondary prevention

- In patients diagnosed with CRC attributed to sporadic disease, a colonoscopy should be performed within 1 year of resection. If negative, further surveillance intervals could be spread out to every 3–5 years.
- Prophylactic subtotal colectomy can reasonably be discussed with patients with Lynch syndrome colon cancer. Given the 16% incidence of developing a second CRC within 10 years in Lynch syndrome and the similar quality of life between partial and subtotal colectomy survivors, prophylactic subtotal colectomy can be discussed as an alternative to surveillance colonoscopies every 1–2 years. Functional outcome is worse with the more extensive surgery but, again, overall quality of life has been reported to be similar.
- Consuming four cups per day of coffee in patients with stage III CRC may prevent disease recurrence or mortality (HR 0.59).
- Higher postoperative vitamin D (25-OHD) levels are associated with lower CRC-specific and all-cause mortality. Comparing the highest with the lowest tertile in patients with stage II CRC, HR was 0.44.

Diagnosis

CLINICAL PEARLS
- Unexplained iron deficiency anemia or blood in the stool should raise concern for CRC.
- A digital rectal examination may reveal occult blood or a rectal mass. A clinical evaluation for ascites, hepatomegaly, and lymphadenopathy should be completed.
- If CRC is suspected, colonoscopy can be used to establish diagnosis through biopsy. Once established, serum chemistries, liver function tests, CEA, and imaging (CT, ultrasound, or MRI) of the abdomen, pelvis, and chest complete staging.

Differential diagnosis

Differential diagnosis	Features
Arteriovenous malformation	Appear as cherry-red macules on direct visualization Biopsy shows dilated, ectatic, thin-walled vessels
Carcinoid tumors	Most common in appendix, rectum, and cecum Biopsy shows polygonal cells with finely dispersed chromatin
Diverticular disease	Mesenteric and pericolonic inflammation without lymphadenopathy Involvement of >10 cm of colon
Occult upper gastrointestinal bleed	Findings on upper endoscopy Not detected by stool immunochemical tests

Typical presentation
- Early stage CRC is typically asymptomatic; therefore these patients are identified at screening.
- Location of tumor growth affects signs and symptoms. Rectal and left-sided tumors are more associated with hematochezia, a change in bowel habits including fragmented or narrowed caliber stool, obstructive symptoms, and tenesmus. Right-sided tumors are more likely to cause clinically significant anemia from melena or occult gastrointestinal bleeding.
- Abdominal pain, palpable mass, or weight loss can occur as a result of a tumor at any location in the colon or rectum.

Clinical diagnosis
History
- It is important to obtain a complete screening history including adequacy of preparation and completeness of prior colonoscopies.
- Establishing history of smoking, irritable bowel disease (IBD), radiation exposure, dietary habits, and personal and familial cancer and polyp history are essential in estimating risk.
- Symptoms of local disease should be evaluated by reviewing for presence of changes in bowel habits, dark or red stools, weight loss, and abdominal pain.
- Abdominal distention, early satiety, and lymphadenopathy are symptoms that can indicate metastatic spread.

Physical examination
- Bulging flanks, shifting dullness, a fluid wave or other signs of ascites raise concern for spread to the peritoneum or massive liver metastases causing portal hypertension.
- Digital rectal examination is essential. In addition to the primary tumor, this examination can identify peritoneal implants and assess the feasibility of a low anterior resection.
- Spread to palpable lymph nodes is very rare. Supraclavicular adenopathy, in all patients, is reactive less than 5% of the time and is a finding worrisome for metastatic cancer.

Disease severity classification
See Table 11.2.
- Primary tumor (T)
  - Tis: carcinoma *in situ*: intraepithelial or invasion of lamina propria
  - T1: tumor invades submucosa
  - T2: tumor invades muscularis propria
  - T3: tumor invades through muscularis propria into subserosa or nonperitonealized peri-colic/perirectal tissues
  - T4a: tumor penetrates to surface of visceral peritoneum
  - T4b: tumor directly invades/is adherent to other organs.

Table 11.2 TNM staging.

Stage	T	N	M
0	Tis	N0	M0
I	T1 or T2	N0	M0
IIA	T3	N0	M0
IIB	T4a	N0	M0
IIC	T4b	N0	M0
IIIA	T1–2	N1	M0
	T1	N2a	
IIIB	T3–T4a	N1	M0
	T2–3	N2a	
	T1–2	N2b	
IIIC	T4b	N1–2	M0
	T4a	N2	
	T3	N2b	
IVA	Any T	Any N	M1a
IVB	Any T	Any N	M1b

(Source: Amin MB, et al. AJCC Cancer Staging Manual, 8th edition, 2017.)

- Regional lymph nodes (N)
  - N0: no regional lymph node metastasis
  - N1: metastasis in one to three regional lymph nodes
  - N2a: metastasis in four to six regional lymph nodes
  - N2b: metastasis in seven or more regional lymph nodes.
- Distant metastases (M)
  - M0: no distant metastasis
  - M1a: distant metastasis confined to one organ/site
  - M1b: metastases in more than one organ/site or the peritoneum.

Laboratory diagnosis
List of diagnostic tests
- **CEA:** this tumor marker is most useful as an adjunct to assessment of response to palliative therapy and for surveillance of relapse because of low sensitivity and nondiagnostic specificity.
- **CBC, iron panel:** iron deficiency anemia is often associated with CRC, but is neither sensitive nor specific.
- A biopsy is required to establish the diagnosis.

Pathologic features on biopsy
- The vast majority of tumors of the colon and rectum are adenocarcinomas. Caudal-type homeobox 2 (CSX2) and cytokeratin 20 (CK20) are two of the most sensitive and specific immunohistochemical markers to identify adenocarcinoma originating from the colon.
- MSI, the result of DNA mismatch repair (MMR) deficiency, is the only molecular factor routinely used for clinical decision-making; single agent fluoropyrimidine-based adjuvant chemotherapy is less beneficial, and potentially harmful, for patients with MSI stage 2, particularly stage 2A, colon cancer.
- Testing for mutations in the genes that encode for *RAS* and *BRAF* is indicated for stage IV CRC. *RAS* and *BRAF* are downstream of EGFR in the *RAS-RAF-MEK-ERK* pathway which has been implicated in the transition from adenoma to carcinoma. Therefore, even in the presence of

EGFR blockade with targeted agents such as cetuximab or panitumumab, this pathway can be constitutively activated by mutations in these genes, and these agents rendered ineffective.
- After histologic confirmation of a malignant neoplasm originating from the colon or rectum, all patients should be referred for resection unless unresectable metastatic disease is also present.

Lists of imaging techniques
- **CT of the abdomen and pelvis:** preoperatively, this test evaluates tumor size, nodal disease, distant metastases, and complications such as fistulae, perforation, or obstruction (Figure 11.3).
- **CT of the thorax:** standard practice is to extend the initial staging CT to include the thorax to evaluate for distant metastases, although the frequent finding of indeterminate pulmonary nodules make the clinical benefit of this test unclear.
- **Liver MRI:** contrast-enhanced MRI is more sensitive for hepatic lesions than CT, especially in the setting of fatty liver changes.
- **Rigid sigmoidoscopy:** tumors with a distal edge that is within 18 cm of the anal verge on flexible endoscopy should be referred to a colorectal surgeon for rigid proctoscopy to assess the true distance from the distal tumor to the anal verge: rectal tumors are within 12 cm. The perioperative and surgical management of rectal cancer differs from that of colon cancer (see section on Treatment).
- **Transrectal ultrasound or pelvic MRI:** in patients with rectal adenocarcinoma, these examinations help to define locally advanced (T3/4 or N1) disease.

Potential pitfalls/common errors made regarding diagnosis of disease
- In approximately 25% of colonoscopies, poor bowel preparation causes the study to be inadequate. This leads to an increase in the miss rate and risk of complications.
- Adults of any age with a change in bowel habits should be referred for diagnostic (as opposed to screening) colonoscopy.

Treatment
Treatment rationale
- Disease stage guides the treatment approach. Localized CRC can only be cured by removal with either radical surgery or, for selected patients with T1 tumors, endoscopic resection.
- Neoadjuvant (preoperative) chemotherapy and radiation is recommended for working stage II and III rectal cancers to optimize local failure-free survival.
- CRC appropriate for resection should be treated with partial colectomy and removal of regional lymph nodes. A minimum of 12 lymph nodes need to be pathologically assessed to secure pathologic N stage.
- Surgery is the cornerstone of curative therapy for both rectal and colon adenocarcinoma, but surgical approaches can differ significantly for the goal of achieving histologically negative margins.
- After potentially curative resection, adjuvant (postoperative) chemotherapy is used to reduce recurrence rates by eradicating micrometastases, generally 6–8 weeks after surgery. This has shown the most benefit in stage III disease. Web-based tools such as Adjuvant! Online help clinicians weigh the risks and benefits of adjuvant treatment based on MMR deficiency, histologic grade, patient age, soluble tumor marker levels, and other factors and can be of particular use in managing patients with stage IIA disease.
- In patients with limited metastatic disease, surgery is potentially curative in combination with chemotherapy. However, most patients with metastatic disease are not surgical candidates and receive palliative chemotherapy, which has been shown to prolong survival, improve quality of life, and relieve symptoms.

Table of treatment

Treatment	Comments
Conservative	
BSC	Treatment is recommended in nearly all patients, even those with incurable metastatic disease. In these patients, chemotherapy increases a median OS from about 5 months to over 2 years
Medical	
Cytotoxic agents Fluoropyrimidines • 5-FU • Capecitabine Topoisomerase I inhibitors • Irinotecan (IRI) Platinum-based agent • Oxaliplatin (OX) Nucleoside analog • Trifluridine-tipiracil (TAS 102) *Biological targeted agents* Anti-EGFR monoclonal antibodies • Cetuximab • Panitumumab Anti-VEGF agents • Bevacizumab • Aflibercept Anti-VEGF receptor agents • Ramucirumab • Regorafenib Combination regimens: • FOLFOX (OX plus short-term infusional 5-FU and LV) • FOLFIRI (IRI plus short-term infusion FU and LV) • CAPOX (capecitabine plus OX)	Common side effects of fluoropyrimidines include diarrhea, myelosuppression, nausea, stomatitis, and hand-foot syndrome. Important rare side effects include Prinzmetal angina (improves with exertion) and Takotsubo cardiomyopathy Leucovorin (LV) is usually given with 5-FU to enhance its effect Bevacizumab increases the activity of any active cytotoxic regimen but is expensive with modest benefit Regorafenib is orally available and may be used as a single agent in patients with metastatic disease refractory to or intolerant of cytotoxic, anti-EGFR, and anti-VEGF therapy. TAS-102 may be used in the same population, or after regorafenib Initial combination chemotherapy is appropriate for most patients with advanced disease These chemotherapy doublets have shown similar outcomes as first line regimens for nonoperable metastatic disease, and therefore treatment choice is made based on expected toxicities
Surgical	
Colon resection • Laparoscopic-assisted • Open Liver and/or lung metastatectomy	Laparoscopic-assisted is preferred over open for uncomplicated CRC without history of extensive prior abdominal surgery The surgical specimen should contain at least 12 lymph nodes for evaluation Metastatectomy is appropriate for curative intent in patients with resectable disease and adequate predicted post-resection functional reserve
Radiologic	
	In combination with chemotherapy, radiotherapy is used in rectal cancer in the neoadjuvant or adjuvant setting for rectal cancer

Prevention/management of complications

- Bevacizumab is associated with impaired wound healing. Therefore, surgery should be avoided within 4–6 weeks of treatment.
- Oxaliplatin causes a dose-dependent acute neurotoxicity in up to 85% of patients. A cumulative ($>680\,mg/m^2$) sensory neuropathy is dose-limiting and can cause discontinuation despite disease response.

CLINICAL PEARLS
- Cure is only possible with surgery and may be obtained in patients with stage I–III disease and select patients with oligometastatic stage IV CRC.
- Rectal cancer has special treatment considerations which otherwise would not apply to all CRCs: neoadjuvant chemoradiation for working stage II and III disease.
- In the adjuvant setting, oxaliplatin-containing regimens are recommended for stage III patients aged 70 and younger.
- A chemotherapy doublet (CAPOX, FOLFIRI, or FOLFOX) with bevacizumab is first line therapy for stage IV disease.

Special populations
Pregnancy

- CRC during pregnancy raises numerous challenges regarding management of the mother and fetus. A colon cancer diagnosis or treatment that is delayed during pregnancy may worsen maternal prognosis. Conversely, treatments including surgery, often in combination with potentially teratogenic chemotherapy or radiotherapy, poses increased maternal–fetal risk and can be detrimental to normal fetal development. In these difficult clinical situations, a multidisciplinary approach is imperative to formulate plans to optimize outcomes for pregnant patients.

Children

- While CRC is one of the common malignancies in adults, it is a much rarer diagnosis in children. Based on 2008–2012 Surveillance, Epidemiology, and End Results Program (SEER) data, only 0.1% of the number of new cases of CRC occurred at an age under 20 in the USA. However, for unclear reasons, when compared with adults, children present at a later disease stage, have more unfavorable histology, and an overall poorer prognosis. Children with certain familial syndromes are also at increased risk for CRC (see section on Familial syndromes). Staging and treatment of CRC in children are based on adult management principles.

Elderly

- Similar to the clinical approach of all other cancers, the treatment plan must be tailored to the individual. This is especially true for elderly patients, which includes assessing performance status, emotional and physical comorbidities, and overall clinical impression of each patient given that the median age at diagnosis is 71. These factors need to be considered when discussing treatment options.

Others
Familial syndromes

- Lynch syndrome or HNPCC: autosomal dominant disorder which causes mutations in genes that code for DNA mismatch repair enzymes, causing microsatellite instability. Patients with Lynch syndrome have a lifetime risk of colon cancer of approximately 70–80%. Other primary malignancies associated with Lynch syndrome include breast, gastrointestinal system, pancreas, ovarian, endometrial, and genitourinary cancers. Genetic testing and counseling is recommended for individuals deemed to be high risk.

- FAP: autosomal dominant disorder resulting in germline mutations of *APC* gene (tumor suppressor gene). FAP accounts for up to 1% of all colon cancers. These patients can develop hundreds to thousands of colon polyps, and will almost inevitably transform into colon cancer if left untreated.

Adolescents and young adults

- Patients younger than 35 years of age who are diagnosed with CRC should be referred for genetic counseling. In a recent retrospective study, 19% of hereditary syndromes were diagnosed in patients in this age group without a family history of CRC. Recent data suggest that the incidence of colon cancer is increasing in adults younger than 50 for unknown reasons, but may result in changes to future screening guidelines.

Prognosis

CLINICAL PEARLS

- Pathologic stage at time of diagnosis is the most important prognostic indicator. Other adverse factors include lymphovascular invasion, undifferentiated histology, mucinous or signet-ring features, elevated preoperative serum CEA, and residual tumor after definitive therapy.
- Regional lymph node involvement strongly predicts a worse outcome following surgical resection.
- Current 5-year survival rates for CRC based on SEER data from 2005 to 2011: localized 90.1%; regional 70.8%; distant 13.1%; unstaged 34.5% (Figure 11.1).
- Molecular factors
  - Oncogene mutations located downstream of the EGFR signaling pathway, mainly *BRAF*-activating mutations, particularly V600E, and RAS mutations (*KRAS* and *NRAS*) have a poorer prognosis
  - Loss of heterozygosity at the long arm of chromosome 18 (18q) is associated with a poorer prognosis.

Natural history of untreated disease

- If left untreated, over a 10–15 year period, a precancerous adenomatous colon polyp can undergo sequential mutations, grow within the bowel lumen, and potentially cause local symptoms including obstruction. It can also invade the lymphovascular system and spread to regional and distant sites, most commonly the liver and lungs.

Prognosis for treated patients

- Approximately 40% of stage II and III patients have recurrence after initial therapy, with most recurrences happening in the first 3 years (over 90% within the first 5 years).
- Adjuvant platinum-based chemotherapy in stage II or III patients shows a disease-free survival benefit, especially in the first 2 years after surgery. The OS benefit was recently confirmed over a 10-year period.
- Adjuvant 5-FU/leucovorin in stage II patients shows absolute survival benefit (3.6%) when compared with observed patients, demonstrated in the QUASAR trial.

Follow-up tests and monitoring

- Intensive surveillance increases identification of operable metachronous relapses. After initial treatment, patients should have a full history, physical examination, and CEA level every 3–6 months for 2 years, then every 6 months afterward for a total of 5 years. In general, patients should also have a colonoscopy at 1 year, repeated at 3 years and at 5 years. Surveillance CT imaging can be performed every 6–12 months for 5 years based on the individualized risk for recurrence.

Reading list

André T, de Gramont A, Vernerey D, et al. Adjuvant fluorouracil, leucovorin, and oxaliplatin in stage II to III colon cancer: updated 10-year survival and outcomes according to BRAF mutation and mismatch repair status of the MOSAIC Study. J Clin Oncol 2015;33:4176–4187.

Brenner H, Kloor M, Pox CP. Colorectal cancer. Lancet 2014;383:1490–1502.

Howlader N, Noone AM, Krapcho M, et al., eds. SEER Cancer Statistics Review, 1975–2012, National Cancer Institute. Bethesda, MD, http://seer.cancer.gov/csr/1975_2012/, based on November 2014 SEER data submission, posted to the SEER website, April 2015.

Hyngstrom JR, Hu CY, Xing Y, et al. Clinicopathology and outcomes for mucinous and signet ring colorectal adenocarcinoma: analysis from the National Cancer Data Base. Ann Surg Oncol 2012;19(9):2814–2821.

Sargent D, Sobrero A, Grothey A, et al. Evidence for cure by adjuvant therapy in colon cancer: observations based on individual patient data from 20,898 patients on 18 randomized trials. J Clin Oncol 2009;27:872–877.

Sauer R, Liersch T, Merkel S, et al. Preoperative versus postoperative chemoradiotherapy for locally advanced rectal cancer: results of the German CAO/ARO/AIO-94 Randomized Phase III Trial after a median follow-up of 11 years. J Clin Oncol 2012;30:1926–1933.

Suggested websites

AJCC Cancer Staging References: http://cancerstaging.org/references-tools/deskreferences/Pages/default.aspx

NCCN Guidelines: http://www.nccn.org/professionals/physician_gls/f_guidelines.asp#site

SEER Cancer Data: http://seer.cancer.gov/statfacts/html/colorect.html

Guidelines
National society guidelines

Title	Source	Date and weblink
NCCN Guidelines	National Comprehensive Cancer Network, evidence-based, consensus-driven management algorithms	2017 (Version 2.2017) https://www.nccn.org/professionals/physician_gls/pdf/colon.pdf
ASCO Clinical Practice Guidelines	American Society of Clinical Oncology, guides on specific clinical scenarios and tests including familial syndromes and molecular biomarkers	2013–2017 http://jco.ascopubs.org/site/misc/specialarticles.xhtml#GASTROINTESTINAL_CANCER
AJCC Cancer Staging Manual, 7th edition	American Joint Committee on Cancer staging guidelines	2009 https://cancerstaging.org/references-tools/quickreferences/documents/colonmedium.pdf

International society guidelines

Title	Source	Date and weblink
ESMO	European Society of Medical Oncology, current for metastatic disease only	2016 http://www.esmo.org/Guidelines/Gastrointestinal-Cancers/Management-of-Patients-with-Metastatic-Colorectal-Cancer

Evidence

Type of evidence	Title	Date and weblink
Phase 3 study, RCT	Adjuvant 5-fluorouracil/leucovorin was superior to 5-fluorouracil/levamisole in high risk AJCC stages II and III disease	2005 http://jco.ascopubs.org/content/23/34/8671.full.pdf
RCT	MOSAIC Trial – addition of oxaliplatin to 5-fluorouracil/leucovorin was superior to 5-fluorouracil/leucovorin alone in the adjuvant setting	2004 http://www.nejm.org/doi/full/10.1056/NEJMoa032709 2015 (updated) http://jco.ascopubs.org/content/early/2015/10/26/JCO.2015.63.4238.full
RCT	QUASAR Trial – adjuvant 5-fluorouracil/leucovorin in stage II patients shows absolute survival benefit (3.6%) when compared with observed patients	2007 http://www.thelancet.com/pdfs/journals/lancet/PIIS0140-6736%2807%2961866-2.pdf
Phase 3 study, RCT	CORRECT Trial – regorafenib improves OS in previously treated metastatic colorectal cancer patients when compared with placebo	2013 http://www.thelancet.com/journals/lancet/article/PIIS0140-6736%2812%2961900-X/fulltext

Images

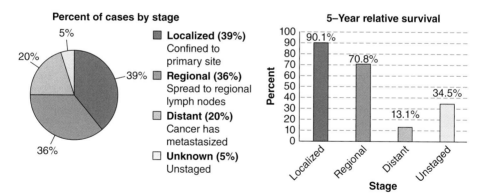

SEER 18 2005–2011, all races, both sexes by SEER summary stage 2000

Figure 11.1 Percentage of cases and 5-year relative survival by stage at diagnosis: colon and rectum cancer. (Source: Howlader N, *et al.* Reproduced from SEER Cancer Statistics Review, 1975–2012, National Cancer Institute.)

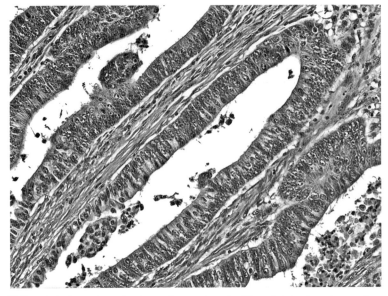

Figure 11.2 Pathologic specimen showing well to moderately differentiated colon adenocarcinoma. See color version on website.

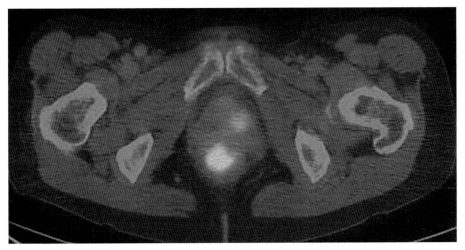

Figure 11.3 Hypermetabolic areas (bright yellow–red) lesions on PET/CT imaging consistent with rectal cancer. (Source: Reproduced with authors' permission.) See color version on website.

Additional material for this chapter can be found online at: www.wiley.com/go/oh/mountsinaioncology

This includes advice for patients, a case study, ICD codes, and multiple choice questions. The following images are available in color: Figures 11.2 and 11.3.

CHAPTER 12

Gastric Cancer

Sofya Pintova

Icahn School of Medicine at Mount Sinai, New York, NY, USA

OVERALL BOTTOM LINE
- Gastric adenocarcinoma is an aggressive form of cancer which encompasses a heterogeneous range of tumors with varying biologic behavior.
- Although stomach cancers often present at more advanced stages with symptoms such as vomiting, abdominal pain, anorexia, and weight loss, screening is routinely performed only in countries with a high incidence and in high risk populations such as those with hereditary syndromes.
- Locoregional disease should be treated by a multidisciplinary team with surgical resection as well as chemotherapy or chemoradiotherapy.
- Metastatic disease is incurable. Systemic therapy can prolong life.

Background
Definition of disease
- Gastric cancer is the fifth most common malignancy worldwide. The disease can be further subclassified into:
  - **Intestinal type:** tends to occur more frequently in men and older individuals.
  - **Diffuse type:** tends to exhibit a more aggressive biologic behavior.

Disease classification
The diagnosis is made by biopsy with pathology revealing adenocarcinoma.

Incidence/prevalence
- In the USA it is estimated that the number of new cases of stomach cancer is 7.4 per 100 000 per year according to the SEER database and approximately 3.4 per 100 000 deaths occur per year (https://seer.cancer.gov/statfacts/html/stomach.html).
- Worldwide, the incidence of stomach cancer is much higher than in North America, making it the fifth most common malignancy worldwide.
- In Eastern Asia, the incidence of gastric cancer reaches 24 per 100 000 cases and in areas of Eastern Europe up to 20 new cases per 100 000 per year are diagnosed.

Mount Sinai Expert Guides: Oncology, First Edition. Edited by William K. Oh and Ajai Chari.
© 2019 John Wiley & Sons Ltd. Published 2019 by John Wiley & Sons Ltd.
Companion Website: www.wiley.com/go/oh/mountsinaioncology

Etiology/pathogenesis
- The sequence of molecular pathogenesis is not completely understood.
- The pathogenesis of the diffuse type of gastric cancer appears to be linked to a germline mutation in the *CDH-1* gene (cell adhesion protein E-cadherin).
- The intestinal type of gastric cancer is hypothesized to follow a sequence of events that results in a precancerous process which eventually transforms into invasive adenocarcinoma. It is thought that the carcinogenic process begins with the development of superficial gastritis and then transforms into chronic nonatrophic gastritis → chronic atrophic gastritis → intestinal metaplasia and finally dysplasia.

Risk factors

Risk factor	Odds ratio
Salt or salt-preserved foods	2–3
Nitroso compounds	1.42
Obesity	1.22
Smoking	1.53
Helicobacter pylori	2.8–49
Gastric surgery	1.66
Abdominal irradiation	11.2
Previous chemotherapy	3.2–7.6
Pernicious anemia	2–6
Occupational exposure (e.g. rubber, nickel)	2–3
Hereditary syndromes	Variable

Prevention

BOTTOM LINE/CLINICAL PEARLS
- Eradication of *H. pylori* infection has been shown to decrease the incidence of gastric cancer.
- Other protective factors include diets high in fresh fruit, vegetables, and fiber; NSAIDs; and reproductive hormones, with later onset of menopause being protective against the development of gastric cancer.

Screening
- Upper endoscopy is the preferred method for screening. Upper endoscopy is more sensitive than upper gastrointestinal series in the detection of gastric cancers: 69% vs. 36.7%. Specificity of both tests is 96%.
- Universal screening is recommended in some countries with a high incidence of gastric cancer such as Japan and Korea.
- Screening can also be considered in high risk groups including patients with gastric adenomas, gastric intestinal metaplasia, pernicious anemia, and hereditary syndromes.

Primary and secondary prevention
- Primary prevention should be directed at eradication of *H. pylori* infection.
- Prophylactic gastrectomy can be considered in patients with hereditary syndromes.

Diagnosis

> **CLINICAL PEARLS**
> - Early stage tumors infrequently cause symptoms and many patients present at a more advanced stage. Gastric cancer is suspected with symptoms of abdominal pain, anorexia, nausea, dysphagia, early satiety, and weight loss. Vomiting or dysmotility can be observed in the case of gastric outlet obstruction or if the tumor affects Auerbach's plexus resulting in pseudoachalasia symptoms.
> - If the disease has spread, physical examination can suggest sites of metastases. Lymphadenopathy can sometimes be palpated on examination in the supraclavicular region (Virchow node), periumbilical node (Sister Mary Joseph node), or axillary lymphadenopathy (Irish node). Hepatomegaly or jaundice can suggest hepatic metastases. Ascites and abdominal distension can be a sign of peritoneal carcinomatosis.
> - Microcytic anemia can be observed on CBC. Radiologic studies may suggest a gastric mass and/or sites of disease spread. Endoscopy with biopsy of a gastric mass or percutaneous biopsies of distant sites are the best methods to confirm the diagnosis (Figure 12.1).

Differential diagnosis

Differential diagnosis	Features
Neuroendocrine tumor	Carcinoid symptoms such as flushing, diarrhea, and palpitations
Lymphoma	Fevers and night sweats
Gastrointestinal stromal tumor	Similar to those of gastric adenocarcinoma

Typical presentation
- Early tumors are typically asymptomatic and may be found incidentally or during surveillance in areas where surveillance is implemented.
- Frequently, the disease is found when a patient presents with gastrointestinal bleeding or when anemia is discovered on a CBC which prompts further evaluation with endoscopy. Patients may also present with new symptoms of gastroesophageal reflux disease (GERD), abdominal pain, weight loss, and early satiety.
- In more advanced or metastatic disease, patients present with more significant abdominal pain, ascites, lymphadenopathy, jaundice, or symptoms of bowel obstruction.

Clinical diagnosis
History
- New onset of GERD, abdominal pain, anemia, nausea, weight loss – especially in older individuals – should prompt further evaluation and consideration for endoscopy referral.

Physical examination
- Tenderness on palpation of the abdomen.
- Ascites.
- Hepatomegaly.
- Lymphadenopathy.
- Jaundice.
- Gastrointestinal bleeding.

Disease severity classification
Disease severity can be better understood by the TNM staging system (Table 12.1).

Table 12.1 TNM, based on AJCC/UICC TNM schema (7th edn)

Stage	Tumor	Node	Metastasis
Stage 0	Tis	N0	M0
Stage IA	T1	N0	M0
Stage IB	T2	N0	M0
	T1	N1	M0
Stage IIA	T3	N0	M0
	T2	N1	M0
	T1	N2	M0
Stage IIB	T4a	N0	M0
	T3	N1	M0
	T2	N2	M0
	T1	N3	M0
Stage IIIA	T4a	N1	M0
	T3	N2	M0
	T2	N3	M0
Stage IIIB	T4b	N0 or N1	M0
	T4a	N2	M0
	T3	N3	M0
Stage IIIC	T4b	N2 or N3	M0
	T4a	N3	M0
Stage IV	Any T	Any N	M1

Laboratory diagnosis
List of diagnostic tests
- CBC and iron studies to evaluate for iron deficiency anemia.
- Comprehensive metabolic panel to assess renal and hepatic function.
- Tumor markers such as CEA and CA19-9 to determine if they can aide in following management of the cancer.
- Biopsy specimens should be tested for HER2.

Lists of imaging techniques
- CT of the chest, abdomen, and pelvis to look for distant metastases.
- PET-CT and MRI can also be used to further assess the primary tumor and metastatic sites of disease.
- EUS is frequently employed to evaluate the depth of tumor invasion in the stomach and locoregional nodal involvement.
- Diagnostic laparoscopy is used to assess both the primary tumor and peritoneal carcinomatosis. Laparoscopy is also an opportunity to perform peritoneal cytology to investigate the presence of microscopic peritoneal metastases (Table 12.2).

Potential pitfalls/common errors made regarding diagnosis of disease
- Symptoms of gastric cancer can be nonspecific such as vague abdominal pain, GERD, and anorexia. Especially in older individuals and patients with risk factors, there should be a low threshold for referral for endoscopy and further evaluation.

Table 12.2 Diagnostic and staging investigations in gastric cancer.

Procedure	Purpose
Routine blood tests	Check for evidence of iron-deficiency anaemia Check hepatic and renal function to determine appropriate therapeutic options
Endoscopy + biopsy	Obtain tissue for diagnosis, histologic classification and molecular biomarkers, e.g. HER-2 status
CT of the thorax + abdomen ± pelvis	Staging of tumor – particularly to detect local/distant lymphadenopathy and metastatic disease sites
EUS	Accurate assessment of T and N stage in potentially operable tumors Determine proximal and distal extent of the tumor
Laparoscopy + washings	To exclude occult metastatic disease involving the diaphragm/peritoneum
Positron emission tomography (PET, if available)	May improve detection of occult metastatic disease in some cases

(Source: Waddell et al. 2014. Reproduced with permission from Elsevier.)

Treatment (Algorithm 12.1)

Treatment rationale

- Treatment depends on the stage of the cancer. Patients should be managed by a multidisciplinary team.
- Early gastric cancers such as T1a tumors may be amenable to endoscopic resection or, if endoscopic resection is not possible, surgical resection.
- Surgical resection offers the best chance of cure. However, risk of recurrence still remains high. Adjuvant therapies with chemotherapy and/or radiation can decrease the risk of recurrence in stages >IA.
- For locoregional disease, perioperative chemotherapy is an option. Surgical resection followed either by adjuvant chemoradiation or adjuvant chemotherapy in cases where a D2 dissection was performed is also acceptable.

Algorithm 12.1 Management of gastric cancer.

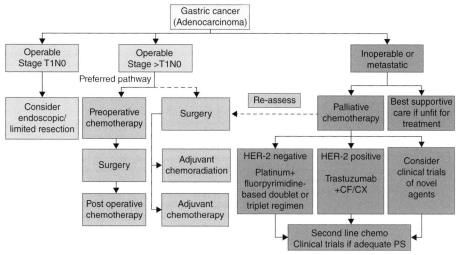

(Source: Waddell et al. 2014. Reproduced with permission from Elsevier.)

- For advanced or metastatic disease, generally systemic chemotherapy is the best option to prolong survival. For HER2-positive tumors, trastuzumab should be added to chemotherapy.

When to hospitalize

- Many reasons prompt hospitalization in patients with gastric cancer. Some common events that result in hospitalizations are significant gastrointestinal bleeding, pain, infectious complications of treatment, and inability to tolerate oral intake.

Table of treatment

Treatment	Comments
Conservative	For patients with poor performance status, best supportive care may be an appropriate option for management
Medical/radiologic	
Locoregional disease Neoadjuvant chemo-RT	For esophagogastric junction tumors neoadjuvant chemo-RT with weekly carbo/taxol concurrently with radiation can be utilized with evidence of improved outcomes over surgery alone (CROSS trial)
Perioperative chemotherapy	Survival benefit was demonstrated in the MAGIC trial with perioperative ECF. Alternative options include EOX, ECX, EOF, and FOLFOX in patients with poorer performance status
Adjuvant chemotherapy following gastrectomy with D2 lymph node dissection	Some trials such as the CLASSIC trial have demonstrated improved disease-free survival with adjuvant cape-ox
Adjuvant chemo-radiation	McDonald regimen demonstrated superior OS in patients receiving adjuvant chemoradiotherapy with 5-FU/LV over surgery alone. Controversy exists whether adjuvant chemoradiation offers improved outcomes over adjuvant chemotherapy in the setting of R0 resection and D2 LN dissection. There may be a benefit to adjuvant chemo-RT especially in patients with LN+ tumors as demonstrated in the ARTIST trial
Metastatic disease Tumors should be tested for HER2 and, if present, trastuzumab should be added to the chemotherapy regimen	Choices of chemotherapy in this setting include triplet, doublet, and single agent combinations. Examples of options: DCF, ECF, FOLFOX, +/− trastuzumab, FOLFIRI, CF +/− trastuzumab, carboplatin + paclitaxel, paclitaxel + ramucirumab and ramucirumab as single agent
Surgical	
Partial gastrectomy Total gastrectomy	Choice of partial or total gastrectomy depends on patient and tumor-related factors
D2 LN dissection	D2 LN dissection is recommended in medically fit patients
Radiologic	
	See Medical section

Prevention/management of complications

- Inability to tolerate oral intake may require management with a nutritionist and implementation of artificial nutrition therapies such as total parenteral nutrition (TPN) and intestinal feeding through jejunal tubes.
- Gastric outlet obstruction is suspected with inability to tolerate oral intake and significant vomiting. Endoscopic stenting, gastrojejunostomy, and decompression intestinal tubes help alleviate symptoms and improve nutrition.

CLINICAL PEARLS

- For very early disease, endoscopic resection or surgical resection should be considered.
- For stage IB and higher, treatment modalities in addition to surgery should be considered. Many prefer perioperative chemotherapy with EOX in younger and more fit patients and FOLFOX in older patients or those with poorer performance status.
- Adjuvant chemotherapy with cape-ox or FOLFOX following a gastrectomy with D2 LN dissection is an option.
- Adjuvant radiation with concurrent chemotherapy especially in patients with LN involvement is an appropriate option.
- For advanced or metastatic disease it is generally preferable to use a doublet rather than a triplet combination because of significant toxicity from three-drug regimens. In HER2-positive tumors trastuzumab should be added to chemotherapy.

Special populations
Elderly
- In the elderly, therapy should be selected based on performance status and comorbidities.

Prognosis

BOTTOM LINE/CLINICAL PEARLS

- Gastric adenocarcinoma is an aggressive tumor.
- Surgical resection with adjuvant therapies for localized disease offer a possibility of cure. Even with improved chemotherapies, radiotherapy, and surgical techniques, 5-year survival for all stages is about 30% in the USA.
- Metastatic disease is incurable. The goal of therapy is to prolong life. With treatment for stage IV disease average survival is approximately 1 year.
- Prognosis depends on stage and appears to be better in Asian patients.

Natural history of untreated disease
- Advanced or metastatic stomach cancer generally progresses rapidly and average life expectancy for untreated disease is about 6 months.

References and reading list

Bang YJ, Van Cutsem E, Feyereyslova A, et al. Trastuzumab in combination with chemotherapy versus chemotherapy alone for treatment of HER2-positive advanced gastric or gastro-oesophageal junction cancer (ToGA): a phase III, open-label randomized controlled trial, Lancet 2010;376:1302.

Bang YJ, Kim YW, Yang HK, et al. Adjuvant capecitabine and oxaliplatin for gastric cancer after D2 gastrectomy (CLASSIC): a phase 3 open-label randomized controlled trial. Lancet 2012;379:315–321.

Cunningham D, Allum WH, Stenning SP, et al. Perioperative chemotherapy versus surgery alone for resectable gastroesophageal cancer, N Engl J Med 2006;355:11–20.

Cunningham D, Starling N, Rao S, et al. Capecitabine and oxaliplatin for advanced esophagogastric cancer. N Engl J Med 2008;358:36–46.

Macdonald JS, Smalleu SR, Benededtti J, et al. Chemoradiotherapy after surgery compared with surgery alone for adenocarcinoma of the stomach or gastroesophageal junction. N Engl J Med 2001;345:725–730.

Park SH, Sohn TS, Lee J, et al. Phase III trial to compare adjuvant chemotherapy with capecitabine and cisplatin versus concurrent chemoradiotherapy in gastric cancer: final report of the adjuvant chemoradiotherapy in stomach tumors trial, including survival and subset analyses, J Clin Oncol 2015;33:3130–3136.

Van Hagen P, Hulshof MC, van Lanschott JJ, et al. Preoperative chemoradiotherapy for esophageal or junctional cancer. N Engl J Med 2012;366:2074–2084.

Waddell T, Verheij M, Allum W, et al. Gastric cancer: ESMO–ESSO–ESTRO Clinical Practice Guidelines for diagnosis, treatment and follow-up. Radiother Oncol 2014;110:189–194.

Zhu WG, Xua DF, Pu J, et al. A randomized, controlled, multicenter study comparing intensity-modulated radiotherapy plus concurrent chemotherapy with chemotherapy alone in gastric cancer patients with D2 resection. Radiother Oncol 2012;104:361–366.

Guidelines
National society guidelines

Title	Source	Date and weblink
National Comprehensive Cancer Network Section on Gastric Cancer	NCCN	2014 https://www.nccn.org/

Image

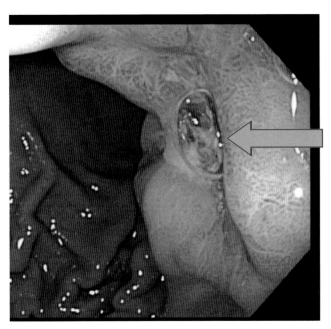

Figure 12.1 Endoscopic view of an ulcerated gastric mass. See color version on website.

Additional material for this chapter can be found online at: www.wiley.com/go/oh/mountsinaioncology

This includes advice for patients, a case study, ICD codes, and multiple choice questions. The following image is available in color: Figure 12.1.

CHAPTER 13

Esophageal Cancer

Madhuri Rao[1] and Andrea S. Wolf[2]
[1] University of Minnesota, Minneapolis, MN, USA
[2] Icahn School of Medicine at Mount Sinai, New York, NY, USA

OVERALL BOTTOM LINE

- The incidence of esophageal cancer has increased in certain populations (e.g. adenocarcinoma in patients with undertreated reflux esophagitis) without much improvement in survival over the past three decades. Five-year survival for all stages is 18%.
- Esophageal cancer bears a large financial burden on the healthcare system, with $1.6 billion spent in 2014 on patients with esophageal cancer in the USA.
- The management of esophageal cancer from initial diagnosis through completion of treatment requires a multidisciplinary approach, involving gastroenterologists, surgeons, and medical and radiation oncologists.
- Multimodality treatment for locally advanced disease generally involves chemoradiation with or without esophagectomy. Additional adjuvant chemotherapy and/or radiation is considered in certain cases.
- Surgical and nonsurgical options may be appropriate depending on the depth of tumor and/or extent of disease. For example, endoscopic treatment such as endomucosal resection or ablation are appropriate for some early stage tumors.

Background
Definition of disease
- Esophageal cancer is a malignancy of any portion of the esophagus from the cricopharyngeus down to the gastroesophageal junction (GEJ), including tumors of the gastric cardia that extend to the GEJ.
- Adenocarcinoma and squamous cell carcinoma are the most common histologic types.
- Rare histologies include choriocarcinoma, lymphoma, melanoma, sarcoma, and small cell cancer.

Incidence/prevalence
- There were approximately 16 980 new cases in 2015 (1% of all cancers).
- There were an estimated 15 590 deaths from esophageal cancer in 2015.
- Prevalence: the reported 35 781 people were living with esophageal cancer in the USA in 2012 (Figure 13.1).

Economic impact
The NCI estimated the cost of treating esophageal cancer in the USA in 2014 was $1.6 billion.

Mount Sinai Expert Guides: Oncology, First Edition. Edited by William K. Oh and Ajai Chari.
Companion Website: www.wiley.com/go/oh/mountsinaioncology

Etiology

Squamous cell carcinoma is associated with the following risk factors:

- Smoking or chewing tobacco
- Excessive alchohol intake
- Diet: *N*-nitroso compounds, hot beverages, areca nut, beetle nut
- Underlying esophagitis (e.g. achalasia, lye ingestion, eosinophilic esophagitis)
- Human papilloma virus
- Atrophic gastritis
- Bisphosphonates.

Adenocarcinoma:

- Increased esophageal acid exposure: GERD, drugs that reduce lower esophageal sphincter pressures, Zollinger–Ellison syndrome
- Smoking
- Obesity.

Pathology/pathogenesis

Squamous cell carcinoma

- Squamous cell carcinomas (SCCs) are usually located in the proximal or mid third of the esophagus.
- Submucosal invasion at an early stage is common.
- An area of chronic epithelial irritation or injury may be the etiology of an infiltrating and/or ulcerated mass.
- As the draining lymphatics are located relatively superficially in the lamina propria (in contrast to the deeper muscularis mucosa), early local lymph node invasion is frequent.
- Thirty percent of patients have distant metastases at presentation.

Adenocarcinoma

- Adenocarcinomas are most commonly located in the GEJ or distal third of the esophagus.
- They often develop in or are associated with Barrett's metaplasia, which is a condition in which the columnar mucosa of the distal esophagus develops squamous metaplastic changes in response to chronic reflux.
- The pattern of lymphatic and metastatic spread is similar to that seen in SCC.

Predictive/risk factors

In the USA, the major risk factors for SCC of the esophagus are smoking and alcohol consumption. Additional risk factors have been described: poor nutrition, low intake of fruits and vegetables, and consumption of very hot beverages. The major risk factors for adenocarcinoma of the esophagus are Barrett's esophagus, GERD, smoking, and high BMI.

Risk factor	Odds ratio
GERD	43.5 (adenocarcinoma) for patients with long standing and severe GERD symptoms as compared with asymptomatic patients
Smoking (60+ pack-years)	2.7 (adenocarcinoma); 5.7 (SCC)
Abdominal diameter	3.47 (adenocarcinoma) for abdominal diameter of >25 cm as compared with <20 cm

Prevention

> **BOTTOM LINE/CLINICAL PEARLS**
> - Esophageal cancer is often detected at advanced stage.
> - Smoking cessation, weight loss, and treatment and close follow-up of reflux disease or other chronic esophageal conditions such as achalasia can prevent the development of esophageal cancer.

Screening
- Some have advocated performing screening in areas of high incidence of esophageal cancer, such as in certain Asian countries.
- Chromoendoscopy with Lugol iodine has been shown to detect early esophageal cancer.
- Current guidelines recommend strict surveillance of patients with Barrett's esophagus, although studies have not conclusively demonstrated benefit in preventing the development of esophageal adenocarcinoma (Algorithm 13.1).

Algorithm 13.1 Management of Barrett's esophagus

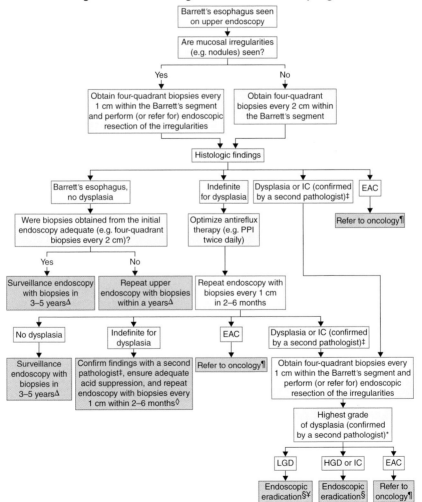

(Source: UptoDate: Barrett's Esophagus-Surveillance and Management.)

Primary prevention

- Avoidance of tobacco and alcohol.
- Treatment and surveillance of Barrett's esophagus.
- GERD management.
- Avoidance of esophageal injury (e.g. lye ingestion).
- Anti-inflammatory drugs: several epidemiologic studies have found an association between aspirin or NSAIDs and decreased risk of developing or dying from esophageal cancer. A meta-analysis demonstrated an odds ratio of 0.57 (95% CI 0.47–0.71).

Secondary prevention

- Guidelines for post-treatment surveillance for recurrent esophageal cancer are detailed in the section on treatment.

Diagnosis (Algorithm 13.2)

Algorithm 13.2 Diagnosis, initial evaluation, and clinical staging of esophageal cancer

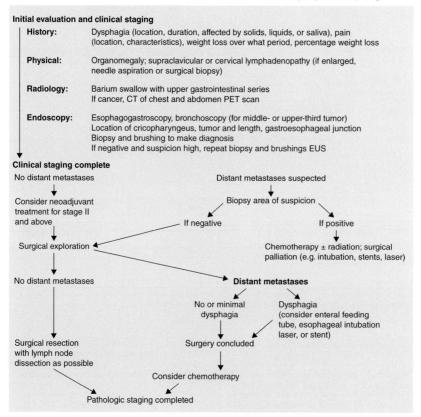

(Source: Shields TW. General Thoracic Surgery, 7th edition, Fig. 158.13. Reproduced with permission from Lippincott Williams and Wilkins.)

- History should focus on symptoms such as dysphagia, odynophagia, weight loss, reflux, regurgitation, vomiting, or (rarely without other symptoms) black tarry stools. A detailed social history of smoking, alcohol consumption, and dietary intake is important.

- Physical examination should evaluate for cachexia, anemia, cervical or supraclavicular adenopathy, abdominal masses, hepatomegaly, or fluid wave, with the abdominal findings listed reflecting intra-abdominal metastases.
- An esophagram is useful in all patients presenting with dysphagia.
- The diagnosis of esophageal cancer requires esophagogastroduodenoscopy (EGD) with biopsies of tumor or abnormal mucosa.
- Staging is appropriate for all cases of diagnosed esophageal cancer.
- Staging includes EUS, PET-CT, and, if symptoms suggest brain metastases, brain MRI.

Differential diagnosis

Differential diagnosis	Features
Achalasia	EGD: no evidence of tumor Manometry: aperistalsis, nonrelaxation of lower esophageal sphincter Esophagram may be confusing
Chronic esophagitis	EGD and biopsies: edema, inflammatory cells
Benign esophageal stricture	EGD and biopsies: inflammatory cells, difficult to differentiate Imaging: smooth tapering, more symmetric narrowing (malignant – abrupt narrowing, asymmetric)
Esophageal diverticulum	Barium swallow: filling of diverticulum
Extrinsic esophageal compression–aortic aneurysm, ectopic left subclavian artery, double aortic arch, intrathoracic thyroid, mediastinal tumor, mediastinal lymph node enlargement	Imaging (CT/MRI): will delineate vascular and mediastinal pathology EGD: no actual obstruction/intraluminal lesion

Typical presentation
- Patients usually present with symptoms of dysphagia (difficulty swallowing) or odynophagia (painful swallowing). Nevertheless, occasionally, the disease is diagnosed in patients undergoing EGD for other symptoms, such as reflux, anemia, or abdominal pain.
- Patients with more advanced disease can present with aspiration, regurgitation, vomiting, weight loss, and cachexia.
- Physical examination can reveal supraclavicular or cervical lymphadenopathy or an abdominal mass suggesting intra-abdominal metastases.
- Occasionally, patients present with gastrointestinal bleeding from friable tumor or invasion of local vascular structures, such as the left atrium or the aorta.
- Finally, patients can present with perforation or fistulization to the tracheobronchial tree.

History
Early detection is critical and it is important to have a high index of suspicion in a patient with symptoms. The patient history should focus on recent changes in diet and any reflux-related symptoms, such as heartburn, chest pain, sour water-brash taste, or regurgitation. Social history should include information on smoking, alcohol intake, and chewing tobacco. An elderly patient with dysphagia should be considered to have esophageal cancer unless proven otherwise.

Dysphagia that has progressed from intolerance of solid food only to intolerance of liquids suggests at least a locally advanced tumor. Weight loss, general malaise, and odynophagia are concerning for even more advanced stage. Symptoms of hoarseness resulting from recurrent laryngeal nerve involvement or recurrent aspiration from a fistula or esophageal obstruction should be elicited.

Physical examination
- A full physical examination is appropriate. General examination findings of jaundice, cachexia, and temporal wasting can be found in patients with advanced stage and/or metastatic tumors.
- One should perform a head and neck examination looking for lymphadenopathy and evidence of other synchronous head and neck tumors, particularly in patients with a significant smoking and/or tobacco history.
- Chest and respiratory examinations are usually nonspecific.
- Abdominal examination can reveal ascites and/or umbilical lymphadenopathy in metastatic disease.
- The extremities should be examined for edema or other evidence of deep vein thrombosis.

Disease severity classification
This is based on the 7th edition of the American Joint Commission on Cancer Staging for Esophageal Cancer. The most important update in the 7th edition system is the inclusion of grade and separation of adenocarcinoma and squamous cell carcinoma.

List of diagnostic tests
- Laboratory investigations: a complete blood count and a basic metabolic panel will help detect anemia in a patient with a bleeding tumor and electrolyte disturbances in a patient with dysphagia and poor oral intake. Liver function tests including albumin levels will reflect nutritional status and may expose metastatic involvement of the liver.
- Pulmonary function tests should be performed prior to esophagectomy to assess the patient's ability to tolerate single-lung ventilation if needed for chest surgery.
- Upper endoscopy/EGD with biopsies is the gold standard for diagnosis.
- EUS with or without biopsies is recommended for staging if the EUS scope can pass.

Lists of imaging techniques
- A barium swallow (esophagram) is generally the first imaging test ordered in a patient presenting with dysphagia. A filling defect and/or apple appearance to the contrast image suggests a malignancy (Figure 13.2).
- A CT scan of the chest, abdomen, and pelvis can help define the local and distant extent of disease.
- PET-CT should be performed in any patient with a diagnosis of esophageal cancer to evaluate for PET-avid nodal disease that may be missed on regular CT.
- In any patient with symptoms (or those with advanced disease), MRI or CT with contrast of the brain should be performed to evaluate for intracranial metastases as these are poorly evaluated on PET-CT.

Potential pitfalls/common errors made regarding diagnosis of disease
- The most dangerous pitfall is missing or delaying diagnosis by not suspecting the diagnosis and/or not performing an accurate or adequate biopsy if the lesion is early stage.

- Another common error is understaging a patient. Clinical understaging can lead to a patient undergoing surgery when induction chemoradiation or systemic chemotherapy would be in the patient's best interest.

Treatment (Algorithm 13.3)

Algorithm 13.3 Management of esophageal cancer

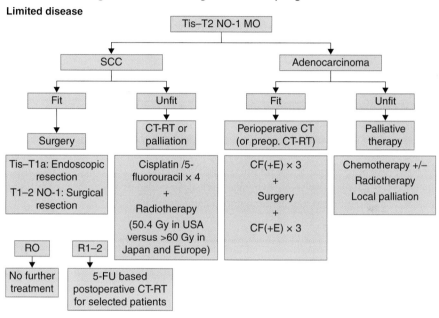

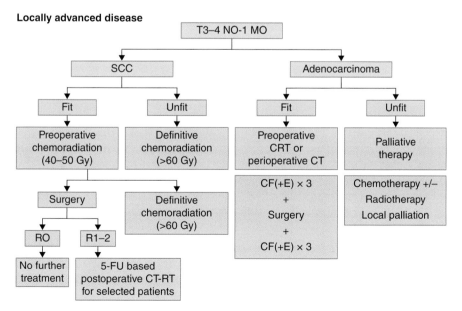

(Source: ESMO Clinical Guidelines. Ann Oncol 2010;21(Suppl 5):46–49. Reproduced with permission from OUP.)

Treatment rationale

- For medically fit patients with T1 tumors, the historic standard of care had been esophagectomy. Currently, however, endoscopic resection is recommended for tumors that are amenable to this therapy. Patients who undergo endoscopic therapies require strict follow-up.
- For patients with T2/3 and/or N1/2 disease, multimodality treatment is the standard of care (see section on Evidence). The best form of multimodality therapy, however, has not been established. Double-agent platinum-based chemotherapy with concurrent radiation is recommended. Surgical resection following induction is recommended if there is no evidence of advanced disease following neoadjuvant therapy. However, there is some controversy and it is not clear that esophagectomy following chemoradiation confers survival benefit over chemoradiation alone for SCC.
- The surgical approach for esophagectomy is based on anatomic tumor location (see Table of treatment). Most clinicians do not perform routine staging laparoscopy. For patients who are not medically fit to undergo surgery or those with T4 (unresectable) tumors, definitive chemoradiation is the standard of care.
- For certain carefully selected patients who undergo definitive chemoradiation and have documented residual disease and/or recurrence, salvage esophagectomy can be considered depending on the extent of disease at the time of updated staging.
- For inoperable patients with severe dysphagia, palliative procedures, such as a stent or feeding tube, should be performed to maintain nutrition and hydration.

When to hospitalize

- **Dehydration:** patients undergoing chemotherapy and/or radiation and those with dysphagia resulting from locally advanced disease can become hypovolemic as a result of poor oral intake. This can lead to severe metabolic disarray and requires hospitalization for hydration as well as correction of severe electrolyte abnormalities.
- **Malnutrition:** patients with dysphagia can become severely malnourished, requiring hospitalization to establish alternate methods of nutrition (stent, feeding tube, intravenous access for parenteral nutrition).
- **Upper gastrointestinal bleeding:** esophageal tumors can cause upper gastrointestinal bleeding. A patient with a brisk acute bleed can require hospitalization for hemodynamic stabilization. Most patients with bleeding, however, present with chronic blood loss anemia and require hospitalization for transfusion and/or local therapy to reduce the bleeding. Patients undergoing chemotherapy are at highest risk for anemia resulting from chemotherapy-related hematopoietic suppression and while many patients with chemotherapy-related anemia can be transfused in the ambulatory setting, those who are also bleeding are more likely to require hospitalization.
- **Aspiration:** patients with severe dysphagia, particularly those with tumors in the mid esophagus or higher, are at risk for aspiration and resultant pneumonitis and/or pneumonia. Symptomatic aspiration requires hospitalization and recurrent aspiration requires hospitalization to attempt therapy to reduce the patient's risk, particularly if it is caused by malignant stricture. Patients with locally advanced disease with recurrent aspiration pneumonia should also be evaluated for possible esophageal–tracheobronchial fistula as this would manifest as recurrent "aspiration" pneumonia.

Managing the hospitalized patient

- Hypovolemic and/or malnourished patients require fluid resuscitation and correction of metabolic disarray.
- Enteral nutrition should be reinstituted whenever feasible. Options include an endoscopic stent to re-establish oral feeds, nasogastric feeds, or placement of a "permanent" feeding tube. For

patients who are surgical candidates in need of a feeding tube, jejunostomy is preferred over gastrostomy. Gastrostomy is avoided in these patients to minimize risk of complication related to use of the stomach as a gastric conduit (often caused by disruption of the gastroepiploic vascular supply to the anastomosis).
- Parenteral nutrition through central intravenous access is a less preferred option if enteral nutrition is not possible or if the interval of nutritional supplementation is short.
- In patients with acute or chronic anemia from bleeding, hemodynamic stability is established. Once hemodynamically stable, these patients can be considered for local therapy in the form of endoscopic ablation/cauterization/resection, radiation, or even palliative esophagectomy.
- Esophageal perforation resulting from advanced (T4) tumor is an emergency and requires immediate medical attention and hospitalization. Generally, this is considered unresectable disease, and many clinicians have stabilized patients with endoscopic stents, but surgery is indicated in certain cases.

Table of treatment

Treatment	Comments
Palliative	Extensive metastatic disease/multiple comorbidities with minimal life expectancy
Medical	Chemotherapy: neoadjuvant, adjuvant, or palliative
Surgical	Trans-hiatal: patients with poor pulmonary function tests, early stage nonbulky disease without significant nodal involvement Ivor Lewis: tumors in the mid distal esophagus (Figure 13.3) McKeown/three-hole: tumors in the upper third of the esophagus Left thoracoabdominal: GEJ tumors with extension into cardia, for which total gastrectomy may be indicated
Radiologic	Radiation therapy: neoadjuvant, adjuvant, or palliative
Psychosocial	Smoking and alcohol cessation programs, support groups for patients with esophageal cancer

Prevention/management of complications
- Each treatment modality is associated with side effects and risks of complications.
- Chemotherapy has a number of risks. Treatment can result in malnutrition or metabolic disarray from anorexia, nausea, and/or vomiting in patients already vulnerable to malnutrition. Other side effects include anemia, leukopenia, and thrombocytopenia resulting from bone marrow suppression, alopecia, and peripheral neuropathy depending on the agent used. Each of these entities is treated accordingly.
- Radiation likewise is associated with a variable incidence of side effects, such as nausea and vomiting, esophagitis that could lead to esophageal strictures, neurotoxicity, and pulmonary toxicity. Most of these are temporary and can be managed with specific medications such as antiemetics and steroids for nausea, local anesthetic sprays for esophagitis, and so on. The more complex problems such as esophageal stricturing may need more invasive treatments such as dilation and stenting. Rarely, patients undergoing chemoradiation for SCC in the mid esophagus develop tracheoesophageal fistula, with higher risk for patients with an indwelling esophageal stent, as the tumor responds to treatment. Management of this complex issue is determined on a case-by-case basis and is beyond the scope of this chapter.
- Esophagectomy is associated with several risks, ranging from minor (postoperative atrial arrhythmia) to major, including anastomotic leak, chyle leak, recurrent laryngeal nerve injury, gastric conduit necrosis, venous thromboembolism, pneumonia, or pyloric obstruction. Several

of these are risks of any thoracic surgical procedure and are managed accordingly. For patients with an anastomotic leak, treatment includes drainage, antibiotics, with or without stenting or repair. Rarely, diversion (with cervical esophagostomy) is required for patients in extremis because of an uncontrolled leak and/or gastric necrosis.

CLINICAL PEARLS
- Neoadjuvant therapy is recommended for patients with a tumor T2 or higher and/or nodal disease.
- Multimodality treatment with surgery, chemotherapy, and radiation yields the best survival results for locally advanced esophageal cancer.
- Definitive chemoradiation is a reasonable strategy for patients without metastases who are not fit to undergo esophagectomy.

Special populations
Pregnancy
- Esophageal cancer in the pregnant patient is a rare and complex situation. Endoscopic resection and surgery can be performed with caution when indicated.
- For patients with advanced disease, it may be possible to delay chemotherapy and radiation if the patient is close to term but the risk a prolonged delay in oncologic treatment must be measured, recognizing that progression of disease and/or malnutrition will result in both maternal and fetal compromise.

Children
- Generally, esophageal cancer is not seen in children. Other, rarer, esophageal tumors do occur in children and should be treated accordingly. For example, sarcomas of the esophagus should be managed with esophagectomy.

Elderly
- Any elderly patient with dysphagia should be considered to have esophageal cancer until proven otherwise. This population is also at higher risk for dehydration and malnutrition.
- Advanced age alone does not preclude treatment for esophageal cancer, and many patients over 80 years have been successfully managed with chemotherapy, radiation, and surgery.

Prognosis

BOTTOM LINE/CLINICAL PEARLS
- Overall 5-year survival for all patients with esophageal cancer is close to 20% with earlier stages having a much better prognosis.
- 5-year survival >80% is seen in patients with tumors that do not invade the submucosa.
- According to the SEER database, between 2009–2015, 5-year survival for localized disease was 47%, regional disease 25%, and distant disease was 5%.

Natural history of untreated disease
- Untreated disease generally leads to obstruction, inability to tolerate oral intake and eventually one's own secretions, progression of malignancy (with likely metastases), and death. Most untreated patients will need palliative treatment for dysphagia or odynophagia.

Follow-up tests and monitoring

Surveillance after treatment of early stage cancer

- **Following endoscopic ablation/resection:** EGD every 3 months for the first year, every 4–6 months for the second year, and then annually for at least 3 years.
- **Following esophagectomy:** CT of the chest and abdomen or PET/CT every 4–12 months for 3 years and then every 6–12 months for 2 years, then annually; EGD and/or esophagram as clinically indicated.

Advanced stage

- Surveillance imaging every 3–6 months the first year, every 6–9 months thereafter for the next 2 years; PET/CT is recommended over CT.

Reading list

Griffith Pearson F, Alexander Patterson G. Pearson's Thoracic and EsophagealSurgery. Churchill Livingstone, 2008.

Shields TW, LoCicero J, Reed CE, et al., eds. General Thoracic Surgery. Lippincott Williams & Wilkins, 2011.

Suggested websites

www.cancer.gov
www.nccn.org
www.cochrane.org

Guidelines
National society guidelines

Title	Source	Date and weblink
Principles of surgery	NCCN guidelines, version 3	2015 http://www.nccn.org/professionals/physician_gls/pdf/esophageal.pdf
Primary treatment for medically fit patients	NCCN guidelines, version 3	2015 http://www.nccn.org/professionals/physician_gls/pdf/esophageal.pdf

Evidence

Type of evidence	Title and comment	Date and weblink
Prospective RCT	Preoperative chemoradiotherapy for esophageal or junctional cancer **Comment:** Preoperative chemoradiotherapy improved survival among patients with potentially curable esophageal or EGJ cancer	2012 https://www.ncbi.nlm.nih.gov/pubmed/22646630
Prospective RCT	Perioperative chemotherapy versus surgery alone for resectable gastroesophageal cancer **Comment:** In patients with operable gastric or lower esophageal adenocarcinomas, a perioperative regimen of ECF decreased tumor size and stage and significantly improved PFS and OS	2006 https://www.ncbi.nlm.nih.gov/pubmed/16822992

Images

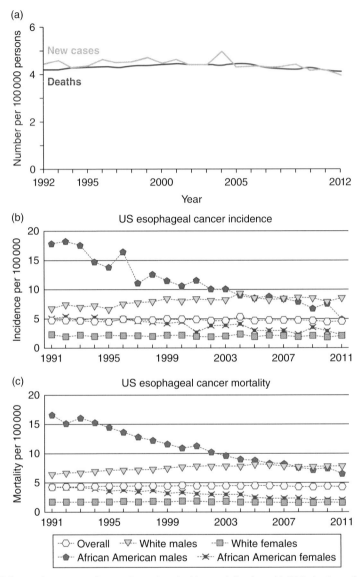

Figure 13.1 Prevalence: SEER. (Source: Reproduced with permission from (a) SEER database, (b,c) www.cancer.gov.)

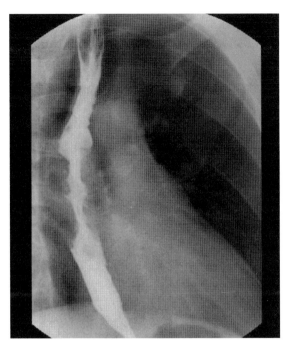

Figure 13.2 Esophagram showing mid esophageal apple core type filling defect that proved to be a squamous cell carcinoma on biopsy. (Courtesy of Andrea Wolf, personal collection.)

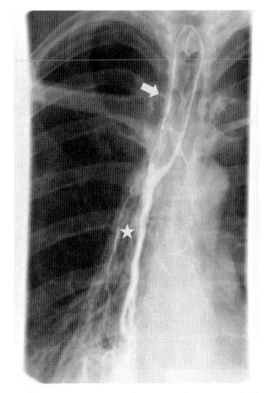

Figure 13.3 Esophagram following Ivor Lewis esophagectomy depicting proximal esophagus (arrow) and gastric conduit (star). (Courtesy of Andrea Wolf, personal collection.)

Additional material for this chapter can be found online at:
www.wiley.com/go/oh/mountsinaioncology

This includes advice for patients, a case study, ICD codes, and
multiple choice questions.

CHAPTER 14

Anal Cancer

Ashley J. D'Silva, Danielle S. Seiden, and Peter S. Kozuch
Icahn School of Medicine at Mount Sinai, New York, NY, USA

OVERALL BOTTOM LINE

- The incidence of anal cancer has been increasing over the past 30 years.
- Close association with human papillomavirus (HPV) infection and HIV. HPV anal infection also increases significantly in cases of concomitant HIV infection: HPV prevalence was 45% for any HPV genotypes in 305 HIV-infected men who have sex with men (MSM) in Taiwan compared with 18% ($p < 0.001$) in HIV-uninfected MSM ($p < 0.001$).
- Concurrent radiotherapy with infusional 5-FU and mitomycin is the standard of care and cure is possible in the majority of patients with preservation of the anal sphincter. Based on limited trial data supporting its efficacy and favorable tolerability, capecitabine is increasingly being substituted for 5-FU. A study evaluated 66 patients treated with mitomycin at 12 mg/m^2 on day 1, week 1 with median capecitabine dose of 825 mg/m^2 orally twice daily on radiation days. Capecitabine dose reductions because of toxicity were recorded for 13 patients (20%). At a median follow-up of 20 months, 94% of patients with squamous cell histology had no evidence of relapse.
- Surgery (abdominoperineal resection) is reserved for those with recurrent or persistent disease after chemoradiotherapy and offers a chance for long-term disease control and survival.

Background
Definition of disease

- Anal cancer can be divided into two categories based on histopathologic region: the anal canal and the anal margin (Figure 14.1).
- In clinical practice, anal cancers are further classified based upon treatment modality and physical location of origin:
  - Well-differentiated anal margin cancers that are T1N0 can be managed surgically if the anal canal is uninvolved
  - Anal canal lesions are the most common type of anal cancer and should be managed with chemoradiation
  - SCC of the rectum should be treated as if they are SCC of the anal canal
  - SCC of the perianal skin, which is often treated with chemoradiation, can be treated with local excision if the lesion is discrete from the anal verge
  - Other rare types of anal cancer include adenocarcinoma, melanoma, sarcoma, and lymphoma; these types are beyond the scope of this chapter.
- SCC that arises from the squamocolumnar junction can be further characterized as keratinizing (basaloid) or nonkeratinizing (cloacogenic).

Mount Sinai Expert Guides: Oncology, First Edition. Edited by William K. Oh and Ajai Chari.
© 2019 John Wiley & Sons Ltd. Published 2019 by John Wiley & Sons Ltd.
Companion Website: www.wiley.com/go/oh/mountsinaioncology

Disease classification

While the anal canal can be defined histologically, anatomically, and functionally, as of 2016 the management of epithelial cancers that involve the anal canal is the same. It is the region defined by the sphincter muscles, composed primarily of squamous epithelium, which has a superior border of a 1–2 cm zone between the rectal and anal epithelium. The inferior border is the anal verge, where epidermoid epithelium of the anal margin begins. Anal margin, including the perianal skin, is a 5–6 cm radius extending from the squamous mucocutaneous junction.

Incidence/prevalence

- There are 1.8 per 100 000 new cases of anal cancer, accounting for 0.2% of all cancer deaths.
- An estimated 7270 new cases were expected in 2015, with a lifetime risk of 0.2% (http://seer .cancer.gov/statfacts/html/anus.html).
- In the HIV population, the incidence has increased from 19 per 100 000 in 1992–1995 to 78.2 during 2000–2003, and 131 per 100 000 for HIV-positive MSM in North America. The reason for this is partially attributable to the survival benefit achieved by highly active antiretroviral therapy (HAART) and also to its lack of impact on the development of precancerous lesions.

Economic impact

- HPV vaccination is still very much in its infancy, but it is hypothesized that with the reduction of HPV infection, the incidence of HPV-driven anal cancer will be reduced.
- Anal Papanicolaou (Pap) smears with subsequent high-resolution anoscopy for abnormal findings should be performed for high risk populations. New York State guidelines recommend including HIV patients aged 60–74 who are MSM, have a history of anal condylomas, and women with abnormal cervical and/or vulvar histology. This annual practice can lead to identification and treatment of high grade anal intraepithelial neoplasia (AIN).
- The anal Pap smears enable identification of high grade squamous intraepithelial lesions (HSIL). Early identification allows patients to have a choice between topical ablative therapy or active monitoring. A large phase 3 randomized control trial examining time to anal cancer amongst those receiving topical or ablative therapy versus active monitoring will be completed in 2022. This trial will help elucidate whether topical or ablative treatment versus active monitoring can help prevent patients from developing anal cancer.

Etiology

- Squamous carcinomas of the anus are primarily HPV derived, in particular high risk HPV such as HPV 16 and 18. Based on a study in Denmark and Sweden, it was estimated that 84% of anal carcinoma was attributable to HPV.
- When the immune system is suppressed by immunosuppressive agents or by HIV infection, HPV infection is more likely to persist in the anal region.
- High grade AIN may be a precursor to anal carcinoma. It can be identified by cytology, biopsy, high-resolution anoscopy, DRE, or HPV testing. Progression rates to cancer may be low, and the regression rate is unknown; however, various treatments can have substantial benefits. Treatment with electrocautery, which is superior in intra-anal lesions, has been shown to have the ability to control disease in up to 80% of patients. Treatment with superficial topical imiquimod, which has better response in perianal, widespread, multifocal disease, can result in pathologic resolution in HIV-positive MSM who are on HAART. Preliminary data concerning use of topical 5-FU have been shown to result in an overall response rate of 57%. Regardless, routine screening in low risk individuals remains controversial.

Pathology/pathogenesis

- While several subclassifications of SCC of the anus have been identified, no significant difference in outcomes have been identified and these histologies are collectively referred to and managed as SCC of the anal canal.
- HPV infection of the anal canal with oncogenic strains (HPV 16) denotes a link between sexual activity and anal cancer. There is a close association noted in the premalignant and malignant lesions with not only the anogenital tract, but also with oropharyngeal cancers. HPV infection can manifest clinically as condylomata or a subclinical entity. High grade AIN is thought be the precursor of anal cancer and progression to invasive carcinoma is multifactorial and has a correlation with HIV seropositivity, low CD4 counts, type of HPV, and the quantity of high risk HPV in the anal canal.
- Chronic immunosuppression associated with active HIV, immunosuppression resulting from solid organ transplant or chronic immunosuppressive treatment for autoimmune diseases are all correlated with higher rates of progression of AIN to SCC.

Predictive/risk factors

Risk factor	Odds ratio
HPV	HPV is the largest risk factor for anal cancer, though there are no odds ratios pertaining to this risk because HPV infection is not typically known prior to discovery of a lesion related to HPV (CIN, AIN, etc.)
HIV	28.8
Men who are not exclusively heterosexual	17.3
Women with history of cervical intraepithelial neoplasia	16.4
≥15 sexual partners in lifetime	Men: 5.3; Women: 11.0
Organ transplant recipients	5.9
Smoking	3.9
History of genital warts	3.1
Anal receptive sex	2.3

Prevention

CLINICAL PEARLS
- HPV vaccination can prevent disease occurrence. The Centers for Disease Control (CDC) currently recommends quadrivalent HPV vaccination for all girls and boys aged 11–12. It is also recommended that any female between 13 and 26 years who has not been previously vaccinated receive the vaccine. Any male from 13 to 21 years who has not been previously vaccinated is also recommended to receive the vaccine. MSM or those who are immunosuppressed are recommended to have the vaccine up until age 26. Early data shows that the HPV vaccination can prevent development of cervical lesions related to HPV in up to 98% of women. A study in the *Journal of Infectious Disease* has shown that the vaccination has reduced the prevalence of HPV by 56% among women aged 14–19. There are not yet any

specific data concerning the HPV vaccine and its effect on anal cancer, but evidence from the studies previously mentioned can be extrapolated until more data matures.
• Preliminary data from an ongoing clinical trial studying the use of an antiviral drug, ranpirnase, for treatment of HPV has shown promise. The drug may have the ability to eradicate anal condylomas completely, which have been significantly associated with development of anal cancer. Further investigation will be necessary to prove this drug's application in the context of anal cancer.

Screening
• Although there are no national or international screening guidelines for anal cancer, there are New York State Department of Health guidelines for anal cytology screening in HIV-infected individuals.
• Anal cytology screening should be completed annually in HIV-infected patients who (i) are MSM; (ii) have a history of anogenital condylomas; (iii) are women with abnormal cervical and/or vulvar histology (http://www.hivguidelines.org/clinical-guidelines/adults/anal-dysplasia-and-cancer/).

Primary prevention
• Use of condoms and education about proper use of condoms has been shown to reduce incidence of HIV infection by 80%. Given that HIV is a risk factor for anal cancer (odds ratio 28.8), use of condoms can be a factor in the reduction of rates of anal cancer.
• Vaccination against HPV has been proven to prevent cervical lesions caused by HPV. Given that the vast majority of anal cancers are HPV derived (similar to cervical cancer rates), administration of the HPV vaccine can prevent the formation of anal cancer, although we do not yet have specific data.

Secondary prevention
• DRE should be performed 8–12 weeks after completion of definitive treatment. Those with persistent disease should be examined again 4 weeks later (clinical response can be noted up to 6 months after completion of CRT) to assess for further regression.
• DRE, anoscopy, and inguinal node palpation every 3–6 months.
• For those with slow regression or locally advanced disease (stage III based on TNM staging), annual chest, abdominal, and pelvic imaging is recommended for 3 years.

Diagnosis (Algorithm 14.1)

BOTTOM LINE/CLINICAL PEARLS
• It is important to ask patients with known risk factors about any history of rectal bleeding, anorectal pain, or fecal incontinence.
• Patients who endorse symptoms of rectal bleeding, anorectal pain or pruritus, a self-detected anal mass, or fecal incontinence should have complete physical examination that includes a DRE and directed biopsies or Pap smear for cytology.
• Patients who have masses identified on DRE should have follow-up anoscopic or protoscopic evaluation and biopsies, and appropriate surveillance and follow-up of any cytologic atypia.

Algorithm 14.1 Diagnosis of anal cancer

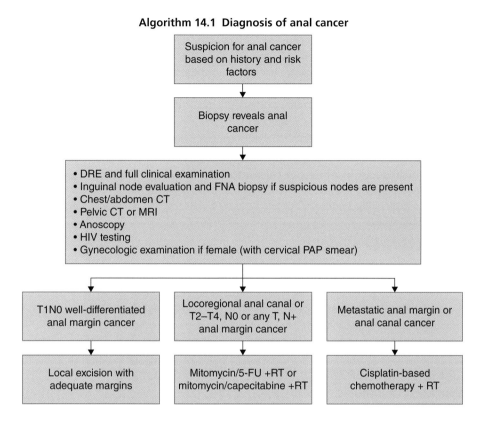

Differential diagnosis

Differential diagnosis	Features
Hemorrhoids	Bleeding
Anal fissure	Pain and bleeding
Polyps	Mass on examination

Typical presentation

The typical patient with anal cancer will present with rectal bleeding with or without anorectal discomfort or pain. Rectal bleeding occurs in nearly half of patients, while 30% have symptoms of pain or sensation of a mass, and the remaining 20% have no tumor-associated symptomatology. A history of anorectal condyloma is present in approximately half of homosexual men with SCC and one-third of women, which is significantly higher than the general population.

Clinical diagnosis

History

- Assess for signs and symptoms of impending bowel obstruction (exceptionally rare in anal cancer) and anemia and document any new or evolving genitourinary or bowel dysfunction. Ask about anal discharge, irritation, pruritus, or tenesmus.
- Assess for known risk factors (receptive anal intercourse, HIV positivity, IV drug use, cigarette smoking, immunosuppression).

Physical examination

- Careful inspection of perianal skin looking for tumor-associated fistulas to the perianal skin or direct extension to the perianal skin. Patients with anal canal cancers may also have concurrent condylomas. Also inspect and palpate genitals looking for additional condylomata or lesions suspicious for neoplasia.
- DRE assessing for sphincter tone and function and estimate of tumor mass and tethering or fixation to deep structures (prostate, seminal vesicles). Assess for inguinal lymphadenopathy.
- Women should have a gynecologic evaluation including screening for cervical cancer.

Useful clinical decision rules and calculators

- If inguinal adenopathy is noted, a FNA of the node is recommended.
- PET imaging should be performed for any T2–4,N0 lesion, or any size primary with suspected lymph node metastases.
- HIV and CD4 testing is encouraged.

Disease severity classification

- The AJCC and the International Union Against Cancer (IUAC) TNM system for anal carcinoma is based on tumor size, invasion of adjacent structures, nodal and distant metastases.
- The tumor's size and nodal involvement are the main prognostic indicators.
- In patients with AJCC stage I, the 5-year OS is 70%, while the OS for stage IV disease is 19%.
- OS and locoregional failure are also adversely correlated with palpable adenopathy and male sex.

Laboratory diagnosis

List of diagnostic tests

- Complete blood count.
- Complete metabolic panel.
- Consider HIV testing with CD4 count in patients at high risk.

Lists of imaging techniques

- CT of chest/abdomen/pelvis.
- MRI of abdomen and pelvis as an alternative to CT of abdomen and pelvis.
- PET/CT: MRI/CT is suboptimal in detecting inguinal nodal metastases (which can be <5 mm), as well as occult metastatic disease. Completion of PET/CT results in an upstaging in approximately one-third of patients indicating higher dose radiotherapy to the groin.

Potential pitfalls/common errors made regarding diagnosis of disease

- Rectal bleeding or perianal pruritus or even identified masses can be attributed to hemorrhoids thus delaying diagnosis.
- SCC of the perianal skin (anal margin) should be staged and classified as skin cancers. T1,N0 patients can be treated with wide local excision with adjuvant radiation for high risk histologic features. Patients with T2 lesions or nodal involvement should be treated with definitive chemoradiation.
- Anal canal cancers that are resected or identified at the time of hemorrhoidectomy should still be treated with curative intent chemoradiation, even if the resection margin is uninvolved. These cancers can still be associated with regional (perirectal or inguinal) nodal metastases. Local resection of even small (<1 cm) SCC of the anal canal is insufficient treatment.

Treatment (Algorithms 14.2 and 14.3)

Algorithm 14.2 Management of anal cancer

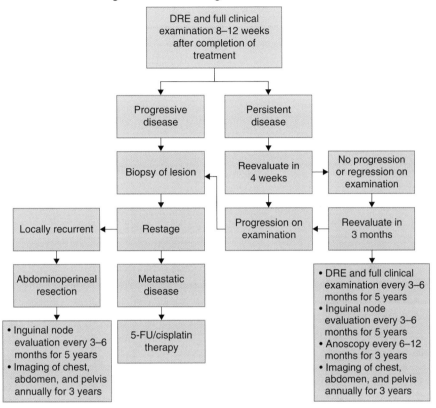

Algorithm 14.3 Management of recurrence of anal cancer

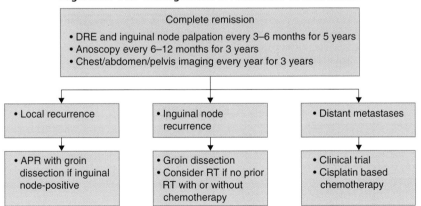

Treatment rationale

- **Localized disease:** radiation with concurrent infusional 5-FU 1000 mg/m^2 on days 1–4 and 29–32, plus mitomycin 10 mg/m^2 on days 1 and 29. A reasonable alternative is capecitabine 825 mg/m^2 PO twice daily given on Monday–Friday throughout radiation plus mitomycin

10 mg/m^2 IV on days 1 and 29. For elderly patients, and for those patients with poorly controlled HIV, there is a dearth of data. Expert opinion, however, suggests dose reduction of mitomycin ranging from 5 to 8 mg/m^2 has efficacy with decreased toxicity along with either 5-FU or capecitabine.

- **Locally advanced disease:** T3/T4 primary tumors or N2/N3 disease are treated similarly to localized disease, but with a 10–14 Gy radiotherapy boost given in 2-Gy fractions (55–59 Gy vs. 45 Gy for localized disease).
- **Recurrent/persistent disease:** should be salvaged with curative surgery (abdominoperineal resection) though there is significant morbidity. Long-term disease control is achieved in only 25–40% of patients. The efficacy of nonsurgical salvage is not known.
- **Metastatic disease:** infusional 5-FU 1000 mg/m^2/day continuous days 1–5 with cisplatin 75–100 mg/m^2 on day 2, repeat cycle every 4 weeks or modified FOLFOX 6 which consists of oxaliplatin 85 mg/m^2 IV, bolus and 46-hour infusional 5-FU 400 mg/m^2 and 2400 mg/m^2, respectively, along with biomodulating leucovorin 20 mg/m^2, cycles repeated every 2 weeks until disease progression.
- Akin to metachronous metastatic relapse of colorectal cancer, isolated liver metastases treated surgically or with local ablative procedures – or in the case of para-aortic disease radiation – may benefit a subset of patients.
- Ongoing phase 2 International Multicenter InterAACT study is comparing cisplatin with 5-FU to carboplatin with paclitaxel in patients with inoperable locally recurrent or metastatic SCC of the anus. The aim of this trial is to compare response rates, but it is also measuring PFS, OS, toxicity, and overall quality of life in these patients. No regimens thus far have demonstrated efficacy once metastatic disease has progressed on cisplatin-based therapy.

Table of treatment

Treatment	Comments
Conservative *Local excision*	Perianal SCC <2 cm can be managed with local excision with postoperative radiation or CRT for high risk features or inadequate margins
Medical *Local with concurrent radiotherapy* 5-FU 1000 mg/m^2 continuous infusion days 1–4 and 29–32 with mitomycin 10 mg/m^2 on days 1 and 29 *or* Capecitabine 825 mg/m^2 PO twice daily Mon–Fri given throughout radiation with mitomycin 10 mg/m^2 IV on days 1 and 29 *or* Capecitabine 825 mg/m^2 PO twice daily x 6 weeks with mitomycin 12 mg/m^2 IV on day 1 *Metastatic disease* 5-FU 1000 mg/m^2 continuous infusion on days 1–5 with cisplatin 100 mg/m^2 IV on day 2, repeat cycle every 4 weeks	ACT I trial confirmed that chemo-RT with 5-FU and mitomycin was more effective in controlling local disease than RT alone (relative risk 0.54; 95% CI 0.42–0.69; $p < 0.0001$) In a phase 3 intergroup study, patients receiving chemo-RT with the combination of 5-FU and mitomycin had a lower colostomy rate (9% vs. 22%; $p = 0.002$) and a higher 4-year disease-free survival (73% vs. 51%; $p = 0.0003$) than patients receiving chemo-RT with 5-FU alone Capecitabine, an oral fluoropyrimidine prodrug, is an accepted alternative to 5-FU in the treatment. Data is retrospective, but patients had less grade 3–4 hematologic toxicity HPV- and/or p16-positivity are prognostic for improved OS in patients with anal carcinoma Conflicting data, however, suggest patients with HIV may have higher local relapse rates and greater skin toxicity, but there is no difference in complete response or OS at 5 years

(*Continued*)

Treatment	Comments
Surgical *Abdominoperineal resection (APR)*	Patients with persistent or recurrent disease can have long-term disease control with salvage APR
Radiologic CT of the chest/abdomen/pelvis MRI of the abdomen/pelvis PET/CT scan	All patients should have a CT of the chest and either a CT or MRI of the abdomen/pelvis PET scan should be carried out for all patients as nodal staging is often adjusted after PET imaging
Psychologic Treatment can be difficult with significant pain and bowel and genitourinary toxicity resulting in hospitalization	Aggressive pain control and recognition of toxicities of treatment can help optimize compliance and potentially lead to better outcomes

Prevention/management of complications

- Diarrhea: can be quite significant and require aggressive supportive measures with loperamide and diphenoxylate.
- Oral mucositis from 5-FU: pain control, monitor for infection.
- Erythema/desquamation: topical lidocaine, stool softeners titrated to soft, comfortable bowel regimens, silver sulfadiazine cream (this must be applied several hours after each RT fraction), topical lidocaine, sitz baths, and oral analgesia including narcotic analgesia.
- 3D-CRT and IMRT are newer treatment modalities that can achieve high degrees of accuracy while reducing risks of radiation toxicity related to healthy tissue exposure, such as femoral head necrosis.
- There have been reports of hemolytic–uremic syndrome related to mitomycin C therapy. This can occur at any time during therapy. Most cases, however, occur with cumulative lifetime exposure to 60 mg/m^2 or more.
- There have been rare occurrences of Takotsubo cardiomyopathy related to mitomycin C administration as well as very infrequent cases with 5-FU and capecitabine administration. Additionally, there can be an association between 5-FU use and Prinzmetal angina. Patients should seek immediate medical attention if they experience signs and symptoms related to cardiac dysfunction.

Special populations
Pregnancy

- Chemotherapy and radiation are typically delayed in a pregnant patient found to have anal cancer. Shared decision-making concerning the patient's choices is the best approach to this unique situation.

Elderly

- Consider using capecitabine instead of infusional 5-FU to reduce grade 3 or 4 hematologic toxicity (provide supporting data and efficacy/toxicity outcomes).
- Dose reduction in mitomycin to 7–8 mg/m^2 (provide supporting data and efficacy/toxicity outcomes).

Others
HIV-positive patients

- In general, HIV-positive patients who are stable on antiretroviral therapy should exhibit good responses to standard treatment. However, there are reports that patients with low CD4 counts

or histories of HIV/AIDS-related complications may have difficulty tolerating full-dose therapy or mitomycin treatment. Dose adjustment may be necessary in these patients.
- CD4 counts should be monitored within 2–3 weeks of starting therapy and then every 6–8 weeks until normalized.
- HIV-positive patients will also require prophylaxis for opportunistic infections while undergoing treatment.

Prognosis

> **BOTTOM LINE/CLINICAL PEARLS**
> - The overall 5-year survival rate in the USA is 60% for men and 78% for women.
> - Prognosis is inversely related to disease stage, thus early detection is very important in anal cancer.
> - Studies have found that the following factors have been associated with worse OS: male gender, increased tumor diameter, positive lymph nodes, and cigarette smoking.

Natural history of untreated disease
- If left untreated, anal cancer can spread through direct invasion of adjacent structures, lymphatic dissemination through perirectal, inguinal, and pelvic lymph nodes, as well as hematogenous spread to distant organs.

Prognosis for treated patients
- Prognosis largely depends upon TNM staging. Patients who are diagnosed with stage I anal cancer have overall 5-year survival rates of 70%. Having stage II disease decreases that rate to 59%, stage III to 41%, and stage IV disease is associated with a 19% 5-year survival rate.
- The most recent data from RTOG 9811 has shown that patients treated with radiotherapy plus 5-FU/mitomysin have OS rates of 78.3% and DFS rates of 67.8%. Patients treated with RT plus 5-FU/cisplatin have OS rates of 70.7% and DFS rates of 57.8%.

Follow-up tests and monitoring
- For all patients who have achieved complete remission, the following should be performed every 3–6 months for 5 years:
  - DRE
  - Anoscopic evaluation (with re-biopsy if persistent lesion, and anal cytology to confirm lesion clearance)
  - Inguinal node palpation.
- For those patients who had been staged at T3/T4 or had positive inguinal nodes upon diagnosis, imaging of the chest/abdomen/pelvis should be completed annually for 3 years.

Reading list
Ahmed S, Eng C. Optimal treatment strategies for anal cancer. Current Treat Options Oncol 2014;15:443–455.
Ajani JA, Winter KA, Gunderson LL, et al. Prognostic factors derived from a prospective database dictate clinical biology of anal cancer. Cancer 2010;116:4007–4013.
Baricevic I, He X, Chakrabarty B, et al. High-sensitivity human papilloma virus genotyping reveals near universal positivity in anal squamous cell carcinoma: different implications for vaccine prevention and prognosis. Eur J Cancer 2015;51:776–785.
Cheng SH, Chu FY, Lin YS, et al. Influence of age and CD4+ T cell counts on the prevalence of genital human papillomavirus infection among HIV-seropositive men who have sex with men in Taiwan. J Med Virol 2012;84:1876–1883.

Clark MA, Hartley A, Geh JI. Cancer of the anal canal. Lancet Oncol 2004;5:149–157.

Daling JR, Madeleine MM, Johnson LG, et al. Human papillomavirus, smoking, and sexual practices in the etiology of anal cancer. Cancer 2014;101:270–280.

Flejou JF. An update on anal neoplasia. Histopathology 2015;66:147–160.

Klas JV, Rothenberger DA, Wong WD, et al. Malignant tumors of the anal canal: the spectrum of disease, treatment, and outcomes. Cancer 1999;85:1686–1693.

Mitchell MP, Abboud M, Eng C, et al. Intensity-modulated radiation therapy with concurrent chemotherapy for anal cancer: outcomes and toxicity. Am J Clin Oncol 2014;37:461–466.

Shridhar R, Shibata D, Chan E, et al. Anal cancer: current standards in care and recent changes in practice. CA Cancer J Clin 2015;65:139–162.

Suggested websites

American Cancer Society: http://www.cancer.org/cancer/analcancer/detailedguide/anal-cancer-what-is-anal-cancer

Guidelines
National society guidelines

Title	Source and comment	Date and weblink
NCCN Clinical Practice Guidelines in Oncology for Anal Carcinoma	National Comprehensive Cancer Network **Comment:** Investigation and management of squamous cell anal carcinoma	2012 http://www.nccn.org/professionals/physician_gls/pdf/anal.pdf
Practice Parameters for Anal Squamous Neoplasms	Standards Practice Task Force of the American Society of Colon and Rectal Surgeons **Comment:** Guidelines for the evaluation and treatment of squamous cell anal carcinoma	2012 https://www.fascrs.org/sites/default/files/downloads/publication/practice_parameters_for_anal_squamous_neoplasms.21.pdf

International society guidelines

Title	Source and comment	Date and weblink
Anal Cancer: ESMO-ESSO-ESTRO Clinical Practice Guidelines	European Society for Medical Oncology **Comment:** Clinical practice guidelines for diagnosis, management, and follow-up for squamous cell anal carcinoma	2014 https://www.esmo.org/Guidelines/Gastrointestinal-Cancers/Anal-Cancer

Evidence

Type of evidence	Title and comment	Date and weblink
RCT	Epidermoid anal cancer: results from the UKCCCR randomized trial of radiotherapy alone versus radiotherapy, 5-fluorouracil, and mitomycin	1996 https://www.ncbi.nlm.nih.gov/pubmed/8874455

(Continued)

Type of evidence	Title and comment	Date and weblink
	Comment: This landmark trial (ACT I) confirmed that the standard treatment for anal cancer should be radiotherapy in combination with infused fluorouracil and mitomycin	
RCT	Role of mitomycin in combination with fluorouracil and radiotherapy, and of salvage chemoradiation in the definitive nonsurgical treatment of epidermoid carcinoma of the anal canal: results of a phase III randomized intergroup study **Comment:** This study confirmed the importance of mitomycin in the standard chemoradiation treatment regimen for anal cancer.	1996 https://www.ncbi.nlm.nih.gov/pubmed/?term=DOI%3A+10.1200%2FJCO.1996.14.9.2527
RCT	Fluorouracil, mitomycin, and radiotherapy vs. fluorouracil, cisplatin and radiotherapy for carcinoma of the anal canal: a randomized controlled trial **Comment:** This trial confirmed that mitomycin is superior to cisplatin for use in combination with fluorouracil and radiation	2008 https://www.ncbi.nlm.nih.gov/pubmed/18430910
RCT	Mitomycin or cisplatin chemoradiation with or without maintenance chemotherapy for treatment of squamous-cell carcinoma of the anus (ACT II): a randomised, phase 3, open-label, 2 × 2 factorial trial **Comment:** This trial (ACT II) was a follow up to ACT I that confirmed that the treatment regimen should remain the same	2013 https://www.ncbi.nlm.nih.gov/pubmed/23578724
Clinical trial	5-FU and cisplatin combination chemotherapy for metastatic squamous-cell anal cancer **Comment:** This trial of a fluoruracil with cisplatin found that the combination resulted in a high response rate in patients with metastatic anal cancer	1999 https://www.ncbi.nlm.nih.gov/pubmed/10572237

Image

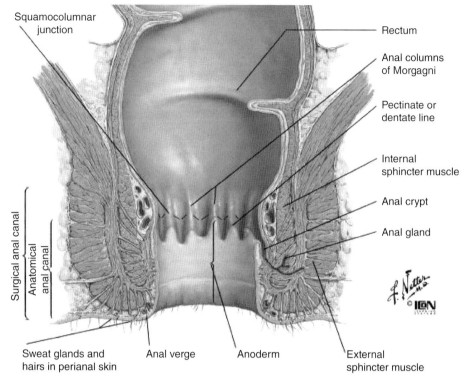

Squamocolumnar junction

Rectum

Anal columns of Morgagni

Pectinate or dentate line

Internal sphincter muscle

Anal crypt

Anal gland

Surgical anal canal

Anatomical anal canal

Sweat glands and hairs in perianal skin

Anal verge

Anoderm

External sphincter muscle

Figure 14.1 Anatomy of the anal canal. The anal canal is divided by the dentate or pectinate line, which marks the transition from glandular or columnar epithelial cells of the rectal mucosa to squamous epithelial cells of the anal mucosa. This line is also known as the transitional zone. The anal verge corresponds to the transition from squamous mucosa to epidermal-lined perianal skin. Most anal cancers arise from the transitional zone or the squamous cell mucosa. (Source: Netter FH. Atlas of Human Anatomy. Philadelphia, PA: Saunders/Elsevier, 2006: 373. Reproduced with permission.)

Additional material for this chapter can be found online at: www.wiley.com/go/oh/mountsinaioncology

This includes advice to patients, a case study, ICD codes, and multiple choice questions.

CHAPTER 15

Invasive Epithelial Ovarian Cancer

Brittney S. Zimmerman[1], Jeannette Guziel[2], and Amy Tiersten[1]
[1] Icahn School of Medicine at Mount Sinai, New York, NY, USA
[2] Southern California Permanente Medical Group, Woodland Hills, CA, USA

OVERALL BOTTOM LINE
- Ovarian cancer is the leading cause of death from gynecologic cancer in the USA and the fifth most common cause of cancer mortality in females.
- The incidence of ovarian cancer increases with age. The average age at diagnosis of ovarian cancer in the USA is 63 years. The age at diagnosis of ovarian cancer is younger among women with a hereditary ovarian cancer syndrome.
- The majority of ovarian cancers are diagnosed at an advanced stage: confined to primary site (15%); regional lymph nodes (17%); distant metastases (61%); and unstaged (7%).
- Ovarian cancer is a very chemo-responsive disease and advances in therapies have resulted in improved survival.

Background
Definition of disease
- Ovarian cancer is a type of cancer that begins in the ovaries. The majority of ovarian cancers arise from the epithelium (outer lining) of the ovary.
- This chapter focuses mainly on epithelial ovarian cancer (EOC).

Disease classification
- Epithelial ovarian malignancies include serous, mucinous, endometrioid, and clear cell tumors. Serous is the most common subtype.
- Other ovarian cell types are germ cell tumors and sex cord-stromal tumors.
- Serous carcinoma is regarded as closely related to fallopian tube and peritoneal serous carcinoma, based upon similarities in histology and clinical behavior.
- Borderline ovarian tumors do not invade underlying stroma and are of low malignant potential. Prognosis is excellent and surgical resection is the treatment of choice. Stage III disease has 80% survival at 5 years. If it recurs or invades, then treat with systemic therapy.

Incidence/prevalence
- Worldwide, 225 000 women were diagnosed with ovarian cancer and 140 000 died from this disease in 2008.
- In the USA, approximately 22 000 cases were diagnosed in 2018 with 14 000 deaths. This makes ovarian cancer the second most common gynecologic malignancy, the most common cause of gynecologic cancer death, and the fifth leading cause of cancer death in women.
- The lifetime risk of developing ovarian cancer is 1.4%.

Mount Sinai Expert Guides: Oncology, First Edition. Edited by William K. Oh and Ajai Chari.
© 2019 John Wiley & Sons Ltd. Published 2019 by John Wiley & Sons Ltd.
Companion Website: www.wiley.com/go/oh/mountsinaioncology

Ovarian cancer pathology[a]	Frequency (%)
Epithelial carcinoma	90
Germ cell neoplasms	2
Stromal tumors	7
Miscellaneous	1

[a]This chapter focuses on investigation, diagnosis, and treatment of invasive epithelial ovarian cancer.

Epithelial ovarian cancer	Frequency (%)
Serous	46
Endometrioid	16
Mucinous[a]	13
Clear cell[a]	7
Undifferentiated	18

[a]Poorer prognosis and poor response to chemotherapy than serous.

Etiology

- It is unclear what causes ovarian cancer but age (>50 years), reproductive factors, and genetic factors all have a role.

Predictive/risk factors

Risk factor	Relative risk
Increasing age	
Late age at menopause (>52 years vs. <45 years)	1.46
Infertility	2.76
Endometriosis	2.04–3.05
Polycystic ovarian syndrome	2.16
Use of an intrauterine device	1.76
Cigarette smoking (for mucinous carcinomas)	2.1
Genetic factors: *BRCA1, BRCA2, BRIP1, RAD51C, RAD51D*, Mismatch Repair Mutations	

- **Lifetime risk if positive family history:** one second degree relative (3%), one first degree relative (5%), two first degree relatives (11%).
- **Genetics:** several susceptibility genes have been identified for epithelial ovarian cancer (10–15% of ovarian cancer) (Figure 15.1; Boxes 15.1 and 15.2).
  - ***BRCA1:*** 70% of hereditary ovarian cancer (lifetime risk of ovarian cancer 40–60%)
  - ***BRCA2:*** 20% of hereditary ovarian cancer (lifetime risk 15–25%)

- *Mismatch repair genes (HNPCC):* 2% of hereditary ovarian cancer (lifetime risk 6–20%)
- The likelihood of identifying a *BRCA1/2* mutation in a woman with ovarian cancer at any age is approximately 13–18%.
- Per the most recent NCCN guidelines, any patient at any age diagnosed with ovarian cancer should undergo testing for BRCA1/2 mutations and genetic risk evaluation.

BOX 15.1 US PREVENTIVE SERVICES TASK FORCE (USPSTF) RECOMMENDATIONS ON WHO SHOULD BE OFFERED GENETIC TESTING FOR *BRCA* MUTATIONS*

For non-Ashkenazi Jewish women:
- Two first degree relatives with breast cancer, one of whom was diagnosed at age 50 or younger
- A combination of three or more first or second degree relatives with breast cancer regardless of age at diagnosis
- A combination of both breast and ovarian cancer among first and second degree relatives
- A first degree relative with bilateral breast cancer
- A combination of two or more first or second degree relatives with ovarian cancer, regardless of age at diagnosis
- A first or second degree relative with both breast and ovarian cancer at any age
- History of breast cancer in a male relative

For women of Ashkenazi Jewish descent:
- Any first degree relative (or two second degree relatives on the same side of the family) with breast or ovarian cancer

* These recommendations do not apply to women with a family history of breast or ovarian cancer that includes a relative with a known deleterious *BRCA* mutation.

BOX 15.2 RISK ASSESSMENT CRITERIA FOR HEREDITARY BREAST–OVARIAN CANCER SYNDROME

Referral should be considered for any individual with a personal history of or first degree relative with:
- Breast cancer diagnosed at or before age 50
- Triple negative breast cancer diagnosed at or before age 60
- Two or more primary breast cancers in the same person
- Ovarian, fallopian tube, or primary peritoneal cancer
- Ashkenazi Jewish ancestry and breast or pancreatic cancer at any age
- Male breast cancer
- Individuals with a family history of three or more cases of breast, ovarian, pancreatic, and/or aggressive prostate cancer (Gleason score ≥7)

Prevention

BOTTOM LINE/CLINICAL PEARLS
- **Protective factors** (factors that reduce the risk): multiple parity, history of breastfeeding, oral contraceptives, and tubal ligation.

Screening

- Women at average risk for ovarian cancer should *not* undergo screening. Data from the Prostate, Lung, Colorectal, and Ovarian (PLCO) Cancer Screening trial in the USA show no change in the stage of cancer detected by screening and no decrease in cancer-specific or overall mortality for women who underwent annual screening (4 years of transvaginal ultrasound [TVUS] and 6 years of CA-125 serum levels). More trials are underway.
- Recently, in the UK Collaborative Trial of Ovarian Cancer Screening, 46 237 women, aged 50 years or older, underwent incidence screening by using the multimodal strategy in which annual serum CA-125 was interpreted with the risk of ovarian cancer algorithm (ROCA). ROCA is a computerized algorithm that calculates the risks and benefits for women to be screened for ovarian cancer and divides women into three risk groups – low, intermediate, and high – based on changes in the CA-125 level. The algorithm accurately detected 86% of women with ovarian cancer, and ruled out almost 100% of women who were cancer-free. High risk women are tested further with TVUS and CA-125.
- Women with a family history of ovarian cancer or familial ovarian cancer syndromes are at higher risk of the disease and screening may be appropriate.
- For women with identified hereditary ovarian cancer syndromes, the Society of Gynecologic Oncology (SGO) and the NCCN recommend screening every 6 months with CA-125 and TVUS beginning between the ages of 30 and 35 years or 5–10 years earlier than the earliest age of first diagnosis of ovarian cancer in the family.

Primary prevention

- Avoiding risk factors and increasing protective factors may help to prevent cancer.
- Risk-reducing salpingo-oophorectomy (80% risk reduction) is recommended for women who have inherited *BRCA1* or *BRCA2* genes or have an inherited ovarian cancer syndrome as soon as childbearing is completed or by age 35–40. It can also decrease breast cancer risk in premenopausal *BRCA*-positive women.

Diagnosis

BOTTOM LINE/CLINICAL PEARLS
- Imaging of the abdominal cavity and measurement of the CA-125 level are obtained for diagnosis.
- Laparotomy with total abdominal hysterectomy/bilateral salpingo-oophorectomy (TAH/BSO) with comprehensive staging (inspection of all peritoneal surfaces, biopsy of suspicious areas/adhesions, omentectomy, pelvic and para-aortic lymph node dissection and maximal cytoreduction) is the primary procedure to establish diagnoses, assess disease extent, and to achieve maximal tumor cytoreduction.
- No gross residual disease is the goal of primary cytoreductive surgery. Optimal debulking is considered to be residual disease <1 cm maximum diameter or thickness and is strongly associated with OS.
- Cytology is performed on pelvic washings and the surface of the diaphragm; omentectomy is also performed.
- Less frequently (≈20%), the diagnosis is based upon tissue or fluid obtained via image-guided biopsy, paracentesis, or thoracentesis.

Differential diagnosis

Features	Differential diagnosis
Extraovarian mass	Ectopic pregnancy Hydrosalpinx or tubo-ovarian abscess Paraovarian cyst Peritoneal inclusion cyst Pedunculated fibroid Diverticular abscess Appendiceal abscess or tumor Fallopian tube cancer Inflammatory or malignant bowel disease Pelvic kidney
Ovarian mass	Simple or hemorrhagic physiologic cysts (e.g. follicular, corpus luteum) Endometrioma Theca lutein cysts Benign, malignant, or borderline neoplasms (e.g. epithelial, germ cell, sex-cord) Metastatic carcinoma (e.g. breast, colon, endometrium)

Typical presentation
- Often, symptoms do not appear until the cancer has spread.
- Acute presentation: typically patients with advanced disease present with a condition that requires urgent care and evaluation (e.g. pleural effusion, bowel obstruction).
- Subacute fashion: adnexal mass, pelvic or abdominal pain, bloating, dysuria, feeling full/early satiety, difficulty eating.
- Can be discovered at the time of surgery performed for another indication.

Clinical diagnosis
History
- Assess for symptoms of abdominal pain, bloating, and difficulty eating.
- Assess for a family history of cancer with special attention to a history of gynecologic or breast malignancies.

Physical examination
- Increasing abdominal girth/ascites.
- Pelvic mass.
- Pleural effusions.

Useful clinical decision rules and calculators
- EOC is surgically staged according to the Joint International Federation of Gynecology and Obstetrics (FIGO)/TNM classification system.
- FIGO Ovarian Cancer Staging (Tables 15.1–15.4).

Disease severity classification
- Prognostic factors: age, stage, volume of residual disease (<1 cm correlated with better OS), histologic grade and type, and performance status.

Table 15.1 Stage I: cancer confined to the ovaries.

IA	Tumor limited to one ovary, capsule intact, no tumor on surface, negative washings
IB	Tumor involves both ovaries otherwise like IA
IC	Tumor limited to one or both ovaries
IC1	Surgical spill
IC2	Capsule rupture before surgery or tumor on ovarian surface
IC3	Malignant cells in the ascites or peritoneal washings

Table 15.2 STAGE II: tumor involves one or both ovaries with pelvic extension (below the pelvic brim) or primary peritoneal cancer.

IIA	Extension and/or implant on uterus and/or fallopian tubes
IIB	Extension to other pelvic intraperitoneal tissues

Table 15.3 STAGE III: tumor involves one or both ovaries with cytologically or histologically confirmed spread to the peritoneum outside the pelvis and/or metastasis to the retroperitoneal lymph nodes.

IIIA	Positive retroperitoneal lymph nodes and/or microscopic metastasis beyond the pelvis
IIIA1	Positive retroperitoneal lymph nodes only IIIA1(i) Metastasis ≤10 mm IIIA1(ii) Metastasis >10 mm
IIIA2	Microscopic, extrapelvic (above the brim) peritoneal involvement ± positive retroperitoneal lymph nodes
IIIB	Macroscopic, extrapelvic, peritoneal metastasis ≤2 cm ± positive retroperitoneal lymph nodes Includes extension to capsule of liver/spleen
IIIC	Macroscopic, extrapelvic, peritoneal metastasis >2 cm ± positive retroperitoneal lymph nodes Includes extension to capsule of liver/spleen

Table 15.4 STAGE IV: distant metastasis excluding peritoneal metastasis.

IVA	Pleural effusion with positive cytology
IVB	Hepatic and/or splenic parenchymal metastasis, metastasis to extra-abdominal organs (including inguinal lymph nodes and lymph nodes outside of the abdominal cavity)

- Limited stage (stage I and II) risk groups:
  - **Low risk:** grade 1 disease, intracystic disease, no extraovarian disease, negative peritoneal disease, no ascites. Associated with a 10% chance of recurrence. *No benefit to adjuvant therapy.*
  - **High risk:** grade 2–3 disease, extracystic disease, extraovarian disease, positive peritoneal cytology, ascites. Associated with a 40% chance of recurrence. *Adjuvant platinum-based therapy is recommended.*

Laboratory diagnosis
List of diagnostic tests
- Increased CA-125 in 20% of early stage disease and 80% of advanced stage disease.

Lists of imaging techniques

- Ultrasound and/or abdominal pelvic CT/MRI and/or PET-CT as clinically indicated or to monitor response to treatment.

Treatment
Treatment rationale
Early stage disease = stage I (limited to ovaries) and II (limited to pelvis)

- Stage IA/B:
  - Grade 1: no adjuvant chemotherapy
  - Grade 2: consider IV taxane/carboplatin for 3–6 cycles
  - Grade 3/clear cell: IV taxane/carboplatin for 3–6 cycles.
- Stage IC: adjuvant IV taxane/carboplatin for 3–6 cycles.
- Stage II: adjuvant IV taxane/carboplatin for 6 cycles.

Advanced stage disease = stage III (intraperitoneal or nodal spread) and IV (distant disease)

- Adjuvant chemotherapy after maximal attempt at surgical cytoreduction is the standard of care treatment for advanced disease.
- IV paclitaxel/carboplatin with AUC 6 every 3 weeks became the standard adjuvant chemotherapy based on the following studies:
  - Paclitaxel/cisplatin is superior to cyclophosphamide/cisplatin. GOG 111 demonstrated a HR of 0.61 (95% CI 0.47–0.79) for OS favoring paclitaxel/cisplatin. This survival benefit was confirmed in the EORTC-NCIC OV10 trial.
  - Carboplatin/paclitaxel is at least equivalent in efficacy to cisplatin/paclitaxel with improved toxicity profile (AGO Trial, GOG 158).
- Weekly paclitaxel with carboplatin has been shown to improve OS when compared with every 3-week paclitaxel/carboplatin in addition to having better quality of life (QOL) and toxicity profile. Using weekly paclitaxel (vs. every 3 weeks) in combination with carboplatin is therefore also considered standard of care adjuvant therapy.
  - Japanese Trial (Katsumata et al. 2009): conventional carboplatin/paclitaxel (every 3 weeks, AUC 6) vs. dose dense (weekly paclitaxel, AUC 6), carboplatin/paclitaxel showed a PFS of 17 vs. 28 months ($p = 0.0014$) and a 65% vs. 72% 3-year OS ($p = 0.03$) all favoring dose dense therapy. Grade 3–4 anemia was more common in dose dense arm but other toxicities were not significant.
  - A confirmatory European trial ASCO 2013 (LBA 5501) comparing weekly carboplatin/paclitaxel with every 3 week regimen showed no difference in PFS but better QOL and toxicity with weekly paclitaxel.
  - GOG 262 reported at ESMO 2013 (weekly vs. every 3 week paclitaxel/carboplatin, bevacizumab optional) showed a better PFS in the weekly group (14 vs. 10 months; HR 0.60, 95% CI) if the patients did not receive bevacizumab, but there was no difference in survival.
  - A weekly carboplatin + weekly paclitaxel regimen based on the MITO-7 phase 3 trial may also be considered in poor performance status patients or patients with multiple comorbidities. Weekly carboplatin/paclitaxel yielded a similar PFS to standard of care with less toxicity and better QOL.
- Intraperitoneal (IP) chemotherapy is standard of care for small volume residual disease as issued by the NCI with the advantage of maximal drug delivery and an OS benefit.

- Three large randomized, phase 3 clinical trials of IP chemotherapy (GOG 104, 114, and 172) clearly demonstrated a superior PFS and OS with IP chemotherapy compared with IV chemotherapy.
- GOG 172 showed a 68 vs. 50 month median OS advantage for IP cisplatin/IP+IV paclitaxel vs. IV cisplatin/IV paclitaxel in optimally debulked stage III ovarian cancer.
- IP therapy is associated with greater grade 3–4 toxicities (myelosupression, metabolic abnormalities, catheter complications, bowel complications, abdominal pain), decreased compliance, and decreased QOL. However, at 12-month follow-up, the groups experienced no difference in QOL, except that paresthesias were more likely to persist in the IP arm.
- **IP therapy is therefore recommended only if there is a trained staff to administer it and only after careful patient selection with a discussion of risks and benefits.**
- The ongoing GOG 252 trial has enrolled patients with minimal residual disease ≤1 cm and will hopefully determine the optimal treatment in terms of efficacy and toxicity for advanced ovarian cancer incorporating both dose dense schedules and IP vs. IV regimens in the adjuvant setting. Treatment arms are as follows:
  - Paclitaxel 80 mg/m^2 IV weekly + carboplatin AUC 6 IV + bevacizumab
  - Paclitaxel 80 mg/m^2 IV weekly + carboplatin AUC 6 IP + bevacizumab
  - Paclitaxel 135 mg/m^2 IV over 3 hours day 1, cisplatin 75 mg/m^2 IP on day 2, paclitaxel 60 mg/m^2 IP on day 8 + bevacizumab.

Maintenance therapy in newly diagnosed advanced ovarian cancer (Table 15.5):
- Maintenance bevacizumab:
  - Bevacizumab can be added to adjuvant chemotherapy with an additional PFS benefit. If bevacizumab is given in the neoadjuvant setting, it should be held for 6 weeks prior to debulking surgery so as not to interfere with wound healing.
  - GOG 218 and ICON 7 showed a PFS advantage for the addition of bevacizumab to IV carboplatin/paclitaxel followed by bevacizumab maintenance, but no clear OS advantage.
- Maintenance pazopanib:
  - Pazopanib is an oral multi-kinase inhibitor against VEGF. In a phase III trial of 940 patients, maintenance pazopanib prolonged PFS compared with placebo, with no difference in OS.
- Maintenance PARP-inhibition:
  - In a recent study published in December 2018 for patients with advanced BRCA1/2 mutated high grade serous or endometroid ovarian cancer with complete or partial response to platinum based therapy, maintenance olaparib showed improved PFS, with a 70% lower risk of disease progression or death when compared with placebo.

Table 15.5 Summary of options for consolidation/maintenance after front-line therapy

Therapy	Trial (s)	Results	Conclusion
Bevacizumab Maintenance vs. placebo	GOG 218 ICON-7	Median PFS 14.1 vs. 10.3 months (GOG 218) No OS benefit (ICON-7)	Improvement in PFS No OS benefit
Pazopanib Maintenance vs. placebo	JCO 2014	Median PFS 17.9 vs 12.3 months	Improvement in PFS No OS benefit
Olaparib Maintenance vs. placebo (BRCA+patients)	SOLO1	Freedom from disease progression or death at 3 years, 60% vs. 27%; HR 0.30	Improvement in PFS (70% lower risk of disease progression or death)

Recurrent epithelial ovarian cancer

- The risk of recurrence after primary treatment:
  - Early stage, low risk = 10%
  - Early stage, high risk = 20% (after adjuvant therapy)
  - Low volume residual disease = 60–70%
  - Large volume residual disease = 80–85%.
- Most recurrences occur within the first 3 years.
- Each subsequent line of therapy in the recurrent setting is associated with shorter disease-free intervals.
- Treatment of recurrent disease is based on the platinum-free interval (PFI) and is dichotomized to:
  - **Platinum-sensitive = PFI >6 months**
  - **Platinum-resistant = PFI ≤6 months.**
  The PFI predicts the expected response rate and duration of response.
- Treatment is determined by response to first line therapy and PFI.
- There is no advantage to receiving early treatment based on a rising CA-125. Treatment should be based on progressive disease found on imaging or physical examination findings. CA-125 can, however, trigger further studies and/or imaging.
- **Platinum-sensitive disease:** retreat with carboplatin-based doublet (RR ≈ 60%, survival is 30+ months). Treat until progression of disease, unacceptable toxicity, or complete clinical response.
  - Oceans Trial in platinum-sensitive recurrent disease: improvement in median PFS (12.4 vs. 8.4 months) for carboplatin/gemcitabine + bevacizumab with bevacizumab maintenance vs. carboplatin/gemcitabine alone
  - All three PARP-inhibitors (olaparib, rucaparib, niraparib) are FDA approved for platinum-sensitive recurrent ovarian cancer regardless of BRCA status.
- **Platinum-resistant disease:** treat with alternative drug therapy (RR ≈ 12–32%, survival 8+ months). Treat until progression of disease, unacceptable toxicity, or complete clinical response. Single agent sequential therapies (i.e. paclitaxel, pemetrexed, 5-FU-LV) is preferred to combination because it may offer a potential balance between efficacy of treatment and an acceptable toxicity profile (Tables 15.6 and 15.7).
  - Can consider adding bevacizumab to chemotherapy (AURELIA trial)
  - Targeted agents: bevacizumab, olaparib, rucaparib

Table 15.6 Combination therapies in platinum-sensitive EOC.

Phase III Trial	Regimen	Median PFS (months)	Median OS (months)
ICON-4	Carboplatin vs. carboplatin/paclitaxel	9 vs. 12	24 vs. 29
AGO-AVAR	Carboplatin vs. carboplatin/gemcitabine	5.8 vs. 8.6	Not powered for OS
CALYPSO	Carboplatin/paclitaxel vs. carboplatin/pegylated liposomal doxorubicin	9.4 vs. 11.3	30.7 vs. 33
OCEANS	Carboplatin/gemcitabine vs. carboplatin/gemcitabine+ bevacizumab followed by bevacizumab maintenance	8 vs. 12	33 vs. 35

Table 15.7 Response rates to single
agent drugs in platinum-resistant
disease.

Drug	Response
Oral etoposide	11/42 (27%)
Topotecan	9/67 (24%)
Tamoxifen	10/77 (13%)
Ifosfamide	5/41 (12%)
Gemcitabine	6/27 (22%)
Liposomal doxorubicin	9/34 (29%)
Vinorelbine	5/24 (21%)

- Consider tamoxifen or aromatase inhibitors in cases of asymptomatic recurrence/rise in CA-125 (tamoxifen ~13% response rate, letrozole ~15% response rate).
- Bevacizumab in platinum-resistant recurrent disease:
  - AURELIA Trial: chemotherapy (investigator's choice) + bevacizumab vs. chemotherapy showed a PFS advantage of 3 months for the addition of bevacizumab in addition to improved RR (11.8% chemotherapy vs. 27.3% chemotherapy + bevacizumab).
- **PARP-inhibitors in platinum-resistant recurrent disease:**
  - Olaparib in *BRCA1* and *BRCA2* patients with chemo-refractory disease: approved for patients with advanced ovarian cancer who have received treatment with ≥3 lines of chemotherapy and who have a germline *BRCA* mutation.
  - FDA approved single agent olaparib in 2014 based on a study of 134 patients with germline BRCA mutations who had an ORR of 34% and median duration of response of 7.9 months.
  - An additional study by Kaufman et al. (2015) showed a response rate of 31% and 40% of patients had stable disease >8 weeks for patients with germline *BRCA* mutated ovarian cancer receiving single agent olaparib.
  - FDA approved single agent rucaparib in 2016 for the treatment of patients with deleterious *BRCA* mutation (germline and/or somatic) associated advanced ovarian cancer who progressed after ≥2 lines of chemotherapy. This was based on an ORR of 54% and median duration of response of 9.2 months.
  - FDA approved BRACAnalysis CDx (Myriad), a companion diagnostic that will detect the presence of *BRCA* mutations in blood samples from patients with ovarian cancer as well as FoundationFocus CDx BCRA test (Foundation Medicine, Inc) for detection of presence of BRCA mutations in tumor tissue.

Therapies under investigation

- PI3K/AKT inhibition
  - Overactivation of the PI3K/AKT pathway is implicated in carcinogenesis and has been shown to be activated in 45% of high grade serous ovarian cancer.
  - Novel AKT inhibitors have shown response rates ~30% in patients with platinum resistant ovarian cancer in combination with chemotherapy.
  - Phase II trials of AKT-inhibitors in combination with chemotherapy are ongoing.
- Immunotherapy
  - Presence of high tumor infiltrating lymphocytes has been associated with improved prognosis in patients with recurrent ovarian cancer. Over 60% of epithelial ovarian tumors stain strongly positive for PD-L1 which may provide an active target for therapy.

- Phase Ib-II trials have investigated the activity and safety of anti-PD1 or anti-PD-L1 mono-clonal antibodies in platinum-resistant epithelial ovarian cancer. ORR have ranged from 5.9% to 15%.
- Recent data published in 2019 showed some anti-tumor effect of pembrolizumab in advanced metastatic or pre-treated PD-L1 + ovarian cancer with RR 11.5% (KEYNOTE-028).
- Vaccine trials and trials of immunotherapy alone or in combination with chemotherapy or biologic agents are ongoing.

When to hospitalize

- Bowel obstruction.
- Febrile neutropenia.
- Dehydration.
- Pleural effusions.

Table of treatment (see also Table 15.8)

Treatment	Comments
Medical	
Chemotherapy following surgery Limited stage (I and II) Low risk: observation High risk: IV carboplatin/paclitaxel	
Advanced stage (III and IV) IV paclitaxel 175 mg/m^2/3 hours IV carboplatin AUC 6 Repeat every 3 weeks x 6 cycles *or* IV paclitaxel (80 mg/m^2/1 hour) weekly IV carboplatin AUC 6 every 3 weeks 21 day cycle x 6 cycles	*Can consider:* Addition of bevacizumab IP therapy in small volume disease Consolidation therapy
Recurrent or persistent disease Platinum-sensitive disease Carboplatin + (PLD/gemcitabine/paclitaxel) + /–bevacizumab PARP-inhibitors approved regardless of BRCA status	
Platinum-resistant disease Single agent sequential therapy	
BRCA1/BRCA2 mutation with chemorefractory disease Olaparib	
Surgical	
Primary cytoreduction: laparotomy with TAH/BSO and pelvic washing with the goal of optimal debulking (<1 cm residual disease)	Surgery can be performed before or after neoadjuvant chemotherapy in bulky stage IIIC or IV disease.
Secondary cytoreduction: performed in the setting of recurrence if no gross disease in the abdomen is an obtainable goal No evidence to support second look surgery Palliative surgery: individualized	The EORTC-GCG/NCIC-CTG trial (Vergote et al. 2010) showed that neoadjuvant chemotherapy followed by interval debulking surgery was not inferior to primary debulking surgery followed by chemo. HR for death was 0.98 (90% CI 0.84–1.13; $p = 0.01$). Complete resection of all macroscopic disease (at primary or interval surgery) was the strongest independent variable in predicting OS

Table 15.8 Acceptable recurrence therapies for epithelial ovarian cancer.

	Cytotoxic therapy (alphabetical)		Targeted therapy
	Platinum sensitive	Platinum resistant	
Preferred agent	Carboplatin/gemcitabine	Docetaxel	Bevacizumab Olaparib Rucaparib
	Carboplatin/gemcitabine/bevacizumab	Etoposide (oral)	
	Carboplatin/liposomal doxorubicin	Gemcitabine	
	Carboplatin/paclitaxel	Liposomal doxorubicin	
	Carboplatin/paclitaxel/bevacizumab	Liposomal doxorubicin + bevacizumab	
	Cisplatin/gemcitabine	Paclitaxel (weekly) +/− pazopanib	
		Paclitaxel (weekly) + bevacizumab	
		Topetecan	
		Topetecan + bevacizumab	

(Source: Adapted from NCCN guidelines version 1.2019.)

Prevention/management of complications

- The treatment of ovarian cancer includes chemotherapies that more commonly cause drug reactions: carboplatin, cisplatin, oxaliplatin, paclitaxel, docetaxel, and liposomal doxorubicin.
- Taxanes tend to be infusion-related drug reactions (hot flushing, rash), often attributed to cremophor in the formulation, and tend to occur within the first few cycles of treatment, although can occur at any time.
- Platinum drugs tend to produce a true hypersensitivity allergic reaction (shortness of breath, hives/itching, changes in blood pressure) and tend to occur following re-exposure to the drug.
- Providers, nurses, and patients should be familiar with the symptoms of a drug reaction and comply with appropriate premedications/intervention medications when necessary. Desensitization protocols may be appropriate to give the drug again.

CLINICAL PEARLS
- Optimal debulking with none to minimal gross residual disease is the goal of primary cytoreductive surgery and is the standard of care.
- IV carboplatin/paclitaxel (given every 3 weeks or weekly) is standard adjuvant therapy for high risk limited stage disease and for advanced disease after primary cytoreduction.
- Intraperitoneal chemotherapy is standard of care for small volume residual disease as issued by the NCI but requires expertise in administration and can be more toxic.
- Treatment choice and response to therapy is determined by the platinum-free interval (platinum-sensitive or platinum-resistant) in the recurrent setting.
- All patients with ovarian cancer should be tested for germline *BRCA1* and *BRCA2* mutations and can be considered for PARP-inhibitor therapy when the patient has progressed on multiple therapies in the recurrent setting.
- There are a growing number of targeted therapies (bevacizumab, pazopanib, etc.), which have shown a significant PFS, but no OS in ovarian cancer yet.

Special populations
Elderly
- Patients with advanced disease who are elderly, have poor prognosis, and have comorbidities may not tolerate standard IP or IV combinations of chemotherapy. Single agent platinum agents may be appropriate for these patients.

Prognosis

> **BOTTOM LINE/CLINICAL PEARLS**
> - Survival from ovarian cancer is related to the stage at diagnosis; 5-year survival is over 90% for the minority of women with stage I disease. This number drops to about 75–80% for regional disease and 25% for those with distant metastases.
> - There are long-term survivors: 10-year survival is 30–40% for small volume disease and 15–20% for large volume disease.
> - Patients with *BRCA* mutations may have a better prognosis because of increased sensitivity to platinum-based chemotherapy.
> - Ovarian cancer is a very chemo-sensitive disease. The lack of OS benefit for newer targeted agents that show a significant PFS advantage may be a result of the many subsequent lines of treatment received throughout the disease process.

References and reading list

Aghajanian C, Blank SV, Goff BA, et al. OCEANS: a randomized, double-blinded, placebo-controlled phase III trial of chemotherapy with or without bevacizumab (BEV) in patients with platinum-sensitive recurrent epithelial ovarian (EOC), primary peritoneal (PPC), or fallopian tube cancer (FTC). J Clin Oncol 2012;30:2039–2045.

Balasubramaniam S, Beaver JA, Horton S, et al. FDA Approval Summary: Rucaparib for the treatment of patients with deleterious *BRCA* mutation-associated advanced ovarian cancer. Clin Cancer Res. 2017;23:7165–7170.

Blagden SP, Hamilton AL, Mileshkin L, et al. Phase IB dose escalation and expansion study of AKT inhibitor afuresertib with carboplatin and paclitaxel in recurrent platinum-resistant ovarian cancer. Clin Cancer Res 2018:OF1–OF7.

Cancer Genome Atlas Research Network. Integrated genomic analyses of ovarian carcinoma. Nature 2011;474:609–615.

du Bois A, Floquet A, Kim JW, et al. Incorporation of pazopanib in maintenance therapy of ovarian cancer. J Clin Oncol 2014;32:3374–3382.

Gadducci, A, Guerrieri M. Immune Checkpoint inhibitors in gynecological cancers: update of literature and perspectives of clinical research. Int J Cancer Res Treat 2017;37:5955–5965.

Katsumata, N, Yasuda M, Takahashi F, et al. Dose-dense paclitaxel once a week in combination with carboplatin every 3 weeks for advanced ovarian cancer: a phase 3, open-label, randomised controlled trial. Lancet 2009;374:1331–1338.

Kaufman B, Shapira-Frommer R, Schmutzler RK, et al. Olaparib monotherapy in patients with advanced cancer and a germline BRCA1/2 mutation. J Clin Oncol 2015;33:244–250.

Kim G, Ison G, McKee AE, et al. FDA approval summary: olaparib monotherapy in patients with deleterious germline BRCA-mutated advanced ovarian cancer treated with three or more lines of chemotherapy. Clin Cancer Res 2015;21:4257–4261.

Ledermann J, Harter P, Gourley C, et al. Olaparib maintenance therapy in platinum-sensitive relapsed ovarian cancer. N Engl J Med 2012;366:1382.

Markman M, Iseminger KA, Hatch KD, et al. Tamoxifen in platinum-refractory ovarian cancer: a Gynecologic Oncology Group Ancillary Report. Gynecol Oncol 1996;62:4–6.

Mirza MR, Monk BJ, Herrstedt J, et al. Niraparib maintenance therapy in platinum-sensitive, recurrent ovarian cancer. N Engl J Med 2016;375:2154–2164.

Moore K, Colombo N, Scambia B, et al. Maintenance olaparib in patients with newly diagnosed advanced ovarian cancer. N Engl J Med 2018;379:2495–2505.

Papadimitriou CA, Markaki S, Siapkaras J, et al. Hormonal therapy with letrozole for relapsed epithelial ovarian cancer. Long-term results of a phase II study. Oncology 2004;66:112–117.

Parmer MK, Ledermann JA, Colombo N, et al. Paclitaxel plus platinum-based chemotherapy versus conventional platinum-based chemotherapy in women with relapsed ovarian cancer: the ICON4/AGO-OVAR-2.2 trial. Lancet 2003;361:2099–2106.

Pfisterer J, Plante M, Vergote I, et al. Gemcitabine plus carboplatin compared with carboplatin in patients with platinum-sensitive recurrent ovarian cancer: an intergroup trial of the AGO-OVAR, the NCIC CTG, and the EORTC GCG. J Clin Oncol 2006;24:4699–4707.

Pujade-Lauraine E, Mahner S, Kaern J, et al. A randomized, phase III study of carboplatin and pegylated liposomal doxorubicin versus carboplatin and paclitaxel in relapsed platinum-sensitive ovarian cancer (OC): CALYPSO study of the Gynecologic Cancer Intergroup (GCIG). J Clin Oncol 2009;27.

Pujade-Lauraine E, Hilpert F, Weber B, et al. AURELIA: a randomized phase III trial evaluating bevacizumab (BEV) plus chemotherapy (CT) for platinum (PT)-resistant recurrent ovarian cancer (OC). J Clin Oncol 2012;30.

Swisher EM, Lin KK, Oza AM, et al. Rucaparib in relapsed, platinum-sensitive high-grade ovarian carcinoma (ARIEL2 Part 1): an international, multicentre, open-label, phase 2 trial. Lancet Oncol 2017;18:75–87.

Toss A, Cristofanilli M. Molecular characterization and targeted therapeutic approaches in breast cancer. Breast Cancer Res 2015;17:60.

Toss A, Tomasello C, Razzaboni E, et al. Hereditary ovarian cancer: not only BRCA1 and 2 genes. BioMed Res Int 2015:1–11.

Varga A, Piha-Paul S, Ott PA, et al. Pembrolizumab in patients with programmed death ligand 1-positive advanced ovarian cancer: analysis of KEYNOTE-028. Gynecol Oncol 2019;152:243–250.

Vergote I, Trope CG, Amant F, et al. Neoadjuvant chemotherapy or primary surgery in stage IIIC or IV ovarian cancer. N Engl J Med 2010;363:943–953.

Wagner U, Marth C, Largillier R, et al. Final overall survival results of phase III GCIG CALYPSO trial of pegylated liposomal doxorubicin and carboplatin vs paclitaxel and carboplatin in platinum-sensitive ovarian cancer patients. Br J Cancer 2012;107:588–591.

Suggested websites

American Society of Clinical Oncology (ASCO): www.asco.org

National Comprehensive Cancer Network (NCCN): http://www.nccn.org (requires professional login)

Guidelines

National society guidelines

Title	Source	Date and weblink
	National Comprehensive Cancer Network (NCCN)	2019 NCCN Clinical Practice Guidelines in oncology: ovarian cancer. (March 8, 2019)
	Society of Gynecologic Oncology (SGO)	2009–2017 SGO Guidelines: ovarian cancer. www.sgo.org

International society guidelines

Title	Source	Date and weblink
	International Federation of Gynecologists and Obstetrics (FIGO)	2014 FIGO ovarian cancer staging guidelines. www.figo.org

Image

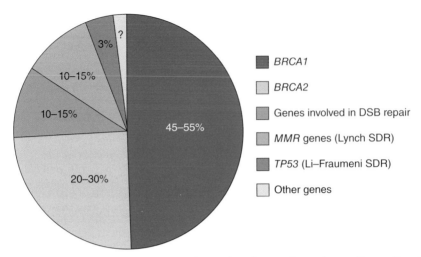

Figure 15.1 Susceptibility genes and their prevalence in hereditary ovarian syndromes. (Source: Toss et al. Review article: Hereditary ovarian cancer: not only BRCA1 and 2 genes. Available from https://www.ncbi.nlm .nih.gov/pmc/articles/PMC4449870/.)

Additional material for this title can be found online at:
www.wiley.com/go/oh/mountsinaioncology

CHAPTER 16

Endometrial Cancer

Jamal Rahaman and Carmel J. Cohen
Icahn School of Medicine at Mount Sinai, New York, NY, USA

OVERALL BOTTOM LINE
- Endometrial carcinoma is the most frequent gynecologic cancer in the USA with over 50 000 new cases diagnosed each year.
- Over 80% have the classic estrogen-dependent endometrioid histology with a favorable prognosis (type I cancers).
- Type II cancers have a different molecular profile associated with more virulent disease and diminished survival and include uterine papillary serous carcinomas (UPSC) and clear cell carcinomas.
- Surgery, where possible, constitutes the definitive primary treatment.
- Primary radiation therapy and primary hormonal therapy are alternatives for inoperable patients.
- Paclitaxel (T), carboplatin (C), cisplatin (P), and doxorubicin (A) are the most active single agents, with TC and TAP being the most effective combination chemotherapy regimens.

Background
Definition of disease
- Endometrioid adenocarcinoma is the most common of the endometrial cancer histologies characterized by the disappearance of stroma between abnormal glands that have enfolding of their linings into the lumens, disordered nuclear chromatin distribution, nuclear enlargement, and a variable degree of mitosis, necrosis, and hemorrhage. It accounts for 80–95% of the adenocarcinomas.
- Other less common histologies include UPSC, clear cell carcinoma, endometrial papillary adenocarcinoma, and adenosquamous carcinoma.

Disease classification
- Type I cancers represent over 80% of endometrial cancers and have the classic estrogen-dependent endometrioid histology with a favorable prognosis.
- Type II endometrial cancers have a distinct phenotype and now are recognized to also have a different molecular profile associated with more virulent disease and diminished survival and includes UPSC and clear cell carcinomas.

Incidence/prevalence
- In 2015, 54 870 new cases of uterine corpus cancer were diagnosed in the USA and 10 170 women died from this cancer. Endometrial carcinoma occurs most often in the sixth and seventh decades of life, with an average age at onset of 60 years, and a lifetime risk of 2.6%.

Mount Sinai Expert Guides: Oncology, First Edition. Edited by William K. Oh and Ajai Chari.
© 2019 John Wiley & Sons Ltd. Published 2019 by John Wiley & Sons Ltd.
Companion Website: www.wiley.com/go/oh/mountsinaioncology

- Compared with white women, black women have a lower incidence of endometrial carcinoma but with less favorable histologies, more advanced stages of disease, more poorly differentiated tumors, and higher mortality.

Etiology
- Endogenous or exogenous exposure to estrogen is believed to be an important risk factor for the development of endometrial hyperplasia and type I endometrial cancers. Estrogens not opposed by progestins lead to increased mitotic activity of endometrial cells, resulting in more frequent errors in DNA replication and somatic mutations.
- Type II tumors are estrogen independent and include high grade endometrioid and serous histologies and are characterized by a high mutational rate of TP53, have high copy numbers, and are microsatellite stable tumors.

Pathology/pathogenesis
- Tumor growth may be confined to the endometrium, invade the underlying myometrium, penetrate to the uterine serosal surface or adjacent bladder or rectum, or extend into the cervical canal and invade cervical glands or stroma.
- Lymphatic spread occurs primarily to pelvic and para-aortic lymph nodes, and occasionally involves inguinal nodes.
- Peritoneal disease spreads via transmigration from the fallopian tubes or through serosal penetration.
- Hematogenous spread is not uncommon but usually occurs late.

Predictive/risk factors

Risk factor	Relative risk
Increasing age	Women 50–70 years have a 1.4% risk, the overall lifetime risk is 2.6%
Obesity	2–10
Unopposed estrogen therapy	2–10
Lynch syndrome – genetic mutations MLH1, MSH2, MSH6, PMS2	20–70% lifetime risk
Race	White 1.6 times Asian
Tamoxifen therapy	2.5–7.5
Nulliparity	2
Late menopause (after age 55)	2
Polycystic ovary syndrome	3
Cowden syndrome (PTEN mutation)	13–19% lifetime risk
Estrogen secreting tumor	NA
Diabetes mellitus	2
Early menarche	NA

Prevention

> **BOTTOM LINE/CLINICAL PEARLS**
> - Factors that reduce circulating estrogen levels (weight loss/exercise, cigarette smoking) appear to be protective.
> - Progestins antagonize the effects of estrogen on the endometrium and prevent the development of hyperplasia and cancer and can reverse precancerous complex atypical endometrial hyperplasia.
> - Prior use of oral contraceptives also appears to be protective.

Screening
- The relatively low prevalence of endometrial carcinoma in the population (5 per 1000 women >45 years) makes standardized screening inefficient.
- The American College of Obstetrics and Gynecology (ACOG) and the SGO do not recommend routine screening of patients for uterine cancer.
- The American Cancer Society (ACS) does recommend annual endometrial biopsies starting at age 35 for women known to have or be at risk for HNPCC and/or Lynch syndrome.

Primary prevention
- The increased risk of endometrial carcinoma associated with unopposed estrogens means that women with an intact uterus should rarely, if ever, be prescribed estrogen-only replacement therapy.
- The use of the estrogen–progesterone oral contraceptive pill decreases the risk by 50% and the protective effect persists for more than 10–20 years after cessation.
- Progestin-only contraception and therapy including depot-medroxyprogesterone acetate, progestin implants, and progestin-releasing intrauterine devices provide protection against development of endometrial cancer.

Diagnosis (Algorithm 16.1)

Algorithm 16.1 Surgical management of endometrial carcinoma

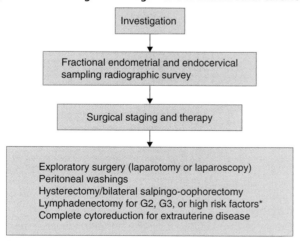

*< 50% myoinvasion, clear cell or papillary serous histology, adnexal metastasis, lymph-vascular space invasion and/or cervical invasion, > 50% uterine cavity involved, suspicious nodes.

> **BOTTOM LINE/CLINICAL PEARLS**
> - Over 75% of patients with endometrial carcinoma present with the classic symptom of postmenopausal bleeding or abnormal uterine bleeding. Additionally, patients with endometrial carcinoma present with vaginal discharge or have a thickened endometrium incidentally noted on ultrasound, CT scan or MRI performed for another reason.
> - Some patients present with abnormal cervical cytology findings including endometrial cells in women aged over 40, atypical glandular cells, or adenocarcinoma.
> - Pathologic evaluation of the endometrium provides histologic diagnosis and can identify other etiologies of bleeding such as chronic endometritis, atrophy, polyps, cervical cancer, or unusual histologic variants. This can be achieved by an office endometrial biopsy or a dilatation and curettage (D&C) under anesthesia.
> - Hysteroscopy has been advocated as an adjuvant to D&C to improve detection of pathology in the evaluation of postmenopausal bleeding.

Differential diagnosis

Differential diagnosis	Features
Benign endometrial polyps	Abnormal bleeding and a thickened endometrial stripe on sonography – carcinoma can only be excluded by complete polypectomy at hysteroscopy
Endometrial hyperplasia	Abnormal bleeding and a thickened endometrial stripe on sonography – carcinoma can only be excluded by thorough global curettage – 25–40% of complex atypical endometrial hyperplasia will have an associated endometrial cancer
Uterine fibroids	Fibroids (especially submucous) can develop with heavy vaginal bleeding (menorrhagia). Prior to hysterectomy, all women with abnormal uterine bleeding should have endometrial sampling to exclude an endometrial cancer
Endocervical carcinoma	Can produce identical symptoms including menorrhagia, postmenopausal bleeding, and abnormal cytology on a Pap smear
	A fractional curettage to assess the endocervical mucosa should be included in the preoperative evaluation and cervical biopsies and cone biopsy considered in select cases
	The appropriate management is surgery with a radical hysterectomy for early stages I and IIA and chemo-radiation for advanced stages of endocervical cancer
Uterine sarcoma	Uterine sarcomas (especially leiomyosarcomas and endometrial stromal sarcomas) can develop with abnormal bleeding and an enlarging uterus and have negative findings on D&C
	The diagnosis is sometimes only established by a hysterectomy

Typical presentation
- Patients with endometrial carcinoma typically present with abnormal uterine bleeding. It is most commonly found in women who are postmenopausal and with increasing age in pre-menopausal women.
- Incidental finding on imaging – a thickened endometrial lining is sometimes found incidentally on ultrasound, CT, or MRI performed for another indication.

- Some patients present with abnormal cervical cytology findings including endometrial cells in women aged over 40, atypical glandular cells, or adenocarcinoma.
- Incidental finding at hysterectomy – endometrial carcinoma or hyperplasia is sometimes discovered incidentally when hysterectomy is performed for benign disease. Prior to hysterectomy, all women with abnormal uterine bleeding should have endometrial sampling.

Clinical diagnosis
History
Because patients with endometrial carcinoma typically present with abnormal uterine bleeding the following bleeding patterns should prompt endometrial evaluation.
- **Postmenopausal women:** any bleeding, including spotting or staining. Three to 20% of women with postmenopausal bleeding are found to have endometrial carcinoma and another 5–15% have endometrial hyperplasia.
- **Age 45 to menopause:** any abnormal uterine bleeding, including intermenstrual bleeding in women who are ovulatory, frequent (interval between the onset of bleeding episodes is less than 21 days), heavy (total volume of >80 mL), or prolonged (longer than 7 days). In addition, endometrial neoplasia should be suspected in women with prolonged periods of amenorrhea (6 months or more) in women with anovulation.
- **Younger than 45 years:** abnormal uterine bleeding that is persistent, occurs in the setting of a history of unopposed estrogen exposure (obesity, chronic anovulation) or failed medical management of the bleeding, or in women at high risk of endometrial cancer (e.g. Lynch and Cowden syndromes).

Physical examination
Prior to treatment, a complete pelvic and general physical examination should be performed, with particular attention to the size and mobility of the uterus and the presence of extrauterine masses or ascites; potential sites of nodal metastases should also be examined (e.g. supraclavicular nodes).

Because surgical staging is the preferred definitive management, a thorough physical examination for preoperative clearance for major surgery is required.

Useful clinical decision rules and calculators
Endometrial carcinoma is a histologic diagnosis based upon the results of evaluation of an endometrial biopsy, curettage sample, or hysterectomy specimen.
- **Negative endometrial sampling:** the sensitivity for endometrial sampling is 90% or higher. Risk factors for false negative endometrial sampling include a personal history of colorectal cancer, endometrial polyps, and morbid obesity.
- Women with an endometrial biopsy result that has insufficient endometrial cells should have sampling repeated with a D&C as well as a hysteroscopy to assure thorough evaluation.
- **Persistent or recurrent bleeding:** if bleeding persists or recurs after endometrial sampling with benign findings, further evaluation is required with a hysteroscopy or, if necessary, a hysterectomy.

Disease severity classification
Endometrial carcinoma is surgically staged according to the joint 2010 FIGO/TNM classification system (Table 16.1).

Table 16.1 Staging of endometrial carcinoma.

TNM categories	FIGO[a] stages	Definition
Primary tumor (T)		
TX		Primary tumor cannot be assessed
T0		No evidence of primary tumor
Tis[b]		Carcinoma *in situ* (preinvasive carcinoma)
T1	I	Tumor confined to the corpus uteri
T1a	IA	Tumor limited to the endometrium or invades less than half of the myometrium
T1b	IB	Tumor invades half or more of the myometrium
T2	II	Tumor invades stromal connective tissue of the cervix but does not extend beyond the uterus[c]
T3a	IIIA	Tumor involves serosa and/or adnexa (direct extension or metastasis)[d]
T3b	IIIB	Vaginal involvement (direct extension or metastasis) or parametrial involvement[d]
	IIIC	Metastasis to pelvic and/or para-aortic lymph nodes[d]
T4	IVA	Tumor invades bladder mucosa and/or bowel (bullous edema is not sufficient to classify a tumor as T4)
Regional lymph nodes (N)		
NX		Regional lymph nodes cannot be assessed
N0		No regional lymph node metastasis
N1	IIIC1	Regional lymph node metastasis to pelvic lymph nodes (positive pelvic nodes)
N2	IIIC2	Regional lymph node metastasis to para-aortic lymph nodes, with or without positive pelvic lymph nodes
Distant metastasis (M)		
M0		No distant metastasis
M1	IVB	Distant metastasis (includes metastasis to inguinal lymph nodes, intraperitoneal disease, or lung, liver, or bone. It excludes metastasis to para-aortic lymph nodes, vagina, pelvic serosa, or adnexa)

[a] Either G1, G2, or G3.
[b] FIGO no longer includes stage 0 (Tis).
[c] Endocervical glandular involvement only should be considered as stage I and no longer as stage II.
[d] Positive cytology has to be reported separately without changing the stage.

Laboratory diagnosis

List of diagnostic tests

- Women of reproductive age with suspected endometrial hyperplasia or carcinoma should have urine or serum human chorionic gonadotropin testing to exclude pregnancy as an etiology of abnormal uterine bleeding and to ensure that endometrial sampling will not disrupt a pregnancy.
- Preoperative blood testing should include a CBC, type and screen, and metabolic profile.
- Measurement of the serum tumor marker CA-125 is a clinically useful test for predicting extrauterine spread of endometrial carcinoma.

Lists of imaging techniques

- For women with suspected endometrial carcinoma or hyperplasia, pelvic sonography is often the first line imaging study to evaluate for other etiologies of abnormal uterine bleeding.
- In the infrequent situation in which a patient is staged clinically, contrast-enhanced MRI appears to be the best radiographic modality for detecting myometrial invasion or cervical involvement when compared with nonenhanced MRI, ultrasound, or CT.
- MRI is also the best imaging modality, compared with CT or PET with or without CT, for detecting lymph node metastases.
- A chest radiograph should be performed as part of the initial assessment.
- For patients with advanced or recurrent disease, a metastatic investigation should include a CT scan or MRI of the chest, abdomen, and pelvis.
- PET scans have utility in detecting occult lesions.

Potential pitfalls/common errors made regarding diagnosis of disease

- Prior to hysterectomy, all women with abnormal uterine bleeding should have endometrial sampling to exclude an associated endometrial carcinoma.
- All patients having a hysterectomy for complex endometrial hyperplasia should have a frozen section taken to exclude an associated endometrial cancer (25–40% risk). If cancer is discovered, a staging procedure can be performed immediately, with a BSO, pelvic and para-aortic lymphadenectomy and omentectomy (for serous and clear cell cancers).

Treatment (Algorithm 16.2)

Algorithm 16.2 Postoperative management of endometrial carcinoma

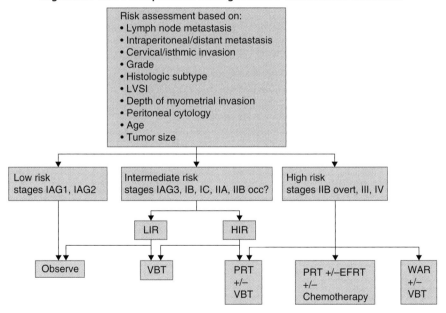

EFRT, extended field radiotherapy; HIR, high intermediate risk based on GOG-99; LIR, low intermediate risk; LVSI, lymph-vascular space invasion; PRT, pelvic radiotherapy; VBT, vaginal brachytherapy; WAR, whole abdominopelvic radiotherapy. Age: <50, three factors; 50–70, two factors; >70, one factor. High risk factors were LVSI, outer 1/3 invasion, and Grade 2–3.

Treatment rationale

All women with endometrial cancer should undergo surgical staging, especially if the disease is not suspected to be metastatic. Surgical staging defines the extent of disease and largely defines the risk of recurrence. Adjuvant therapy for stage I disease is determined by age, depth of myometrial invasion, lymph–vascular space invasion, and tumor grade.

Surgery, where possible, constitutes the definitive primary treatment for most patients with endometrial carcinoma (Figures 16.1 and 16.2). Primary radiation therapy and primary hormonal therapy are alternatives for inoperable patients.

- Women with low grade (grade 1 or 2) endometrioid cancers confined to the endometrium (a subset of stage IA disease) are classified as having **low-risk endometrial cancer**. Because their prognosis following surgery is excellent, no adjuvant treatment is required.
- Women with endometrial cancer that invades the myometrium (stage IA or IB) or demonstrates occult cervical stromal invasion (stage II) have **intermediate-risk** disease. These patients are candidates for adjuvant radiation therapy. Although there is no clear role for chemotherapy as part of an adjuvant treatment strategy, some clinicians recommend chemotherapy to women with high intermediate-risk disease.
- Women who have any of the following features have **high-risk endometrial cancer:** stage III disease, regardless of histology or grade; and/or uterine serous carcinoma or clear cell carcinoma of any stage. Women with high risk disease often receive chemotherapy with or without radiation therapy given their high risk of both distant and locoregional relapse.

Table of treatment

Treatment	Comments
Conservative/hormonal	Women with apparent stage IA grade 1 endometrial carcinoma who wish to preserve fertility can opt to avoid hysterectomy/BSO and undergo progestin therapy. These women should undergo hysterectomy/BSO after completion of childbearing, even in cases with demonstrated tumor regression
Medical	For patients with early high risk, advanced, and recurrent disease chemotherapy is recommended. Paclitaxel (T), carboplatin (C), cisplatin (P) and doxorubicin (A) are the most active single agents with TC and TAP being the most effective combination chemotherapy regimens
Surgical	A total extrafascial hysterectomy with BSO with pelvic and para-aortic lymph node dissection is the standard staging procedure for endometrial carcinoma
	Abdominal, vaginal, laparoscopic, or robot-assisted approaches are possible
	An omentectomy is frequently carried out for patients with serous or clear cell histology
	Cytoreduction is performed when metastases are evident
Radiation	Radiation therapy can be administered as primary definitive management for inoperable patients
	Adjuvant vaginal cuff brachytherapy with or without whole pelvic radiotherapy is recommended for patients with intermediate or high risk stage I and II cancer
	For advanced stages and recurrent cancer whole pelvic and extended field (to include para-aortic nodes) is appropriate
	Targeted radiation to painful bony metastasis is a useful option

---

CLINICAL PEARLS
- Surgery constitutes the definitive primary treatment for most patients with endometrial carcinoma.
- Primary radiation therapy and primary hormonal therapy are alternatives for inoperable patients.
- For women with low risk endometrial cancer no additional treatment is needed after surgery because their prognosis is excellent.
- Women with intermediate-risk disease are candidates for adjuvant radiation therapy.
- Women with high risk disease may require chemotherapy with or without radiation therapy.

Special populations
Elderly

Older age has been associated with higher rates of clinical failure and survival in several studies. The association between age and prognosis can be illustrated by data from the Gynecologic Oncology Group (GOG) protocol 33, in which 5-year relative survival rates for women with clinical stage I and II endometrial cancer stratified by age were as follows:

- ≤40 years – 96%
- 41–50 years – 94%
- 51–60 years – 87%
- 61–70 years – 78%
- 71–80 years – 71%
- ≥80 years – 54%.

Prognosis

BOTTOM LINE/CLINICAL PEARLS
- The prognosis of endometrial carcinoma is determined primarily by disease stage and histology (including both grade and histologic subtype). Fortunately, most women with endometrial carcinoma have a favorable prognosis, because the majority of patients have endometrioid (usually good prognosis) and present with early stage disease because of abnormal uterine bleeding.
- Other histologic types of endometrial carcinoma (e.g. serous, clear cell) as well as other types of uterine cancer are associated with a poorer prognosis. In general, the rate of 5-year survival for stage I disease is approximately 80–90%, for stage II it is 70–80%, and for stages III and IV it is 20–60% (Table 16.2).

Prognosis for treated patients
- This is included in the survival data from both the FIGO report and the SEER data.

Follow-up tests and monitoring
- Post-treatment surveillance is aimed at the early detection of recurrent disease. For women with endometrial carcinoma, surveillance consists mainly of monitoring for symptoms and physical examination.
- There is no high-quality evidence that any specific post-treatment surveillance strategy is associated with improved outcomes. In the absence of data, we agree with the consensus-based

Table 16.2 Uterine carcinoma: FIGO surgical stage and OS.

FIGO stage	OS (%)		
	2 years[a]	5 years[a]	5 years[b]
IA	97	91	90
IB	97	91	78
IC	94	85	–
II	–	–	74
IIA	93	83	–
IIB	85	74	–
IIIA	80	66	56
IIIB	62	50	36
IIIC	75	57	–
IIIC1	–	–	57
IIIC2	–	–	49
IVA	47	26	22
IVB	37	20	21

[a] Data from: FIGO for patients treated in 1999–2001, using the original 1988 FIGO surgical staging classification (from Int J Gynaecol Obstet 2006;95:S105).
[b] Data from: SEER database for patients treated in 1988–2006, staged according to the 2010 FIGO staging system (from Obstet Gynecol 2010;116:1141).

guidelines from the US National Comprehensive Cancer Network (NCCN) and the SGO, which include the following.
- Review of symptoms and physical examination including speculum and bimanual pelvic examination every 3–6 months for 2 years, then every 6 months or annually. The frequency of examinations depends upon the risk of persistent or recurrent disease. Although surveillance using vaginal cytology is recommended by the NCCN, the SGO does not support this.
- When planning the post-treatment surveillance strategy, care should be taken to limit the number of CT scans, given concerns about radiation exposure and the risk for secondary malignancies.
- CT and MRI should be performed for patients who are symptomatic or have abnormal findings on physical examination.
- PET as a modality for the evaluation of a suspected recurrence has a sensitivity and specificity of 95% and 93%, respectively.

Reading list

Bokhman JV. Two pathogenetic types of endometrial carcinoma. Gynecol Oncol 1983;15:10–17.
Boruta DM 2nd, Gehrig PA, Fader AN, et al. Management of women with uterine papillary serous cancer: a Society of Gynecologic Oncology (SGO) review. Gynecol Oncol 2009;115:142–153.
Cancer Genome Atlas Research Network, Kandoth C, Schultz N, Cherniack AD, et al. Integrated genomic characterization of endometrial carcinoma. Nature 2013;497:67–73.
Cohen CJ, Rahaman J. Endometrial cancer: management of high risk and recurrence including the tamoxifen controversy. Cancer 1995;76:2044–2052.
Gusberg SB. Precursors of corpus carcinoma, estrogen and adenomatous hyperplasia. Am J Obstet Gynecol 1947;54:905–927.

Olawaiye AB, Boruta DM 2nd. Management of women with clear cell endometrial cancer: a Society of Gynecologic Oncology (SGO) review. Gynecol Oncol 2009;113:277–283.

Ramirez PT, Frumovitz M, Bodurka DC, et al. Hormonal therapy for the management of grade 1 endometrial adenocarcinoma: a literature review. Gynecol Oncol 2004;95:133–138.

Rahaman J, Cohen CJ. Endometrial cancer. In: Kufe DW, Pollock RE, Weichselbaum RR, et al., eds. Holland-Frei Cancer Medicine, 8th edition, 2010.

Suggested websites

http://www.nccn.org/professionals/physician_gls/f_guidelines.asp

Guidelines
National society guidelines

Title	Source	Date and weblink
NCCN Clinical practice guidelines in oncology	NCCN	2019 http://www.nccn.org/professionals/ physician_gls/f_guidelines.asp
Post-treatment surveillance and diagnosis of recurrence in women with gynecologic malignancies: Society of Gynecologic Oncologists recommendations	Society of Gynecologic Oncologists	2011 https://www.ncbi.nlm.nih.gov/pubmed/ 21752752

Evidence

Type of evidence	Title and comment	Date and weblink
RCT	A phase III trial of surgery with or without adjunctive external pelvic radiation therapy in intermediate risk endometrial adenocarcinoma: a Gynecologic Oncology Group study **Comment:** The GOG 99 is the only randomized trial to evaluate the value of RT in well-staged patients with intermediate risk	2004 https://www.ncbi.nlm.nih.gov/ pubmed/14984936
RCT	Surgery and postoperative radiotherapy versus surgery alone for patients with stage-1 endometrial carcinoma: multicentre randomised trial. PORTEC Study Group. Post Operative Radiation Therapy in Endometrial Carcinoma	2000 https://www.ncbi.nlm.nih.gov/ pubmed/10791524
RCT	Vaginal brachytherapy versus pelvic external beam radiotherapy for patients with endometrial cancer of high-intermediate risk (PORTEC-2): an open-label, non-inferiority, randomised trial	2010 https://www.ncbi.nlm.nih.gov/ pubmed/20206777
RCT	Randomized phase III noninferiority trial of first line chemotherapy for metastatic or recurrent endometrial carcinoma: a Gynecologic Oncology Group Study **Comment:** This GOG 209 study established taxol/carboplatin combination chemotherapy as a better tolerated and equivalent therapeutic option to taxol/doxorubicin/cisplatin	2012 https://www.gynecologi concology-online.net/article/ S0090-8258(12)00228-4/ fulltext doi:10.1016/j.ygyno. 2012.03.034

(Continued)

(*Continued*)

Type of evidence	Title and comment	Date and weblink
RCT	Phase III trial of doxorubicin plus cisplatin with or without paclitaxel plus filgrastim in advanced endometrial carcinoma: a Gynecologic Oncology Group Study. **Comment:** Demonstrated that TAP was superior PFS to AP but associated with more toxicity.	2004 https://www.ncbi.nlm.nih.gov/pubmed/15169803
RCT	Randomized phase III trial of pelvic radiotherapy versus cisplatin-based combined chemotherapy in patients with intermediate- and high risk endometrial cancer: a Japanese Gynecologic Oncology Group study	2008 https://www.ncbi.nlm.nih.gov/pubmed/17996926
RCT	Randomized phase III trial of whole-abdominal irradiation versus doxorubicin and cisplatin chemotherapy in advanced endometrial carcinoma: a Gynecologic Oncology Group Study	2006 https://www.ncbi.nlm.nih.gov/pubmed/16330675
RCT	Phase III trial of doxorubicin with or without cisplatin in advanced endometrial carcinoma: a Gynecologic Oncology Group Study	2004 https://www.ncbi.nlm.nih.gov/pubmed/15459211
Prospective cohort study	Surgical pathologic spread patterns of endometrial cancer. A Gynecologic Oncology Group Study	1987 https://www.ncbi.nlm.nih.gov/pubmed/3652025
Prospective cohort study	Relationship between surgical-pathological risk factors and outcome in clinical stage I and II carcinoma of the endometrium: a Gynecologic Oncology Group Study	1991 https://www.ncbi.nlm.nih.gov/pubmed/1989916

Images

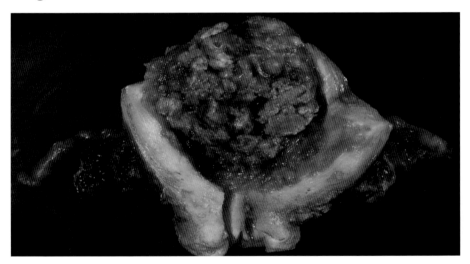

Figure 16.1 Endometrial cancer. (Courtesy of Dr. Tamara Kalir, Department of Pathology, Icahn School of Medicine at Mount Sinai.) See color version on website.

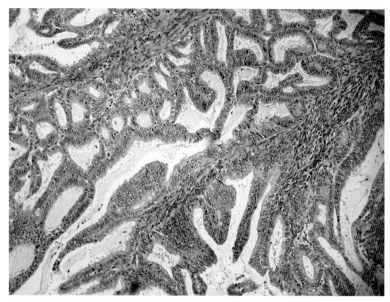

Figure 16.2 Photomicrograph of a well-differentiated endometrioid endometrial adenocarcinoma. (Courtesy of Dr. Tamara Kalir, Department of Pathology, Icahn School of Medicine at Mount Sinai.) See color version on website.

Additional material for this chapter can be found online at: www.wiley.com/go/oh/mountsinaioncology

The following images are available in color: Figures 16.1 and 16.2.

CHAPTER 17

Cervical Cancer

Navya Nair, Ann Marie Beddoe, and Peter Dottino
Icahn School of Medicine at Mount Sinai, New York, NY, USA

OVERALL BOTTOM LINE
- Cervical cancer is a major source of morbidity and mortality worldwide, with most cases occurring in developing nations.
- With screening and treatment of preinvasive disease, cervical cancer can be prevented.
- Most cervical cancers are the end result of a long process that begins with HPV infection.
- Vaccines against HPV can prevent preinvasive disease that leads to cervical cancer.
- Treatment of cervical cancer is dependent on stage and includes surgery, radiation therapy, and chemotherapy.

Background
Definition of disease
Cancer arising from the cervix (lower segment of the uterus) as a result of abnormal growth of cells that have the potential to invade neighboring tissue and spread.

Disease classification
- The majority of cervical cancers are squamous cell type (75–80%).
- Most of the remainder are adenocarcinomas.

Incidence/prevalence
- In the USA, it is estimated that there are 12 900 new cases of cervical cancer and 4100 cervical cancer deaths annually.
- Worldwide, cervical cancer is the fourth most common cancer in women with 528 000 new cases and 266 000 deaths in 2012 (Figure 17.1).

Economic impact
- Economic impact is most significant in low and middle-income countries.
- In 2008, cervical cancer accounted for $1.3 billion lost in disability-adjusted life years.

Etiology
- Cervical cancer is typically the end result of a process that begins with infection with HPV.
- Chronic HPV infection leads to cervical dysplasia (preinvasive disease) and subsequently cervical cancer.
- HPV strains 16 and 18 account for over 70% of cervical cancer cases.

Mount Sinai Expert Guides: Oncology, First Edition. Edited by William K. Oh and Ajai Chari.
© 2019 John Wiley & Sons Ltd. Published 2019 by John Wiley & Sons Ltd.
Companion Website: www.wiley.com/go/oh/mountsinaioncology

Pathology/pathogenesis
- Presenting symptoms including abnormal vaginal bleeding (including postcoital bleeding) and/or abnormal vaginal discharge.
- Symptoms of advanced disease include hematuria, rectal bleeding, referred leg or flank pain, and lymphedema.

Predictive/risk factors

Risk factor	Odds ratio
HPV infection	81.3 (95% CI 42.0–157.1)
HIV	12.2 (95% CI 9.4–15.6)[a]
Cigarette smoking	1.5 (95% CI 1.0–2.2)

[a] Standard rate ratio: observed cases in HIV population to general population.

Prevention

> **BOTTOM LINE/CLINICAL PEARLS**
> - Papanicolaou smear screening, treatment of pre-invasive disease, and HPV vaccination can prevent development of cervical cancer.

Screening
- Papanicolaou smear screening in adult women.
- Papanicolaou smear screening with HPV co-testing in adult women 30 years and older.
- Cobas HPV screening in adult women.

Primary prevention
- Cervical cancer screening has been shown to decrease the incidence of cervical cancers.
- Treatment of high grade cervical dysplasia decreases rate of progression to cervical cancer.
- HPV vaccination decreases rates of cervical dysplasia.

Diagnosis (Algorithm 17.1)

Algorithm 17.1 Diagnosis of cervical cancer

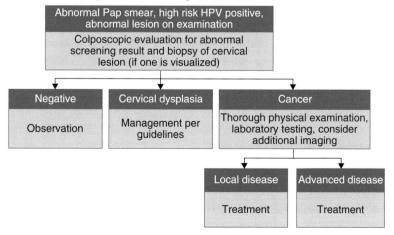

> **BOTTOM LINE/CLINICAL PEARLS**
> - History of no prior cervical cancer screening or untreated prior cervical dysplasia.
> - Examination findings can be variable: visible exophytic polypoid friable mass, barrel-shaped cervix on palpation, visible ulcerative lesion.
> - Biopsy must be carried out to confirm diagnosis. Staging is performed clinically and includes thorough physical examination and additional evaluation as needed (cystoscopy, proctoscopy, chest X-ray, intravenous pyelogram).

Differential diagnosis

Differential diagnosis	Features
Cervical polyp or nabothian cyst	On examination, a benign polyp or cyst is uniform with smooth edges; however, pathology will confirm diagnosis
Ulcerative lesion	Infections such as herpes in the cervix will typically present with multiple vesicles and tender ulcers
Other malignancies	Bladder cancer, endometrial cancer, rectal cancer can infiltrate the cervix

Typical presentation
- The most common presenting symptoms include abnormal vaginal bleeding and vaginal discharge. Women can also be asymptomatic; abnormal Papanicolaou screening results or a lesion seen on routine examination prompts further investigation with a biopsy for definitive diagnosis.
- As the tumor enlarges, it can cause symptoms of pelvic pain. If the tumor starts to invade towards the bladder or rectum, symptoms of issues with urination and/or defecation can develop. In advanced cases, back pain, and lower extremity swelling can be present.

Clinical diagnosis
History
- Key factors that must be elicited from the history are prior abnormal Papanicolaou smears, chronic HPV infection, and history of cervical dysplasia.
- History of immunosuppression including HIV (cervical cancer is an AIDS defining illness in HIV patients), history of organ transplant, chronic use of steroids or other immunomodulators place patients at higher risk of developing cervical cancer.
- Additional risk factors that must be ascertained include: smoking history, history of oral contraceptive use, multiple sexual partners, early age of first intercourse.

Physical examination
- A clinician skilled in evaluating patients for cervical cancer must perform the physical examination. Examination includes a speculum examination to visualize the mass and its extent as well as a rectovaginal examination to evaluate for spread of disease to the parametria and/or pelvic side walls (Figures 17.2 and 17.3). Other areas that must be examined are the superficial inguinal, femoral, and supraclavicular lymph nodes.

Laboratory diagnosis
List of diagnostic tests
- **Biopsy of the abnormal lesion:** to confirm the diagnosis.
- **CBC:** to evaluate for anemia. Thrombocytosis can also be present in a fraction of patients.

- **Serum chemistry:** specifically, creatinine level to evaluate the kidney function. Abnormal kidney function can be a sign of advanced stage disease. Assessment of kidney function is also important in patients who will need platinum chemotherapy.

Lists of imaging techniques
- FIGO system for staging of cervical cancer is based on clinical evaluation. The key portion of the evaluation is a thorough physical examination.
- Chest X-ray and IVP can be performed if there is clinical suspicion but are not required.
- CT, PET, and MRI can be performed to assess extent of disease, measure treatment response, and evaluate for recurrence but are not essential to FIGO staging.

Potential pitfalls/common errors made regarding diagnosis of disease
- Inexperienced examiner not skilled in recognizing the disease.
- Lesion missed on examination/biopsy.
- Delay in seeking care.

Treatment (Algorithm 17.2)

Algorithm 17.2 Treatment of cervical cancer, based on stage of disease

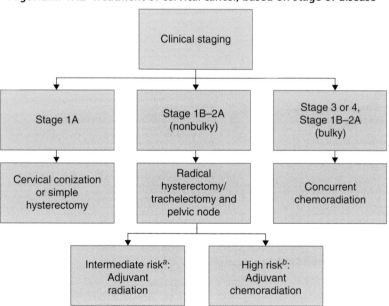

[a] Intermediate risk based on Sedlis criteria (lymphovascular space invasion and deep one-third cervical stromal invasion and tumor of any size, lymphovascular space invasion and middle one-third stromal invasion and tumor size ≥ 2 cm, lymphovascular space invasion and superficial one-third stromal invasion and tumor size ≥ 5 cm, no lymphovascular space invasion with deep or middle one-third stromal invasion and tumor size ≥ 4 cm).
[b] High risk based on Peter's criteria (positive surgical margins, pathologically confirmed involvement of pelvic lymph nodes, microscopic involvement of parametrium).

Treatment rationale
- Early stage disease is treated with surgery or radiation. Bulky and advanced stage disease are mainly treated with radiation with cisplatinum given concurrently as a radiosensitizer.
- Stage 1A1 disease is treated by cervical conization or simple hysterectomy.
- Stage 1A2 disease can be treated by modified radical hysterectomy or trachelectomy with or without pelvic and para-aortic lymph node dissection.
- Early stage (1B–2A), nonbulky disease is treated by radical hysterectomy or trachelectomy with pelvic and para-aortic lymph node dissection or external beam radiotherapy with chemotherapy.
- Bulky early stage and advanced stage disease are treated with external beam radiotherapy with concurrent cisplatin chemotherapy and intracavitary brachytherapy.
- For patients with metastatic disease at diagnosis, systemic chemotherapy (carboplatin, paclitaxel, bevacizumab) is recommended.

When to hospitalize
- Patients must be hospitalized following radical surgery (hysterectomy, trachelectomy) for postoperative care.
- Patients who have active heavy bleeding from their tumor or are severely anemic must be hospitalized.
- Patients with treatment-related complications must be hospitalized.

Managing the hospitalized patient
- Close observation for postoperative complications.
- Transfusion of blood products for anemic patients.
- Emergency radiation therapy for patients actively bleeding, requiring urgent hemostasis.
- Antibiotic therapy for infections.

Table of treatment

Treatment	Comments
Conservative	Cervical conization can be considered for treatment of stage 1A disease in patients who desire to preserve fertility
Medical	Chemotherapy (cisplatin) given concurrently with radiation therapy is standard treatment for those with advanced stage or bulky early stage disease Chemotherapy (carboplatin, paclitaxel, +/– bevacizumab) is primary treatment for metastatic disease
Surgical	Stage 1A: cervical conization or simple hysterectomy Stage 1B or 2A (nonbulky): radical hysterectomy or trachelectomy with pelvic and para-aortic lymph node dissection
Radiologic	External beam radiation therapy with intracavitary brachytherapy has been shown to be most effective in treating advanced stage and bulky early stage disease. Cisplatin is given concurrently to sensitize the cancer cells to radiation treatment

Prevention/management of complications
- Complications of surgery include infection, blood loss, and damage to nearby structures. Complications of radical surgery include postoperative vesicovaginal or ureterovaginal fistula formation, ureteral strictures, bladder dysfunction, lymphedema, lymphocyst formation.

- Infection: surgical infection can be prevented with preoperative antibiotics, adherence to sterile technique
- Blood loss and damage to nearby structures: risk is lower with experienced surgeons
- Vesicovaginal fistulas can be managed conservatively with continuous drainage of urine from bladder and treatment of existing urinary tract infection. Ureterovaginal fistulas can be managed with ureteral stent placement or percutaneous nephrostomy tube placement to drain the urinary system
- Ureteral stricture can be managed by placement of ureteral stents and/or nephrostomy tube placement
- Bladder dysfunction can be managed with bladder training, intermittent self-catheterization, prolonged catheter placement, or medical therapy
- Lymphedema is treated with supportive care
- Lymphcysts can be managed with observation or drainage.
- Complications of chemotherapy include nephrotoxicity, peripheral neuropathy, and bone marrow suppression. Nephrotoxicity can be prevented with adequate hydration with chemotherapy. Neuropathy can be managed by dose reduction and/or drug therapy for more severe neuropathy. Colony stimulating factors can be used to treat bone marrow suppression. Bone marrow suppression can place patients at risk for neutropenic sepsis, which is managed by intravenous antibiotics.
- Complications of radiation therapy can be acute or chronic and include radiation proctitis, radiation cystitis, and vaginal stricture. Radiation proctitis and cystitis can be prevented with minimizing exposure of nearby structures to radiation field. Dilators are used for treatment of vaginal stricture.

CLINICAL PEARLS
- Accurate clinical staging is essential to treatment in cervical cancer.
- Treatment of cervical cancer is dependent on stage of disease.
- Early stage disease is treated with surgery.
- Advanced stage disease is treated with concurrent chemo-radiation.

Special populations
Pregnancy
- The majority of cervical cancers diagnosed in pregnancy are stage 1 disease. Patients <20 weeks gestation should be offered immediate treatment (resulting in pregnancy termination). Patients >20 weeks gestation can opt to delay treatment until fetal lung maturity is documented and then undergo Cesarean section with radical surgery.

Elderly
- In patients who are frail or have numerous comorbid conditions, treatment with concurrent chemo-radiation is preferable to radical surgery.

Others
- HIV patients: treatment of HIV is important in maintaining the immune system to decrease rates of recurrence of cancer and/or dysplasia.

Prognosis

BOTTOM LINE/CLINICAL PEARLS
- Cervical cancer spreads through direct extension and through lymphatic channels.
- Untreated disease can lead to invasion of surrounding structures and subsequently patients can develop life-threatening complications such as renal failure and rectal obstruction.
- Prognostic factors include stage, tumor size, tumor volume, margin status, nodal status, and lymphovascular space invasion.

Natural history of untreated disease
- Untreated disease will spread locally and through lymphatic channels.
- Disease can spread to neighboring organs such as the bladder and/or rectum.
- Disease can spread through lymphatic channels to the pelvic and para-aortic lymph nodes.

Prognosis for treated patients
- Early stage disease: 5-year survival 58–93%.
- Advanced disease: 5-year survival 15–35%.

Follow-up tests and monitoring
- Following treatment of cervical cancer, patients should undergo surveillance every 3–6 months based on stage of disease.
- Surveillance should include a review of symptoms, physical examination, Papanicolaou testing, and imaging as indicated.

Reading list

Chemoradiotherapy for Cervical Cancer Meta-Analysis Collaboration. Reducing uncertainties about the effects of chemoradiotherapy for cervical cancer: a systematic review and meta-analysis of individual patient data from 18 randomized trials. J Clin Oncol 2008;26:5802–5812. doi: 10.1200/JCO.2008.16.4368.

Koh WJ, Greer BE, Abu-Rustum NR, et al. Cervical Cancer, Version 2.2015. J Natl Compr Canc Netw 2015;13:395–404.

Massad LS, Einstein MH, Huh WK, et al. 2012 updated consensus guidelines for the management of abnormal cervical cancer screening tests and cancer precursors. J Low Genit Tract Dis 2013;17: S1–S27.

Randall ME, Fracasso PM, Toita T, et al. Cervix. In: Barakat RR, Berchuck A, Markman M, et al., eds. Principles and Practice of Gynecologic Oncology. Philadelphia: Wolters Kluwer Health/Lippincott Williams & Wilkins, 2013:598–660.

Saslow D, Solomon D, Lawson HW, et al. American Cancer Society, American Society for Colposcopy and Cervical Pathology, and American Society for Clinical Pathology screening guidelines for the prevention and early detection of cervical cancer. J Low Genit Tract Dis 2012;16:175–204.

Schiffman MH, Bauer HM, Hoover RN, et al. Epidemiologic evidence showing that human papillomavirus infection causes most cervical intraepithelial neoplasia. J Natl Cancer Inst 1993;85:958–964.

Suggested websites

www.asccp.org
https://www.cancer.org/cancer/cervical-cancer/html
https://www.cdc.gov/cancer/cervical/

Guidelines
National society guidelines

Title	Source	Date and weblink
Cervical cancer screening	American Society for Colposcopy and Cervical Pathology	2012 https://www.ncbi.nlm.nih.gov/pubmed/22418039
Management of abnormal cervical cancer screening results	American Society for Colposcopy and Cervical Pathology	2013 https://www.ncbi.nlm.nih.gov/pubmed/23519301
Treatment of cervical cancer	National Comprehensive Cancer Network	2015 https://www.ncbi.nlm.nih.gov/pubmed/25870376
Surveillance	Society of Gynecologic Oncology	2011 https://www.ncbi.nlm.nih.gov/pubmed/21752752

Evidence

Type of evidence	Title and comment	Date and weblink
Randomized controlled trial	A randomized trial of pelvic radiation therapy versus no further therapy in selected patients with stage IB carcinoma of the cervix after radical hysterectomy and pelvic lymphadenectomy: a Gynecologic Oncology Group Study **Comment:** Gynecologic Oncology Group trial 92 established the role of adjuvant postoperative pelvic radiation in intermediate risk patients at reducing recurrence of disease	1999 https://www.ncbi.nlm.nih.gov/pubmed/10329031
Prospective surgical/ pathologic study	A prospective surgical pathological study of stage I squamous carcinoma of the cervix: a Gynecologic Oncology Group Study **Comment:** Gynecologic Oncology Group trial 49 found that pelvic nodal metastasis, tumor size, lymphovascular space invasion, and depth of cervical stromal invasion were significant predictive factors in cervical cancer recurrence	1989 https://www.ncbi.nlm.nih.gov/pubmed/2599466
Randomized controlled trial	Concurrent chemotherapy and pelvic radiation therapy compared with pelvic radiation therapy alone as adjuvant therapy after radical surgery in high risk early-stage cancer of the cervix **Comment:** Gynecologic Oncology Group trial 109 showed that concurrent chemotherapy with radiation therapy improves PFS and OS in patients with high risk, early-stage disease who have been treated surgically for cervical cancer	2000 https://www.ncbi.nlm.nih.gov/pubmed/10764420
Randomized controlled trial	A phase III trial of adjuvant chemotherapy following chemoradiation as primary treatment for locally advanced cervical cancer compared to chemoradiation alone: The OUTBACK TRIAL **Comment:** The OUTBACK trial is ongoing and its objective is to evaluate if adjuvant chemotherapy in addition to chemoradiation improves OS	2012 http://ascopubs.org/doi/abs/10.1200/jco.2014.32.15_suppl.tps5632

Images

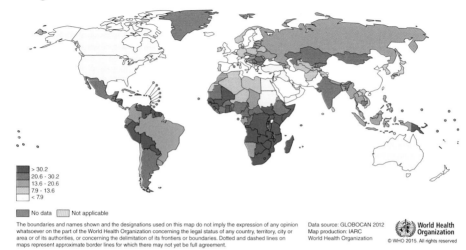

> 30.2
20.6 - 30.2
13.6 - 20.6
7.9 - 13.6
< 7.9

☐ No data   ☐ Not applicable

The boundaries and names shown and the designations used on this map do not imply the expression of any opinion whatsoever on the part of the World Health Organization concerning the legal status of any country, territory, city or area or of its authorities, or concerning the delimitation of its frontiers or boundaries. Dotted and dashed lines on maps represent approximate border lines for which there may not yet be full agreement.

Data source: GLOBOCAN 2012
Map production: IARC
World Health Organization

World Health Organization

Figure 17.1 Global distribution of cervical cancer cases. (Source: GLOBOCAN 2012 v1.0, Cancer Incidence and Mortality Worldwide: IARC CancerBase No. 11. Lyon, France: International Agency for Research on Cancer; 2013. Available from: http://globocan.iarc.fr, accessed on 11/24/2015.)

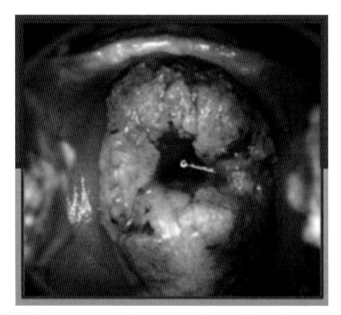

Figure 17.2 Cervical cancer seen on speculum examination (personal collection). See website for color version.

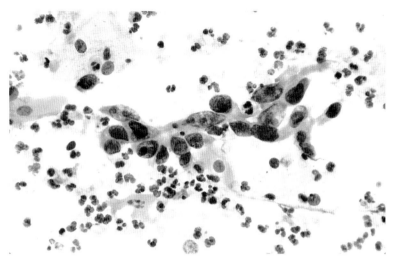

Figure 17.3 Cytologic specimen showing cervical cancer. (Image courtesy of National Cancer Institute: public domain.) See website for color version.

Additional material for this chapter can be found online at:
www.wiley.com/go/oh/mountsinaioncology

This includes advice for patients, a case study, multiple choice questions, and ICD codes. The following images are available in color: Figures 17.2 and 17.3.

CHAPTER 18

Melanoma

Philip Friedlander and Corazon B. Cajulis
Icahn School of Medicine at Mount Sinai, New York, NY, USA

OVERALL BOTTOM LINE
- Melanoma accounts for less than 2% of all skin cancers but causes the most mortality among skin cancers.
- Sun avoidance measures help prevent the development of melanoma.
- The majority of melanomas select for activation of the mitogen activated protein kinase (MAPK) signaling pathway by selecting for an activating mutation in *BRAF* (50% of melanomas) or *NRAS* (15% of melanomas).
- Treatment and management depends on the stage of disease with local and regional (stages I–III) melanomas managed surgically with wide excision and consideration of sentinel lymph node biopsy.
- Recently, there has been a significant advance in the systemic management of stage IV melanoma through the use of immunotherapy (CTLA4 and PD-1 inhibitors) and MAPK targeted therapy (*BRAF* and *MEK* inhibitors).

Background
Definition of disease
- Melanoma is a neoplasm that develops in melanocytes or is a cancer of melanocytes.
- It accounts for <2% of skin cancers but causes a high percentage of skin cancer mortality.

Disease classification
- There are four major histologic subtypes of cutaneous melanoma:
  - **Superficial spreading:** accounts for approximately 70% of all melanomas. Most arise de novo with one-fourth developing in association with a pre-existing nevus. Growth is horizontal (radial growth phase) initially and followed by invasive vertical growth (vertical growth phase).
  - **Lentigo maligna:** accounts for 10–15% of melanomas and commonly arises on areas of sun-damaged skin in older individuals. The melanoma often appears as a tan–brown macule which gradually grows in size and becomes darker and asymmetric.
  - **Acral lentiginous:** accounts for 5% of melanomas and is the most common type of melanoma in Asian and dark-skinned individuals. It arises on palmar, plantar, and subungual surfaces.
  - **Nodular:** accounts for 15–30% of all melanomas. Lesions appear darkly pigmented (although nonpigmented lesions exist, they are less frequent). They contain a vertical growth phase but lack a radial growth phase. The average depth of invasion (Breslow thickness) at the time of diagnosis is greater than that of superficial spreading melanomas.

Mount Sinai Expert Guides: Oncology, First Edition. Edited by William K. Oh and Ajai Chari.
© 2019 John Wiley & Sons Ltd. Published 2019 by John Wiley & Sons Ltd.
Companion Website: www.wiley.com/go/oh/mountsinaioncology

- Cutaneous melanomas are classified as being localized to the primary site (stage I or II), regional with spread to draining lymph nodes or dermal lymphatics (stage III), or distantly metastatic (stage IV).
- Less than 10% of melanomas are not cutaneous and arise on mucosal surfaces or are ocular (uveal melanomas). In approximately 5% of patients with melanoma the primary site is not detected (melanoma of unknown primary).

Incidence/prevalence
- The lifetime risk of developing melanoma is 2.4% for Caucasians, 0.1% for black people, and 0.5% for Hispanics (American Cancer Society, Melanoma Skin Cancer 2015).
- The median age at the time of melanoma diagnosis is 59 years (National Comprehensive Cancer Network v2.2016).
- In 2015, it was estimated that 73 870 cases of melanoma were diagnosed with 9940 people dying from the malignancy (American Cancer Society, Melanoma Skin Cancer 2015).

Economic impact
- The average annual cost per person with melanoma rose 106% from $2320 in 2002–2006 to $4780 a year in 2007–2011.
- The CDC estimate a loss of approximately $413 000 in future earnings for a person who died from melanoma with a translated total cost of $3.5 billion attributed to melanoma deaths.
- An incremental total cost increase is associated with a progressively higher stage of disease, ranging from $4448.48 for *in situ* tumors to $159 808.17 for stage IV melanoma. Surveillance accounts for 25% of the total medical cost over 5 years.

Etiology
Although the precise etiology of melanoma is unknown, melanoma has been linked to ultraviolet radiation exposure both naturally via sun exposure or artificially through tanning bed use. The association is stronger with ultraviolet B than with ultraviolet A radiation but both are important. Evidence from epidemiologic studies support this relationship.

Pathology/pathogenesis
- Ultraviolet B radiation damages the DNA in melanocytes creating cyclobutane pyrimidine dimers leading to the formation of cytosine to thymine transitions. This mechanism is not dependent on melanin.
- Ultraviolet A radiation also creates cyclobutane pyrimidine dimers but in a manner that is dependent on melanin and reactive oxygen species.
- Melanin is oxidized by reactive oxygen species from ultraviolet, normal metabolic processes, or inflammatory responses generating an increase of redox-active tautomer, intracellular redox cycling with melanosomal and DNA damage, transcription factor activation and enhancement, and the activation antiapoptotic phenotype of the melanocytes. The increased intracellular reactive oxygen species lead to DNA damage.
- The majority of acquired melanocytic nevi contain mutant *BRAF* which activates the MAPK pathway leading to cellular senescence. Selection for additional genetic alterations which are not well defined leads to transformation of nevus cells to melanoma. Loss of expression of the tumor suppressor p16 is believed to have an important role as is activation of the PI3K signaling pathway via loss of PTEN expression.
- The expression of programmed death ligand 1 (PD-L1) on the surface of metastatic melanoma cells inhibits the cytotoxic activity of PD-1 (programmed death 1) expressing T cells which infiltrate the tumor.

Predictive/risk factors

- Exposure to ultraviolet radiation through sun exposure, tanning bed use, or psoralen (PUVA) therapy.
- High nevus count on skin surface.
- Dysplastic nevi (atypical moles) present on the skin surface.
- Large congenital melanocytic nevus.
- Family history of melanoma in first degree relative.
- Personal history of a prior melanoma.
- Fair skin, red hair, and skin that freckles easily.
- History of nonmelanoma skin cancer (basal cell or squamous cell carcinoma).
- Immunosuppression (organ transplant recipients, patients with lymphoma or HIV).
- Xeroderma pigmentosum.
- Inherited genetic mutations (e.g. the CDK4 and CDKN2A genes).

Prevention

> **BOTTOM LINE/CLINICAL PEARLS**
> - Sun protection measures that limit ultraviolet ray exposure can decrease the chance of developing melanoma.
> - Avoiding tanning beds will decrease exposure to ultraviolet radiation and decrease the chance of developing melanoma.

Screening

- Skin examination to identify suspicious skin lesions can be performed for individuals with specific risk factors (https://www.uptodate.com/contents/screening-and-early-detection-of-melanoma).
- Dermoscopy, usually performed by a dermatologist, can be used to evaluate further a concerning pigmented lesion.

Primary prevention

- Avoidance of sunburn, sunbathing, and tanning beds.
- Protection of children from excessive sun exposure because severe sunburn in childhood increases the risk for melanoma.
- Generous application of sunscreen with at least SPF 30 to all exposed skin.
- Sun protection measures as such protective clothing, sunglasses, and wide-brimmed hats and seeking shade as needed especially between 10 a.m. and 4 p.m. as sun rays are strongest during these times.
- The slogan 'Slip! Slop! Slap! Wrap!' refers to slipping on a shirt, slopping on sunscreen, slapping on a hat, and wrapping on sunglasses.
- Screening for early detection of suspicious lesions with regular skin self-examination and visits to a dermatologist.

Secondary prevention

- Self-skin examination.
- Regular follow-up with a dermatologist, especially for individuals at increased risk for the development of melanoma.
- Patient and family education on screening and sun protection measures.

Diagnosis (Algorithm 18.1)

Algorithm 18.1 Diagnosis of melanoma

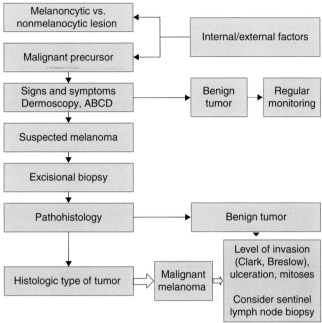

- Ask the patient about prior excessive sun exposure including severe sunburns during childhood, history of melanoma or other skin cancer, PUVA treatment, sun protection measures/practice, family history of cancer (including melanoma or skin cancer), and changes to a skin lesion or mole.
- Perform a skin examination to evaluate or differentiate typical from atypical nevi and assess suspicious lesions using ABCDs (A, asymmetry; B, irregular borders; C, color – very dark black or blue and have variation of color; D, diameter ≥6 mm; Table 18.1). Dermoscopy can be performed to further characterize the skin lesion.
- Biopsy the skin lesion concerning for melanoma. The biopsy optimally should be excisional and diagnosis of melanoma made by the reviewing pathologist.

Table 18.1 ABCD rule.

Criteria	Score X	Factor	Results
A Asymmetry (perpendicular axes: contour, colors, and structures)	0–2	1.3	0–2.6
B Borders (eight segments; abrupt ending of pigment pattern)	0–8	0.1	0–0.8
C Colors (white, red, light brown (tan), dark brown, blue–gray, black)	1–6	0.5	0.5–3.0
D Dermoscopic structures (pigment network, structureless areas, dots, aggregated globules, branched streaks)	1–5	0.5	0.5–2.5
Total score	Benign		<4.76
	Suspicious		4.76–5.45
	Melanoma		>5.45

Differential diagnosis

Differential diagnosis	Features
Squamous cell carcinoma (SCC)	Nonmelanotic skin cancer often pink or red in appearance. An amelanotic melanoma may have a similar appearance
Basal cell carcinoma (BCC)	Nonmelanotic skin cancer arising from basal cells in the skin. A plaque or nodule that may have a shiny pearl-like appearance. An amelanotic melanoma may have such an appearance. Some BCCs contain pigment
Dysplastic nevus	A pigmented atypical mole that is not malignant

Typical presentation
- Individuals typically are fair-skinned with the median age at diagnosis being 59 years. Melanoma can initially be detected by the patient noticing a pigmented lesion on the skin surface that is changing in symmetry, shape, size, or color and then bringing the lesion to medical attention. Some melanomas are first identified by a physician during a physical examination.

Clinical diagnosis
History
- Enquire about new or changing skin lesions. Specific details as to the type of changes and the time course of the changes should be determined. Changes in shape, size, color, and symmetry as well as bleeding or ulcerations should be defined.
- Determine the patient's personal and family history of cancer including but not limited to melanoma and other skin cancers.
- Determine if the patient has a history of dysplastic nevi.
- Inquire about use of sun protection measures such as use of sun block and protective clothing and about extent of prior ultraviolet radiation exposure.

Physical examination
- A full skin body examination (from head to toe) is performed by a dermatologist to assess for lesions concerning for malignancy. Examination should be performed in a well-lit comfortable environment with patient privacy ensured.
- Lymph node basins in the drainage area of the melanoma should be palpated to assess for lymphadenopathy. The locoregional area should be palpated to assess for in-transit metastases.

Disease severity classification
The stage at presentation provides important prognostic information and guides treatment planning. The AJCC melanoma staging system uses pathologic features and patterns of spread from the primary site to determine stage. For a given patient a T, N, and M score is determined. The T score is based upon the vertical depth of invasion (Breslow thickness) and is modified (a or b) based upon the absence or presence of ulceration at the primary site. Thin melanomas (≤ 1 mm thickness) are also modified (a or b) based on the absence or presence of mitoses. The N stage is determined by the number of lymph nodes involved, the presence of in-transit metastases, and the size of involved nodes. The M stage is determined by the location of distant metastases. An elevation in LDH in the blood automatically confers the worst prognostic substage of stage IV melanoma (M1C) irrespective of the location of metastases.

The following is the AJCC TNM staging system for melanoma:

- T stage: tumor size/thickness:
  - Tx: the primary tumor cannot be assessed (i.e. severely regressed melanoma)
  - T0: no evidence of primary tumor
  - Tis: melanoma *in situ*
  - T1–T4:
    - T1: ≤1.0 mm
    - T2: 1.01–2 mm
    - T3: 2.01–4 mm
    - T4: >4 mm.

Thin melanomas (T1) are assigned subcategory a (without ulceration and mitosis < 1/mm^2) or subcategory b (with ulceration or mitosis ≥ 1/mm^2). Deeper melanomas are subcategorized as a or b based on the ulceration status.

- N stage: lymph node analysis includes number of lymph nodes involved and a subcategory (a, b, or c) to denote presence of:
  - a: micrometastasis
  - b: macrometastasis
  - c: in-transit metastases without metastatic node
  - N0: no nodes involved
  - N1: 1 node involved
  - N2: 2–3 nodes involved, in-transit metastases without metastatic nodes
  - N3: 4 or more nodes involved or in-transit metastases plus metastatic nodes.

Micrometastases are usually diagnosed after sentinel lymph node biopsy. Macrometastases often are clinically detectable and confirmed by biopsy.

- M stage: distant spread of the melanoma:
  - a: metastases to skin subcutaneous, or distant lymph nodes
  - b: metastases to lungs
  - c: metastases to all other visceral sites or distant metastases to any site combined with elevated serum LDH.

The TNM scores are combined to determine the overall stage: stage 0 (melanoma *in situ*); stage I (localized melanoma with thickness ≤1 mm or melanoma 1.01–2 mm thick with ulceration); stage II (localized melanoma 1.01–2 mm thickness with ulceration or melanoma thicker than 2 mm); stage III (presence of regional lymph node or in-transit metastases); or stage IV (distant metastases).

Laboratory diagnosis
List of diagnostic tests

- **Biopsy of suspicious cutaneous lesion:** the pathology report will document the diagnosis of melanoma and should include the Breslow thickness, ulceration status, mitotic rate, deep and peripheral margin status, presence or absence of microsatellitosis, and for thin melanomas the Clark level. Pathologists are encouraged to report the location of the tumor and the presence of tumor infiltrating lymphocytes, regression, neurotrophism, and lymphovascular invasion. Often, hematoxylin and eosin staining will be performed in addition to immunohistochemistry.
- **CBC, CMP, and LDH:** have low sensitivity to assess for recurrence in locoregional melanoma and are not performed on a routine basis.
- **Genetic analysis of biopsied melanoma:** to determine if a mutation is present at position 600 of *BRAF*. This information is important for management of patients with stage IV melanoma and should be determined in these patients.

Lists of imaging techniques
- MRI of brain with or without contrast to define the extent of disease in stage IV melanoma and to follow at intervals for the development of brain metastases. Also consider when a patient develops new or worsening neurologic symptoms or headaches.
- CT CAP or PET scan to define the extent of stage IV melanoma and to monitor interval change over time. Also consider on a case-by-case basis in patients with stage III or deep stage II melanoma for surveillance or for evaluation of symptoms. There is no proven survival benefit to surveillance imaging in patients with stage I–III melanoma.

Potential pitfalls/common errors made regarding diagnosis of disease
- Inaccurate pathology assessment.
- Inaccurate dermatologic assessment of a cutaneous lesion.

Treatment (Algorithm 18.2)

Algorithm 18.2 Treatment of melanoma

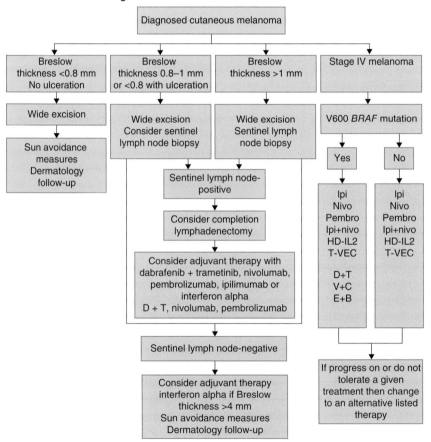

B, binimetinib; C, cobimetinib; D, dabrafenib; E, encorafenib; HD-IL-2, high dose interleukin 2; Ipi, ipilimumab; nivo, nivolumab; pembro, pembrolizumab; T, trametinib; V, vemurafenib.

Treatment rationale
- Manage localized melanomas surgically. Recommended margins are 0.5–1 cm (melanoma *in situ*), 1 cm (≤1 mm thick), 1–2 cm (1.01–2 mm thick), and 2 cm (>2 mm thick). Consider sentinel lymph node (SLN) biopsy when the melanoma is >1 mm thick or 0.8–1 mm thick,

or <0.8 mm thick with ulceration or other adverse pathologic features. A lymphadenectomy should be considered when the SLN is involved. Patients presenting with lymphadenopathy should undergo biopsy to confirm melanoma followed by lymphadenectomy.
- Consider adjuvant interferon alpha (stage III or deep stage II melanoma) and nivolumab, pembrolizumab or ipilimumab (stage III melanoma). Consider dabrafenib plus trametinib if V600 BRAF mutation present (stage III melanoma).
- Consider systemic therapy for stage IV melanoma and metastatectomy in select cases of oligometastases. Options for wild-type *BRAF* melanoma include immunotherapy (CTLA4 inhibitor ipilimumab, PD-1 inhibitors nivolumab and pembrolizumab, ipilimumab plus nivolumab, interleukin-2, T-VEC, and dacarbazine). Immunotherapy is preferred over dacarbazine. T-VEC, a modified oncolytic herpes virus producing the immune stimulant granulocyte–macrophage colony stimulating factor, is administered intratumorally. Consider in patients with unresectable cutaneous, subcutaneous, or nodal lesions and limited visceral disease.
- In V600 *BRAF*-mutated melanoma consider *BRAF* (encorafenib, vemurafenib or dabrafenib) and *MEK* (binimetinib, trametinib or cobimetinib) inhibitor treatment. Combined *BRAF* and *MEK* inhibition (encorafenib plus binimetinib, dabrafenib plus trametinib, or vemurafenib plus cobimetinib) confers additional survival benefits. Optimal sequencing of immunotherapy versus *BRAF* inhibition is unknown.

When to hospitalize
- Consider as part of evaluation and management of high grade toxicity form treatment.
- Consider to optimize evaluation and palliation of disease-related symptoms and functional declines.

Table of treatment

Treatment	Comments
Conservative	In patients with stage I–III melanoma: daily sunscreen use, sun avoidance measures, dermatology follow-up for skin checks
Medical	
Interferon alpha Ipilimumab nivolumab, pembrolizumab	Adjuvant therapy for stage III melanoma. Monitor for autoimmune toxicity. Interferon also approved for use in stage II melanoma with T4 thickness
High dose interleukin 2 Ipilimumab Pembrolizumab Nivolumab Ipilimumab plus nivolumab	For patients with stage IV melanoma irrespective of the presence or absence of a *BRAF* mutation
T-VEC	T-VEC is administered intratumorally into soft tissue metastasis or lymph node accessible by ultrasound. Patients should have limited visceral disease
Encorafenib Dabrafenib Vemurafenib Trametinib Cobimetinib Binimetinib, encorafenib plus binimetinib Dabrafenib plus trametinib Vemurafenib plus cobimetinib	Inhibitors of the MAPK signaling pathway Option for patients with melanoma expressing V600 mutated *BRAF*. Concurrent *BRAF* and *MEK* inhibition increases the response rate and survival compared with *BRAF* inhibition alone

(*Continued*)

Treatment	Comments
Surgical	
Wide excision	For patients with primary cutaneous melanoma. Size of margins depends on Breslow thickness
Sentinal lymph node biopsy	Perform when the Breslow thickness of the primary melanoma is >1.0 mm
	Consider when the thickness is 0.8–1.0 mm or <0.8 with ulceration
Completion lymph node dissection	Consider when the sentinel lymph node is positive for melanoma
Radiologic	
PET scan CT of the chest, abdomen, pelvis Brain MRI	To define baseline extent of disease and interval change over time in patients with stage IV melanoma
	Consider in high risk stage II and III melanoma patients to assess for development of metastases or to evaluate a concerning symptom in earlier stage melanoma

Prevention/management of complications
- Autoimmune toxicity caused by CTLA4 and PD-1 inhibitors (examples include rash, colitis, nephritis, uveitis, pneumonitis, endocrine, neurologic, and hepatitis). Management includes holding or discontinuation of treatment and consideration of steroids or other immunosuppressants.
- High fever with *BRAF* inhibitors: management includes consideration of holding treatment, hydration, tylenol, dose reductions, steroids in refractory cases.
- Cutaneous squamous cell carcinoma with *BRAF* targeted therapy: dermatology evaluations, excision of the carcinomas.

CLINICAL PEARLS
- Consider SLN biopsy in melanomas more than 1 mm thick and those 0.8–1 mm thick or <0.8 mm with other adverse pathologic features.
- Consider treatments which inhibit the MAPK pathway (*BRAF* and *MEK* inhibitors) in patients with melanoma expressing mutant *BRAF* but not wild-type *BRAF*.
- Development of high grade autoimmune toxicities can limit treatment with PD-1 and CTLA-4 inhibitors.

Special populations
Others
- Melanoma containing a mutation in *cKIT*: while not FDA approved, can consider use of *KIT* inhibitors such as imatinib as treatment for stage IV melanomas containing *KIT* mutations.
- If brain metastases are detected consider neurosurgical resection and or radiation based treatment approaches.

Prognosis

> **BOTTOM LINE/CLINICAL PEARLS**
> - For stage IV melanoma the 5-year survival rate is 15–20% and the 10-year survival rate is 10–15%.
> - For stage IA melanoma the 5-year survival rate is approximately 97% and the 10-year survival rate 95%.
> - Immunotherapy (CTLA-4 and PD-1 inhibitors) and targeted therapy (*BRAF* and *MEK* inhibitors) have demonstrated survival benefits in stage IV melanoma.

Reading list

Alexandrescu D. Melanoma costs: a dynamic model comparing estimated overall costs of various clinical stages. Dermatol Online J 2009;15:11.

Chapman P, Hauschild A, Robert C, et al. Improved survival with vemurafenib in melanoma with BRAF V600E mutation. N Engl J Med 2011;364:2507–2516.

Curtin JA, Fridlyand J, Kageshita T, et al. Distinct sets of genetic alterations in melanoma. N Engl J Med 2005;353:2135–2147.

Larkin J, Chiarion-Sileni V, Gonzalez R, et al. Combined nivolumab and ipilimumab or monotherapy in untreated melanoma. N Engl J Med 2015;373:23–34.

Meyskens F, Farmer P, Anton-Culver H. Etiologic pathogenesis of melanoma: a unifying hypothesis for the attributable risk. Clin Cancer Res 2004;10:2581–2583.

Robert C, Karaszewska B, Schachter J, et al. Improved overall survival in melanoma with combined dabrafenib and trametinib. N Engl J Med 2015;372:30–39.

Robert C, Schachter J, Long GV, et al. Pembrolizumab versus ipilimumab in advanced melanoma. N Engl J Med 2015;372:2521–2532.

Shain AH, Yeh I, Kovalyshyn I, et al. The genetic evolution of melanoma from precursor lesions. N Engl J Med 2015;373:1926–1936.

Suggested websites

www.nccn.org
www.acs.org
www.aim@melanoma.org
www.up-to-date.com
www.melanomafoundation.org
http://emedicine.medscape.com
www.ncbi.nlm.nih.gov

Guidelines
National society guidelines

Title	Source	Date and weblink
Melanoma	NCCN	2016 www.nccn.org

> **Additional material for this chapter can be found online at:**
> **www.wiley.com/go/oh/mountsinaioncology**
>
> **This includes advice for patients and ICD codes.**

CHAPTER 19

Sarcomas

Robert G. Maki

Northwell Cancer Institute and Cold Spring Harbor Laboratory, Long Island, NY, USA

> ## OVERALL BOTTOM LINE
> - Sarcomas encompass over 70 different types of cancer.
> - Treatment is a function of histology and anatomic site.
> - Defining the treatment plan to cure or palliate is the most important first question of treatment.
> - Adjuvant therapy is given to patients with diagnoses most common in pediatric populations and to some patients with a gastrointestinal stromal tumor.

Background

Definition of disease

- Sarcomas are malignant neoplasms of soft tissue and bone.
- Some soft tissue and bone neoplasms such as desmoid tumor or deep fibromatosis are locally aggressive but do not metastasize or only rarely; these cause death only in rare cases.

Disease classification

- Sarcomas are classified by histology and increasingly by using DNA and/or molecular methods to determine the specific subtype, which can also have therapeutic implications.

Incidence/prevalence

- Approximately 15 000 new diagnoses per year in the USA; 80% soft tissue and 20% bone.
- Sarcomas represent ~15% of pediatric cancers and <1% of adult cancers.
- Gastrointestinal stromal tumor (GIST) is the most common sarcoma in adults; liposarcoma, leiomyosarcoma, and undifferentiated pleomorphic sarcoma are other common adult subtypes.
- Osteosarcoma, Ewing sarcoma, and rhabdomyosarcoma are the three most common sarcomas in children.

Etiology

- Most sarcomas are spontaneous cancers without an obvious inciting cause.
- The most common known cause of sarcomas is prior therapeutic radiation exposure; secondary sarcomas arise in the penumbra of the radiation port at a median of 9 years after radiotherapy is complete.

Pathology/pathogenesis

- Reciprocal translocations between two chromosomes cause many sarcomas under age 40.
- *KIT* or *PDGFRA* mutation is the driving factor for GIST.

Mount Sinai Expert Guides: Oncology, First Edition. Edited by William K. Oh and Ajai Chari.
© 2019 John Wiley & Sons Ltd. Published 2019 by John Wiley & Sons Ltd.
Companion Website: www.wiley.com/go/oh/mountsinaioncology

- Sarcomas are most common over the age of 50 and are usually highly aneuploid, looking much like other adult cancers genomically.

Predictive/risk factors

Risk factor	Odds ratio
Metastatic disease	Fatal in over 90% of patients

Prevention

> **BOTTOM LINE/CLINICAL PEARLS**
> - No interventions other than avoiding therapeutic irradiation have been demonstrated to prevent the development of the disease.

Screening

- There are no screening tests for sarcoma, unless a patient has a genetic syndrome (e.g. familial GIST, Li–Fraumeni syndrome), in which intermittent monitoring for the development of a primary cancer can be considered (NCCN Guidelines).

Diagnosis

> **BOTTOM LINE/CLINICAL PEARLS**
> - Enlarging painless mass.
> - Lipomas (superficial, squishy) are at least 100 times more common than sarcomas.
> - Any mass bigger than a golf ball merits evaluation.
> - Core needle biopsy by a clinician knowledgeable in eventual surgical excision anatomy is usually sufficient for diagnosis whether soft tissue or bony primary tumor.
> - An experience pathologist is critical for the proper diagnosis.

Differential diagnosis

Differential diagnosis	Features
Lipoma	Superficial, subcutaneous, squishy, not changing over years
Enchondroma	In appropriate anatomic site; common benign bone finding

Typical presentation

- A 50-year-old woman presents with an 8-cm mass growing in the left gluteal area over the course of 6 months. It is increasingly uncomfortable to sit on that area of the body.
- An 11-year-old boy presents with antalgic gait and painful swelling about the right knee in the distal femur.

Clinical diagnosis

History

- Length of time the lesion has been noticed.
- If painful, when the pain is most severe.
- Family history of sarcomas or other cancers.

Physical examination
- Identify the size of the mass, as much as possible manually. Is the mass mobile or fixed?
- Is there evidence based on symptoms of other sites of metastatic disease?

Useful clinical decision rules and calculators
- Risk can be calculated based on histology, size, and other factors.

Disease severity classification
- AJCC version 7 sarcoma staging criteria are used for adults with sarcomas.
- Rhabdomyosarcoma in children has its own staging system.

Laboratory diagnosis
List of diagnostic tests
- MRI of primary site (soft tissue primary).
- Plain X-rays in addition to MRI (bony primary).
- Core needle biopsy (by orthopod or interventional radiology).
- Expert pathology review, which includes FISH or other DNA tests.

Lists of imaging techniques
- MRI of primary site.
- Noncontrast CT scan of chest to rule out lung metastatic disease for extremity or uterine primary.
- For GIST, CT of abdomen and pelvis with contrast to complete staging.
- Surgeon should decide on the benefit and/or need for PET.
- Pediatric hematology: oncology should be involved early for any child with a possible sarcoma.

Potential pitfalls/common errors made regarding diagnosis of disease
- Transverse incision across an extremity for diagnostic biopsy; resection of old biopsy site becomes much more difficult.
- Attention must be paid to hemostasis otherwise tumor cells could track with bleeding.
- Multiple biopsies at different sites increase the risk of tumor spread.
- Lack of experience of many pathologists with diagnosis leads to misdiagnosis in as many as 25% of patients.

Treatment
Treatment rationale
- Surgery is nearly always necessary for curative intent.
- Adjuvant radiation therapy is often used for larger soft tissue tumors.
- Adjuvant radiation therapy is not offered for osteosarcoma.
- Systemic therapy before or after surgery is nearly always given to patients with diagnoses more common in children (e.g. Ewing sarcoma, osteosarcoma, and rhabdomyosarcoma).
- The benefit of systemic therapy in the adjuvant setting for most common soft tissue sarcomas in adults is small, if any.
- For GIST, 3 years of adjuvant imatinib is appropriate for higher risk tumors based on a randomized clinical trial.
- Metastatic disease is treated with radiation, chemotherapy, or surgery depending on the nature of the recurrence.
- Some people with sarcoma metastatic to lungs can be cured with surgery. Most other surgery in the metastatic setting is palliative.

When to hospitalize
- Oncologic emergencies (e.g. spinal cord compression, pain crisis, hypercalcemia of malignancy, bowel obstruction).
- Complications of chemotherapy (e.g. febrile neutropenia, sepsis).

Managing the hospitalized patient
- Febrile neutropenic patients must be managed with "stop sepsis" management in mind: blood, urine cultures, other body fluid cultures, and rapid application of antibiotics.
- Spinal cord compression needs rapid surgical debulking; radiotherapy can be considered post-operatively or if surgery is not feasible. Chemotherapy is nearly never appropriate for management of a cord compression.

Table of treatment
Conservative
- For lower risk cancers (after surgery).
- Also appropriate for patients with end-stage disease.

Medical
- Imatinib, sunitinib, regorafenib for GIST.
- Doxorubicin for soft tissue sarcomas.
- Ifosfamide for soft tissue sarcomas.
- Vincristine-doxorubicin-cyclophosphamide for Ewing sarcoma.
- Ifosfamide-etoposide for Ewing sarcoma.
- Vincristine-dactinomycin-cyclophosphamide for pediatric rhabdomyosarcoma.
- Cisplatin-doxorubicin +/− methotrexate for osteosarcoma.

Surgical
- Primary surgery.
- Palliative surgery
  - e.g. impending fracture from metastatic disease − better to operate before the fracture than afterwards.

Radiologic
- Radiation for primary disease to improve cure rate.
- Palliative radiation
  - Traditional palliative radiation schemes
  - Radiosurgical approaches (short course).

Complementary medicine
- Pain medication.
- Antiemetics.
- Other medications for supportive care.

Other
- Immunotherapy is still experimental.
- Interventional radiologic techniques for metastatic disease
  - Embolization of liver
  - Radiofrequency ablation
  - Cryotherapy.

Treatment	Comments
Conservative	For patients with low risk tumors; palliative care only in end-stages
Medical (see text)	Consult medical oncology for details of what to watch for because each diagnosis is different and not amenable to a clinical pearl
Surgical	Primary therapy for soft tissue or bone sarcomas Used much less frequently for palliation
Radiologic	Higher risk patients often receive radiation for extremity sarcomas Radiation can be used for palliation of painful or otherwise symptomatic metastatic lesions
Complementary	Pain and palliative care consultation early in management of metastatic disease, in particular those patients with significant issues with pain that are difficult to manage
Other	Immunotherapy remains experimental
	Interventional radiology techniques or radiosurgery for individual lesions causing morbidity

Prevention/management of complications
- Febrile neutropenia from cytotoxic chemotherapy; track CBC/absolute neutrophil count.
- Nephropathy from ifosfamide; follow creatinine.
- Proteinuria from VEGF inhibitors; monitor by urinalysis or timed urine protein collection, unfolded protein response.

Management/treatment algorithm
Sarcomas involve over 70 diagnoses. It is not possible to provide a management plan other than to say multidisciplinary approaches are paramount for the greatest degree of clinical success. Mishaps in chemotherapy, surgery, and radiation can lead to adverse outcomes. Refer to the NCCN guidelines for considerations of management for diverse clinical scenarios.

CLINICAL PEARLS
- "Stop sepsis" protocols for febrile neutropenia.
- Use antiemetics routinely with appropriate chemotherapy agents.
- Pain medications and antiemetics such as ondansetron cause constipation; be sure patients have appropriate laxatives.
- Be aware of neuropathy from specific chemotherapy agents (e.g. vinca alkaloids, cisplatin).
- Cardiomyopathy is uncommon; nonetheless cardiac function (echo or MUGA) must be monitored for patients receiving anthracycline.

Special populations
Pregnancy
- Chemotherapy is avoided in the first trimester. Certain chemotherapy drugs can be safely administered during the second or third trimester, however, and surgery can be conducted then. Radiation is almost never used in pregnancy.

Children
- Children nearly always receive systemic chemotherapy for their specific sarcoma diagnoses.
- Treatment regimens have been developed for each common pediatric sarcoma (i.e. osteogenic sarcoma, Ewing sarcoma, rhabdomyosarcoma).

- Each sarcoma is common in a unique age group with rhabdomyosarcoma more common between ages 2 and 7, and osteosarcoma and Ewing sarcoma from 10–17 years of age.

Elderly
- Surgery and often radiation therapy are still necessary for curative intent in elderly patients.
- Adjuvant chemotherapy for extremity sarcoma is not given to elderly patients as the risk outweighs potential benefit.
- Adjuvant imatinib can still be considered for elderly patients.

Others
- Surgery is contraindicated in patients who have a high risk of perioperative mortality.
- "Definitive" radiation therapy occasionally can be used when surgery cannot be employed, sometimes with curative intent.
- Chemotherapy, if given to a patient with significant comorbidities, must be tailored to those comorbidities, otherwise the risk of death from drug toxicity is higher.

Prognosis

> **BOTTOM LINE/CLINICAL PEARLS**
> - Sarcoma management varies widely based on histology, anatomic site, age, and patient comorbidities.
> - Surgery is nearly always needed for curative intent.
> - Radiation therapy is often employed for larger tumors, especially in older patients; the concern of long-term radiation side effects makes one circumspect about its use in younger patients.
> - Chemotherapy is essentially mandatory in patients with diagnoses more common in children (e.g. osteogenic sarcoma, Ewing sarcoma, rhabdomyosarcoma).

Natural history of untreated disease
- The death rate from metastatic disease is very high.
- Ignored primary lesions will lead to surgeries that would not have been contemplated otherwise (e.g. amputations). Amputations currently represent under 10% of the surgeries needed for primary control of a sarcoma.

Prognosis for treated patients
Prognosis is a function of histology, stage, and tumor location.

Follow-up tests and monitoring
- Following patients for metastatic disease after primary treatment is commonly conducted every 4–6 months for 3 years or more following treatment of the primary disease, for the average sarcoma. This recommendation varies based on the aggressiveness of the tumor subtype and its ability to recur or metastasize.

Reading list
American Joint Committee on Cancer. AJCC Cancer Staging Manual, 8th edition. New York: Springer, 2017.

Brennan MF, Antonescu CR, Maki RG. Management of Soft Tissue Sarcoma. 2nd edition. New York: Springer, 2017.

Hornick JL. Practical Soft Tissue Pathology: A Diagnostic Approach. Philadelphia: Elsevier, 2013.

Lin PP, Patel S. Bone Sarcoma. New York: Springer, 2013.

Maki RG, Blay JY, Demetri GD, et al. Key issues in the clinical management of gastrointestinal stromal tumors: an expert discussion. Oncologist 2015;20:823–830. PMID: 26070915.

Schöffski P, Cornillie J, Wozniak A, et al. Soft tissue sarcoma: an update on systemic treatment options for patients with advanced disease. Oncol Res Treat 2014;37:355–362. PMID: 24903768.

Suggested websites

https://www.cancer.net/cancer-types/sarcoma-soft-tissue
https://www.cancer.net/cancer-types/bone-cancer
https://www.cancer.gov/types/soft-tissue-sarcoma/hp
https://www.cancer.gov/types/bone
http://www.nccn.org/professionals/physician_gls/PDF/sarcoma.pdf

Guidelines
National society guidelines

Title	Source and comment	Date and weblink
National Comprehensive Cancer Network	NCCN **Comment:** Very good reference for basics on sarcoma management, although it is mostly a document to capture most things physicians do as a backstop for justification for insurance coverage	2019 http://www.nccn.org/professionals/physician_gls/PDF/sarcoma.pdf

Evidence

Type of evidence	Title and comment	Date and weblink
RCT	One vs. three years of adjuvant imatinib for operable gastrointestinal stromal tumor: a randomized trial **Comment:** Adjuvant imatinib is useful for primary GIST therapy	2012 https://www.ncbi.nlm.nih.gov/pubmed/22453568
RCT	Pazopanib for metastatic soft-tissue sarcoma (PALETTE): a randomised, double-blind, placebo-controlled phase 3 trial **Comment:** Pazopanib is useful for advanced sarcomas after failure of other chemotherapy	2012 https://www.ncbi.nlm.nih.gov/pubmed/22595799
RCT	Randomized controlled trial of interval-compressed chemotherapy for the treatment of localized Ewing sarcoma **Comment:** Adjuvant chemotherapy is useful for Ewing sarcoma	2012 https://www.ncbi.nlm.nih.gov/pubmed/23091096
RCT	Doxorubicin alone versus intensified doxorubicin plus ifosfamide for first line treatment of advanced or metastatic soft-tissue sarcoma: a randomised controlled phase 3 trial **Comment:** Doxorubicin and ifosfamide is useful as is doxorubicin in first line metastatic sarcoma	2014 https://www.ncbi.nlm.nih.gov/pubmed/24618336

Additional material for this chapter can be found online at:
www.wiley.com/go/oh/mountsinaioncology

This includes advice for patients, a case study, and ICD codes.

CHAPTER 20

Thyroid Cancer

Aaron M. Etra and Krzysztof Misiukiewicz
Icahn School of Medicine at Mount Sinai, New York, NY, USA

OVERALL BOTTOM LINE
- Thyroid cancer represents a wide spectrum of histologically different malignancies with different biology and prognosis, from relatively indolent, papillary, and follicular, to very aggressive, anaplastic carcinoma.
- Ultrasound of the thyroid with cervical lymph node assessment should be performed for all known and suspected thyroid nodules.
- Ultrasound-guided FNA biopsy, if clinically indicated, is the most accurate method for evaluating thyroid nodules and selecting patients for thyroid surgery.
- Appropriate histologic diagnosis by an experienced pathologist is essential.
- Surgery is the primary mode of therapy for patients with differentiated thyroid cancer. The surgical approach depends upon the extent of the disease, the patient's age, family history, previous radiation exposure, and the presence of comorbid conditions.

Background
Definition of disease
- Thyroid carcinoma is a cancer of the thyroid gland. There are multiple subtypes with vastly different prognoses and treatment options.

Disease classification
- Differentiated thyroid cancer (DTC) can be subdivided into papillary, follicular, and Hurthle subtypes.
- Medullary thyroid cancer (MTC).
- Anaplastic thyroid cancer (ATC).

Incidence/prevalence
- Overall, the incidence of thyroid cancer in the USA is 13.5 cases per 100 000 people (SEER 2015). There is a marked 3 : 1 female preponderance in all but MTC, and the median age of diagnosis is 45–50 years.
- Some 82% of cases are of the papillary subtype, 10–15% are of the follicular subtype, 3% are of the Hurthle subtype, 2–3% are of the medullary subtype, and 2–3% are of the anaplastic subtype.
- Based on current trends, the incidence of thyroid cancer may increase to 89 500 per year by 2023.

Mount Sinai Expert Guides: Oncology, First Edition. Edited by William K. Oh and Ajai Chari.
© 2019 John Wiley & Sons Ltd. Published 2019 by John Wiley & Sons Ltd.
Companion Website: www.wiley.com/go/oh/mountsinaioncology

Economic impact
- Published per patient cost estimates for papillary thyroid cancer patients without metastasis are $34 723 and with metastasis $58 660, with a total cost of $18–21 billion by 2023.

Etiology
- Often, the etiology of these diseases is not known.
- Some patients have a hereditary predisposition to developing papillary thyroid cancer, for example those with Gardner syndrome, Cowden syndrome, and multiple endocrine neoplasia (MEN) syndrome. People without a known syndrome are still at increased risk if they have a family history.
- History of radiation exposure, either iatrogenic or occupational, is a predisposing factor.

Pathology/pathogenesis
- Multiple signaling pathways involved in regulation of the cell cycle have been implicated in development of thyroid cancer.
- Specifically, mutations involving the *MAPK* and *PI3K-AKT* pathways have been observed. The *BRAF* V600E mutation occurs in about 45% of papillary thyroid cancers, and *RAS* mutations are thought to contribute to the evolution of thyroid adenomas to carcinoma.
- Copy number gene variations, most commonly involving EGFR and VEGFR1, are more prevalent in ATC, perhaps contributing to the aggressiveness of this thyroid cancer subtype.
- Epigenetic phenomena, notably hypermethylation, likely contribute to suppression of tumor suppressor gene activation in papillary, follicular, and anaplastic thyroid cancers.

Prevention

> **BOTTOM LINE/CLINICAL PEARLS**
> - Unfortunately, lifestyle modifications have little if any effect on the development of thyroid cancer. However, in light of radiation exposure as a risk factor, unnecessary irradiation of the thyroid gland should be avoided, especially in childhood.

Screening
- Routine screening is not recommended. A large percentage of people are thought to carry a subclinical papillary thyroid cancer that will not contribute to their morbidity or mortality. National sonographic screening programs, notably in Korea, have yielded a dramatic increase in thyroid cancer diagnosis and treatment, without a concurrent decline in cancer-related mortality.
- The role of sonographic thyroid cancer screening remains controversial, even in high risk patients, such as those with Cowden disease, FAP, MEN2, and so on. At the minimum, high risk patients should undergo careful history and physical examination routinely.

Primary prevention
- Minimize exposure to ionizing radiation.

Secondary prevention
- At this time, no interventions have been definitively shown to minimize the risk of cancer recurrence.

Diagnosis (Algorithm 20.1)

Algorithm 20.1 Diagnosis of thyroid cancer

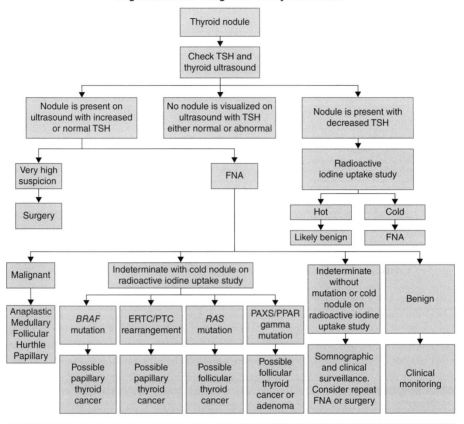

BOTTOM LINE/CLINICAL PEARLS

- Symptoms brought about by mass effect, hyperthyroidism, hypothyroidism, or hypocalcemia can also be present.
- Patients may present with an asymptomatic palpable thyroid nodule, or a nodule can be incidentally noted on chest or neck imaging.
- Further diagnostic evaluation with serum thyroid stimulating hormone (TSH), ultrasound, and FNA biopsy should be performed.
- If the TSH is low, a radioisotope scan should be performed to characterize the thyroid nodule.

Differential diagnosis

Differential diagnosis	Features
Thyroid adenoma	Like a thyroid malignancy, a thyroid adenoma can hypersecrete thyroid hormone (or not). It is primarily differentiated from a thyroid neoplasm via pathologic analysis of an FNA specimen
Colloid nodule	Usually does not generate symptoms, pathologic analysis of FNA tissue will be diagnostic

Typical presentation

- Hoarseness
- Neck mass
- Dysphagia
- Dyspnea.

Clinical diagnosis

History

- Upon presentation, the patient should be asked when they first noted the neck mass, how rapidly it is growing, and whether their ability to breathe or swallow has been compromised. Additionally, the presence of temperature intolerance, hair and nail changes, and perturbations in weight and energy level should be noted. Lastly, the patient should be asked about exposure to ionizing radiation, as well as whether there is a family history of thyroid cancer or a cancer syndrome.

Physical examination

- Physical examination should be carefully performed to ascertain the size and consistency of the thyroid nodule, its adhesion to local structures, as well as to evaluate for the local or distant presence of lymphadenopathy. Additionally, the patient's ability to breathe (i.e. the presence of stridor) and swallow, as well as signs of hypothyroidism or hyperthyroidism should be assessed.

Disease severity classification

- As with many neoplasms, thyroid cancer is staged according to a TNM scheme with stages allocated based on the extent of tumor growth, spread to the lymph nodes, and the presence or absence of metastasis. Additionally, some thyroid cancer subtypes are more treatable than others, with ATC and MTC carrying worse prognoses than follicular or papillary thyroid cancers.

List of diagnostic tests

- If a thyroid nodule is palpated or noted incidentally on imaging, an ultrasound of the neck with cervical lymph node assessment should be performed. Suspicious sonographic findings include hypo-echogenicity, microcalcifications, absence of peripheral halo, irregular borders, solid aspect, intranodular blood flow, and shape (taller than wide).
- If there is sonographic suspicion for thyroid cancer, if the thyroid mass is >1 cm, or if there is a family history or personal history of exposure to ionizing radiation, then the lesion should be biopsied via FNA.
- TSH, FT4, T3, calcitonin, and radioactive iodine (RAI) uptake tests may be considered as well (RAI uptake will need to be ordered if TSH is low).
- Ultrasound and MRI are the preferred modalities for local staging. Iodinated CT contrast can interfere with RAI-based diagnostic tests and therapies. Consultation with a thyroid specialist is warranted to weigh the risks and benefits of different strategies (King 2008).

Lists of imaging techniques

- Ultrasound is the preferred modality for initial assessment of the thyroid gland and local lymph nodes. This test should be ordered whenever a possible thyroid nodule is palpated on physical examination or when one is noted incidentally on CT or MRI.
- If thyroid ultrasound is ambiguous, an FDG-PET scan may be considered but is not routinely required.
- In the event that the patient is thought to have a high likelihood of advanced disease on presentation, CT or MRI assessment with intravenous contrast may be necessary for staging.

Potential pitfalls/common errors made regarding diagnosis of disease
- Some palpable lesions may not correspond to radiologic abnormalities.
- Abnormal lymph nodes adjacent to the thyroid gland can be mistaken for benign nodules in a multinodular thyroid.

Treatment
Treatment rationale
Most of the time, thyroid cancer is initially treated with thyroid lobectomy or total thyroidectomy. Neck dissection may also be required.
- Suppression of TSH with levothyroxine may be considered in some circumstances.
- RAI ablation is employed in some papillary, follicular, and Hurthle cell thyroid cancers either as part of the initial treatment or as a salvage regimen.
- Some thyroid carcinomas are treated with adjuvant or salvage EBRT.
- Sorafenib and lenvatinib are approved by the US FDA for treatment of metastatic DTC that is refractory to radioactive iodine ablation.
- Vandetanib or cabozantinib are approved by the FDA for treatment of unresectable or recurrent MTC.
- There is a role for chemotherapy and EBRT in unresectable ATC.

When to hospitalize
- Post-thyroidectomy bilateral recurrent nerve injury can be immediately life-threatening, causing stridor and dyspnea.
- Additionally, postoperative hypocalcemia can result in tetany, seizures, laryngospasm, or markedly prolonged QT intervals.
- Gastrointestinal perforation, cardiac ischemia/infarction, bleeding, rising liver tests, and abnormal renal function can arise in patients being treated with TKIs.

Managing the hospitalized patient
- For severe recurrent nerve injury, reintubation and tracheostomy may be necessary. Surgical procedures such as laryngoplasty and arytenoid adduction can be considered.
- Continuous intravenous drip with calcium gluconate for severe hypocalcemia.

Table of treatment

Treatment	Comments
Conservative	An active surveillance management approach to papillary microcarcinoma in contrast to immediate surgical resection can be considered but *only in properly selected patients*
Medical	Postoperative thyroid hormone replacement with goal of TSH below 0.5 mU/L DTC: Thyroid remnant ablation with RAI RAI refractory R/M DTC: • Sorafenib 400 mg orally twice daily • Lenvatinib 24 mg orally once daily R/M MTC: • Vandetanib 300 mg orally once daily • Cabozantinib 140 mg orally once daily

(*Continued*)

Treatment	Comments
Surgical	Goal: • To establish histologic diagnosis • Definitive cancer removal Total vs. partial thyroidectomy is dependent on the size of the tumor, family history, and/or history of previous radiation exposure
External beam radiation	External beam radiation is reserved for advanced disease

Prevention/management of complications

RAI:

• Rapid clearance of RAI from the urinary bladder can be enhanced by adequate volume oral hydration.
• Sialadenitis – NSAIDs can be used.
• Fertility counseling should be offered.

TKI:

• Proteinuria: laboratory tests, urine dipstick/urinalysis/24-hour urine collection.
• Q/T prolongation with torsade de pointes and sudden death – baseline ECG.
• Hemorrhagic events: therapy interruption, dosage reduction, or discontinuation may be required.
• Hepatic failure (sometimes fatal) can occur – liver function tests.

CLINICAL PEARLS
• Active surveillance in patients with papillary microcarcinoma can be considered in very highly selected patients.
• Total vs. partial thyroidectomy depends on tumor size, family history, and previous radiation exposure, as well as the patient's comorbidities.
• TKIs are reserved for RAI refractory R/M DTC patients but only with radiographically measurable evidence of progression.
• TKIs cannot be offered to patients with laboratory-only based evidence of progression; calcitonin in MTC and Tb in DTC. Radiographically measurable disease is essential.

Special populations

Pregnancy

• FNA of suspicious thyroid nodules should be performed in euthyroid and hypothyroid pregnant women. Often, FNA biopsy can be deferred until after pregnancy and cessation of lactation.
• Surgery, partial or total thyroidectomy, performed during pregnancy is associated with greater risk of complications, prolonged hospitalization, and higher costs.
• Prognosis of pregnant women treated after delivery compared with nonpregnant women with DTC is similar.
• RAI should not be given to nursing women.

Children

• In 2015, the American Thyroid Association (ATA) issued the first guidelines on the management of pediatric thyroid nodules and differentiated thyroid cancer.

- Pediatric thyroid nodules carry a far greater risk for malignancy than in adults, as approximately 26–36% of patients present with more advanced disease. Therefore, expeditious investigation is recommended.
- Previous radiation exposure remains a major risk factor.
- For the majority of children with papillary thyroid cancer, total thyroidectomy is recommended.
- Thyrogen stimulation followed by RAI for residual avid tumor can be used.
- The prognosis is excellent, with mortality rates of less than 10%.
- As many young pediatric patients have hereditary syndromes, genetic counseling is highly recommended.

Prognosis

BOTTOM LINE/CLINICAL PEARLS
- Papillary cancer: 10-year OS is about 93%.
- Follicular cancer: 10-year OS is about 85%.
- Hurthle cell cancer: 5-year OS is about 93%.
- MTC: lymph node-negative 10-year OS is about 85%; lymph node-positive 10-year OS is 40%.

Natural history of untreated disease
- In highly selected patients with papillary microcarcinoma, active surveillance can be considered.

Prognosis for treated patients
Most patients with papillary cancer do not die of their disease. Several factors have been identified that are associated with a higher risk for tumor recurrence and cancer-related mortality.

Follow-up tests and monitoring
- Physical examination, TSH, Tb, Tb-Ab levels at 6, 12 months then annually if disease free.
- Periodic ultrasound of the neck.
- TSH stimulated RAI scan in high risk patients, with history of previous RAI avid lesions, with abnormal triglyceride levels, elevated Tb-Ab, abnormal ultrasound of the neck TSH simulated triglyceride levels in patients treated with RAI and Tb-Ab.
- For MTC patients calcitonin/CEA every 6–12 months. Central and lateral neck compartment ultrasound can be considered.

References and reading list

American Thyroid Association (ATA) Guidelines Taskforce on Thyroid Nodules and Differentiated Thyroid Cancer, Cooper DS, Doherty GM, Haugen BR, et al. Revised American Thyroid Association management guidelines for patients with thyroid nodules and differentiated thyroid cancer. Thyroid 2009;19:1167.

Brose MS, Nutting CM, Jarzab B, et al., DECISION Investigators. Sorafenib in radioactive iodine-refractory, locally advanced or metastatic differentiated thyroid cancer: a randomised, double-blind, phase 3 trial. Lancet 2014;384:319–328.

King A. Imaging for staging and management of thyroid cancer. Cancer Imaging 2008;8(1):57–69.

Schlumberger M, Tahara M, Wirth LJ, et al. Lenvatinib versus placebo in radioiodine-refractory thyroid cancer. N Engl J Med 2015;372:621.

Schoffski P, Elisei R, Muller S, et al. An international, double-blind, randomized, placebo-controlled phase III trial (EXAM) of cabozantinib (XL184) in medullary thyroid carcinoma (MTC) patients (pts) with documented RECIST progression at baseline. J Clin Oncol 2012;30(suppl):5508.

Wells SA Jr, Robinson BG, Gagel RF, et al. Vandetanib in patients with locally advanced or metastatic medullary thyroid cancer: a randomized, double-blind phase III trial. J Clin Oncol 2012;30:134.

Suggested websites

https://www.thyroid.org
https://www.thyroid.org/professionals/ata-professional-guidelines/#
https://www.cancer.org/cancer/thyroidcancer/
www.thyca.org
http://seer.cancer.gov/statfacts/html/thyro.html

Guidelines
National society guidelines

Title	Source	Date and weblink
2015 American Thyroid Association management guidelines for adult patients with thyroid nodules and differentiated thyroid cancer	American Thyroid Association (ATA)	2015 https://online.liebertpub.com/doi/pdfplus/10.1089/thy.2015.0020
Thyroid carcinoma	National Comprehensive Cancer Network (NCCN)	2019 www.nccn.org

International society guidelines

Title	Source	Date and weblink
Thyroid cancer: ESMO Clinical Practice Guidelines for diagnosis, treatment, and follow-up	European Society of Medical Oncology	2012 http://annoc.oxfordjournals.org/content/23/suppl_7/vii10.long

Evidence

Type of evidence	Title and comment	Date and weblink
RCT	Lenvatinib versus placebo in radioiodine-refractory thyroid cancer **Comment:** Improvement in PFS, RR in patients with R/M RAI refractory DTC. Led to FDA approval in 2015	2015 https://www.ncbi.nlm.nih.gov/pubmed/25671254
RCT	Sorafenib in radioactive iodine-refractory, locally advanced or metastatic differentiated thyroid cancer **Comment:** Improvement in PFS in patients with R/MRAI refractory DTC. Led to FDA approval in 2013	2014 https://www.ncbi.nlm.nih.gov/pubmed/24768112
RCT	Vandetanib in patients with locally advanced or metastatic medullary thyroid cancer **Comment:** Improvement in PFS, RR in patients with R/M MTC. Led to FDA approval	2012 https://www.ncbi.nlm.nih.gov/pubmed/22025146
RCT	An international, double-blind, randomized, placebo-controlled phase III trial (EXAM) of cabozantinib (XL184) in medullary thyroid carcinoma (MTC) patients (pts) with documented RECIST progression at baseline **Comment:** Improvement in PFS, RR in patients with R/M MTC. Led to FDA approval	2012 https://scinapse.io/papers/2328208895

Additional material for this chapter can be found online at:
www.wiley.com/go/oh/mountsinaioncology

This includes advice for patients, a case study, ICD codes, and
multiple choice questions.

CHAPTER 21

Head and Neck Cancer

Le Min Lee and Bruce E. Culliney
Icahn School of Medicine at Mount Sinai, New York, NY, USA

OVERALL BOTTOM LINE
- Choice of therapy in head and neck cancer depends on the specific primary site and stage of disease.
- Treatment planning needs to incorporate a multidisciplinary approach.
- The incidence of human papillomavirus-related oropharyngeal cancers is increasing.
- Human papillomavirus-related oropharyngeal cancers are associated with a better prognosis.

Background
Definition of disease
Head and neck cancers (HNC) consist of a heterogeneous group of malignant tumors of the upper aerodigestive tract.

Disease classification
- Site-specific cancers are delineated by anatomic boundaries: the oral cavity and lip, pharynx, larynx, nasal cavity and paranasal sinuses, thyroid and salivary glands (Figure 21.1).
- Squamous cell carcinoma accounts for 90% of HNCs and is the focus of this chapter.

Incidence/prevalence
- In 2018, approximately 64 690 new cases of HNC were diagnosed, accounting for 3.7% of newly diagnosed cancers in the USA. An estimated 13 740 deaths occurred in 2018.
- The estimated annual global incidence is 400 000–600 000 and the estimated mortality rate is 223 000–300 000 deaths per year.

Economic impact
- The estimate of direct medical costs for HNC totaled $3.64 billion in 2010 and the value of lost productivity from HNC was $3.4 billion.

Etiology
- Tobacco and alcohol use have been the most important predisposing factors and appear to have a multiplicative effect.
- HPV, particularly HPV types 16 and 18, has emerged as an important causative factor of squamous cell oropharyngeal cancers (particularly in the palatine and lingual tonsils, and the base of tongue).

Mount Sinai Expert Guides: Oncology, First Edition. Edited by William K. Oh and Ajai Chari.
© 2019 John Wiley & Sons Ltd. Published 2019 by John Wiley & Sons Ltd.
Companion Website: www.wiley.com/go/oh/mountsinaioncology

- Nasopharyngeal and paranasal sinus cancers are associated with Epstein–Barr virus (EBV) infection.
- Occupational exposures such as nickel, radium, mustard gas, chromium, and by-products of leather tanning and woodworking are associated with tumors of the sinonasal tract.

Pathology/pathogenesis
- HNCs progress through multistep carcinogenesis from normal histology to hyperplasia, dysplasia, carcinoma *in situ*, invasive carcinoma, and metastasis.
- *P53* tumor-suppressor gene alterations represent an early event in progression whereas mutations in the *p16* gene, an inhibitor of cyclin-dependent kinase that is important in regulating the cell cycle, are associated with later stages of tumor progression.
- The loss of heterozygosity of certain chromosomes (3p14, 9p21, 17p13, 8p, 11q, 13q, 14q, 6p, 4q27, and 10q23) and amplification, deletion, up-regulation, or down-regulation of certain oncogenes or tumor suppressor genes such as *EGFR, Rb, p65, COX-2, cyclin D1*, and *PTEN* have been identified as genetic alterations in each of the pathologic stages of HNC.
- HPV viral proteins E6 and E7 inactivate the tumor suppressor protein p53 and pRb, resulting in loss of cell cycle regulation, cellular proliferation, and chromosome instability.

Prevention

> **BOTTOM LINE**
> - No interventions have been demonstrated to prevent the development of the disease.

Screening
- Screening is not recommended.

Primary prevention
- Tobacco and alcohol cessation is essential.
- Counseling in combination with pharmacologic therapy, such as nicotine replacement therapy, is the most effective and leads to the best results in smoking cessation.

Secondary prevention
- Smoking cessation decreases the risk of developing second primary tumors.
- Patients who continue with tobacco and alcohol consumption after the diagnosis of HNC have a lower response rate to treatment and increased risks of recurrence.

Diagnosis (Algorithm 21.1)

> **CLINICAL PEARLS**
> - Signs and symptoms are associated with the specific primary site.
> - Location of pathologic lymph node may suggest the primary site.
> - Initial evaluation of HNC should include a comprehensive head and neck examination, imaging of the primary site and neck, PET/CT, and routine laboratory tests.

Algorithm 21.1 Diagnosis of head and neck cancer

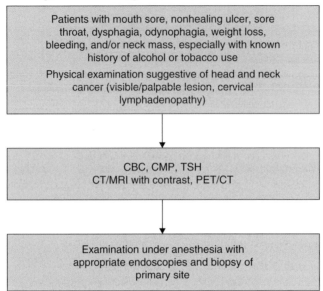

Typical presentation

Signs and symptoms vary with affected anatomic site.

- **Nasopharyngeal cancer:** symptoms such as nasal obstruction, hearing loss, tinnitus, otitis media, and cranial nerves II and VI dysfunction are often caused by extension of tumor into adjacent structures. Patients may present with a painless neck mass resulting from regional lymph node metastasis.
- **Oral cavity cancer:** mouth sore, nonhealing ulcer, dysphagia, odynophagia, weight loss, bleeding, infiltrative and/or exophytic lesion (tongue cancer), and an exophytic or ulcerative lesion (lip cancer).
- **Oropharyngeal cancer:** sore throat, dysphagia, odynophagia and otalgia, regional lymph node metastasis.
- **Hypopharyngeal cancer:** patients often remain asymptomatic and seek medical attention at a more advanced stage with sore throat, dysphagia, odynophagia, and neck mass.
- **Laryngeal cancer:** hoarseness is an early symptom of glottic cancer, hence it is often discovered at an earlier stage whereas supraglottic cancers are often diagnosed later and can occur with airway obstruction or palpable metastatic lymphadenopathy.
- **Sinus cancer:** epistaxis, nasal obstruction, facial pain, and headache.

Clinical diagnosis

History

- One should look out for symptoms suggestive of HNC as detailed in the section on Typical presentation.
- Detailed social history is also important to determine exposure to major risk factors associated with HNC.

Physical examination

- Inspection, palpation, and careful assessment of the primary tumor and surrounding structures should follow. Mirror and fiberoptic examinations are often helpful.

- One should also carefully assess for cervical lymphadenopathy. Metastases to level I cervical nodes (submental and submandibular) are typically associated with cancers of the oral cavity, cancers of the laryngeal cancer typically spread to the upper and mid neck (level II and III). Nasopharyngeal cancer spreads to the upper neck and posterior triangle (level II and V). Lymphadenopathy in the lower part of the neck or supraclavicular area should raise concern about a primary lesion below the clavicles or thyroid cancer.

Disease severity classification
- Disease severity depends on staging of disease. More advanced TNM stages are associated with more severe disease.
- Staging for the primary tumor (T) is based on tumor size and is uniform for the tumor of the lip, oral cavity, and oropharynx. However, T stage for glottis larynx, supraglottic larynx, hypopharynx, and nasopharynx is based on subsite involvement and is specific to each subsite.
- With the exception of nasopharyngeal tumors, regional lymph node involvement (N) and distant metastases (M) have been uniform for all subsites.
- The TNM staging system was revised in the AJCC Cancer Staging, 8th edition, with regard to HPV-mediated (*p16+*) oropharyngeal cancer.
- In general, stage I or II include relatively small primary tumors without nodal involvement. Stage III or IV disease includes larger tumors invading underlying structures and/or regional lymph node involvement and distant metastatic spread.

Laboratory diagnosis
- CBC, CMP, and baseline TSH, prior to radiation.
- HPV testing in the clinical setting can be performed via HPV *in situ* hybridization and a surrogate marker, *p16* immunochemistry, which is more widely available and strongly correlates with HPV status.

List of diagnostic tests
- Examination under anesthesia with appropriate endoscopies performed by experienced surgeons allows direct visualization of mucosal abnormalities, primary tumor tissue biopsy, and evaluation of cancer of unknown primary in patients presenting with a neck mass.

Lists of imaging techniques
- CT or MRI with contrast of the primary site is recommended to demarcate the extent of disease.
- PET/CT is routinely carried out to detect occult cervical nodal and distant metastases, evaluate tumors of unknown primary, synchronous second primary tumors, and establish a pretreatment baseline.

Potential pitfalls/common errors made regarding diagnosis of disease
- Delay in investigation of cervical lymphadenopathy can lead to diagnosis of HNC in a later stage.
- Symptoms such as sore throat and nasal congestion that are prolonged and not responding to sufficient and appropriate treatment should prompt further investigation, especially in smokers and alcoholics at risk of HNC.

Treatment (Algorithm 21.2)
Treatment rationale
- Management of patients with HNC is complex and is best served with a multidisciplinary approach involving surgical, medical and radiation oncologists, dentists, nutritionists, speech and swallowing therapists, physical and occupational therapists.

Algorithm 21.2 Management of head and neck cancer

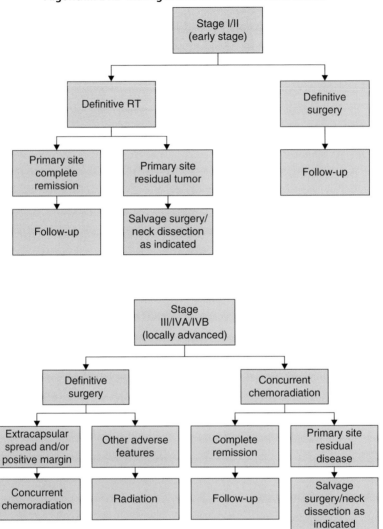

Early stage disease (stage I and II)
- Early stage disease (stage I and II) is typically managed with single modality treatment with curative surgery or definitive RT.
- Surgery may be indicated if a clear margin is technically feasible without causing unacceptable morbidity.
- The type of surgery depends on site and stage of disease.
- Either IMRT or 3D conformal RT is recommended.

Locally advanced disease (stages III, IVA, and IVB)
- Combined modality therapy with surgery and radiation or chemoradiation is generally recommended for treatment of locally advanced disease (stages III, IVA, and IVB).
- For oral cavity subsite, surgery is generally preferred and recommended if feasible.

Algorithm 21.2 (*Continued*)

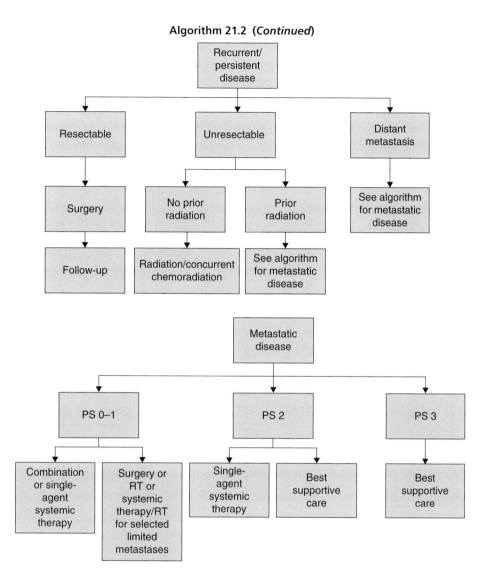

- Surgery followed by adjuvant RT within 6 weeks of resection with or without concurrent chemotherapy based on pathologic risk factors or combined chemoradiation is the standard approach for moderately advanced/resectable locally advanced disease.
- For patients with good performance status (PS of 0 or 1) who have locally advanced disease at diagnosis, curative concurrent chemoradiation is often recommended. Cisplatin 100 mg/m^2 given on day 1, 22, and 43 of radiation is the standard of care. Alternatively, weekly cisplatin 40 mg/m^2 is sometimes recommended. Weekly carboplatin (AUC 1.5–2) is an alternative for patients who are not a candidate for cisplatin-based therapy.
- Concurrent RT and weekly cetuximab, a monoclonal antibody against the EGFR receptor, have been shown to improve locoregional control and reduce mortality without increasing toxicities when compared with RT alone in definitive treatment of locally advanced HNC. It has represented a therapeutic option for patients with locally advanced HNC who are not candidates for

platinum-based regimens (nephrotoxicity, ototoxicity, neuropathy). Based on this result, RTOG 1016 compared radiation with either high dose cisplatin or cetuximab in patients with HPV-related oropharyngeal carcinoma. These results were recently presented. Patients receiving cisplatin plus radiation had superior OS and improved locoregional control. This reinforces the use of high dose cisplatin chemotherapy as the standard of care in this group of patients.

- In recent years, transoral robotic surgery (TORS) has been used for staging and treatment of oropharyngeal carcinoma. TORS can represent the definitive treatment in selected patients with oropharyngeal carcinoma with limited disease and accessible tumors, allows organ preservation, and the possibility to de-intensify adjuvant treatment.
- Postoperative chemotherapy/RT is recommended for adverse pathologic features such as extra-nodal extension and/or positive surgical margins.
- The role of induction chemotherapy is controversial and is not recommended outside of clinical trials.
- It will be important to investigate further de-intensification strategies for HPV-associated tumors.

Cancer of occult primary

- A metastatic neck node without an identifiable primary site after appropriate investigation is defined as cancer of occult primary.
- FNA of the neck node should be performed. FNA is favored over core and open biopsies as the latter can interfere with subsequent treatment.
- Examination under anesthesia with directed biopsy of suspicious mucosa and common locations of occult tumors such as hypopharynx, nasopharynx, and base of tongue is the next step if pathology from the neck node is consistent with squamous cell carcinoma, especially if the lymph node is high in the neck, suggesting a head and neck primary.
- If no identifiable primary is found after appropriate investigation, the patient is treated according to stage of apparent disease and, depending on *p16* status, RT is directed to multiple possible primary sites.

Recurrent/persistent disease

- For recurrent or persistent disease, neck dissection/salvage surgery is recommended if the tumor is resectable. Adjuvant therapy varies depending on the individual patient's risk factors.
- Concurrent chemoradiation is recommended for patients with unresectable recurrent disease, provided that the patient did not receive prior radiation and has a reasonably good performance status.
- Recurrent disease that is not amenable to radiation and surgery is treated as for patients with metastatic disease.

Metastatic disease

- Enrollment in a clinical trial is preferred.
- Palliative RT is sometimes appropriate for selected sites of localized and symptomatic disease.
- Palliative chemotherapy for advanced metastatic disease should be individualized based on patient characteristics and the prior therapies the patient has received. For patients with good performance status (PS 0–1), combination or single agent cytotoxic drugs or targeted therapy are reasonable options.

- Single agent chemotherapy can be used in selected patients with a PS of 2.
- Single agent chemotherapy typically generates a response rate in the range of 15–35%. Combination regimens generally have higher response rates but often do not lead to improved survival.
- Active single agents include cisplatin, carboplatin, 5-fluorouracil, docetaxel, paclitaxel, methotrexate, and cetuximab.
- Active combination regimens include cisplatin or carboplatin plus 5-fluorouracil; cisplatin or carboplatin plus a taxane (docetaxel or paclitaxel); cisplatin with cetuximab.
- The addition of cetuximab to platinum-based chemotherapy with 5-fluorouracil has been shown to significantly prolong PFS and OS in patients with recurrent or metastatic squamous cell carcinoma.
- Most recently, immunotherapy with the PD-1 inhibitors nivolumab and pembrolizumab have shown benefit in patients with recurrent disease who have failed platinum-based chemotherapy. Both drugs are now FDA approved for this indication.
- Supportive care focusing on symptom control with palliative care is appropriate for patients with poor performance status (PS > 2).

Table of treatment

Treatment	Comments
Medical	
Cisplatin 100 mg/m^2 on days 1, 22, and 43	Given with concurrent RT
Cetuximab 400 mg/m^2 loading dose 1 week prior to the initiation of RT then 250 mg/m^2 weekly during the course of RT	Given with concurrent RT
Weekly carboplatin AUC 1.5–2	Given with concurrent RT, for patients who cannot tolerate cisplatin
Weekly cisplatin 40 mg/m^2	Given with concurrent RT

Prevention/management of complications

- Treatment-associated xerostomia and salivary gland dysfunction can cause oral and dental complications such as dental caries, dentoalveolar infection, and osteoradionecrosis.
- Dental evaluation before, during, and after radiation, with tooth extraction 2 weeks before radiation if indicated, and treatment of active dental conditions, using salivary substitutes to decrease dry mouth and using topical fluoride to prevent dental caries can help reduce complications.
- Malnutrition and weight loss secondary to treatment-induced mucositis is common. All patients should receive nutritional evaluation before, during, and after treatment. Prophylactic feeding tube placement is not recommended for all patients but is sometimes required to facilitate treatment. Patients receiving intense multimodality therapy that is anticipated to cause severe side effects such as dysphagia and patients with severe pretreatment weight loss, ongoing dehydration, severe aspiration, and significant comorbidities should have the prophylactic feeding tube placed.
- It is important for all patients to have initial consultation and ongoing follow-up with speech/swallow specialists.

> **CLINICAL PEARLS**
> - Stage I and II disease are treated with single modality treatment with surgery or radiation with curative intent.
> - Stage III and IV disease are treated with combined modality treatment with surgery and radiation or chemoradiation with curative intent.
> - Metastatic and local recurrences are treated with palliative intent.

Special populations
Elderly
- Elderly patients above age 70 may not receive significant benefit from aggressive treatment.

Others
- Comorbidities such as coronary artery disease, congestive heart failure, diabetes, cirrhosis, end-stage renal disease, stroke, dementia, AIDS, and obesity affect performance status and limit chemotherapy options.
- Patients with comorbidities have a worse prognosis than otherwise healthy individuals.

Prognosis

> **BOTTOM LINE/CLINICAL PEARLS**
> - The major prognostic factors for HNC are the presence of locoregional metastasis, vascular or lymphatic invasion, positive surgical margins, and extracapsular spread of tumor cells from involved lymph nodes into soft tissue of the neck.
> - HPV-positive oropharyngeal cancer appears to have improved treatment response, PFS and OS.
> - Synchronous second primary tumors (occurs within 6 months of diagnosis of first primary) occur in about 3–7% of patients with HNC, depending on whether tobacco use is continued.
> - It is thought to be secondary to carcinogen exposure over the entire aerodigestive tract and the exposed mucosa is at risk for development of cancer, a concept called field cancerization.

Follow-up tests and monitoring
- Post-treatment imaging of primary (and neck, if treated) is generally obtained at 12 weeks following treatment.
- History and physical examination including a complete head and neck examination, mirror and fiberoptic examination should be carried out every 1–3 months in the first year, every 2–6 months in the second year, and every 4–8 months in years 3–5 after completion of treatment. Follow-up can then be performed annually.
- Increased TSH levels have been detected in 20–25% of patients who received neck irradiation, so TSH should be checked every 6–12 months if the neck was irradiated.
- Ongoing dental evaluation is recommended for the oral cavity and sites exposed to radiation treatment.
- Nutritional, speech/hearing, and swallowing evaluation and rehabilitation should be performed as clinically indicated.

Reading list
Bernier J, Domenge C, Ozsahin M, et al. Postoperative irradiation with or without concomitant chemotherapy for locally advanced head and neck cancer. N Engl J Med 2004;350:1945–1952.

Bonner JA, Harari PM, Giralt J, et al. Radiotherapy plus cetuximab for squamous-cell carcinoma of the head and neck. N Engl J Med 2006;354:567–578.

Colevas AD. Chemotherapy options for patients with metastatic or recurrent squamous cell carcinoma of the head and neck. J Clin Oncol 2006;24:2644–2652.

Cooper JS, Pajak TF, Forastiere AA, et al. Postoperative concurrent radiotherapy and chemotherapy for high-risk squamous-cell carcinoma of the head and neck. N Engl J Med 2004;350:1937–1944.

Forastiere AA, Goepfert H, Maor M, et al. Concurrent chemotherapy and radiotherapy for organ preservation in advanced laryngeal cancer. N Engl J Med 2003;349:2091–2098.

Pignon JP, Bourhis J, Domenge C, et al. Chemotherapy added to locoregional treatment for head and neck squamous-cell carcinoma: three meta-analyses of updated individual data. MACH-NC Collaborative Group – Meta-Analysis of Chemotherapy on Head and Neck Cancer. Lancet 2000;355:949–955.

Pignon JP, le Maitre A, Maillard E, et al. Meta-analysis of chemotherapy in head and neck cancer (MACH-NC): an update on 93 randomised trials and 17,346 patients. Radiother Oncol 2009;92:4–14.

Vermorken JB, Mesia R, Rivera F, et al. Platinum-based chemotherapy plus cetuximab in head and neck cancer. N Engl J Med 2008;359:1116–1127.

Vokes E, Weichselbaum R, Lippman S, Hong W. Head and neck cancer. N Engl J Med 1993;328:184–194.

Guidelines
National society guidelines

Title	Source	Date and weblink
National Comprehensive Cancer Network Clinical Practice Guidelines in Head and Neck Cancers	NCCN	Version I.2015. http://www.nccn.org/professionals/physician_gls/pdf/head-and-neck.pdf
American Joint Committee on Cancer TNM staging classification, 8th edition	AJCC	2017 http://cancerstaging.org/references-tools/deskreferences/Pages/default.aspx

Image

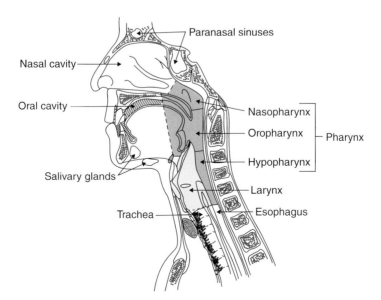

Figure 21.1 Sagittal section of head and neck cancer subsites. (Source: Adapted from Vokes et al. 1993.)

Additional material for this chapter can be found online at:
www.wiley.com/go/oh/mountsinaioncology

This includes a case study and ICD codes.

CHAPTER 22

Brain Tumors

Rebecca M. Brown and Adília Hormigo

Icahn School of Medicine at Mount Sinai, New York, NY, USA

OVERALL BOTTOM LINE

- The most common brain tumors are metastases, most frequently from lung, breast, melanoma, and renal cell cancer.
- There are >120 different types of intracranial tumors. This chapter focuses on the most common: brain metastases, meningiomas, and gliomas.
- Glioblastoma (GBM) represents 17% of all primary brain tumors, and over half of all gliomas.
- Symptoms depend on tumor location, rate of tumor growth, and propensity to hemorrhage.
- Treatment includes gross total resection, radiotherapy, chemotherapy, or biologic agents/targeted therapy.

Background
Definition of disease

- A brain tumor is the abnormal growth of atypical cells in the brain (primary brain tumors), or on the membrane covering the brain (meningioma). Tumors caused by the spread of cancer from another organ are metastases (Figures 22.1–22.7).

Disease classification

- The most widely accepted classification is from the WHO, last revised in 2016. The assignment of grade and classification of primary brain tumors is based on histologic and molecular characteristics.

Incidence/prevalence

- In the USA, 70 000 new primary brain tumors, 120 000 meningiomas, and 200 000 brain metastases are diagnosed annually. It is estimated that 700 000 people in the USA are currently living with a brain tumor.
- Prevalence of meningiomas increases with age, from 1 in 100 000 person-years in the third decade of life to 30 times that number in octogenarians.

Economic impact

- In the USA, brain cancer treatment is the most expensive per patient compared with other cancers. At an estimated overall annual expenditure of $4.47 billion, brain cancer is the eighth highest costing cancer overall.
- Brain tumors create a high burden of morbidity and mortality preventing return to the workforce.

Mount Sinai Expert Guides: Oncology, First Edition. Edited by William K. Oh and Ajai Chari.

© 2019 John Wiley & Sons Ltd. Published 2019 by John Wiley & Sons Ltd.

Companion Website: www.wiley.com/go/oh/mountsinaioncology

Etiology
- Etiology is unknown. Certain genetic syndromes predispose to brain tumor formation (see Risk factors table).
- Irradiation of the head may predispose to meningiomas.

Pathology/pathogenesis
- The cell of origin of gliomas is unknown. Gliomas likely derive from glial progenitor/stem cells versus dedifferentiation and malignant transformation of mature cells.
- Gliomas are subdivided into three categories: astrocytomas, oligodendrogliomas, and ependymomas, according to their histologic features. This does not mean that they originate from that cell lineage.
- GBMs can develop *de novo* or secondarily from a diffuse/anaplastic astrocytoma, even after treatment.
- A grade II oligodendroglioma can transform into an anaplastic grade III oligodendroglioma.
- Meningiomas are thought to derive from arachnoid cap cells.

Predictive/risk factors

Risk factor	Odds ratio
Genetic • **NF1:** astrocytoma, optic nerve glioma • **NF2:** vestibular schwannoma, meningioma, ependymoma • **Tuberous sclerosis:** subependymal giant cell astrocytoma • **Rb mutation:** retinoblastoma, pineoblastoma, malignant glioma • **Li–Fraumeni syndrome:** breast cancer, sarcoma (among other tumors), and malignant glioma • **Turcot syndrome:** GBM and medulloblastoma	Unknown
Occupational exposures: inadequate evidence	Unknown
Ionizing radiation: high level of evidence	Unknown

Prevention

> **BOTTOM LINE/CLINICAL PEARLS**
> - No interventions are known to prevent brain tumors.

Screening
- **NF1:** annual visual field screening to assess for optic pathway glioma until 8 years old and then every other year until 18 years old. Whole body MRI is being investigated.
- **NF2:** annual brain MRI and audiometry with brain auditory evoked response (BAER) testing from age 10 to 30.
- **Li–Fraumeni syndrome:** surveillance per the treating neuro-oncologist and oncologist. Whole body MRI screening is being investigated.
- **Tuberous sclerosis:** brain MRI every 1–3 years until 25 years of age.
- **Turcot syndrome:** surveillance per the treating neuro-oncologist.

Diagnosis (Algorithm 22.1)

Algorithm 22.1 Diagnosis of brain tumors. Concerning neurologic signs or symptoms warrant an MRI of the brain with or without contrast. Small meningiomas are often diagnosed based on imaging alone, but diagnosis of large meningiomas is confirmed with pathology after resection. Gliomas are both diagnosed and graded via pathology with supporting information from genetic markers. Brain metastases in a patient with known widespread metastatic cancer will not require a pathologic diagnosis; however, if metastases appear to be from an unknown primary cancer or are identified in a patient with systemic cancer that has been controlled for a significant period of time, tissue will be required for diagnosis.

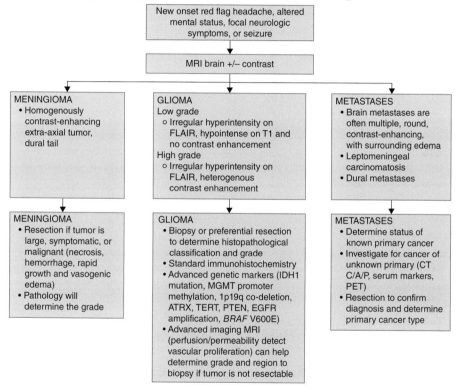

Brain MRI with and without contrast is the gold standard.

Differential diagnosis

Differential diagnosis	MRI features
Abscess	Complete ring enhancement with a hypointense core that is bright on diffusion-weighted imaging and dark on apparent diffusion coefficient
Toxoplasmosis	Patients with HIV/AIDS (see Chapter 32)
Treatment-related changes such as pseudoprogression	Contrast-enhancing mass with a disproportionately large region of edema. Advanced imaging MRI can help with diagnosis
Tumefactive multiple sclerosis	Large lesions with little mass effect/edema. Incomplete ring enhancement

Typical presentation
- Headache is the most common symptom, but it does not help with localization.
- Additional neurologic symptoms are frequently present.
- Focal seizures are a common presentation of low grade gliomas.
- Meningiomas can cause focal neurologic deficits or seizures, depending on tumor location. Small meningiomas are frequently asymptomatic.

Clinical diagnosis
History
- New onset headaches or an abrupt change in headache intensity or quality in someone >45 years of age are important clues. *Red flag* symptoms include early morning onset, headache waking the patient from sleep, nausea/vomiting, and rapidly evolving neurologic symptoms.
- Altered mental status, focal neurologic deficits, or seizures in patients with known active cancer suggests metastasis.

Physical examination
A full neurologic examination can reveal diverse symptoms such as cognitive impairment/aphasia, sensory deficits, hemiparesis/ataxia, or cranial nerve dysfunction.

Useful clinical decision rules and calculators
- Order an MRI of the brain for any patient over 45 years old with "red flag" headache symptoms (see section on History), or any other concerning subacute neurologic symptoms or signs.
- Meningiomas can recur, sometimes rapidly, even after complete resection. Close follow-up imaging is recommended.

Disease severity classification
- Low grade astrocytomas are classified as pilocytic (grade I) or diffuse (grade II), and high grade are anaplastic (grade III) and GBM (grade IV). Oligodendroglial tumors have two grades: oligodendroglioma (grade II) and anaplastic oligodendroglioma (grade III).
- Ependymoma (grades I–III) has a better prognosis than other glial tumors but it can recur after surgery and there is an approximate 10% risk of leptomeningeal infiltration. Anaplastic (malignant) ependymomas are more invasive within the brain parenchyma and leptomeninges.
- Meningiomas are subdivided into grade I (benign), grade II (atypical), and a rare malignant variant grade III (anaplastic).

Pathology

Tumor type	Histologic subtype	Pathology
Meningioma	Numerous types	Commonly, densely packed whorled cells, psammoma bodies
Glioma	Astrocytoma	**Pilocytic (I):** sparse fibrillary infiltrative atypical astrocytic cells, low degree of nuclear atypia. Rosenthal fibers. Eosinophilic granular bodies
		Diffuse (II): higher degree of nuclear atypia, some mitotic figures, diverse cellular morphology
		Anaplastic (III): similar to diffuse, except higher MIB1. May have vascular proliferation
		GBM (IV): highly cellular, cellular and nuclear anaplasia with high MIB1 and necrosis. Pseudopalisading. Glomeruloid neovascularization
	Oligodendroglial tumor	**Oligodendroglioma (II):** uniform "fried egg" cells, calcification, reticular capillaries
		Anaplastic (III): higher cellularity, anaplasia, MIB1, + microvascular proliferation ± necrosis

- Genetic testing of gliomas:
  - **MGMT promoter methylation:** MGMT repairs DNA damage. When its promoter is silenced by methylation, tumor cells are more susceptible to chemotherapy. Patients respond better to treatment and have increased survival.
  - **1p/19q co-deletion:** characteristic of oligodendrogliomas.
  - **IDH1/2 mutation:** present in the majority of low grade gliomas and secondary GBMs.
  - **EGFR amplification and mutation:** indicates primary GBM.
  - **PTEN mutation:** usually a late event in high grade glioma and carries a poor prognosis.
  - **Loss of ATRX expression:** characteristic of astrocytomas.
  - **TERT promoter mutation:** associated with poorer outcome.

Lists of imaging techniques
- MRI:
  - **Metastases:** most commonly multiple, round, variably sized, surrounding edema, frequently found at the gray–white junction.
  - **Meningioma:** uniformly contrast-enhancing, extra-axial, dural tail.
  - **Low grade glioma:** little to no contrast enhancement. Cystic with a mural nodule or diffusely infiltrating.
  - **High grade glioma:** irregular, diffuse, heterogeneously enhancing, $\pm$ microhemorrhage and central necrosis.
  - **Gliomatosis cerebri:** diffuse glioma involving three or more lobes of the brain $\pm$ focal contrast enhancement. No longer a diagnosis in the WHO 2016 guidelines.
  - **Leptomeningeal carcinomatosis:** leptomeningeal contrast enhancement is seen best in the cerebellar folia or cortical sulci.
- **Advanced MRI:** relative cerebral blood volume, perfusion, and permeability modalities.
- MR spectroscopy can differentiate low grade IDH mutant tumors from high grade glioma or other lesions such as tumefactive multiple sclerosis (MS).

Potential pitfalls/common errors made regarding diagnosis of disease
- Gliomas are prone to sampling error. They may have subregions that are of higher grade.
- Lymphoma and GBM can both appear butterfly-shaped, crossing the corpus callosum. Lymphoma is homogenously enhancing.
- Meningiomas can be difficult to distinguish from intraparenchymal gliomas on CT and MRI.
- Do not give steroids if a diagnosis of lymphoma is being considered.
- Consider tumefactive MS before pursuing brain biopsy.

Treatment (Algorithm 22.2)
Treatment rationale
- Metastases:
  - Treatment depends on number of metastases, size, location, and status of systemic cancer (see Algorithm 22.2).
- Meningioma:
  - Observation for small meningiomas versus resection for aggressive, large, or symptomatic tumors. Focal radiation can be considered in some cases.
- Astrocytoma:
  - **Pilocytic:** resection $\pm$ radiation
  - **Diffuse:** resection $\pm$ radiation $\pm$ chemotherapy

- **Anaplastic/GBM:** resection + concurrent chemotherapy with radiation + adjuvant chemotherapy
- **Gliomatosis cerebri:** chemotherapy ± radiation
- Therapies targeted against the tumor's unique molecular profile are undergoing active research.
- Oligodendroglial tumor:
  - **Oligodendroglioma:** resection ± chemotherapy ± radiation
  - **Anaplastic oligodendroglioma:** resection+ chemotherapy+ radiation.

When to hospitalize
- Status epilepticus or for seizure control
- Neutropenic fever
- Clinical deterioration from tumor progression.

Algorithm 22.2 Treatment guidelines for the three most common adult brain tumors

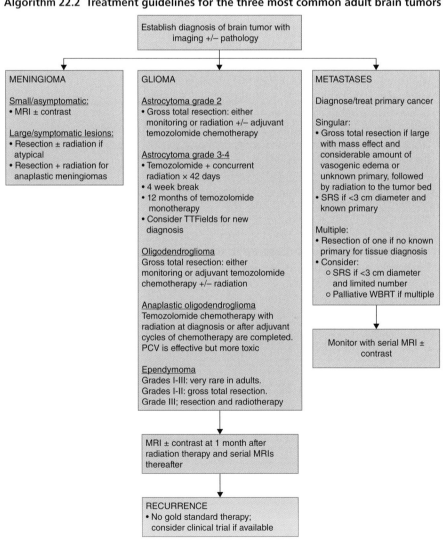

Table of treatment

Treatment	Comments
Surgical	Goal = gross total resection when possible Biopsy if not resectable
Radiotherapy	Glioma: 60 Gy, 5 days/week in 30 fractions Stereotactic radiosurgery for metastases <3 cm diameter Palliative whole brain radiation therapy for multiple metastases but risk of significant cognitive deficits. Stereotactic radiosurgery can be considered
Psychologic	Brain tumors and sequelae of treatment can incur physical and cognitive disability, and depression
Complementary	Avoid vitamins or supplements Avoid enzyme-inducing antiepileptics because of potential interaction with chemotherapy Patients taking CBD/THC marijuana, should be communicated to the patient's physician to ensure that there are no interactions with other medications
Medical	*Temozolomide* (Temodar) Alkylating agent (first line), also thought to be a radiosensitizer Part of the Stupp protocol for GBM (2005) for concurrent chemotherapy and radiation followed by 12 months of adjuvant chemotherapy 75 mg/m^2 PO daily x 42 days with focal radiotherapy • Weekly CBC to monitor for leukopenia, thrombocytopenia • *Pneumocystis* pneumonia prophylaxis can be considered if long-term steroids are required for symptom management 4 weeks off 5/28 cycle of temozolomide, the first cycle at 150 mg/m^2 followed by 200 mg/m^2 if the first is well tolerated • Weekly CBC • Dose adjustment if leukopenia or thrombocytopenia *PCV regimen* Original regimen used for anaplastic oligodendroglioma, but now second line Temozolomide now preferred because of ease of administration (PO) and more favorable side effect profile Procarbazine 100 mg/m^2 PO days 8–21 (daily x 2 weeks) CCNU (1-(2-chloroethyl)-3-cyclohexyl-1-nitrosurea; lomustine) 100 mg/m^2 PO day 1 Vincristine 1.5 mg/m^2 IV days 8 and 29 *BCNU* (bischloroethylnitrosurea; carmustine) Second line for high grade glioma 200 mg/m^2 IV every 8 weeks or 150 mg/m^2 if prior myelosuppression. Maximum cumulative dose 1400–1500 mg/m^2 Implantable carmustine wafers (Gliadel) are not routinely used *TTFields* (tumor-treating fields) Alternating electrical current applied to a shaved head for at least 18 hours/day Used with temozolomide, for newly diagnosed/recurrent GBM Disrupts polymerization of tubulin, preventing mitosis *Bevacizumab* (anti-VEGF biologic therapy) Steroid-sparing agent for symptomatic treatment of high grade glioma 10 mg/kg IV every 2 weeks *Targeted agents* EGFR TKIs are effective for a subset of patients with brain metastases harboring EGFR mutations, particularly with non-small-cell lung cancer and *Her2*-positive breast cancer Capecitabine is a 5-FU precursor chemotherapy effective against breast cancer brain metastases Melanoma brain metastases with *BRAF* V600E mutations respond to vemurafenib Leptomeningeal carcinomatosis can sometimes be treated with intrathecal chemotherapy

Prevention/management of complications
- Monitor CBC for patients on chemotherapy to check for neutropenia and thrombocytopenia.
- Correct electrolyte abnormalities such as hyponatremia that can worsen vasogenic edema.
- Antidiabetic medication for steroid-induced diabetes.
- Bevacizumab can decrease steroid reliance in patients with intolerable side effects.
- Sulfamethoxazole and trimethoprim (Bactrim) for prevention of *Pneumocystis* pneumonia in patients taking chronic steroids >4 weeks.
- Bowel regimen for steroid- and temozolomide-induced constipation.
- Anticoagulants for deep venous thrombosis.
- Monitor blood pressure and urine protein in patients on bevacizumab.

CLINICAL PEARLS
- Grade I meningiomas and low grade astrocytomas can be treated with surgical resection alone.
- Resection followed by radiation therapy and chemotherapy is the mainstay of treatment for high grade gliomas.
- Temozolomide, an oral alkylating agent, is particularly efficacious in MGMT promoter methylated high grade gliomas. It is generally well tolerated. The most serious side effects are bone marrow suppression and rare myelodysplastic syndrome.
- There is no gold standard therapy for recurrent GBM.
- Treatment of brain metastases is dependent upon many factors such as status of the primary cancer, type of cancer, functional status of the patient, and characteristics of the metastases, such as size, number, and mutation profile.

Special populations
Pregnancy
- Management of the pregnant patient with glioma is highly individualized based on patient preference, gestational stage at diagnosis, and tumor progression. Options include monitoring until after birth, surgical resection during pregnancy, or termination of pregnancy for resection and administration of chemotherapy and radiation.

Children
- Gliomas in children and adults differ in characteristic genetic alterations and chemosensitivity.
- Generally, children are more resilient to chemotherapy so that more toxic regimens can be used.
- Children are more sensitive to the effects of radiation therapy on neurocognitive development; therefore, this modality is avoided when possible.

Elderly
- Patients with GBM aged >70 years and with a good performance status can be treated similarly to younger patients. Patients with a poor performance status and comorbidities may benefit from an abbreviated course of radiotherapy alone (for MGMT unmethylated tumors) or temozolomide chemotherapy alone if the tumor is MGMT promoter methylated.

Prognosis

BOTTOM LINE/CLINICAL PEARLS
- Survival in glioma correlates with tumor grade, resectability at diagnosis, methylation of the MGMT promoter, IDH1/2 mutation, 1p19q co-deletion (for oligodendroglioma), and younger age at diagnosis.

- A very small fraction of patients with GBM survive far beyond expectation (>8 years) for unknown reasons.
- Oligodendroglial tumors typically respond better to chemotherapy and radiation and confer a better prognosis than astrocytomas.

Natural history of untreated disease
- Untreated GBM is fatal within weeks to months.

Prognosis for treated patients
- **Pilocytic astrocytoma:**
  - 85–100% 5-year survival.
- **Diffuse astrocytoma:**
  - Average survival is 3–5 years, and 40% of patients survive past 10 years.
- **Anaplastic astrocytoma:**
  - Average survival is 2–3 years, and 25% of patients survive past 5 years.
- **GBM:** ~14.6 months survival (pre-TTFields data)
  - 2-year survival is 30% for patients <45 years old but only 3% for those >65 years, potentially because of less aggressive treatment in the elderly
  - 6% of patients survive past 5 years.
- **Oligodendroglial tumors:** average survival is 4–11 years.
  - Grade II: 66–78% 5-year survival
  - Grade III: 30–38% 5-year survival.
- **Meningiomas:** 80% 5-year survival.

Follow-up tests and monitoring
- Serial neurologic examination and MRI with and without contrast ± advanced imaging for primary brain tumors.

Reading list
Abdulla S, Saada J, Johnson G, Jefferies S, et al. Tumour progression or pseudoprogression? A review of post-treatment radiological appearances of glioblastoma. Clin Radiol 2015;70:1299–1312.

Clarke JL. Leptomeningeal metastasis from systemic cancer. Continuum 2012;18:328–342.

Erkenel M, Hormigo AM, Peak S, et al. Capecitabine therapy of central nervous system metastases from breast cancer. J Neurooncol 2007;85:223–227.

Hegi ME, Diserens AC, Gorlia T, et al. MGMT gene silencing and benefit from temozolomide in glioblastoma. N Engl J Med 2005;10;352:997–1003.

Ostrom QT, Gittleman H, Fulop J, et al. CBTRUS statistical report: primary brain and central nervous system tumors diagnosed in the United States in 2008–2012. Neuro Oncol 2015;17(Suppl 4):1–62.

Stupp R, Taillibert S, Kanner AA, et al. Maintenance therapy with tumor-treating fields plus temozolomide vs temozolomide alone for glioblastoma: a randomized clinical trial. JAMA 2015;314:2535–2543.

Weller M, van den Bent M, Hopkins K, et al. EANO guideline for the diagnosis and treatment of anaplastic gliomas and glioblastoma; European Association for Neuro-Oncology (EANO) Task Force on Malignant Glioma. Lancet Oncol 2014;15:e395–e403.

Suggested websites
Clinical Trials Searchable Database: https://clinicaltrials.gov/
Society for Neuro-Oncology: http://www.soc-neuro-onc.org/
American Brain Tumor Association: http://www.abta.org/
Tumor Treating Fields (TTFields): http://www.optune.com; http://www.novocure.com

Guidelines
National society guidelines

Title	Source	Date and weblink
Central Nervous System Cancers, version 1.2015	National Comprehensive Cancer Network (NCCN)	2015 http://www.nccn.org/professionals/physician_gls/pdf/cns.pdf

International society guidelines

Title	Source	Date and weblink
ESMO: High Grade Malignant Glioma	European Society for Medical Oncology (ESMO)	2014 http://www.esmo.org/Guidelines/CNS-Malignancies/High-Grade-Malignant-Glioma

Evidence

Type of evidence	Title and comment	Date and weblink
RCT	Radiotherapy plus concomitant and adjuvant temozolomide for glioblastoma **Comment:** Radiotherapy+ temozolomide resulted in significantly improved OS when compared with radiotherapy alone	2005 https://www.ncbi.nlm.nih.gov/pubmed/15758009
RCT	MGMT gene silencing and benefit from temozolomide in glioblastoma **Comment:** Demonstrated markedly improved survival benefit of temozolomide compared indirectly with prior chemotherapies, and introduced the clinical importance of the MGMT promoter methylation status in high grade glioma prognostication	2005 https://www.ncbi.nlm.nih.gov/pubmed/15758010
RCT	Maintenance therapy with tumor-treating fields plus temozolomide vs temozolomide alone for glioblastoma: a randomized clinical trial **Comment:** Demonstrates increased survival in recurrent GBM when TTFields are applied in addition to temozolomide	2015 https://www.ncbi.nlm.nih.gov/pubmed/26670971
RCT	Adjuvant procarbazine, lomustine, and vincristine chemotherapy in newly diagnosed anaplastic oligodendroglioma: long-term follow-up of EORTC brain tumor group study 26951 **Comment:** Demonstrates increased OS in patients with grade 3 oligodendroglioma who received adjuvant radiation and PCV regimen, with a trend towards longer survival times in patients with 1p/19q co-deleted tumors	2013 https://www.ncbi.nlm.nih.gov/pubmed/23071237

(Continued)

Type of evidence	Title and comment	Date and weblink
RCT	Radiotherapy for glioblastoma in the elderly **Comment:** Newly diagnosed patients with GBM aged ≥70 years received either focal radiation therapy+supportive care, or supportive care alone. Chemotherapy was not administered. Radiation improved PFS and median OS without affecting cognition or quality of life measures	2007 https://www.ncbi.nlm.nih.gov/pubmed/17429084
RCT	Temozolomide versus standard 6-week radiotherapy versus hypofractionated radiotherapy in patients older than 60 years with glioblastoma: the Nordic randomised, phase 3 trial **Comment:** patients with GBM received standard/hypofractionated radiation or temozolomide. The longest OS in patients >70 years was conferred by temozolomide or hypofractionated radiotherapy	2012 https://www.ncbi.nlm.nih.gov/pubmed/22877848

Images

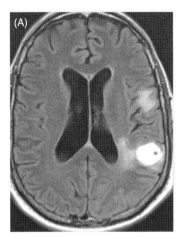 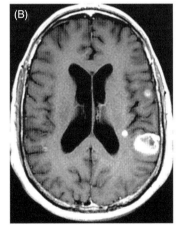

Figure 22.1 Brain metastases. (A) Melanoma metastases are T2 hyperintense on MRI-FLAIR with surrounding edema, and (B) T1+contrast enhancement reveals multiple round enhancing lesions at the gray–white junction.

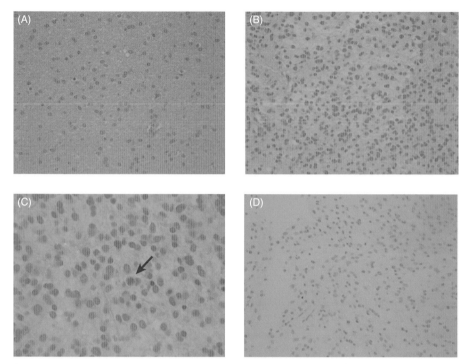

Figure 22.2 Astrocytoma pathology. (A) Low power H&E stain of a grade II astrocytoma. Note the moderate cellularity without pleomorphism or mitoses. (B) Low power H&E stain of a grade III astrocytoma. Cellularity is increased and nuclei demonstrate increasing pleomorphism. (C) High power H&E stain of a grade III astrocytoma with an arrow indicating a mitotic figure. (D) Lack of ATRX staining is indicative of astrocytic gliomas. (Courtesy of Drs. Marco Hefti and Mary Fowkes, Mount Sinai Hospital, Icahn School of Medicine.) See color version on website.

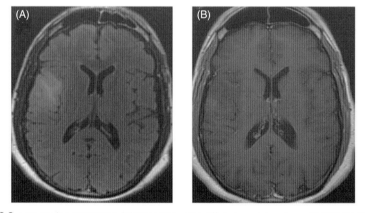

Figure 22.3 Low grade astrocytoma. (A) Frontotemporal diffuse hyperintensity on T2 MRI-FLAIR, and (B) poorly enhancing on T1+ contrast.

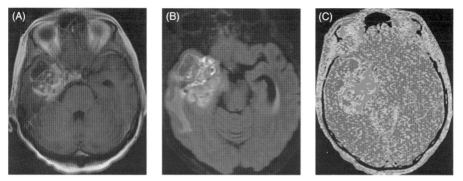

Figure 22.4 GBM. (A) Right anterior and medial temporal heterogeneously enhancing mass on T1+ contrast with regions of focal necrosis; (B) lesions are hyperintense on T2-FLAIR with vasogenic edema; (C) K-trans, advanced MRI that measures capillary permeability, is increased, supporting a high tumor grade. See color version on website.

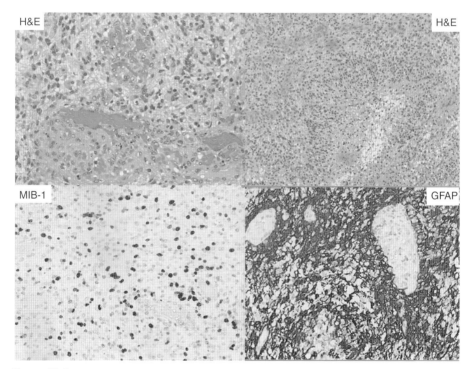

Figure 22.5 GBM histology. Top left: high power H&E: hypercellularity with anaplasia and glomeruloid neovascular proliferation. Top right: low-power H&E: pseudopalisading necrosis. Lower left: MIB-1 index: indicates high rate of mitosis. Lower right: glial fibrillary acidic protein stain: a glial cell lineage marker. (Courtesy of Drs. Marco Hefti and Mary Fowkes, Mount Sinai Hospital, Icahn School of Medicine.) See color version on website.

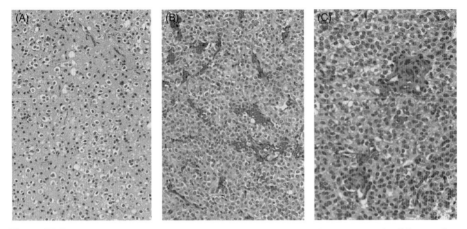

Figure 22.6 Oligodendroglial tumor histology. (A) Grade II oligodendroglioma. Increased cellularity with a "fried egg" appearance. (B) Grade III anaplastic oligodendroglioma, low power. Hypercellularity with pleomorphic nuclei and chicken-wire blood vessels, better depicted on (C). (C) Grade III anaplastic oligodendroglioma, high power. (Courtesy of Drs. Marco Hefti and Mary Fowkes, Mount Sinai Hospital, Icahn School of Medicine.) See color version on website.

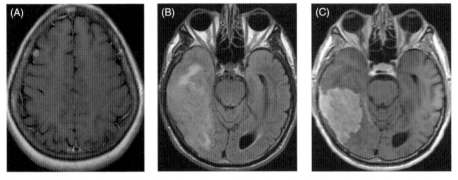

Figure 22.7 Meningioma. (A) Small, incidentally noted right frontal meningioma is uniformly enhancing on T1+ contrast MRI. (B) Large T2 FLAIR hyperintense lesion with surrounding edema harbors an underlying large and aggressive meningioma (C) seen on T1+ contrast with a broad base and dural tail.

Additional material for this chapter can be found online at:
www.wiley.com/go/oh/mountsinaioncology

This includes advice for patients, a case study, ICD codes, and multiple choice questions. The following images are available in color: Figures 22.2, 22.4, 22.5, and 22.6

CHAPTER 23

Neuroendocrine Tumors

Richard R.P. Warner, Jacob A. Martin, and Michelle K. Kim
Icahn School of Medicine at Mount Sinai, New York, NY, USA

OVERALL BOTTOM LINE

- Neuroendocrine tumors are a spectrum of usually slow-growing neoplasms arising mainly from the gastrointestinal tract, pancreas, and the lung.
- They originate from the diffuse neuroendocrine cell system, not the neural crest, and can produce biologically active amines and peptides that, when occurring in excess, can cause a variety of clinical syndromes.
- They all have malignant potential.
- Diagnosis is often delayed and metastases are frequently present by the time the correct diagnosis is established.
- Complete surgical excision is currently the only cure.
- Significant palliation and possible survival benefit are obtained by treatment with somatostatin analogs, an increasingly wide variety of chemotherapy agents, and internal radiation by injected radioemboli or peptide receptor radiotherapy.

Background
Definition of disease

- Neuroendocrine tumors (NETs) are rare, often malignant, but slow-growing endocrine neoplasms usually arising from the gut, pancreas, or lung. They can produce biologically active amines and peptides which, when in excess, cause a variety of endocrine syndromes.

Disease classification

- NETs are generally classified as "carcinoids" when they emanate from the luminal gastrointestinal tract.
- Carcinoids are classified by the embryologic origin of the site from which the tumor arises: foregut, midgut, or hindgut.
- NETs of the pancreas are also known as islet cell tumors.

Incidence/prevalence

- The annual incidence for all NETs based on data from the National Cancer Institute's SEER registry was 3.65 per 100 000 in the US population in the period 2003–2007. This rate is three times the rate from 30 years prior. The prevalence in the USA is estimated at 104 000.

Mount Sinai Expert Guides: Oncology, First Edition. Edited by William K. Oh and Ajai Chari.
© 2019 John Wiley & Sons Ltd. Published 2019 by John Wiley & Sons Ltd.
Companion Website: www.wiley.com/go/oh/mountsinaioncology

- NETs comprise 2% of all malignant tumors of the gastroenteropancreatic system. Approximately 7% of these arise in the pancreas but comprise only 1–2% of all pancreatic neoplasms. The remaining 65% of all NETs are designated carcinoids.
- Approximately 28% of all carcinoids arise from the lung.

Economic impact

The economic impact has not been precisely calculated. It is reasonable to envision a large economic impact because of the long duration of disease, frequently delayed diagnosis or misdiagnosis, the frequent need for surgery, and the frequently fatal outcome.

Etiology

Causes for these tumors are unknown except in a very small minority of cases (less than 4%) in which a genetic cause has been demonstrated. These include paraneoplasic syndromes such as MEN-1, VHL, neurofibromatosis-1, and tuberous sclerosis. Some associations are particularly strong. For example, up to 25% of patients with gastrinoma have MEN-1.

Pathology/pathogenesis

- NETs can be endocrinologically functioning or nonfunctioning or can exhibit symptoms from one or both features. Symptoms can be related to the anatomic site of origin of the tumor or the location of distant metastases. Foregut tumors arise in structures above the diaphragm but also from the stomach and proximal duodenum. Midgut tumors arise in the distal duodenum and small bowel down to the mid transverse colon. Hindgut tumors arise in the more distal colon including the rectum.
- Endocrine functions of the tumor produce symptoms dependent on the hormone produced. Carcinoid syndrome is brought about by serotonin, prostaglandin, bradykinin, and many other vasoactive peptide products. Zollinger–Ellison syndrome is caused by gastrin produced by gastrinomas of pancreatic or duodenal origin. Hypoglycemia is produced by excessive insulin from insulinomas of the pancreas. Many other rare syndromes result from endocrine functioning NETs usually arising in the pancreas but infrequently from the lung or thymus and almost never from the hindgut (see Table 23.1).
- Less than 20% of all carcinoids cause the carcinoid syndrome. Liver metastases are usually required for sufficient unmetabolized hormone to cause the syndrome. However, functioning carcinoids draining into the caval system rather than the portal system can occasionally cause carcinoid syndrome without liver metastases. Most patients with carcinoid syndrome have midgut carcinoids with metastases, but less than 40% of midgut carcinoids result in carcinoid syndrome. Approximately half of pancreatic NETs cause endocrine syndromes.
- Patients with carcinoid syndrome will almost invariably have elevation in 24-hour urinary 5-hydroxyindoleacetic acid (5-HIAA) and/or blood serum serotonin usually accompanied by elevated blood chromogranin A levels. In decreasing order of frequency, the major symptoms of carcinoid syndrome are facial flushing (mostly dry), diarrhea (usually secretory and non-bloody), wheezing resulting from bronchospasm, venous telangiectasia on the face, congestive heart failure (usually right side), and hepatomegaly (from metastases) (see Table 23.2).
- Many of the features of carcinoid syndrome are caused by the excessive circulating serotonin produced by the tumors. 5-HIAA in the urine is the metabolite of serotonin. Serotonin also leads to fibroblast stimulation resulting in fibrosis and also cardiac valve lesions. Increased gut motility with reduced transit time and secretory diarrhea also mainly result from the effects of serotonin. Tryptophan is the precursor from which serotonin is formed but it also is normal substrate for the production of niacin. In very heavily metabolizing carcinoid tumors, tryptophan deficiency can lead to niacin deficiency causing pellagra.

Table 23.1 Neuroendocrine tumor syndromes.

Tumor	Syndrome	Hormone	Clinical features	Site	Malignant (%)	Standard treatment[a]
Carcinoid	Carcinoid syndrome	Serotonin, bradykinin, tachykinins, prostaglandin and others	Facial flushing, diarrhea, bronchospasm, right heart failure, hypotension	GI tract, lung, pancreas, ovary	12.9 overall, >25 midgut carcinoids	Surgery, octreotide, chemotherapy, internal radiotherapy
Insulinoma	Insulinoma	Insulin, proinsulin, C peptide	Hypoglycemia, weight gain	Pancreas	10	Surgery, diet, IV dextrose, chemotherapy, diazoxide
Gastrinoma	Zolinger–Ellison syndrome	Gastrin	Severe peptic ulcer, gastric hypersecretion, diarrhea	70% duodenum, 25% pancreas	60–90	PPI drugs, surgery, octreotide
VIPoma	Verner–Morrison syndrome, pancreatic cholera, WDHA syndrome	Vasoactive intestinal peptide (VIP)	Diarrhea, hypokalemia, achlorhydria, flushing, weight loss	90% pancreas	>50	IV fluids, K+, surgery, octreotide, chemotherapy
Glucagonoma	Glucagonoma syndrome	Glucagon	Diabetes, skin rash, DVT, depression	Pancreas	>50	Surgery, diet, insulin, octreotide, anticoagulant, chemotherapy
Somatostatinoma	Somatostatinoma syndrome	Somatostatin	Diabetes, gallstones, weight loss, steatorrhea	56% pancreas, 44% upper intestine	70–80	Surgery, insulin, pancreatic digestive enzymes
Extremely rare tumors						
ACTHoma	Ectopic Cushing syndrome	ACTH	Hypertension, diabetes, weakness	Pancreas, lung, thymus	>99	Surgery, chemotherapy, octreotide
PTHrPoma	Hyperparathyroidism	Parathyroid hormone-related peptide	Hypercalcemia, nephrolithiasis	Pancreas, lung, thymus	>99	Surgery, chemotherapy
GRFoma	Acromegaly	Growth hormone releasing factor	Acromegaly	Pancreas, lung, thymus	>30	Surgery, chemotherapy, octreotide
Others						
Pheochromocytoma	Pheochromocytoma syndrome	Vasopressors, catecholamines	Hypertension, flushing, palpitations, headache, diaphoresis	Adrenal, sympathetic ganglia		Antihypertension drugs, surgery, chemotherapy, I[131] MIBG

[a] Cytoreduction for all tumor syndromes when metastases are not totally resectable.
(Source: Geschwind & Soulen (eds) Interventional Oncology, 2008. Reproduced with permission of Cambridge University Press.)

Table 23.2   Clinical manifestations of carcinoid syndrome.

Major	Minor
Flushing	Peptic ulcer
Diarrhea	Hypoalbuminemia
Pellagra	Muscle wasting, arthralgias
Venous telangiectasia	Myopathy, fibrosis
Broncospasm	Brawny edema
Cardiac manifestation	Hyperglycemia
Hepatomegaly	

- Tumor products such as prostaglandin, tachykinins, and bradykinin are thought to cause the episodic flushing of carcinoid syndrome.

Special features of carcinoid originating in specific locations
- **Lung:** capable of producing not only carcinoid syndrome but also Cushing syndrome because of adenocorticotropic hormone (ACTH) elaboration. Lung tumors are also capable of producing many of the other peptide hormone syndromes.
- **Thymus:** never produce serotonin or carcinoid syndrome but can cause Cushing syndrome from ACTH production.
- **Stomach:** there are three separate types of gastric carcinoids. They differ greatly in frequency, degree of malignancy, and treatment.
  - **Type I gastric carcinoids:** comprise 70–80% of these stomach tumors and are caused by gastric endocrine cell hyperplasia resulting from hypergastrinemia due to the achlorhydria accompanying atrophic gastritis. Less than 5% of these very slow growing multiple tumors eventually exhibit spread.
  - **Type II gastric carcinoids:** occur in 5% of this group and are also associated with hypergastrinemia accompanying Zollinger–Ellison syndrome. Atrophy of gastric mucosa is not present, and type II usually accompanies MEN-1 syndrome. These tumors have a moderate level of malignancy.
  - **Type III gastric carcinoids:** sporadic, usually solitary lesions, often ulcerated and presenting with bleeding, and sometimes quite large when first discovered. These gastric carcinoids are quite malignant with approximately 50% developing metastases. They are not associated with hypergastrinemia.
- **Duodenal NETs (carcinoids):** these tumors all are similar histologically, usually requiring special staining to be correctly diagnosed. They are of five types: gastrinoma 25%, somatostatinoma 15%, nonfunctioning NET, poorly differentiated ampullary neuroendocrine carcinoma, and gangliocytic paragangliomas. The latter two are particularly rare. All are usually found by endoscopy performed for gastrointestinal bleeding or episodic discomfort.
- **Small bowel carcinoids:** these tumors are often multiple (25%). They usually grow very slowly and are very often overlooked or mistaken for other conditions, leading to a long delay in diagnosis. These are sometimes discovered accidentally at surgery for other conditions or by imaging tests. They often display a measurable increase in the usual carcinoid chemical markers. Tumors over 2 cm in diameter are at greater risk of spread and require more aggressive surgery similar to that for adenocarcinoma.
- **Pancreatic NETs:** these tumors can overproduce peptide substances native to the endocrine cells from which the tumor originates (see Table 23.1) and can be associated with specific clinical syndromes.
- **Appendiceal carcinoids:** usually small and found coincidentally at surgery for acute appendicitis. If the tumor is less than 2 cm, does not show lymphovascular invasion, or extends through

the muscularis propria, simple appendectomy is adequate treatment. Otherwise, right hemi-colectomy is necessary.
- **Rare sites for primary carcinoids**: ovaries, testes, kidney, pancreas, biliary tract, breast, esophagus, prostate, and larynx.

Predictive/risk factors
- The most common primary site in Caucasians is the lung followed closely by the small intestine. In African Americans, Asians, and American Indians the most common primary site is the rectum.
- Overall 5-year survival rates relate to the site of origin and stage of the carcinoid. Rates by site include: appendix 98%; gastric type 1 or 2 81%; rectum 87%; small intestine 60%; and colon 62%.
- T, N, and M status are strong determinants of disease-specific survival.
- Tumor grade also has an impact on survival. Grade is an expression of the degree of differentiation of the tumor. Poorly differentiated tumors have an increased rate of proliferation compared with well-differentiated tumors. Patients with grade 1 tumors tend to survive twice as long as those with grade 2. The patients having lower intermediate grade tumors (grades 1–2) often survive much longer than those with high grade tumors (grades 3–4).

Prevention
No interventions have been demonstrated to prevent the development of most carcinoids/NETs.

Screening
- At present, the only feasible screening method is for heightened awareness of carcinoids/NETs. It is important to include NETs in the differential diagnoses for the wide variety of symptoms these neoplasms can cause but which are usually ascribed to more common conditions. "If you do not suspect it, you cannot detect it."

Secondary prevention
- Recurrence of NETs is prevented only by complete resection of the primary tumor and foci of spread.

Diagnosis (Algorithm 23.1)

Algorithm 23.1 Diagnosis of carcinoid/neuroendocrine tumors

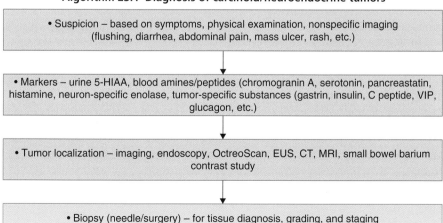

- Suspicion – based on symptoms, physical examination, nonspecific imaging (flushing, diarrhea, abdominal pain, mass ulcer, rash, etc.)

- Markers – urine 5-HIAA, blood amines/peptides (chromogranin A, serotonin, pancreastatin, histamine, neuron-specific enolase, tumor-specific substances (gastrin, insulin, C peptide, VIP, glucagon, etc.)

- Tumor localization – imaging, endoscopy, OctreoScan, EUS, CT, MRI, small bowel barium contrast study

- Biopsy (needle/surgery) – for tissue diagnosis, grading, and staging

---

BOTTOM LINE/CLINICAL PEARLS

- Suspicion of functioning tumors should be aroused by history of recurrent features of their endocrine syndromes (flushing, chronic diarrhea, hypoglycemia, severe gastroduodenal ulceration, atypical asthma, etc.) or in nonfunctioning tumors by recurrent abdominal pain, intestinal obstruction, gastrointestinal bleeding, unexplained abdominal or pulmonary mass, chronic cough, hemoptysis, or recurrent pneumonia.
- Examination may show only normal findings or abdominal tenderness, dry facial flush, telangiectasia, increased bowel sounds, abdominal tenderness, palpable mass, wheezing, enlarged liver, and heart murmur. The findings can be highly varied depending on type, location, and functioning status of the NET.
- Final diagnosis is proven by biopsy. Core biopsy is preferable to fine needle aspiration, but blood and urine chemical "markers" are very helpful in confirming diagnosis. These include 24-hour urine 5-HIAA and blood serotonin, chromogranin A, gastrin, insulin, VIP, glucagon. Often, even nonfunctioning tumors will cause an increased blood chromogranin A. Somatostatin receptor scintigraphy (SSRS; OctreoScan) is positive in greater than 80% of NETs (except for insulinomas).

Differential diagnoses

Because of the wide variety of location and endocrine syndromes these tumors can produce, the differential diagnosis varies greatly dependent upon these factors.

Differential diagnosis	Features
Other abdominal malignancies	Masses suspected of being NETs cannot be diagnosed confidently without biopsy. NETs cannot be distinguished from lymphomas or adenocarcinomas based on imaging alone
Non-neoplastic masses	Biopsy can reveal non-neoplastic causes of masses including tuberculosis, sarcoidosis, and sclerosing mesenteritis
Irritable bowel syndrome (IBS)	Though often silent for years, small bowel carcinoids can eventually cause intermittent change in bowel habits with gradual worsening episodes of pain. In the absence of thorough evaluation, these patients are often managed as IBS for years before a more severe acute intestinal obstruction, bleeding, or symptoms of carcinoid syndrome prompt intervention and hence the discovery of the correct diagnosis
Inflammatory bowel disease (IBD)	The same symptoms are sometimes felt to be caused by Crohn disease and this mistaken diagnosis can be perpetuated by nonspecific abnormalities visualized on small bowel X-ray studies

Typical presentation

Presentation of gastrointestinal tract carcinoid depends on location, presence of metastases, and endocrine function. NETs are frequently silent and found fortuitously. The most common scenario for small bowel carcinoids is chronic intermittent worsening abdominal pain and episodic diarrhea. Sometimes, acute intestinal obstruction is the first clinical presentation. Abdominal mass caused by metastases or gastrointestinal bleeding can be the initial presentation. Occasionally, carcinoid syndrome is the initial presenting feature. Pancreatic NETs often occur as silent small masses incidentally seen on imaging studies or as a palpable upper abdominal mass or with symptoms caused by the specific hormone produced (e.g. gastrin insulin, glucagon, VIP).

Clinical diagnosis

History

- These patients often have a strong family history of other types of malignancy and 25% of carcinoid patients also have a history of metachronous cancer (breast, colon, prostate, lung). Recently described is a hereditary form of small intestinal carcinoid associated with a germline mutation in inositol polyphosphate multikinase which may account for up to one-third of cases previously considered sporadic.
- Patients with chronic vague abdominal symptoms and history of IBS without radiographic, endoscopic, and laboratory studies to exclude other diseases should be suspected for carcinoid or related diarrhea-producing NETs. Patients with IBD symptoms without biopsy confirmation and with poor response to standard treatment should also be suspected.
- A careful detailed history of gastrointestinal symptoms and treatment is essential and should include change in bowel habits, relationship of diarrhea and abdominal pain to eating, timing, and character of loose stools (symptoms after eating; passage of undigested food; greasy floating, bloody stools; nocturnal diarrhea).
- The character of facial flush must be determined. Facial flush from carcinoid syndrome is usually dry, rapidly provoked by alcohol or adrenergic stimuli, and usually involving only the face and anterior neck. It is often accompanied by hypotension, palpitations, and mild dyspnea.
- Hypoglycemic symptoms suggest consideration of insulinoma and history of severe recurrent upper gastrointestinal ulcer disease supports Zollinger–Ellison syndrome (gastrinoma).

Physical examination

- Flush, facial telangiectasia (carcinoid syndrome).
- Rash (necrolytic migratory erythema – glucagonoma).
- Abdominal mass.
- Increased bowel sounds.
- Systolic heart murmur, signs of right heart failure.

Useful clinical additional material

- Small bowel carcinoids are multiple in 25% of cases.
- On rare occasions, flush from carcinoid syndrome can be accompanied by hypertension and then must be differentiated from pheochromocytoma.
- Functioning carcinoids have venous drainage via the portal system (small bowel colon, pancreas) requiring liver metastases to cause carcinoid syndrome. Carcinoids arising from sites draining via the caval system do not require liver metastases to produce carcinoid syndrome.
- Only a small minority of all carcinoids cause carcinoid syndrome.

Disease severity classification

- Grading of NETs indicates their level of aggressiveness, which is related to their degree of cellular differentiation and is objectively determined by the number of mitoses and the presence or absence of necrosis as well as their proliferation index (Ki-67) on microscopic examination. NETS are graded as low grade (grade 1), intermediate grade (grade 2), or high grade (grades 3–4), with high grade having greater than 10 mitoses per 10 high-powered fields and Ki-67 proliferation index greater than 20%. Tumors of high grade have the poorest prognosis. Low grade has less than 2 mitoses per 10 high-powered fields, no necrosis, and a Ki-67 proliferation index of less than 3%.

- American and European governing bodies on cancer have separately defined staging guidelines that are similar for many sites but differ notably at the pancreas and appendix. These guidelines have been validated to different degrees and consequently they have not yet been universally accepted or utilized.

Laboratory diagnosis

Most NETs, including those that are nonfunctioning, will cause some increase in measurable levels of their amine or peptide products. These biomarkers can be tumor nonspecific ([a]) or specific ([b]) for each particular tumor type:

- Carcinoid
  - 24-hour urine 5-HIAA[b]
  - Serotonin[b]
  - Chromogranin A[a]
  - Pancreastatin[b]
- Insulinoma
  - Glucose[a]
  - Insulin[b]
  - Proinsulin[b]
  - C-peptide[b]
- Gastrinoma
  - Gastrin[a]
  - Chromogranin A[a]
  - Gastric HCl (increased)[b]
- VIPoma
  - VIP[b]
- Glucagonoma
  - Glucagon[b]
  - Zinc (decreased)[a]
  - Amino acid profile (decreased)[a]
- Somatostatinoma
  - Somatostatin[b]
- PPoma (non-functioning pancreatic NET)
  - Pancreatic polypeptide[a].

Lists of imaging techniques

- X-ray of abdomen and of chest (can show mass or evidence of intestinal obstruction).
- Obstructive series of the abdomen.
- Ultrasound scan of the abdomen (delineate hepatic masses or other mass lesions).
- MRI with IV contrast.
- CT scan with IV contrast.
- Endoscopy.
- Endoscopic ultrasound.
- Wireless capsule endoscopy.
- Double balloon enteroscopy.
- Barium contrast studies.
- SSRS (OctreoScan): this imaging test is the most specific for NETs. Notably, approximately half of insulinomas do not visualize by this technique. Visualization does not depend upon endocrine function of the NET.

- Gallium 68 scan: still experimental. Is more sensitive and likely to replace OctreoScan in the future.
- Standard FDG-PET scan. It is not as sensitive for slow growing NETs as it is for more aggressive malignancies.

Potential pitfalls/common errors made regarding diagnosis of disease

- Currently over 90% of NET patients are initially misdiagnosed and treated for the wrong disease.
- The most common diagnostic errors are misdiagnosing midgut carcinoid as IBS or IBD.
- The average time to correct diagnosis is 5–7 years from the first symptoms in approximately 50% of cases of midgut carcinoid. The diagnosis is not made until metastases to the liver are present in this large group.
- Flushing in women is often first attributed to menopause. Other etiologies for chronic episodic flushing are VIPoma, medullary carcinoma of the thyroid, pheochromocytoma, diabetic autonomic neuropathy, epilepsy, panic attacks, mast cell disease, hypomastia and mitral valve prolapse, reaction to drugs, allergy, and male hypogonadism.

Treatment (Algorithm 23.2)

Algorithm 23.2 Treatment of neuroendocrine tumors

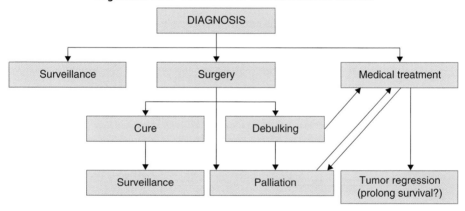

Treatment rationale

- The primary goal of treatment is cure. At present, complete surgical resection of the tumor is the only cure.
- The secondary goals of treatment are palliation and prolongation of survival. In the past, there was little to offer the patient with advanced disease. However, currently many types of treatment are available along with significant advances in surgery. Hence, "wait and see" is no longer appropriate. Patients today should benefit from advances in palliation and prolongation of survival. Unlike more aggressive malignancies, carcinoids/NETs respond well to therapy.
- In advanced surgically unresectable carcinoids/NETs, the best treatment usually involves sequential multimodal therapy. The selection and timing of treatments are determined by the type and location of the NET, its grade/stage, level of endocrine function, age of the patient, and presence of comorbidities.
- The treatment of carcinoids/NETs and carcinoid syndrome can be categorized as supportive, surgical, or antiproliferative (see Algorithm 23.2)

- Somatostatin analogs (including octreotide and lanreotide) are the keystone of treatment for symptoms of carcinoid syndrome, VIPoma, and Zollinger–Ellison syndrome (the latter in conjunction with proton pump inhibitors). Also, octreotide and lantreotide have been demonstrated to inhibit progression of growth in midgut carcinoids.

When to hospitalize
- Dehydration
- Symptomatic hypotension, arrhythmia
- Progressing heart failure
- Gastrointestinal bleeding
- Intestinal obstruction
- Severe malnutrition
- Severe abdominal pain (possibly impending perforation, cholecystitis)
- Uncontrolled diabetes
- Uncontrolled hypoglycemia
- Progressing jaundice
- Deep venous thrombosis
- For certain chemotherapy protocols
- For radiofrequency ablation or hepatic artery (chemo) embolization treatment.

Managing the hospitalized patient
- Multidisciplinary collaboration should be obtained early.
- Monitor vital signs frequently in patients with functioning tumors.
- In order to prevent carcinoid crisis, administer periprocedural supplements of regular immediate-release octreotide in carcinoid syndrome patients undergoing any painful or invasive procedure.

Table of treatment
For treatment of carcinoid NETs, see Tables 23.1 and 23.3.

Table 23.3 Treatment of carcinoid/NETs.

Surgery	Medical supportive	Antiproliferative
Biopsy	Antidiarrheal	Biotherapy
Resection for cure	Somatostatin analogs	Octreotide
Debulking	Traditional drugs	• Lanreotide
Palliation	• Cholestyramine	Radiotherapy
Radiofrequency ablation	• Pancreatic extract	• External beam
Arterial embolization	• Cyproheptadine	• I_{131} MIBG
Chemoembolization	• Opiates	• Y_{90} octreotide
Heart valve replacement	Nutritional supplements	• LU_{177} octreotate
Stents	• Protein	• Y_{90} microspheres
Liver transplant	• Niacin	Cytotoxic chemotherapy
	• MCT oil	• Platinum-based
	Hematinics	• Etoposide
	Electrolytes	• 5-FU
	H_1 and H_2 blockers	• Streptozocin
		• Temozolamide
		New molecular targeted drugs
		• mTOR inhibitors
		• Multityrosine kinase inhibitors
		• Antiangiogenesis agents

Table 23.4 Octreotide types.

Drugs	Adverse effects
Octreotide immediate-release 100–600 µg SC every 6–8 hours and IV bolus for carcinoid crisis followed by continuous IV infusion 100–500 µg/hour	Cramps, steatorrhea, nausea, bradycardia, arrhythmias, gallstones, hyper- or hypoglycemia, pain at injection sites, and granuloma formation (LAR)
Depot long-acting repeatable (LAR) 10–60 mg deep IM in gluteus muscle every 28 days	
Lantreotide depot (somatuline) 60–120 mg deep SC injection every 28 days	

Complications of carcinoid/NETs
- Gastrointestinal bleed resulting from varices, ulcer, tumor erosion, coagulopathy.
- Fever with or without pain caused by tumor necrosis.
- Jaundice resulting from biliary obstruction by calculi (a complication of chronic octreotide therapy), and other side effects of medication.
- Carcinoid crisis: this potentially fatal event requires immediate treatments with O_2, IV fluids, IV octreotide 200–500 µg, and corticosteroids (see Table 23.4).

Prevention/management of complications
- Carcinoid crisis (abrupt severe blood pressure perturbation, usually hypotension and shock, flush, dyspnea, mental changes, bronchospasm, tachycardia, fever, diarrhea) is most often precipitated by anesthesia, surgery, or adrenergic stimuli. It is best prevented by prophylactic subcutaneous injection of octreotide within 1 hour of procedure. Carcinoid crisis can occur even in carcinoid patients not having manifested carcinoid syndrome symptoms if they do have increased levels of markers. Patients with known carcinoid syndrome should be given preprocedural and periprocedural continuous IV octreotide, IV fluids, and IV corticosteroids at least once.
- Tumor necrosis (spontaneous or secondary to treatment) can produce carcinoid crisis, pain, fever, and rarely intraluminal hemorrhage, and abscess formation. Antibiotics (pre- and postoperative), supplemental octreotide, and surgery should be used as needed. Tumor fever can occur chronically.
- Complications of tumor-associated fibrosis include: intestinal obstruction, obstructive uropathy, ischemic bowel with acute infarction, or chronic abdominal angina. This is best treated with appropriate surgery as needed in each case.

CLINICAL PEARLS
- Selective serotonin reuptake inhibitor (SSRI) drugs have the potential to precipitate carcinoid syndrome with flushing and diarrhea occurring in the undiagnosed untreated obscure case.
- Usually only one or two of the symptoms of carcinoid syndrome are present in any given carcinoid case and carcinoid must therefore be included in the differential diagnosis of all patients with any of these symptoms or with unconfirmed IBD, IBS, or recurrent intestinal obstruction.

Special populations
- Carcinoid/NETs can occur in all age groups from newborn to the very elderly, but have greatest frequency in both men and women in their early sixties and occur almost equally in both the

sexes. The most common primary tumor sites in Caucasians are the gastrointestinal tract and the lung, and the rectum in African Americans. Octreotide is not approved for use in pregnant women or children.

Prognosis

> **BOTTOM LINE/CLINICAL PEARLS**
> - Prognosis depends on many factors: grade, size of primary tumor at diagnosis, presence and site of metastasis, age of patient.
> - The range of survival duration varies widely but, including the commonly long delay in diagnosis, OS from the first symptoms averages more than a decade in untreated patients.
> - Recent observations suggest that somatostatin analog treatment (even in nonsyndrome patients) prolongs survival.
> - Treated patients with an endocrine syndrome now appear to live as long as nonsyndrome patients, with most patients of either group dying from either complications of liver metastasis or widespread NET metastasis.
> - Untreated carcinoid syndrome patients most often die from cardiac causes.
> - Follow-up tests and monitoring: progress of disease is usually followed by periodic imaging (MRI, CT) and chemical markers. Chromogranin A or pancreastatin greater than 1000 pg/mL after treatment indicate an especially poor prognosis.

Reading list

Metz DC, Jensen RT. Gastrointestinal neuroendocrine tumors: pancreatic endocrine tumors. Gastroenterology 2008;135:1469–1492.

Modlin IM, Oberg K, eds. A Century of Advances in Neuroendocrine Tumor Biology and Treatment. Felsenstein CCCP, 2007.

Modlin IM, Oberg K, Chung DC, et al. Gastroenteropancreatic neuroendocrine tumors. Lancet Oncol 2008;9:61–72.

Neklason DW, VanDerslice J, Curtin K, et al. Evidence for a heritable contribution to neuroendocrine tumors of the small intestine. Endocr Relat Cancer 2016;23:93–100.

Nilsson O, Arvidsson Y, Johanson V, et al. New medical strategies for midgut carcinoids. Anticancer Agents Med Chem 2010;10:250–269.

North American Neuroendocrine Tumor Society. Consensus guidelines for the diagnosis and management of neuroendocrine tumors (9 articles, 42 authors). Pancreas 2010;39:705–800.

Raut CP, Kulke MH. Targeted therapy in advanced well-differentiated neuroendocrine tumors. Oncologist 2011;16:286–295.

Sei Y, Zhao X, Forbes J, et al. A hereditary form of small intestinal carcinoid associated with a germline mutation in inositol polyphosphate multikinase. Gastroenterology 2015;149:67–78.

Toumpanakis CG, Caplin ME. Molecular genetics of gastroenteropancreatic neuroendocrine tumors. Am J Gastroenterol 2008;103:729–732.

Turaga KK, Kvols LK. Recent progress in the understanding, diagnosis, and treatment of gastroenteropancreatic neuroendocrine tumors. CA Cancer J Clin 2011;61:113–132.

Vinik AL, Anthony L, Boudreaux JP, et al. Neuroendocrine tumors: a critical appraisal of management strategies. Pancreas 2010;39:801–818.

Vinik AL, Silva MP, Woltering G, et al. Biochemical testing for neuroendocrine tumors. Pancreas 2009;38:876–889.

Warner RRP, Kim MK. Carcinoid and related neuroendocrine tumors. In Geschwind JH, Soulen MC, eds. Interventional Oncology: Principles and Practice. Cambridge University Press, 2008: 290–300.

Yao JC, Hassan M, Phan A, et al. One hundred years after "carcinoid": epidemiology of and prognostic factors for neuroendocrine tumors in 35,825 cases in the United States. J Clin Oncol 2008;26:3063–3072.

Guidelines

Title	Source	Date and weblink
NANETS Consensus Guidelines	North American Neuroendocrine Tumor Society (NANETS)	2013 https://www.ncbi.nlm.nih.gov/pubmed/23591432
ENETS Consensus Guidelines for the management of metastatic neuroendocrine tumors	European Neuroendocrine Tumor Society (ENETS)	2012 https://www.ncbi.nlm.nih.gov/pubmed/22262022
Consensus Guidelines for the standard of care for patients with digestive neuroendocrine tumors	European Neuroendocrine Tumor Society (ENETS)	2009 https://www.ncbi.nlm.nih.gov/pubmed/19902563

Additional material for this title can be found online at:
www.wiley.com/go/oh/mountsinaioncology

PART 2

Malignant Hematology

CHAPTER 24

Myeloproliferative Neoplasms

Sangeetha Venugopal[1], Daniel Aruch[2], and John Mascarenhas[1]
[1] Icahn School of Medicine at Mount Sinai, New York, NY, USA
[2] Virginia Oncologist Associates, Virginia Beach, VA, USA

OVERALL BOTTOM LINE

- Myeloproliferative neoplasms (MPNs) are clonal hematopoietic disorders defined by hyperproliferation of terminally differentiated myeloid cells and classified as *BCR-ABL*[+] chronic myelogenous leukemia and *BCR-ABL*[−] MPNs.
- Chronic myelogenous leukemia (CML) is typified by the presence of the Philadelphia chromosome abnormality t(9;22) resulting in a *BCR-ABL1* fusion, thus providing an actionable target.
- *BCR-ABL*[−] classic MPNs include polycythemia vera, essential thrombocythemia, and primary myelofibrosis, which are complicated by thrombosis, hemorrhage, and evolution to acute myeloid leukemia.
- Less common *BCR-ABL*[−] MPNs include chronic eosinophilic leukemia not otherwise specified (NOS), chronic neutrophilic leukemia, and MPN unclassifiable.

Background
Definition of disease
MPNs are a heterogeneous group of clonal hematopoietic neoplasms mostly characterized by a unique phenotype translating to a distinct risk-based therapeutic approach.

Disease classification
- *BCR-ABL*[+] CML.
- *BCR-ABL*[−] MPNs comprising polycythemia vera (PV), essential thrombocythemia (ET), and primary myelofibrosis (PMF) – which are discussed in detail – as well as the less common entities chronic eosinophilic leukemia not otherwise specified (CEL-NOS), chronic neutrophilic leukemia (CNL), and unclassifiable myeloproliferative neoplasm (MPN-u).

Incidence
Estimated incidences:
- **CML:** 1–2 per 100 000 persons with slight male predominance.
- **PV:** 1–2 per 100 000 persons with slight male predominance.
- **ET:** 2–3 per 100 000 persons with female predominance.
- **PMF:** 1–2 per 100 000 persons.

Mount Sinai Expert Guides: Oncology, First Edition. Edited by William K. Oh and Ajai Chari.
© 2019 John Wiley & Sons Ltd. Published 2019 by John Wiley & Sons Ltd.
Companion Website: www.wiley.com/go/oh/mountsinaioncology

- **CNL:** 1–2 per 10 million persons.
- **CEL-NOS:** 3–4 per 10 million persons.

Etiology
- Rare family clusters exist for patients with Philadelphia chromosome negative MPNs secondary to germline mutations or somatic mosaicism and characterized by polyclonal hematopoiesis.
- Environmental exposure to radiation and benzene can increase risk.

Pathology/pathogenesis
- MPNs are frequently characterized by specific acquired mutations that drive the MPN phenotype.
  - CML is characterized by the fusion of the Abelson murine leukemia (*ABL1*) gene on chromosome 9 with the breakpoint cluster region (*BCR*) gene on chromosome 22 and the resultant oncoprotein BCR-ABL1. The constitutively active BCR-ABL1 tyrosine kinase promotes leukemic cell proliferation through hyperactive downstream signaling pathways.
- PV, ET, and PMF are characterized by the presence of somatic mutations in *JAK2*, *MPL,* or *CALR* and the resultant intemperate JAK-STAT pathway activation.
- CNL is characterized by the presence of CSF3R^{T618I} or other activating CSF3R mutations resulting in a hyperactive JAK-STAT pathway or other pathways including SRC-TNK2 kinase signaling pathway, respectively.

Prevention
Currently, there are no primary screening recommendations or preventative therapeutic interventions available for MPNs.

Clinical diagnosis
History
MPN focused history must include constitutional symptoms (fevers, nights sweats, weight loss), vasomotor symptoms (headache, visual disturbances, paresthesias, erythromelalgia), aquagenic pruritus, splenomegaly related complaints (abdominal distention, early satiety, left-sided dragging pain), thrombotic or hemorrhagic symptoms (bruising, bleeding, phlebitis, arterial/venous thrombosis), gout, cardiovascular risk factors (hypertension, diabetes, smoking history), occupational exposures, obstetric history including early fetal demise and miscarriages, and family history of hematologic conditions.

Physical examination
MPN focused physical examination must include evaluation for facial plethora, conjunctival pallor or injection, lymphadenopathy, skin changes (rash, bruising), gouty arthritis/tophi, and hepatosplenomegaly.

There is no pathognomonic physical finding for MPNs.

Diagnosis (Algorithms 24.1–24.3)
- MPNs are typically diagnosed in the setting of unexplained leukocytosis, thrombocytosis, erythrocytosis, cytopenias, or eosinophilia.
- Key laboratory investigations include complete blood count with differential, chemistries including uric acid and LDH, evaluation of the peripheral smear, bone marrow biopsy and aspiration, cytogenetics, and next generation sequencing or polymerase chain reaction to evaluate for *BCR-ABL1*, *JAK2*, calreticulin [*CALR*], *MPL*, *CSF3R*.

Algorithm 24.1 Diagnosis of leukocytosis

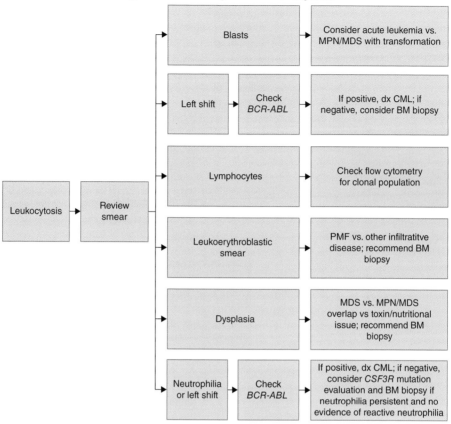

Algorithm 24.2 Diagnosis of thrombocytosis

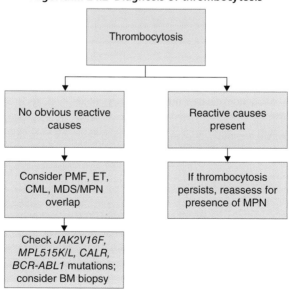

Algorithm 24.3 Diagnosis of erythrocytosis

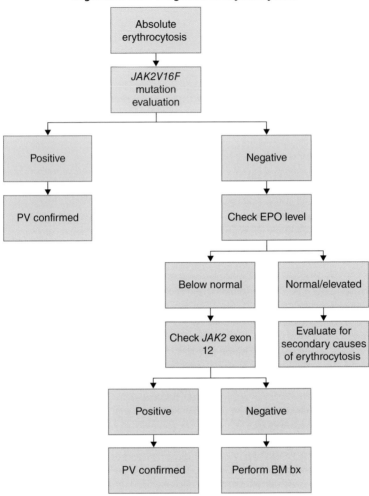

- Each MPN entity is defined by distinct WHO diagnostic criteria, requiring a combination of laboratory parameters, cytogenomic data, and physical examination findings to aid in the definitive diagnosis (Tables 24.1–24.5).
- **CML - Chronic phase:** diagnosis requires presence of Philadelphia chromosome (t(9;22)). **Accelerated phase:** see Table 24.1.
- **Blast phase:** ≥20% peripheral blood or bone marrow blasts, large foci or clusters of blasts on the bone marrow biopsy, or presence of extramedullary blastic infiltrates.
- **PV:** requires erythrocytosis, typical bone marrow morphology, and the presence of *JAK2V16F* or *JAK2* exon 12 mutation. In the absence of JAK2 mutation, PV is diagnosed by erythrocytosis, bone marrow morphology, and low erythropoietin levels (Table 24.2).
- **ET:** presence of thrombocytosis, exclusion of other myeloid malignancies particularly PMF, CML, and PV, typical bone marrow morphology, and a clonal mutation (50% *JAK2*, 30% *CALR*, or 10% *MPL*); reactive causes of thrombocytosis must be excluded in the absence of a clonal marker (Table 24.3).

Table 24.1 WHO criteria for accelerated phase of CML.

Hematologic/cytogenetic criteria	• Persistent or increasing WBC (>10 × 10⁹/L) or splenomegaly or thrombocytosis (>1000 × 10⁹/L) unresponsive to therapy • Persistent thrombocytopenia (<100 × 10⁹/L) unrelated to therapy • 20% or more basophils in the PB • 10–19% blasts in the PB and/or BM • Additional clonal chromosomal abnormalities in *BCR-ABL1*⁺ cells at diagnosis that include "major route" abnormalities (second Ph, trisomy 8, isochromosome 17q, trisomy 19), complex karyotype, or abnormalities of 3q26.2 • Any new clonal chromosomal abnormality in Ph⁺ cells that occurs during therapy
"Provisional" response-to-TKI criteria	• Hematologic resistance to the first TKI (or failure to achieve a complete hematologic response to the first TKI) or • Any hematological, cytogenetic, or molecular indications of resistance to two sequential TKIs or • Occurrence of two or more mutations in *BCR-ABL1* during TKI therapy
Diagnosis	Diagnosis if accelerated phase CML requires one or more of the hematologic/cytogenetic criteria or response-to-TKI criteria

Table 24.2 WHO 2016 diagnostic criteria for *BCR-ABL*⁻ myeloproliferative neoplasms: PV.

Major criteria	1. Hemoglobin >16.5 g/dL in men or >16.0 g/dL in women
	   a or hematocrit >49% in men or >48% in women
	   b or increased red cell mass (RCM) (more than 25% above mean normal predicted value)
	 2. BM biopsy showing hypercellularity for age with trilineage growth (panmyelosis) including prominent erythroid, granulocytic, and megakaryocytic proliferation with pleomorphic, mature megakaryocytes (differences in size)
	 3. Presence of *JAK2V617F* or *JAK2* exon 12 mutation

Minor criteria	Subnormal serum erythropoietin level
Diagnosis	Requires meeting either all three major criteria, or the first two major criteria and the minor criterion

Table 24.3 WHO 2016 diagnostic criteria for *BCR-ABL*⁻ myeloproliferative neoplasms: essential thrombocythemia (ET).

Major criteria	1. Platelet count >450 × 10⁹/L 2. BM biopsy showing proliferation mainly of the megakaryocyte lineage with increased numbers of enlarged, mature megakaryocytes with hyperlobulated nuclei. No significant increase or left shift in neutrophil granulopoiesis or erythropoiesis and very rarely minor (grade 1) increase in reticulin fibers 3. Not meeting WHO criteria for PV, PMF, myelodysplastic syndromes, or other myeloid neoplasms or *BCR-ABL*⁺ CML 4. Presence of *JAK2, CALR, or MPL* mutation
Minor criteria	Presence of a clonal marker or absence of evidence for reactive thrombocytosis
Diagnosis	Requires meeting all four major criteria or the first three major criteria and the minor criterion

- **PMF:** classified as pre PMF or overt PMF. Common to both include exclusion of other myeloid malignancies particularly PV, CML, MDS; clonal mutation (50% *JAK2*, 30% *CALR*, and 10% *MPL*), anemia, elevated LDH, palpable splenomegaly. In the absence of a clonal marker, *ASXL1, EZH2, TET2, IDH1/IDH2, SRSF2, SF3B1* mutations should be tested. Pre PMF is characterized by bone marrow morphology without reticulin fibrosis >grade 1. Overt PMF exhibits leukoery-throblastosis in peripheral smear (dacrocytes, nucleated red blood cells, and left shift of myeloid series) and reticulin or collagen fibrosis grade >2 or 3 (Table 24.4).

Table 24.4 WHO 2016 diagnostic criteria for *BCR-ABL⁻* myeloproliferative neoplasms: pre PMF and overt PMF.

Criteria	Pre PMF	PMF
Major	1. Megakaryocytic proliferation and atypia, without reticulin fibrosis >grade 1, accompanied by increased age-adjusted BM cellularity, granulocytic proliferation, and often decreased erythropoiesis 2. Not meeting the WHO criteria for PV, ET, myelodysplastic syndromes, or other myeloid neoplasms or *BCR-ABL⁺* CML 3. Presence of *JAK2, CALR,* or *MPL* mutation or in the absence of these mutations, presence of another clonal marker (*ASXL1, EZH2, TET2, IDH1/IDH2, SRSF2, SF3B1*) or absence of minor reactive BM reticulin fibrosis	1. Presence of megakaryocytic proliferation and atypia, accompanied by either reticulin and/or collagen fibrosis grades 2 or 3 2. Not meeting the WHO criteria for PV, ET, myelodysplastic syndromes, or other myeloid neoplasms or *BCR-ABL⁺* CML 3. Presence of *JAK2, CALR,* or *MPL* mutation or in the absence of these mutations, presence of another clonal marker (*ASXL1, EZH2, TET2, IDH1/IDH2, SRSF2, SF3B1*) or absence of minor reactive BM reticulin fibrosis
Minor	Presence of at least one of the following, confirmed in two consecutive determinations: a. Anemia not attributed to a comorbid condition b. Leukocytosis >11 × 10⁹/L c. Palpable splenomegaly d. LDH increased to above upper normal limit of institutional reference range	Presence of at least one of the following, confirmed in two consecutive determinations: a. Anemia not attributed to a comorbid condition b. Leukocytosis >11 × 10⁹/L c. Palpable splenomegaly d. LDH increased to above upper normal limit of institutional reference range e. Leukoerythroblastosis
Diagnosis	Diagnosis of pre PMF requires meeting all three major criteria, and at least one minor criterion	Diagnosis of overt PMF requires meeting all three major criteria, and at least one minor criterion

- **CNL:** neutrophilic leukocytosis, typical bone marrow changes in the absence of dysplasia, exclusion of other myeloid malignancies including CML, ET, PV, PMF, presence of *CSF3RT618I* or other activating *CSF3R* mutation. In the absence of *CSF3R* mutation, clonality of myeloid cells must be substantiated once reactive neutrophilia is ruled out (Table 24.5).

Table 24.5 WHO diagnostic criteria for chronic neutrophilic leukemia.

All of the following must be met:	
Peripheral blood	White blood cells (WBCs) >25 000/μL
	Segmented neutrophils and bands >80% of WBCs
	Immature granulocytes <10% of WBCs (i.e. promyelocytes, metamyelocytes, myelocytes)
	Myeloblasts <1% of WBCs
	No dysplasia
	Monocytes <1000/μL
Bone marrow	Hypercellular bone marrow
	Neutrophilic granulocytes increased in percentage and number and normal granulocytic maturation
	Myeloblasts <5%
	No dysplasia
Other criteria	Not meeting the WHO criteria for PV, ET, myelodysplastic syndromes, or other myeloid neoplasms or *BCR-ABL*+ CML
	No rearrangement of *PDGFRA, PDGFRB,* or *FGFR1*, or *PCM1-JAK2*
	Presence of *CSF3RT618I* or other activating *CSF3R* mutation or In the absence of a *CSFR3R* mutation, persistent neutrophilia (at least 3 months), splenomegaly, and no identifiable cause of reactive neutrophilia including absence of a plasma cell neoplasm or, if present, demonstration of clonality of myeloid cells by cytogenetic or molecular studies

- **CEL:** eosinophilia; morphologic abnormalities in the bone marrow; rule out *PDGFR* α/β and *FGFR*1 *PCM1-JAK2* rearrangements; rule out other hematologic malignancies such as inv (16) AML or accompanying lymphoid malignancy; evaluate for end organ damage (echocardiogram, troponin, vitamin B12 level, EKG).

Differential diagnosis

Finding	Differential diagnosis
Leukocytosis	Reactive (infection, malignancy, etc.) or related to primary hematopoietic malignancies including CML, PMF, CNL, acute leukemias
Erythrocytosis	Primarily due to PV or secondary due to smoking, high affinity hemoglobins, erythropoietin secreting tumors, or spurious polycythemia as a result of Gaisböck syndrome
Thrombocytosis	Reactive (infection, malignancy, iron deficiency, etc.) or secondary to primary hematopoietic neoplasms such as ET, CML, PMF, PV
Unusual thrombosis (intra-abdominal, cerebral sinus, etc.)	Inherited thrombophilia, paroxysmal nocturnal hemoglobinuria, ET, PV, PMF

(Continued)

(Continued)

Finding	Differential diagnosis
Cytopenias	PMF, myelodysplastic syndromes (MDS), CML, MDS/MPN overlap syndromes, nutritional deficiencies, other hematologic malignancies (acute leukemia, myeloma, non-Hodgkin lymphoma, etc.), infiltrative disease (solid tumors, storage diseases, infections, etc.)
Bone marrow fibrosis	PMF, other hematologic malignancies (hairy cell leukemia, other lymphoid neoplasms), metastatic carcinoma, drug related, autoimmune disease, infection, hyperparathyroidism
Eosinophilia	CEL, acute myeloid leukemia (AML), myeloid/lymphoid neoplasms with rearrangement of *PDGFRA, PDGFRB, FGFR1*, or *PCM1-JAK2* lymphoid malignancy, Churg–Strauss, parasitic infections, reactive related to drug reaction (drug rash with eosinophilia and systemic symptoms; DRESS), allergies
Splenomegaly	MPNs, hairy cell leukemia, storage diseases, portal hypertension, splenic lymphoma, autoimmune disease (including hemolytic anemia/immune thrombocytopenic purpura), Felty syndrome

Disease severity classification

Chronic myelogenous leukemia

- Sokal, Hasford, and European Treatment and Outcome Study (EUTOS) predictive risk scores were established in different eras of CML therapy and these scores predicts CML prognosis at the time of its diagnosis before starting therapy. Currently, these scores are of limited usefulness outside of clinical trials.
- In general, low and intermediate risk patients per Sokal score can be started on standard dose imatinib, and high risk patients should be considered for second generation TKIs and closely monitored for cytogenetic and molecular response.

Prognostic risk prediction in *BCR-ABL⁻* MPNs

- The initial management of patients with PV and ET is predominantly dictated by the risk of thrombotic complications, the leading cause of preventable death in this population:
  - High risk PV: history of thrombosis at any age or age above 60 years; this subgroup needs cytoreductive therapy.
- ET thrombotic risk prediction is based on the International Prognostic Score of thrombosis in WHO essential thrombocythemia (IPSET-thrombosis) score:
  - High risk disease: history of thrombosis at any age and/or age >60 with a *JAK2 V617F* mutation
  - Intermediate risk disease: age >60, no *JAK2* mutation detected, and no history of thrombosis
  - Low risk disease: age ≤60 with *JAK2* mutation and no history of thrombosis
  - Very low risk disease: age ≤60, no *JAK2* mutation detected, and no history of thrombosis.

High and intermediate risk patients with ET require cytoreductive therapy. Low and very low risk disease is managed with low dose aspirin and observation, respectively.

Currently, there is no consensus on the best prognostic score for PMF, and the preferred model may depend on physician or institutional preference. Given the expanding molecular understanding, cytogenetic and molecular data incorporated models are more effective in predicting OS and leukemia-free survival (LFS) in PMF than those that utilize clinical features alone. However, in the absence of nonavailability of molecular techniques, it is acceptable to use models that are based solely on clinical features and/or karyotype.

GIPSS (genetically inspired prognostic scoring system) is a karyotype-based risk predictive model that incorporates a limited number of mutations to predict OS and LFS:

- Very high risk (VHR) karyotype comprises of single or multiple abnormalities of −7, i(17q), inv(3)/3q21, 12p–/12p11.2, 11q–/11q23, or other autosomal trisomies not including +8/+9 (e.g. +21, +19).
- Favorable: normal karyotype or sole abnormalities of +9, 13q–, 20q–, chromosome 1 translocation/duplication, or sex chromosome abnormality including –Y and unfavorable karyotype includes all other abnormalities.
- High molecular risk (HMR) mutations include *ASXL1, SRSF2,* and *U2AF1Q157.*
- Absence of type 1-like *CALR* mutation.

VHR karyotype is scored 2 points and the rest at 1 point each. GIPSS effectively distinguished 5-year OS and median OS (respectively, in parentheses):

- Low risk: zero points (94%, 26.4 years)
- Intermediate 1 (Int-1): 1 point (73%, 10.3 years)
- Int-2: 2 points (40%, 4.6 years)
- High risk: ≥3 points (14%, 2.6 years).

MIPSS70+ v2.0 (mutation-enhanced international prognostic scoring system plus karyotype, version 2.0) is a complex model that utilizes three clinical risk factors, five HMR mutations, karyotype and absence of type 1-like CALR mutation to risk stratify patients into five categories:

- Clinical risk factors include severe anemia (men: hemoglobin [Hgb] <9 g/dL; women: Hgb <8 g/dL), moderate anemia (men: Hgb 9–10.9 g/dL; women: Hgb 8–9.9 g/dL), circulating blasts ≥2%, and constitutional symptoms.
- Apart from the *ASXL1, SRSF2, U2AF1Q157* HMR mutations, MIPSS70+V2.0 also includes *EZH2, IDH1/2.*

MIPSS70+ v2.0 established an additional very high risk category with a 10-year OS of <3% and a median survival of 1.8 years. MIPSS70+ v2.0 score may be used to refine int-1 and int-2 risk categories by GIPSS. Dynamic international prognostic scoring system (DIPSS) is a dynamic prognostic tool that can be applied at any time point in the clinical course of PMF and in settings where neither cytogenetics nor molecular analysis is available. DIPSS is based entirely on clinical features (age, leukocyte count, hemoglobin, circulating blasts, and constitutional symptoms).

DIPSS-Plus adds three additional prognostic features vis-a-vis transfusion, unfavorable karyotype, and platelet count <100 000/μL.

Hemoglobin <10 g/dL is weighted 2 DIPSS points and the rest are weighted 1 point in both DIPSS and DIPSS-plus (Table 24.6).

List of imaging techniques

Imaging is not required for diagnostic purposes.

Table 24.6 Dynamic international prognostic scoring system (DIPSS).

DIPSS point count	DIPSS risk category	DIPSS-Plus points
0	Low risk	0
1–2	Intermediate-1 risk	1
3–4	Intermediate-2 risk	2
5–6	High risk	3

Potential pitfalls/common errors in diagnosis

- Masked PV is characterized by an elevated hematocrit that does not meet WHO criteria but has typical bone marrow findings and a *JAK2* mutation:
  - About 20% of patients do not meet all WHO criteria.
- "True" ET must be differentiated from pre PMF as this distinction has significant prognostic implications.
- Unusual thrombosis, even without laboratory abnormalities:
  - Abdominal vein, hepatic, and venous sinus thrombosis should prompt an evaluation for MPNs, including a bone marrow evaluation, even in the absence of laboratory abnormalities, particularly in young individuals.
- Chronicity of abnormal laboratory findings:
  - Laboratory tests should be repeated to confirm elevation given the cost and anxiety regarding evaluation of these disorders.
- Leukocytosis:
  - Even mild elevations in the white blood count or platelets can represent an early phase of MPN.
- Review of the peripheral blood smear is an important step in the evaluation of patients with MPNs to look for myeloid and erythroid precursors, including blast forms, as well as morphologic changes, including nucleated red blood cells, giant platelets, and dysplastic features.

Treatment

Chronic myelogenous leukemia

Characterization of disease phase is paramount (i.e. chronic phase, accelerated phase, or blast crisis).

Chronic phase

- Administration of TKI
  - Imatinib (first generation TKI)
    - Dosage: 400 mg/day orally
    - Side effects: nausea, diarrhea, skin rash, hypothyroidism, cytopenias, edema
  - Nilotinib (second generation TKI)
    - Dosage: 300 mg orally twice daily
    - Side effects: nausea, diarrhea, skin rash, hypothyroidism, hyperlipidemia, elevated amylase or lipase, prolonged QTc
  - Dasatinib (second generation TKI)
    - Dosage: 100 mg/day orally
    - Side effects: nausea, diarrhea, skin rash, fluid retention, pleural effusion, pulmonary hypertension, prolonged QTc.
- Monitoring for response (Table 24.7)
  - Disease monitoring with blood counts, FISH, and PCR
  - Monitor for complete hematologic response (CHR). If CHR is achieved, monitor for cytogenetic response (CyCR), which is measured by FISH or conventional cytogenetics. If CyCR is achieved, monitor for complete molecular response (CMR), then major molecular response (MMR).
  - Loss of molecular response alone does not constitute treatment failure but should increase monitoring for cytogenetic or hematologic failure.
  - If evidence of resistance, can increase dosage of current TKI or change to alternative (i.e. first to second generation TKI).
  - Bosutinib can be used as second line.
  - Ponatinib indicated only for those with *T315I ABL* mutations.

Table 24.7   ELN guidelines on response definition for any first line TKI and second line in case of intolerance, all patients (chronic phase, accelerated phase, or blast crisis).

	Optimal	Suboptimal response	TKI failure
3 months	*BCR-ABL1* ≤10% and/or Ph⁺ ≤35%: partial cytogenetic response (CyR)	*BCR-ABL1* >10% and/or Ph⁺ 36–95%	No complete hematologic remission and/or Ph⁺ >95%
6 months	*BCR-ABL1* <1% and/or Ph⁺ 0% (complete CyR)	*BCR-ABL1* 1–10% and/or Ph⁺ 1–35%	*BCR-ABL1* >10% and/or Ph⁺ 35%
12 months	*BCR-ABL1* ≤0.10%: MMR	*BCR-ABL1* >0.1–1%	*BCR-ABL1* >1% and/or Ph⁺ >0
Then, and at any time	MMR or better	Clonal chromosome abnormalities or Ph⁻ (–7, or 7q–)	Loss of CHR or loss of CCyR or PCyR New *BCR-ABL1* mutations Confirmed loss of MMR CCA/Ph⁺

- Omacetaxine is indicated in chronic phase CML patients with resistance or intolerance to two or more TKIs

Accelerated phase
- Administration of TKI (imatinib, nilotinib, or dasatinib).
- Omacetaxine for TKI refractory disease.
  - Consideration of allogeneic HSCT if response with TKI not achieved.

Blast crisis
- Myeloid blast crisis: treat like AML.
- Lymphoid blast crisis: treat like acute lymphoblastic leukemia.
- Allogeneic HSCT strongly recommended.

Polycythemia vera (Algorithm 24.4)

Algorithm 24.4 Treatment of polycythemia vera

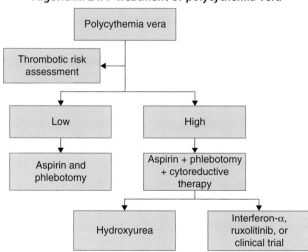

- Therapeutic phlebotomy with goal hematocrit below 45%.
- Antiplatelet therapy with aspirin 81 mg/day orally unless known bleeding diathesis.
- Avoid iron supplementation.

- Optimization of cardiovascular risk factors: avoid smoking; medical optimization of hypertension, obesity, diabetes, hypercholesterolemia.
- High risk and intermediate risk PV.
  - Cytoreductive therapy is strongly recommended.
  - Hydroxyurea is the preferred first line cytoreductive therapeutic agent at present.
    - Starting dose of 500 mg/day orally with titration as tolerated based on blood counts.
    - Key side effects include infertility, mouth sores, skin rash, cytopenias.
  - Pegylated interferon α can also be considered for first or second line.
    - Key side effects include psychiatric manifestations, hypothyroidism, ocular toxicity, and hepatic dysfunction.
  - Ruxolitinib approved for those who are intolerant or resistant to hydroxyurea.
    - Key side effects include cytopenias, increased risk of opportunistic infections (rare).

Essential thrombocythemia (Algorithm 24.5)

Algorithm 24.5 Treatment of essential thrombocythemia

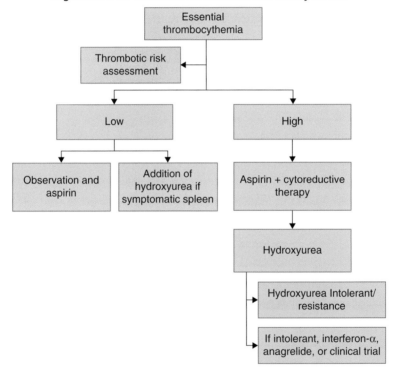

- Antiplatelet therapy with aspirin 81 mg/day orally unless known bleeding diathesis.
- Optimization of cardiovascular risk factors: avoid smoking; medical optimization of hypertension, obesity, diabetes, hypercholesterolemia.
- High risk and intermediate risk ET:
  - Addition of pharmacologic cytoreduction
    - Target platelet count unknown but <600 000 may be considered
  - Hydroxyurea is considered standard of care at this time.
    - Starting dose of 500 mg by mouth daily with titration as tolerated based on blood counts
    - Key side effects include infertility, mouth sores, skin rash, cytopenias.

- Anagrelide may be used for those intolerant or resistant to hydroxyurea.
  - Key side effects include diarrhea, palpitations, dyspnea, and fatigue.
- Pegylated interferon α may also be considered for first or second line.
  - Key side effects include myelosuppression, mood disorders, hypothyroidism, ocular toxicity, and hepatic dysfunction.

Primary myelofibrosis (Algorithm 24.6)

Algorithm 24.6 Treatment of primary myelofibrosis

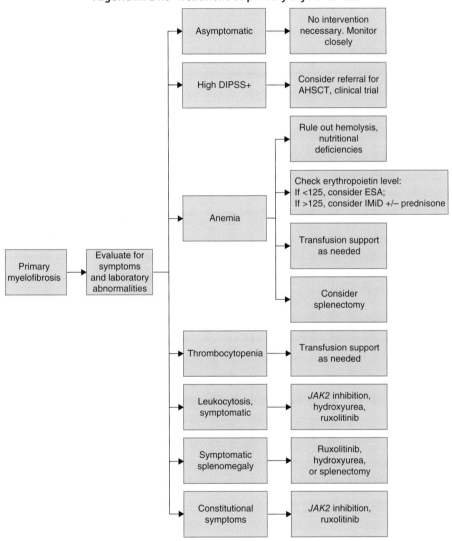

- Treatment based on individual manifestations (i.e. constitutional symptoms, anemia, thrombocytopenia, symptomatic splenomegaly).
- Ruxolitinib:
  - *JAK2* inhibitor approved for treatment of symptomatic splenomegaly and constitutional symptoms in patients with intermediate/high risk disease

- Evidence suggests it may provide a modest improvement in survival
- Key side effects: worsening of cytopenias, herpes zoster, hepatitis-B reactivation and non-melanoma skin cancers.
- Thalidomide, lenalidomide, pomalidomide:
  - May be used to treat anemia in combination with prednisone
  - Key side effects: fatigue and somnolence, increased risk of thrombosis, neuropathy, constipation, leukopenia.
- Hydroxyurea:
  - May be used to treat splenomegaly or extreme leukocytosis/thrombocytosis
  - Key side effects: worsening of cytopenias, mucositis, medial malleolar leg ulcers.
- Splenectomy:
  - Currently considered for those with symptomatic splenomegaly refractory to ruxolitinib or resistant cytopenias.
- Allogeneic HSCT:
  - For eligible patients with a matched sibling or unrelated donor with intermediate or high risk MF by DIPSS criteria
  - Curative potential balanced by significant risk of morbidity and mortality.

Chronic neutrophilic leukemia

- Currently, no standard of care treatment options are available for CNL.
- Consider hydroxyurea for cytoreduction to mitigate symptomatic splenomegaly and hyper-leukocytosis.
- Consider ruxolitinib in the presence of activating *CSF3R* mutation.
- Consider allogeneic HSCT at the earliest as it provides the best option for cure in this high risk but rare MPN.

Special populations
Pregnancy

- Those with childbearing potential should be counseled on teratogenicity of medications (hydroxyurea, TKIs) and the potential complications of pregnancy (thrombosis, bleeding, fetal complications such as IUGR).
- Those receiving these medications should seek nonestrogen containing contraceptive methods particularly in ET and PV.
- A high risk obstetrics specialist should be involved in the care of all pregnant patients with MPN.
- Men should consider sperm banking prior to starting hydroxyurea.
- CML:
  - TKIs should be discontinued in those planning pregnancy to or are pregnant as their safety has not been demonstrated
  - Interferon α can be considered.
- PV and ET
  - All PV patients should be treated with therapeutic phlebotomy to maintain Hct <45% and low dose aspirin
  - Strong consideration should be given for prophylactic low molecular weight heparin for 6 weeks postpartum if no contraindications
  - Risk stratification as per nonpregnant patients with additional high risk features:
    - History of thrombosis or MPN related hemorrhage
    - Those with previous pregnancy complications (i.e. IUGR, stillbirth, or intrauterine death, placental abruption)

- ▪ peripartum hemorrhage
- ▪ severe pre-eclampsia
- ▪ multiple first trimester miscarriages
- ▪ platelets over 1500×10^9/L.
- Those with high risk features should be considered for pharmacologic therapy with interferon α.

Children
- These diseases are very unusual in children but would be managed similarly to adults.

Elderly
- Should be treated and risk stratified as previously stated.
- Frailty should be assessed.
- Oral busulfan or melphalan with intermittent dosing can be considered in place of hydroxyurea or interferon α for patients with poor performance status and limited life expectancy.

Surgical
- For PV and ET, perioperative management should focus on medical optimization of:
  - Hct <45%.
  - Cytoreductive therapy for platelets to goal less than 1×10^9/L perioperatively to reduce risk of bleeding.
  - Preoperative discontinuation of aspirin. Low molecular weight heparin can be given preoperatively after discontinuation in those considered high risk if there are no contraindications.
  - Perioperative monitoring for bleeding complications with consideration of platelet transfusion if excessive bleeding occurs even if normal platelet quantity.
  - Postoperative early ambulation and consideration of 6 weeks of deep vein thrombosis prophylaxis if no contraindications.
- CML
  - No specific recommendations regarding TKI discontinuation perioperatively though TKI therapy is associated with increased risk of thrombosis.
- PMF
  - Transfusional support for those with thrombocytopenia or anemia per standard guidelines or if symptomatic.

Prognosis

> **BOTTOM LINE/CLINICAL PEARLS**
> - Heterogeneity between and within each diagnosis.
> - CML chronic phase greatly improved with TKIs, the prototype of molecularly directed therapy.

Natural history of untreated disease
- See section on disease severity classification for additional details.
- Philadelphia negative MPNs.
- CML: prior to TKIs, 8-year survival was ≤50%.

Prognosis for treated patients
- The BCR-ABL - MPNs are prone for increased risk for thrombotic complications, bleeding, and transformation to acute myeloid leukemia (AML). Patients with PV and ET also have a risk of progression to secondary myelofibrosis (MF), and eventual evolution to AML (Table 24.7).

Table 24.8 Evolution of classic MPNs.

	Thrombosis risk per year (%)	Transformation to PMF at 20 years (%)	Evolution to AML at 20 years (%)
PV	5–10	20–25	5–10
ET	1–2	<10	<5
PMF	1–2	N/A	50

- PV/ET
  - No therapy proven to prevent transformation to PMF or AML
  - Aspirin, phlebotomy, and, when indicated, cytoreduction reduces risk of thrombotic events.
- PMF
  - No therapy proven to prevent transformation to AML (see section on disease severity classification for additional details).
- CML
  - Since 2001, chronic phase, 8-year survival ~90%, and accelerated phase ~75%.
  - Prognosis remains poor in blast crisis with an average survival of 6 months in absence of allogeneic HSCT.

Follow-up tests and monitoring
- **PV/ET:** monitoring for signs or evidence concerning for transformation to PMF/AML (new constitutional symptoms, cytopenias, blasts on peripheral smear) and continued reassessment of thrombotic risks.
- **PMF:** monitoring for signs or evidence concerning for transfusion dependence, need for *JAK2* inhibitor treatment, and evolution to AML (new constitutional symptoms, cytopenias, blasts on peripheral smear).
- **CML:** see section on Treatment: CML, Treatment response.

Reading list
Elliott MA, Tefferi A. Chronic neutrophililc leukemia: update on diagnosis, moleclar genetics, and management. Am J Hematol 2014;89: 651–658.

Gambactori-Passerini C, Piazza R. How I treat newly diagnosed chronic myeloid leukemia in 2015. Am J Hematol 2015;90:156–161.

James C, Ugo V, Le Couédic JP, et al. A unique clonal JAK2 mutation leading to constitutive signaling causes polycythaemia vera. Nature 2005;434:1144–1148.

Klion AD. How I treat hypereosinophilic syndromes. Blood 2015;126:1069–1077.

Mascarenhas J, Mesa R, Prchal J, et al. Optimal therapy for polycythemia vera and essential thrombocythemia can only be determined by the completion of randomized clinical trials. Haematologica 2014;99: 945–949.

Pardanani A. Systemic mastocytosis in adults: 2015 update on diagnosis, risk stratification, and management. Am J Hematol 2015;90:250–262.

Stein BL, Gotlib J, Arcasoy M, et al. Historical views, conventional approaches, and evolving management strategies for myeloproliferative neoplasms. J Natl Compr Canc Netw 2015;13:424–434.

Swerdlow SH Campo E, Harris NL, et al., eds. WHO Classification of Tumours of Haematopoietic and Lymphoid Tissues. Lyon, France: IARC, 2008.

Tefferi A, Barbui T. Polycythemia vera and essential thrombocythemia: 2015 update on diagnosis, risk-stratification and management. Am J Hematol 2015;90:162–173.

Tefferi A, Vannucchi AM, Barbui T. Polycythemia vera treatment algorithm 2018. *Blood Cancer J.* 2018;8:3. doi:10.1038/s41408-017-0042-7

Venugopal S, Mascarenhas J. Chronic Neutrophilic Leukemia: Current and Future Perspectives, Clinical Lymphoma Myeloma and Leukemia 2019; 19(3)129–134. doi.org/10.1016/j.clml.2018.11.012

Verstovsek S, Mesa RA, Gotlib J, et al. A double-blind, placebo-controlled trial of ruxolitinib for myelofibrosis. N Engl J Med 2012;366:799–807.

Guidelines

Title	Source	Date and weblink
European LeukemiaNet recommendations for the management of chronic myeloid leukemia: 2013	ELN	2013 http://www.ncbi.nlm.nih.gov/pubmed/23803709
Revised response criteria for myelofibrosis: International Working Group-Myeloproliferative Neoplasms Research and Treatment (IWG-MRT) and European LeukemiaNet (ELN) consensus report	ELN and IWG-MRT	2013 http://www.ncbi.nlm.nih.gov/pubmed/23838352
Revised response criteria for polycythemia vera and essential thrombocythemia: an ELN and IWG-MRT consensus project	ELN and IWG-MRT	2013 http://www.ncbi.nlm.nih.gov/pubmed/23591792
Philadelphia-negative classical myeloproliferative neoplasms: critical concepts and management recommendations from European LeukemiaNet	ELN	2011 http://www.ncbi.nlm.nih.gov/pubmed/21205761
2016 revision to the World Health Organization classification of myeloid neoplasms and acute leukemia	WHO	https://www.ncbi.nlm.nih.gov/pubmed/27069254/

Additional material for this chapter can be found online at:
www.wiley.com/go/oh/mountsinaioncology

This includes advice for patients, a case study, ICD codes, and multiple choice questions.

CHAPTER 25

Myelodysplastic Syndromes

Thomas U. Marron and Lewis R. Silverman
Icahn School of Medicine at Mount Sinai, New York, NY, USA

OVERALL BOTTOM LINE
- Myelodysplastic syndromes (MDS) are characterized clinically by a hyperproliferative bone marrow and peripheral blood cytopenias caused by ineffective hematopoiesis.
- MDS represents a spectrum of diseases, clonal in origin, that are often thought to represent a preneoplastic or preleukemic state; however, about two-thirds of patients die from complications of MDS without evolving to AML.
- Treatment of MDS is guided by prognosis, determined by multiple factors including severity of cytopenias, percentage of blasts in the bone marrow, and cytogenetic abnormalities.
- Supportive therapies such as erythropoietin and transfusions are the mainstay of treatment for lower risk MDS, while hypomethylating agents and stem cell transplantation (SCT), for suitable candidates, form the basis of treatments for patients with higher risk disease.

Background
Definition of disease
MDS is a heterogeneous group of primary or secondary disorders of the bone marrow typically associated with clonal proliferation of aberrant stem cells resulting in a hyperproliferative marrow space filled with dysplastic cells, leading to ineffective cellular differentiation, and one or more peripheral blood cytopenias. Presence of increased blasts and evolution of a "preleukemic" MDS into AML represents a subset of these disorders, though death from this malignant condition is more commonly brought about by progressive cytopenias and subsequent infection, bleeding, and complications from iron overload.

Disease classification
Initially incorporated into the French–American–British (FAB) classifications of hematologic disorders in 1976, the most recent classification put forth by the WHO in 2001 recognizes six distinct categories of MDS:
- Refractory anemia with ringed sideroblasts (RARS), or without ringed sideroblasts (RA).
- Refractory cytopenia with multilineage dysplasia (RCMD), with or without ringed sideroblasts.
- Refractory anemia with excess blasts (RAEB):
  - RAEB-I (6–10% blasts)
  - RAEB-II (11–19% blasts).
- 5q-syndrome.
- Chronic myelomonocytic leukemia (CMML) (MDS/MPN).
- Myelodysplastic syndrome, unclassifiable.

Mount Sinai Expert Guides: Oncology, First Edition. Edited by William K. Oh and Ajai Chari.
© 2019 John Wiley & Sons Ltd. Published 2019 by John Wiley & Sons Ltd.
Companion Website: www.wiley.com/go/oh/mountsinaioncology

With the exception of 5q-syndrome, these classifications are based entirely on morphologic analysis of the bone marrow, and prognostic scoring systems (see section on Diagnosis) which place more importance on cytogenetic analysis and are more predictive of disease progression, and are typically used as the inclusion criteria for clinical trials.

Incidence/prevalence

It is estimated that 10 000–20 000 new cases of MDS are diagnosed annually in the USA, almost twice the incidence of AML, although the actual incidence is likely significantly higher given the nonspecific symptoms typically associated with more low risk or indolent disease (Rollison et al. 2008).

Economic impact

Stem cell transplantation (SCT) is the only curative therapy for MDS, and is typically only offered to high risk patients with good performance status. Although in some cases curative, the cost typically exceeds $300 000, five times that of supportive care (SC). The cost of newer therapies such as hypomethylating agents and immunomodulatory agents lie in the middle and, although not curative, significantly improve quality of life and survival.

Etiology

Although etiology cannot be identified in most patients with MDS, in some, exposure to radiation, chemicals, or drugs, typically chemotherapeutics, can be implicated to both MDS and AML.

- **Radiation:** well documented in survivors of nuclear bombs, radiation is thought to increase the genetic instability as seen in structural and numerical chromosomal anomalies long after initial exposure. This has also been seen in cancer patients who have received therapeutic radiation.
- **Chemical:** while there are case reports suggesting a variety of environmental chemical exposures predisposing a patient to the development of MDS or AML, petrochemicals, particularly benzene, have been most clearly implicated.
- **Chemotherapy:** a multitude of chemotherapies have been implicated in the development of chromosomal abnormalities and subsequent MDS or AML.

Pathology/pathogenesis

Chromosomal damage and specific mutations in key cell cycling and epigenetic pathways have been implicated in the development of MDS, and there is a substantial body of knowledge that confirms the clonal origin. Furthermore, there is evidence that these disorders can originate from pluripotent stem cells given the frequency with which the lymphoid lineage (B or T cell) has been found to demonstrate aberrant activity in these cells, as well as reports of patients with MDS developing biphenotypic and lymphoid leukemias. We commonly document progressive accumulation of mutations in genes important for trophic signaling pathways and key epigenetic modifying pathways during the course of the disease which may explain the evolution of symptoms and disease severity over time from a lower risk to a higher risk phenotype.

Prevention

BOTTOM LINE/CLINICAL PEARLS
- While there are known risk factors, most importantly exposure to chemotherapy and petrochemicals, there is no known intervention other than avoidance of these toxic exposures that has been demonstrated to prevent the development of MDS.

Screening

There is no evidence supporting regular screening in patients with these toxic exposures.

Diagnosis

> **BOTTOM LINE/CLINICAL PEARLS**
> - Prior to a bone marrow biopsy all other possible etiologies of cytopenias should be excluded.
> - Bone marrow analysis is the mainstay to diagnose MDS, prognosticate, and determine treatment course.
> - International Prognostic Scoring System, Revised (IPSS-R), which incorporates the extent of cytopenias, blast count, and cytogenetic abnormalities, helps in prognostication at the time of diagnosis, and can also be used dynamically during treatment given the not uncommon evolution of the disease and development of new cytogenetic abnormalities.
> - DNA mutation panels are not yet incorporated into diagnostic and treatment algorithms; however, given the high number of mutations in key trophic and epigenetic pathways, which often accrue during the natural course of the disease, this analysis will likely become important in determining not only prognosis, but also treatment as more targeted therapies are developed.

Differential diagnosis

Differential diagnosis	Features
Aplastic anemia	Can be difficult to distinguish from hypoplastic variant of MDS. Cytogenetic abnormalities seen in MDS can help differentiate between the two. This said, hypoplastic MDS can be treated in a similar fashion
Paroxysmal nocturnal hemoglobinuria (PNH)	Flow cytometry can identify clonal population lacking CD55 or CD59, diagnostic of PNH
Large granular lymphocytic leukemia (LGL)	Patients have cytopenias suggestive of MDS, but without any cytogenetic abnormalities or dysmorphic changes. Flow cytometry and T-cell receptor and immunoglobulin gene rearrangement studies can be informative
Overlap syndrome with MPN	Some patients present with overlap syndromes with laboratory tests and bone marrow biopsies suggestive of both MDS and a MPN. Marrow may be hyperproliferative with both dysplasia and evidence of fibrosis peripheral blood leukocytosis seen in advanced MPN. Classic mutation in *JAK2, MPL,* or *Calreticulin* can help further refine the diagnosis
AML	Depending on the classification schema, the defining point between MDS and AML depends on blasts in the peripheral blood *or* bone marrow, whichever is greater. The WHO considers AML to have 20% blasts while the authors typically consider 30% to be the defining barrier

Typical presentation

Though it may be initially diagnosed from incidental findings of a cytopenia on a CBC, patients with MDS commonly present with symptomatic anemia, bleeding, or infection caused by single or multilineage cytopenia in the absence of another explanation such as hemorrhage, toxin and/or drug-exposure, infection, or a biochemical cause such as vitamin deficiency. Depending on the stage, excess blasts can be present in peripheral blood or bone marrow biopsy.

Clinical diagnosis

History

Important history includes familial history of hematologic disorder, symptomatic history, and historic laboratory tests suggestive of cytopenias. It is also important to document any history of exposures given the strong correlation between MDS and exposure to toxins or history of cancer treated with chemotherapy and/or radiation.

Physical examination

Physical examination findings typically correlate with extent of cytopenias in the peripheral blood, including palor, petechiae, and infections.

Useful clinical decision rules and calculators

Most studies of approved drugs were performed using the IPSS which split patients into four risk categories: low, intermediate-1, intermediate-2, and high risk. IPSS-R is a scoring system with five prognostic groups which is also based on percentage of bone marrow blasts, cytogenetics, and degree of cytopenias (Tables 25.1–25.3). It carries a predictive value for both survival and risk of transformation to AML both at the time of diagnosis and also at any time point during the course of the disease. Validation studies demonstrate a close correlation with higher risk and shorter OS. There are additional prognostic classifications not listed here that may also be of use, including that from the WHO (WHO Classification-Based Prognostic Scoring System, WPSS).

Table 25.1 **Risk determined by cytogenetic abnormalities, for use with IPSS-R in Table 25.2.**

Cytogenetic risk	Chromosomal anomaly
Very good	-Y, del(11q)
Good	del(5q), del(12p), del(20q) Normal
Intermediate	del(7q), +8, +19, i(17q) All other abnormalities
Poor	−7, inv(3)/t(3q)/del(3q) Complex (3 abnormalities)
Very poor	Complex (≥3 abnormalities)

Table 25.2 **Scoring system for IPSS-R.**

Prognostic variable points	0	0.5	1	1.5	2	3	4
Cytogenetics (see Table 25.1)	Very good		Good		Intermediate	Poor	Very poor
Bone marrow blast (%)	≤2		2–5		5–10	>10	
Hemoglobin	≥10		8–10	<8			
Platelets	≥100	50–100	<50				
Absolute neutrophil count (ANC)	≥0.8	<0.8					

Table 25.3 IPSS-R risk stratification and median survival per category.

Risk category	Total score	Median OS (months)
Very low	≤1.5	60.8
Low	>1.5–3	58.6
Intermediate	>3–4.5	26
High	>4.5–6	15.8
Very high	>6	5.9

Laboratory diagnosis

List of diagnostic tests

- Bone marrow aspirate and biopsy sent for:
  - Flow cytometry to confirm blast populations
  - Cytogenetics
  - Mutational panels.
- Vitamin B12 and folate.
- PNH screen (CD55 and 59 by flow cytometry).
- Iron studies.
- Depending on presentation, it may also be necessary to exclude other hematologic processes such as multiple myeloma or MPN.

Potential pitfalls/common errors made regarding diagnosis of disease

Though the presence of mutations associated with MDS and AML can eventually become important in decisions about prognosis and treatment, they are not diagnostic and the identification of mutations common to MDS, including *ASXL1, DNMT3A,* and *TET2* without morphologic features in the peripheral blood or bone marrow, is not sufficient to establish a diagnosis.

Treatment (Algorithm 25.1)

Algorithm 25.1 IPSS-R based initial treatment, and subsequent lines of therapy upon progression of disease (PD)

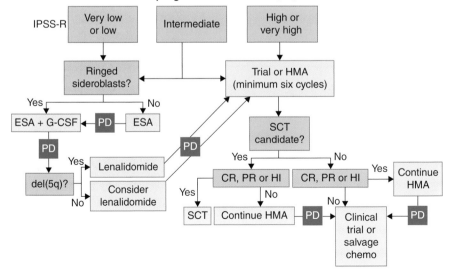

Treatment rationale

Treatment is guided on three key factors: symptoms, performance status, and IPSS-R defined risk. Algorithm 25.1 demonstrates the stratification and decision-making challenges based on IPSS-R of complete remission (CR) achieved with treatment, and following progression of disease (PD).

When to hospitalize

Supportive care and most treatments other than SCT can be managed in the outpatient setting. These patients are typically neutropenic, and if febrile often require hospitalization and intravenous antibiotics. In chronically neutropenic patients the authors typically prescribe prophylactic antibiotics such as quinolones, with Gram-negative bacterial coverage.

Table of treatment

Treatment	Agents	Population clinical effect
Supportive care (SC)	Erythropoiesis stimulating agents (ESAs) ESA + granulocyte colony-stimulating factor (G-CSF)	**All patients, typically use only SC in patients with good prognosis** ESAs are considered the first line therapy for all patients with MDS, alone or in combination depending on prognosis. ESA in combination with G-CSF should be used in patients with sideroblastic anemia up-front, while G-CSF can be added to ESA if a patient does not have a response to ESA alone
Hypomethylating agents (HMA)	Azacitidine	**Approved for use in all risk groups** Only proven to alter natural history of MDS in patients with intermediate or high risk disease Delayed time to progression (vs. SC) Increased OS (vs. SC) Reduced risk of transformation to AML (vs. SC) Symptomatic relief Trend towards higher rates of remission with less toxicity (vs. classic AML induction chemotherapy)
	Decitabine	**Approved for patients with intermediate-1 and worse prognostic groups. Typically used in patients with proliferative disease with high white counts given this therapy is more myelosuppressive** No change in OS in studies, but improved measures such as QoL and transfusion independence
Immunomodulators	Lenalidomide	**Patients with del(5q), typically those with low risk disease without other cytogenetic anomalies** Red cell transfusion independence in 67% of patients, likely increased OS. Approved for use in low risk patients with primarily anemia and normal platelets, given the risk of neutropenia and thrombocytopenia **Also studied in patients without del(5q)** Trial results demonstrated 26.9% of patients achieved transfusion independence, with predicted complication of neutropenia and thrombocytopenia

(Continued)

(*Continued*)

Treatment	Agents	Population clinical effect
Chemotherapy	Anthracycline-based combination chemo FLAG/FLAG-IDA Ara-C monotherapy Clofarabine monotherapy	**For patients who have failed HMA therapy, given data that demonstrates superiority to classic AML-like combinatorial chemotherapy or single agent therapy in those unable to tolerate classic induction** Compared with de novo AML, typically achieves lower CR rates, remission duration, and more prolonged periods of aplasia that occurs with AML
Curative therapy	Allogeneic SCT	**The only curative therapy for MDS, allo-SCT is limited by performance status, and typically to patients who can achieve CR with induction** Based on International Blood and Marrow Transplant Research data, should only be offered to patients with higher risk disease, as in this patient population there is improved OS, while in lower risk patients the mortality associated with the SCT results in a worse OS compared with BSC and other therapies.

Prevention/management of complications

- **Antibiotics:** though no randomized data are available, the authors typically initiate daily pro-phylactic antibiotics with Gram negative bacteria coverage, such as levofloxacin, in patients with prolonged periods of profound neutropenia and an ANC of <200 000/μL.
- **Iron chelation:** given the high transfusion requirements, patients with MDS are at high risk for iron overload including organ dysfunction and infection, and iron accumulation can also have a role in transformation to AML. Per NCCN 2016 guidelines, iron chelation therapy should be started in patients with ferritin >2500 ng/mL or following 25 units of RBCs, particularly patients with lower risk disease. Those with higher risk disease should be considered if they respond to primary therapy.

CLINICAL PEARLS
- Lower risk patents should initially be treated with SC such as ESA and transfusions. If they become transfusion dependent, symptomatic, or their disease is progressing, then initiate more definitive treatment.
- Higher risk patients should be treated at diagnosis. Patients with adequate performance status who are able to achieve CR should be evaluated for allogeneic SCT.
- Patients whom have failed HMA should be considered for a clinical trial given the low response rates and high toxicity of most salvage chemotherapy regimens and the poor prognosis for patients who fail an HMA.

Special populations

- Hypocellular MDS is a rare subset of MDS thought to have an immunologic component. A small percentage of these patients have a PNH clone present alongside dysplastic marrow with classic findings of MDS, while most resemble aplastic anemia. Similar to aplastic anemia, there are reports of using immunosuppression such as cyclosporine and antithymocyte globulin in this group with varying success.

Prognosis

> **BOTTOM LINE/CLINICAL PEARLS**
> - Prognosis is determined by the diagnostic IPSS-R algorithm in Algorithm 25.1, and this has been validated for use both at diagnosis and during the course of disease when the patient undergoes restaging upon progression of disease.
> - Given the heterogeneity of the disease, the natural history is highly variable. Patients with low risk disease can be maintained on SC, and even remain transfusion independent for years, some for decades, while those with high risk disease run the risk of progression to AML, which is difficult to treat, or succumbing to bleeding or infection because of severe cytopenias.
> - The presence of certain mutations appear to be associated with worse OS, but at present p53 mutations are the only ones that are conclusively associated with poor OS and poorer response to all lines of therapy including SCT.

Follow-up tests and monitoring

- Bone marrow biopsy should be performed if the patient appears to have evolving disease with worsening transfusion dependence or cytopenias (if on SC) or if they appear to be progressing on therapy.
- Every time a bone marrow biopsy is performed it should be sent for cytogenetic testing to evaluate for the appearance of any new abnormalities.
- Given the rapidly increasing body of knowledge on driver mutations affecting growth and epigenetic modification, the authors suggest sending for mutational panels at the time of diagnosis and progression, ideally on bone marrow specimens, in order to assess for presence of actionable targets. These are also likely to have a role in future prognostic algorithms.

References and reading list

Cogle CR, Ortendahl JD, Bentley TG, et al. Cost-effectiveness of treatments for high-risk myelodysplastic syndromes after failure of first-line hypomethylating agent therapy. Expert Rev Pharmacoecon Outcomes Res 2016;16:275–284.

Ma X, Does M, Raza A, Mayne ST. Myelodysplastic syndromes: incidence and survival in the United States. Cancer 2007;109:1536–1542.

Rollison DE, Howlader N, Smith MT, et al. Epidemiology of myelodysplastic syndromes and chronic myeloproliferative disorders in the United States, 2001–2004, using data from the NAACCR and SEER programs. Blood 2008;112:45–52.

Suggested websites

For practitioners: www.nccn.org – section on MDS

For practitioners and patients: www.mds-foundation.org; http://www.cancer.gov/types/myeloproliferative/patient/myelodysplastic-treatment-pdq

Guidelines

Title	Date and weblink
NCCN Clinical Practice Guidelines in Oncology (NCCN Guidelines) Myelodysplastic Syndromes	2016 http://www.nccn.org/professionals/physician_gls/pdf/mds.pdf
Myelodysplastic Syndromes: ESMO Clinical Practice Guidelines	2014 http://www.esmo.org/Guidelines/Haematological-Malignancies/Myelodysplastic-Syndromes

(Continued)

(*Continued*)

Title	Date and weblink
Diagnosis and treatment of primary myelodysplastic syndromes in adults: recommendations from the European LeukemiaNet	2013 http://www.bloodjournal.org/content/122/17/2943?sso-checked=true

Evidence

Type of evidence	Title and comment	Date and weblink
Scoring system	Revised International Prognostic Scoring System for Myelodysplastic Syndromes **Comment:** delineates the IPSS-R discussed above, and the correlative survival data	2012 http://www.bloodjournal.org/content/120/12/2454.long
RCT	Lenalidomide in the myelodysplastic syndrome with chromosome 5q deletion **Comment:** demonstrated for the first time the use of lenalidomide in patients with del(5q)	2006 http://www.nejm.org/doi/full/10.1056/NEJMoa061292
RCT	Randomized controlled trial of azacitidine in patients with the myelodysplastic syndrome: a study of the cancer and leukemia group B **Comment:** demonstrated significantly higher response rates, improved quality of life, reduced risk of leukemic transformation, and improved survival compared with SC	2002 http://jco.ascopubs.org/content/20/10/2429.long
	Efficacy of azacitidine compared with that of conventional care regimens in the treatment of higher-risk myelodysplastic syndromes: a randomised, open-label, phase III study **Comment:** demonstrated increased OS in patients with higher risk MDS vs. BSC	2009 http://www.thelancet.com/journals/lanonc/article/PIIS1470-2045%2809%2970003-8/references
Single-arm trial	Intensive chemotherapy is not recommended for patients aged >60 years who have myelodysplastic syndromes or acute myeloid leukemia with high risk karyotypes **Comment:** elderly and high risk patients do not benefit from conventional AML-like chemotherapy regimens	2007 http://onlinelibrary.wiley.com/doi/10.1002/cncr.22779/full
Model system, retrospective data	A decision analysis of allogeneic bone marrow transplantation for the myelodysplastic syndromes: delayed transplantation for low risk myelodysplasia is associated with improved outcome **Comment:** model developed was used to determine that allo-SCT should only be pursued in high risk patients, as the risk of morbidity and mortality in low risk patients overwhelms any benefit given their longer OS and higher quality of life	2004 http://www.bloodjournal.org/content/104/2/579.long?sso-checked=true

Additional material for this chapter can be found online at:
www.wiley.com/go/oh/mountsinaioncology

This includes advice for patients, a case study, ICD codes, and
multiple choice questions.

CHAPTER 26

Multiple Myeloma and Plasma Cell Disorders

Siyang Leng[1] and Ajai Chari[2]
[1] Columbia University Irving Medical Center, New York, NY, USA
[2] Icahn School of Medicine at Mount Sinai, New York, NY, USA

OVERALL BOTTOM LINE

- Plasma cell disorders (PCDs) can present pleiotropically, but are all united by the presence of clonal plasma cell.
- Diagnosis of PCDs requires a comprehensive set of laboratory, pathologic, and radiographic tests.
- Treatment and prognosis of these disorders has improved significantly over the past 15 years because of the introduction of immunomodulatory agents and proteasome inhibitors. Next generation versions of these agents, and immunotherapies, will likely continue to revamp therapy and prognosis in the coming years.

Background
Definition of disease

- PCDs are characterized by a clonal proliferation of plasma cells which can cause end organ complications.

Disease classification

Differential diagnosis	End-organ damage	Symmetric neuropathy	Monoclonal (M) protein	Clonal cells in bone marrow	Comments
Monoclonal gammopathy of undetermined significance (MGUS)	−	−[a]	+ (<3 g/dL)	+ (<10%)	[a]Generally no neuropathy but some patients have antibodies to nerve antigens (e.g. MAG or SGPG)
Smoldering multiple myeloma (SMM)	−	−	+ (≥3 g/dL)	+ (10–60%)	No MM symptoms or biomarkers indicated below
Multiple myeloma (MM)	+	Sensory or sensorimotor	+ (≥3 g/dL)	+ (≥10%)	CRABI symptoms (see section on Diagnosis), >1 MRI lesion, FLC ratio >100

Mount Sinai Expert Guides: Oncology, First Edition. Edited by William K. Oh and Ajai Chari.
Companion Website: www.wiley.com/go/oh/mountsinaioncology

(Continued)

Differential diagnosis	End-organ damage	Symmetric neuropathy	Monoclonal (M) protein	Clonal cells in bone marrow	Comments
Plasma cell leukemia	+	+/−	+	+	>20% circulating plasma cells and/or >2 × 10^9/L plasma cells
Plasmacytoma	+	−	−	−	Medullary or extramedullary
Waldenström macroglobulinemia	+	Distal, sensory or sensorimotor, progressive	+ (IgM only)	+ (≥10%)	Lymphoplasmacytic cells
Primary (or AL) amyloidosis	+	Distal, sensory and autonomic, painful, progressive	+ (usually small)	+/−	Deposition into end organs such as heart, kidney, gastrointestinal tract, liver, thyroid, adrenal, nerves leading to organ dysfunction; must distinguish from other types of amyloid using techniques such as mass spectrometry
Light chain disease	+	+/−	+	+/−	Deposition pattern of light chains is different from AL amyloid
Heavy chain disease	+	−	+	+/−	Deposition pattern of heavy chains is different from AL amyloid
POEMS	+	Proximal and distal, sensorimotor, progressive areflexia	+	+	Polyneuropathy, organomegaly, endocrinopathy, M-protein, skin changes (POEMS); refer to Mayo Clinic diagnostic criteria; VEGF elevated
TEMPI syndrome	+	−	+	+ (<10%)	Telangiectasias, elevated erythropoietin, monoclonal gammopathy, perinephric fluid collection, intrapulmonary shunting (TEMPI)
Schnitzler syndrome	+	−	+ (IgM only)	+/−	Chronic urticarial rash, monoclonal gammopathy, and at least two of the following: periodic fever, joint/bone pain, lymphadenopathy or hepatomegaly or splenomegaly, increased ESR, neutrophilia, abnormal bone imaging
Acquired Fanconi syndrome	+	−	+	+/−	Monoclonal gammopathy is one cause for acquired Fanconi syndrome

Incidence/prevalence
- The incidence and prevalence of MGUS varies by age and ethnicity – prevalence estimated to be 3–4% in Caucasians over the age of 50, and 6–8% in African Americans.
- MM represents ~1.6% of new cancer cases in the USA.
- In 2012, there were an estimated 89 658 people living with MM in the USA.

Economic impact
- PCDs have very high economic impact on both patients and the healthcare system because of the length of treatment (usually years) and the high costs of treatment modalities which include drugs (up to $27 422 per month in 2015), radiation, and stem cell transplant (median cost $99 899 in 2013).

Etiology
- Familial MM is rare and no single associated gene has been identified.
- Exposure to radiation and chemicals (e.g. pesticides, dioxin) have been linked to increased risk of MM.

Pathology/pathogenesis
- PCDs arise from the malignant transformation of postgerminal center plasma cells.
- Each patient's myeloma is comprised of multiple malignant plasma cell clones at time of diagnosis (Figure 26.1). Over time and with exposure to therapy, new mutations and clones emerge, and the relative abundance of clones changes, with the development of an increasingly drug resistant phenotype.
- Dysregulation of the bone marrow microenvironment is believed to have an important role in pathogenesis.

Predictive/risk factors
Note: applies to MM only.

Risk factor	Odds ratio
Age	9 (for age 65–74 compared with 35–44)
African American ethnicity	2–3 (compared with Caucasians)
Asian ethnicity	0.6 (compared with Caucasians)
Male gender	1.4
First degree relative with MM	3.7

Prevention

BOTTOM LINE/CLINICAL PEARLS
- There is no known way to prevent the development of PCDs.
- There is significant interest in preventing SMM from developing into MM, as risk stratification of patients with SMM and therapeutic options have both improved. While innately attractive, additional studies are needed to demonstrate that early treatment improves survival and has acceptable tradeoffs in terms of quality of life and cost effectiveness before it can be widely adopted.

Diagnosis (Algorithm 26.1)

Algorithm 26.1 Diagnosis of MM, SMM, and MGUS

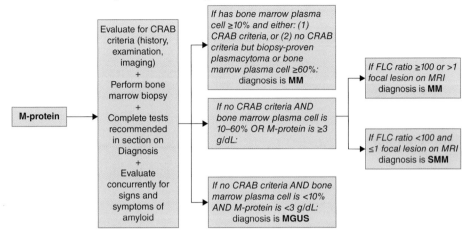

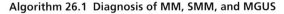

BOTTOM LINE/CLINICAL PEARLS
- **For MM:** look for symptoms, signs, laboratory test results, and imaging consistent with CRABI (hypercalcemia, renal failure, anemia, bone pain or lytic bone lesions, infection).
- **For amyloid:** look for any organ dysfunction (e.g. congestive heart failure, nephrotic syndrome) and M-protein.

Differential diagnosis

Differential diagnosis	Comments
Cold agglutinin disease	Generally IgM monoclonal protein; associated with hemolytic anemia; not associated with hypercalcemia, renal failure, or bone pain
Cryoglobulinemia	Cold urticaria, purpura of lower limbs, Raynaud phenomenon
Polyclonal gammopathies	Caused by presence of reactive plasma cells; many disorders, e.g. hepatitis B or C, HIV, other chronic infections, liver disease, connective tissue disorders
Metastatic carcinoma	No monoclonal protein in serum; bone biopsy would not demonstrate clonal plasma cells
Non-Hodgkin lymphomas	Biopsy of affected tissues demonstrates clonal B cells, not plasma cells
Post-transplant lymphoproliferative disorder	Biopsy of affected tissues demonstrate clonal B cells, not plasma cells
Scleromyxedema	Generally IgGλ; diffuse skin thickening, obstructive lung disease, pulmonary hypertension

Typical presentation
- Refer to section on disease classification.
- For MM:
  - Increased plasma cells in bone marrow (96%)
  - M-protein (93%)
  - Anemia (73%)
  - Lytic bone lesions (67%)
  - Renal failure (19%)
  - Hypercalcemia (13%)
  - Infection.

Clinical diagnosis
History
- CRABI features.
- Refer to section on disease classification.

Physical examination
- A general physical examination should be performed, with particular attention to the musculoskeletal and neurologic systems.
- Patients with amyloid can have macroglossia, signs of heart failure, a shoulder pad sign, hepatomegaly, carpal tunnel syndrome, ecchymoses, and subcutaneous nodules.

Disease severity classification
- The International Staging System (IPSS; recently revised to the IPSS-R) has become the preferred staging system (over the Durie Salmon) because of its ease of use and lack of subjectivity.

Laboratory diagnosis
List of diagnostic tests
- The following tests should be ordered for all patients undergoing an evaluation for a PCD:
  - CBC.
  - Chemistry.
  - Serum protein electrophoresis (SPEP), serum immunofixation (SIFE), serum free light chain analysis (FLC).
  - Bone marrow biopsy with immunohistochemistry or immunophenotyping, cytogenetics, and plasma cell-specific FISH, and possibly gene expression profiling. Can be omitted for patients with M-protein less than 1.5 g/100 mL and clinical picture of MGUS.
  - Skeletal imaging: see lists of imaging techniques.
- Additional tests that are useful in some circumstances:
  - 24-hour urine collection for electrophoresis (UPEP) and immunofixation (UIFE). Should be checked for patients suspected of having amyloid and for all patients with renal abnormalities.
  - Erythrocyte sedimentation rate (ESR), C-reactive protein (CRP), LDH, albumin, and β2-microglobulin are used to stage MM and assess disease activity.
  - Targeted biopsy of a bone lesion, especially for a solitary plasmacytoma.
  - Serum viscosity, especially if IgG >7 k, A >5 k, M >3 k.
  - Fat pad aspirate to evaluate for amyloid. Alternatively, any organ thought to be affected can be biopsied (e.g. heart, kidney, tongue, rectum).

Lists of imaging techniques

- Start with skeletal survey to evaluate for lytic bone lesions. If negative and bone pain or neurologic deficits, follow up with more sensitive tests (low dose whole body CT, PET/CT, or MRI of the entire spine and bony pelvis).
- Consider bone densitometry, particularly in patients receiving bisphosphonates.

Potential pitfalls/common errors made regarding diagnosis of disease

- The SIFE and FLC are frequently omitted during evaluation, but they should be checked as they increase the sensitivity for detecting a monoclonal protein.
- Approximately 1% of MM patients are nonsecretory: they have plasma cell proliferation but these plasma cells do not secrete M-protein. These patients need to be diagnosed and followed using bone marrow biopsies and imaging (PET/CT or MRI).

Treatment (Algorithm 26.2)

Algorithm 26.2 Management of multiple myeloma

Diagnosis	Stem cell transplant candidate?	Yes	Induction chemotherapy		Consider maintenance	Relapse	Salvage therapies: • Chemotherapy • SCT • Clinical trial
		No	Induction chemotherapy	Stem cell harvest and transplant			

Treatment rationale

- Patients with symptomatic MM are typically treated with a combination chemotherapy regimen containing a steroid medication and either a proteasome inhibitor (PI) or an immunomodulatory imide drug (IMiD) or both. Additionally, a traditional chemotherapy agent is sometimes added.
- Patients who are eligible and wish to undergo high dose melphalan with autologous stem cell transplantation (ASCT) typically receive 4–6 months of chemotherapy, and then undergo autologous stem cell harvesting followed by ASCT, which confers a median PFS of ~24–36 months. If maintenance therapy with lenalidomide is used, median PFS is ~48 months.
- ASCT is sometimes performed at the time of relapsed disease rather than as part of the initial treatment, although early ASCT likely confers a greater PFS benefit.
- Treatment of plasmacytomas is typically with radiation and steroids. Upon completion of radiation, patients are followed up by observation.
- Primary amyloidosis is typically treated with chemotherapy similar to that used for MM, albeit dose attenuated. ASCT is an effective modality, and patients who are eligible should be referred.
- Patients with Waldenström macroglobulinemia only warrant treatment when they develop symptoms or certain laboratory test changes. Treatment typically is with rituximab and one or more chemotherapy agents, or the newly approved agent ibrutinib. Patients with hyperviscosity warrant plasmapheresis.

When to hospitalize

- Acute renal failure.
- Symptoms or signs of cord compression.
- Severe infection.
- Chemotherapies that are associated with a high risk of tumor lysis or other complications or require continuous IV administration in the absence of a central line.

Table of treatment

Note: this table is most applicable to MM, although the agents listed are generally used to treat other PCDs as well.

Medical treatments	Comments
Proteasome inhibitors: • Bortezomib (V) – SQ • Carfilzomib (K) – IV • Ixazomib (I) – PO	All patients should receive prophylaxis against herpes zoster Dose limiting toxicities: • V – neuropathy • K – hypertension • I – GI and rash
Immunomodulatory drugs – all PO: • Thalidomide (T) • Lenalidomide[a] (R) • Pomalidomide (P)	Potential for fetal harm – REMS program All increase risk for DVT – aspirin, coumadin or other systemic anticoagulation is required T associated with more neuropathy, constipation, and sedation than other IMiDs R and P are more associated with myelosuppression
Chemotherapy – all IV: • Carmustine[a] • Cyclophosphamide • Doxorubicin • Etoposide[a] • Bendamustine • Melphalan[a]	With exception of cyclophosphamide, no longer first line More myelosuppressive than other classes of agents and oral melphalan impairs stem cell harvest Risk of alopecia
Histone deacetylase inhibitor: • Panobinostat (pano) – PO	Given orally Gastrointestinal side effects depend on choice of partnering agent (and if V, route of administration)
Steroids: • Prednisone – PO • Dexamethasone (D/d) – PO or IV	Weekly dexamethasone preferred over 4 day pulses (unless acute renal failure or spinal cord compression)
Monoclonal antibodies – all IV: • Daratumumab (Dara) • Elotuzumab (E)	Infusion reactions more common with Dara than E but overall very well tolerated Dara affects RBC typing
Bisphosphonates – all IV: • Pamidronic acid[a] • Zoledronic acid[a] • Denosumab	Dental clearance needed prior to initiation because of increased risk for osteonecrosis of jaw

[a] Use with caution in renal failure

Common treatment regimens	Regimens and comments
Induction	VRd, KRd, VCd are preferred though VTd, VD, Rd are options ASCT is often performed after initial chemo
Relapsed/refractory disease	Consider ASCT or any above unused regimen VPd, CRd, CPd, V/pano/d, R/pano/d, clinical trial

Other treatments	Comments
Analgesia	For bone pain
Prophylaxis	Ensure patients have up-to-date pneumococcal (13,23 serotypes) and influenza vaccinations Consider IV immunoglobulin in patients who have recurrent infections and are hypogammaglobulinemic

(*Continued*)

Other treatments	Comments
Radiotherapy	For plasmacytomas causing compressive symptoms
Surgical: • Rod stabilization • Kyphoplasty • Vertebroplasty	Stabilizes the spine and reduces pain

Prevention/management of complications
- **Pathologic fractures:** surgical modalities, bisphosphonates, calcium and vitamin D, analgesia.
- **Renal failure:** chemotherapy, avoid NSAIDs, adequate hydration, dialysis, equivocal data for plasmapheresis if high light chain burden.
- **Hypercalcemia:** hydration, steroids, bisphosphonates, calcitonin, dialysis in severe cases, denosumab.
- **Hyperviscosity:** plasmapheresis.
- **Anemia:** supportive transfusions if indicated; iron, vitamin B12, folate if indicated.
- **Neutropenia:** filgrastim or PEG-filgrastim, reduce or hold chemotherapy.
- **Neuropathy:** reduce or hold chemotherapy, carnitine/B12/B6 in deficient patients, duloxetine.
- **Infections:** antimicrobials as appropriate, hold chemotherapy.

CLINICAL PEARLS
- Patients with certain PCDs – MGUS, SMM, and often Waldenström macroglobulinemia – can be observed without treatment.
- Prior to treatment it is important to risk stratify patients, and to assess their eligibility for ASCT.
- Treatment of PCDs is typically with a chemotherapy regimen incorporating either a PI or IMiD or both as the backbone, along with a steroid. Patients who are eligible undergo ASCT.

Special populations
Elderly
- ASCT is not an option for frail elderly (with published guidelines to calculate frailty).
- IMiDs and PIs are generally well-tolerated, but dose reductions are often needed.

Renal
- See Treatment table for drugs requiring dose modification.
- Plasmapheresis can be considered for markedly elevated FLC leading to renal failure, although its role is unclear in an era with rapid and deep responses with novel agents.

Prognosis

BOTTOM LINE/CLINICAL PEARLS
- Prognosis is highly variable by disease. Within each disease, prognosis can be further stratified based upon the presence or absence of certain risk factors.
- For MM, current estimated median survivals: low risk disease ≥10 years, standard risk disease 7 years, high risk disease 2 years. Similarly, MGUS and SMM can be subdivided into low, intermediate, and high risk groups.

- For MM, commonly accepted markers of high risk disease are ISS stage, LDH, and FISH t(14;16), t(14;20), or del17p13. These can all be identified by FISH performed on the bone marrow. Gene expression profiling, when available, offers additional prognostic information. t(4;14) was previously considered high risk but is now considered intermediate risk with the use of PIs.
- For amyloidosis, current estimated median survivals by Revised Mayo stage: stage I 55 months; stage II 19 months; stage III 12 months; stage IV 5 months.

Reading list

Chng WJ, Dispenzieri A, Chim CS, et al. IMWG consensus on risk stratification in multiple myeloma. Leukemia 2014;28:269–277.

Kyle RA, Rajkumar SV. Criteria for diagnosis, staging, risk stratification and response assessment of multiple myeloma. Leukemia 2009;23:3–9.

Rajkumar SV. Multiple myeloma: 2014 Update on diagnosis, risk-stratification, and management. Am J Hematol 2014;89:999–1009.

Rajkumar SV, Dimopoulos MA, Palumbo A, et al. International Myeloma Working Group updated criteria for the diagnosis of multiple myeloma. Lancet Oncol 2014;15:e538–e548.

Terpos E, Morgan G, Dimopoulos MA, et al. International Myeloma Working Group recommendations for the treatment of multiple myeloma-related bone disease. J Clin Oncol 2013;31:2347–2357.

Suggested websites

International Myeloma Working Group: imwg.myeloma.org

Multiple Myeloma Research Foundation: www.themmrf.org

Guidelines
National society guidelines

Title	Source	Date and weblink
Evaluation, diagnosis and management of MM	NCCN	2015 https://www.nccn.org/professionals/physician_gls/PDF/myeloma.pdf
For amyloidosis	NCCN	2015 https://www.nccn.org/professionals/physician_gls/pdf/amyloidosis.pdf
For Waldenström	NCCN	2015 https://www.nccn.org/professionals/physician_gls/pdf/waldenstroms.pdf

International society guidelines

Title	Source and comment	Date and weblink
International Myeloma Working Group updated criteria for the diagnosis of multiple myeloma	IMWG **Comment:** Diagnosis of MM	2014 https://www.ncbi.nlm.nih.gov/pubmed/25439696
International uniform response criteria for multiple myeloma	IMWG **Comment:** Criteria for assessing the response to therapy for MM	2006 https://www.ncbi.nlm.nih.gov/pubmed/16855634

Image

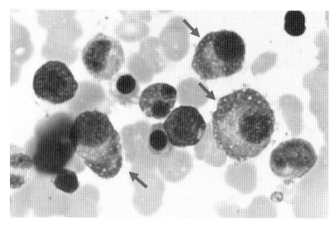

Figure 26.1 Malignant plasma cells (arrows): key features are the eccentric nucleus, basophilic cytoplasm, and pale zone (containing the Golgi apparatus) adjacent to the cytoplasm. (Courtesy of Dr. Julie Teruya-Feldstein.) See website for color version.

Additional material for this chapter can be found online at: www.wiley.com/go/oh/mountsinaioncology

This includes advice for patients, a case study, ICD codes, and multiple choice questions. The following image is available in color: Figure 26.1.

CHAPTER 27

Acute Myeloid Leukemia

Kevin Barley and Shyamala C. Navada
Icahn School of Medicine at Mount Sinai, New York, NY, USA

OVERALL BOTTOM LINE
- Acute myeloid leukemia (AML) is a rare and heterogeneous hematologic neoplasm that is rapidly progressive and fatal without treatment but curable with meticulous care in many patients.
- Risk stratification using cytogenetic and molecular markers is essential to the proper management of patients with AML.
- Enrollment in clinical trials is recommended, when available, for most patients.

Background
Definition of disease
AML is a hematologic neoplasm of myeloid precursors defined as the presence of ≥20% myeloid blasts in the blood or bone marrow or <20% blasts and the presence of t(8;21), inv(16), t(16;16), or t(15;17) (Figure 27.1).

Disease classification
The current classification schema is based upon the identification of recurrent cytogenetic abnormalities rather than morphology, which was used in the French–American–British classification M0–M7 system.
- Acute promyelocytic leukemia (APL; Figure 27.2), formerly M3: identified by FISH for PML-RARA, t(15;17), or PCR for PML-RARA, APL is highly curable, but patients are at high risk of bleeding complications and death early in their course and require urgent treatment with all-trans-retinoic acid (ATRA).
- AML with recurrent cytogenetic abnormalities is discussed further in the section on Prognosis.
- AML transformed from MPNs: identified by prior diagnosis or mutations in *JAK2 V617F* or *calreticulin*, this form of AML has a dismal prognosis and unclear benefit from conventional chemotherapy.
- AML with MDS related changes: these patients are rarely cured by standard therapy and die from consequences of bone marrow failure, but can often obtain disease control with hypomethylating agents.

Incidence/prevalence
The incidence of AML is approximately 4 per 100 000 but significantly increases with age with a total of 20 000 cases per year in the USA.

Mount Sinai Expert Guides: Oncology, First Edition. Edited by William K. Oh and Ajai Chari.
© 2019 John Wiley & Sons Ltd. Published 2019 by John Wiley & Sons Ltd.
Companion Website: www.wiley.com/go/oh/mountsinaioncology

Etiology
- AML can be caused by exposure to anthracyclines, topoisomerase inhibitors, chemicals such as benzene, or result from transformation of MDS or MPNs, but in most cases the etiology of AML is unknown.
- AML is frequently associated with chromosomal abnormalities and recurrent somatic mutations; however, the prevalence of these mutations in the general population increases with age, and while they increase one's risk for developing hematologic malignancies, the vast majority of patients with these mutations do not develop leukemia.

Pathology/pathogenesis
- Cytogenetic abnormalities or somatic mutations frequently affect myeloid transcription factors or other regulators of differentiation.
- There is a failure of maturation or arrest of differentiation of myeloid blasts leading to a rapid proliferation of blasts in the bone marrow.
- Infiltration of the bone marrow results in ineffective or lack of hematopoiesis of normal white cells, red cells, and platelets resulting in immunodeficiency, anemia, and thrombocytopenia.

Predictive/risk factors

Risk factor	Odds ratio
Myelodysplastic syndrome	Varies based upon IPSS-R score
Myeloproliferative neoplasm	Varies based upon DIPSS score
Alkylating agents, topoisomerase inhibitors	Varied reports. 0.8–6.3% prevalence of MDS or AML at 20 years
Adjuvant breast cancer chemotherapy	0.6% absolute risk increase at 10 years
Crude oil exposure	Relative risk 2.89
Chemical exposure: benzene or garment industry related	Hazard ratio 1.15–2.54
HIV	Relative risk 2.5–4.2
Radiation	Dose dependent, peak 5 years after exposure
Cigarette smoking	Odds ratio 1.45

Prevention

> **BOTTOM LINE/CLINICAL PEARLS**
> - The only risk reduction measures available are to minimize exposure to the risk factors mentioned in the table Predictive/risk factors.

Diagnosis

> **BOTTOM LINE/CLINICAL PEARLS**
> - AML should be suspected in patients with profound leukocytosis, significant peripheral blast count, or pancytopenia.

- Initial history should focus on signs of AML secondary to chemotherapy, MDS, or MPNs, exposure to known risk factors as well as signs of complications of AML such as infection or bleeding.
- Physical examination should focus on the bleeding and infectious complications of AML. Patients may have skin manifestations, such as leukemia cutis. They may have petechiae in the setting of low platelet counts.
- Diagnosis is based upon evidence of ≥20% myeloid blasts in the blood or bone marrow or <20% blasts and the presence of either t(8;21), inv(16), t(16;16), or t(15;17).
- Initial evaluation should include an assessment for disseminated intravascular coagulation with prothrombin time (PT), activated partial thromboplastin time (aPTT), fibrinogen, and D-dimer, which can provide early evidence for APL and allow early treatment with ATRA. This should be quickly followed by bone marrow evaluation.

Differential diagnosis

Differential diagnosis	Features
Myelodysplastic syndrome	Evidence of dysplasia with <20% blasts
Myeloproliferative neoplasms	*JAK2 V617F, calreticulin*, or significant fibrosis on marrow evaluation
Aplastic anemia	Marrow will show aplasia
Biphenotypic acute leukemia	Has features of both AML and ALL but is best treated with ALL-type regimens
Acute lymphoblastic leukemia (ALL)	Differentiate with immunophenotype
Chronic myelogenous leukemia in blast phase	Philadelphia chromosome positive

Typical presentation

Patients typically present with an acute illness with symptoms of bone marrow failure (bleeding, bruising, fatigue, infection), leukocytosis (confusion, congestive heart failure), or disseminated intravascular coagulation (DIC). There may be a prior history of chemotherapy, chemical exposure, MDS, or MPN.

Clinical diagnosis

History

- Most patients will present with fatigue, bruising, or infection.
- History should explore for secondary AML, risk factors and chemical exposures, family history, and the bleeding and infectious complications of AML, as well as for signs of leukostasis such as neurologic dysfunction, tinnitus, congestive heart failure, myocardial ischemia, or limb ischemia.

Physical examination

- Often normal other than conjunctival pallor or petechiae.
- Evaluate for splenomegaly, which can suggest preceding MPN.
- Assess for signs of extramedullary disease such as leukemia cutis or nodal involvement, which is more common in patients with myelomonocytic subtypes.
- Evaluate for signs of leukostasis, particularly neurologic deficits, evidence of ischemia, or congestive heart failure.

Table 27.1 Disease severity classification.

Prognosis	Cytogenetics/FISH	Molecular profiling
Favorable	t(8;21) inv(16) t(16;16)	NK* with negative *FLT3-ITD* and mutant *NPM1* or double mutant *CEBPA*
Intermediate	Trisomy 8	t(8;21) with *c-KIT* mutation NK with negative *FLT3-ITD* and single mutant *CEBPA* or negative *NPM1*
Unfavorable	Complex karyotype Monosomy 5 or 7 Abnormalities of 3q, 11q, or 17p	NK with *FLT3-ITD*

Disease severity classification
- Risk is classified by cytogenetic, FISH, and mutational analysis; however, the prognosis of post-MPN and post-MDS AML is worse than de novo AML.
- Acute promyelocytic leukemia (PML-RARA, t(15;17)) is separately stratified because of its favorable prognosis. Risk in this group is stratified: good risk WBC <10 k/µL and platelets >40 k/µL; intermediate risk WBC <10 k/µL and platelets <40 k/µL; poor risk WBC >10 k/µL (Table 27.1).

Laboratory diagnosis
List of diagnostic tests
- CBC with manual differential and peripheral smear; bone marrow biopsy and aspirate: ≥20% blasts.
- Electrolytes, renal and liver function tests, LDH, PT, aPTT, fibrinogen, D-dimer.
- Flow cytometry, FISH, and cytogenetics.
- Molecular studies to evaluate for recurrent somatic mutations including *FLT-3, c-KIT, CEBPA,* and *NPM1*.
- Consider testing with an extended gene mutation profile.
- Human leukocyte antigen (HLA) typing should be sent at diagnosis prior to chemotherapy-induced pancytopenia in patients who are potential candidates for stem cell transplant.

Lists of imaging techniques
- Imaging is generally not useful in AML.
- Imaging should be targeted at any symptoms, particularly neurologic, but no routine imaging is required.

Treatment (Algorithm 27.1)
Treatment rationale
- Clinical trials should be offered to all patients when available.
- The optimal management of hyperleukocytosis (WBC >100 k/µL) is the immediate initiation of chemotherapy. If there will be a delay in chemotherapy, cytoreduction can be achieved with hydroxyurea. Due to the risks and lack of well-defined benefit, leukapheresis should be reserved for patients with clear signs of leukostasis, and leukapheresis should never be used if it will delay chemotherapy.

Acute promyelocytic leukemia:
- Low and intermediate risk APL should receive induction with ATRA/arsenic trioxide (ATO) until complete remission and ATRA/ATO based consolidation.

Algorithm 27.1 Treatment of AML

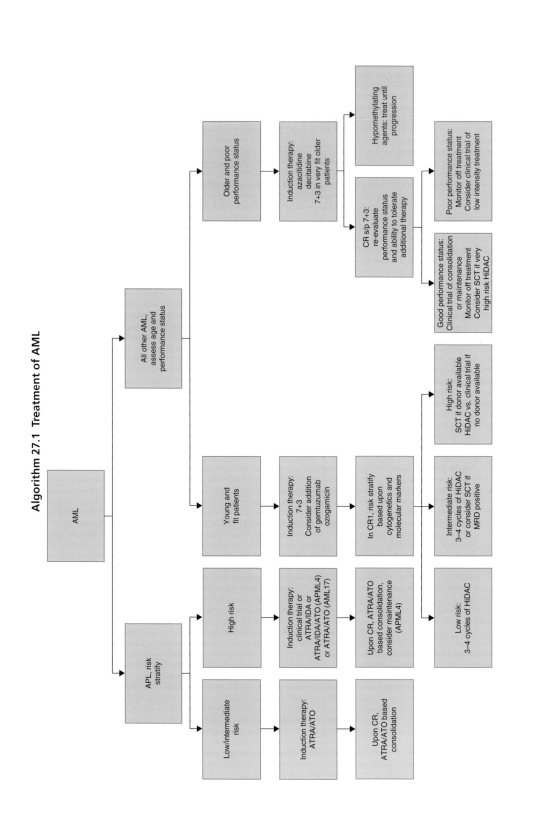

- High risk should be offered clinical trial, ATRA/ATO, ATRA/idarubicin (IDA)/ATO, or the current standard ATRA/IDA induction.

For younger or fit patients with non-APL AML:
- The standard induction regimen is 7 + 3 with 7 day continuous infusion cytarabine (Ara-C) 100–200 mg/m^2/day, and either IDA or daunorubicin (DNR) days 1–3.
  - IDA has superior OS in patients older than 50.
  - DNR 90 mg/m^2 is superior to 45 mg/m^2, but the efficacy of 60 mg/m^2 is less clear.
- The *FLT3* inhibitor midostaurin should be added to standard induction and consolidation for *FLT3* mutant patients as it has been shown to prolong OS and was FDA approved in April 2017.
- Consider the addition of gemtuzumab ozogamicin to 7 + 3. It does not affect complete remission rate, but there is an improvement in remission rate and OS. The improvement in OS was restricted to patients with good or intermediate risk.
- The goal of post-remission therapy is prevention of relapse.
  - For intermediate or good risk patients, high dose Ara-C should be given for 3–4 cycles.
  - For patients >55, evidence does not support the use of post-remission consolidation, but it should be considered in the very fit patient. Clinical trials of consolidation or maintenance therapy should be offered.
- High risk patients should be offered AlloSCT in first compete remission, if a donor is available. If no donor is found, high dose Ara-C or a clinical trial should be offered.

For older or unfit high risk patients with non-APL AML:
- Consider a noncurative intent regimen with azacitidine or decitabine. These regimens are preferably given continuously on a monthly basis, but can also be given for 6–8 cycles followed by a period of observation.

When to hospitalize
- All patients receiving induction chemotherapy require hospitalization.
- Patients who are stable, do not have rapidly rising blast count, and are being treated with hypomethylating agents can be safely managed in the outpatient setting.
- Patients receiving induction chemotherapy can be discharged upon resolution of neutropenia with close follow-up for assessment of transfusion needs and infectious symptoms.
- Patients receiving consolidation chemotherapy can be discharged upon completion of chemotherapy with prophylactic antimicrobials and undergo neutrophil nadir at home, as long as they have close follow-up with 2–3 times weekly blood counts in the outpatient setting.

Table of treatment

Treatment	Comments
Conservative	
Antimicrobial prophylaxis • Acyclovir to prevent herpes zoster reactivation is recommended throughout treatment • Levofloxacin is recommended during periods of severe neutropenia • Posaconazole to prevent invasive mold and fungal infections is recommended throughout treatment	In patients with a history of *Clostridium difficile* infection, alternative or no antibacterial prophylaxis may be preferable Posaconazole, in comparison to fluconazole, prevents more mold and fungal infections and improves OS

(Continued)

(*Continued*)

Treatment	Comments
Transfusion • Platelets should be transfused when the morning platelet count is $<10\,k \times 10^6$ • Patients with APL should receive aggressive transfusion to maintain the platelet count 30–$50\,k \times 10^6$ and fibrinogen 100–150 mg/dL	Prophylactic platelet transfusion reduces major bleeding in AML APL is frequently complicated by DIC, and most early deaths are related to DIC

Medical	
Acute promyelocytic leukemia • **Low risk:** ATRA 45 mg/m²/day in divided doses immediately upon suspicion of the diagnosis and ATO 0.15 mg/kg/day IV until CR followed by consolidation with ATRA and ATO • **High risk:** ATRA 45 mg/m²/day in divided doses immediately upon suspicion of the diagnosis until CR and IDA 12 mg/m² days 2, 4, 6, and 8 followed by consolidation • **High risk alternative APML4:** 45 mg/m²/day in divided doses until CR, IDA 12 mg/m² days 2, 4, 6, 8, and ATO 0.15 mg/kg/day IV starting day 9 until CR followed by consolidation • **High risk alternative AML17:** ATRA 45 mg/m²/day in divided doses until CR, ATO 0.3 mg/kg IV days 1–5 and day 8 until CR followed by consolidation ATRA and ATO Non-APL induction chemotherapy • 7 + 3: 7-day continuous infusion Ara-C 100–200 mg/m²/day and either IDA 12 mg/m²/day or DNR 60–90 mg/m²/day on days 1–3 • **Gemtuzumab ozogamicin:** given with 7 + 3 as 9 mg/m² on day 1 and 14 of induction. Alternative regimens include 3 mg/m² (cap 5 mg) given days 1, 4, and 7 • Azacitidine 75 mg/m² subcutaneously for 7 days of 28-day cycle • Decitabine 20 mg/m² for 10 days repeated every 4–6 weeks Consolidation • HiDAC: Ara-C 3000 mg/m² every 12 hours on days 1, 3, and 5, given for 3–4 cycles	**APL:** all patients require extremely close monitoring for differentiation syndrome and should have a low threshold for initiation of corticosteroids and possibly holding ATRA if symptoms are profound. The APML4 regimen includes prednisone as prophylaxis. All patients require close monitoring for DIC and very aggressive transfusional support. Invasive procedures, including central venous access, should be avoided in high risk patients. ATO requires close monitoring of QTc Higher doses of Ara-C in induction have been studied but not consistently found to be superior The hypomethylating agents azacitidine and decitabine are generally able to be safely administered in an outpatient setting with close follow-up HiDAC has been studied at lower doses of Ara-C and not found to be inferior, but more data are needed. Ara-C 1500 mg/m² is also reasonable. More than four cycles provides no additional benefit, and some studies suggest maximal benefit is achieved at three cycles

Psychologic	
Patients will undergo intensive therapy for months, and a multidisciplinary supportive team is beneficial	

Complementary	
Sperm banking should be offered. The urgency of treatment generally precludes fertility preservation measures in women, but it should be discussed if treatment is not emergent	

Prevention/management of complications

- Patients with AML are at high risk of overwhelming infections, and because of immunosuppression they may be less symptomatic initially, so frequent, diligent evaluation for infectious signs and symptoms is critical.
- Patients with APL have a very high incidence of DIC, and most early deaths are related to bleeding complications. Initiating ATRA immediately upon suspicion of the diagnosis is critical, as is aggressive transfusion support.
- After initiation of therapy for APL, there is a high risk of differentiation syndrome, a syndrome of fever, weight gain, peripheral edema, pulmonary edema, and heart failure. Close monitoring for this complication is needed, and at the first signs, dexamethasone 10 mg twice daily should be started, and in severe cases ATRA may be held.

CLINICAL PEARLS
- New AML with DIC should greatly raise the suspicion for APL. If APL is suspected, ATRA should be started immediately, before a final diagnosis is made.
- Responses to hypomethylating agents can be slow and take as many as 4–6 cycles, so if a patient is tolerating therapy, lack of response after 2–4 cycles is not an indication to change or discontinue treatment.
- Clinical trials of either induction or consolidation therapy remain the best option for many patients with AML.

Special populations
Pregnancy

- The highest risk for fetal loss or malformation is during the first trimester, particularly in the first 3–5 weeks of gestation. Patients who develop AML early in the first trimester should consider termination, but chemotherapy can be given with a 10–20% risk of fetal compromise.
- Patients with APL have a significantly higher risk of fetal malformation with ATRA during the first trimester, and ATRA should be held throughout. If termination is unacceptable, daunorubicin can stabilize the disease until the second trimester and ATRA begun then.
- Patients who develop AML in the second and third trimesters can receive standard therapy with close coordination with maternal–fetal medicine specialists.
- Patients who develop AML late in the third trimester can consider early delivery with post-delivery chemotherapy if feasible from an obstetric perspective.

Children

- AML in children is much rarer than ALL and has a poorer prognosis, although it has also improved in the last decade.
- Treatment is similar to adults with Ara-C/DNR induction and HiDAC consolidation for patients with low or intermediate risk, and stem cell transplantation for higher risk patients once in remission.

Elderly

- Elderly patients frequently have higher risk disease and comorbidities, and they are less able to tolerate intensive therapy, particularly HiDAC consolidation.
- Except in the very fit, superior outcomes can be achieved with a noncurative intent approach with hypomethylating agents; however, clinical trials continue to be an option for patients who are amenable.

Prognosis

> **BOTTOM LINE/CLINICAL PEARLS**
> - Patients with good risk have a CR rate of >80–90% and a relapse rate of 35%.
> - Patients with intermediate risk have approximately a 50–80% response rate with a relapse rate of 50–60%.
> - Patients with poor risk have a <50% risk of CR after first induction and >90% of relapse without stem cell transplantation.

Follow-up tests and monitoring

Patients should be monitored closely during treatment. After treatment, if patients remain in complete remission, periodic monitoring with CBCs and closer follow-up based upon any abnormalities is sufficient.

Reading list

Döhner H, Weisdorf DJ, Bloomfield CD. Acute myeloid leukemia. N Engl J Med 2015;373:1136–1152.

Grossmann V, Schnittger S, Kohlmann A, et al. A novel hierarchical prognostic model of AML solely based on molecular mutations. Blood 2012;120:2963–2972.

Milojkovic D, Apperley JF. How I treat leukemia during pregnancy. Blood 2014;123:974–984.

Patel JP, Gönen M, Figueroa ME, et al. Prognostic relevance of integrated genetic profiling in acute myeloid leukemia. N Engl J Med 2012;366:1079–1089.

Rubnitz JE. How I treat pediatric acute myeloid leukemia. Blood 2012;119:5980–5908.

Suggested websites

https://www.nccn.org/professionals/physician_gls/pdf/aml_blocks.pdf

Guidelines
National society guidelines

Title	Source	Date and weblink
AML treatment	National Comprehensive Cancer Network Guidelines	2019 http://www.nccn.org/professionals/physician_gls/pdf/aml.pdf
Antimicrobial Guidelines	Infectious Disease Society of America Guidelines for Use of Antimicrobial Agents in Neutropenia	2010 http://www.idsociety.org/uploadedFiles/IDSA/Guidelines-Patient_Care/PDF_Library/FN.pdf
BCSH Guidelines	British Society for Standards in Haematology Guidelines	2006 http://www.bcshguidelines.com/documents/aml_bjh_2006.pdf
ELN Guidelines	European Leukemia Network Guidelines	2010 https://www.ncbi.nlm.nih.gov/pubmed/27895058

Evidence

Type of evidence	Title and comment	Date and weblink
RCT	Anthracycline dose intensification in acute myeloid leukemia **Comment:** 7 + 3 with DNR 90 has improved OS compared with DNR 45	2009 https://www.ncbi.nlm.nih.gov/pubmed/19776406

(*Continued*)

Type of evidence	Title and comment	Date and weblink
RCT	Azacitidine prolongs OS compared with conventional care regimens in elderly patients with low bone marrow blast count acute myeloid leukemia **Comment:** Azacitidine compared with best supportive care, low dose cytarabine, or intensive therapy improved OS	2010 https://www.ncbi.nlm.nih.gov/pubmed/20026804
RCT	Superior long-term outcome with idarubicin compared with high-dose daunorubicin in patients with acute myeloid leukemia age 50 years and older **Comment:** IDA compared with DNR has superior outcomes in those older than 50	2013 https://www.ncbi.nlm.nih.gov/pubmed/23248249
RCT	Retinoic acid and arsenic trioxide for acute promyelocytic leukemia **Comment:** In low or intermediate risk APL, ATRA/ATO has superior OS to ATRA/chemotherapy	2013 https://www.ncbi.nlm.nih.gov/pubmed/23841729
Cooperative group	All-trans-retinoic acid, idarubicin, and IV arsenic trioxide as initial therapy in acute promyelocytic leukemia (APML4) **Comment:** APML4; ATRA/IDA/ATO based induction is safe, effective, and has lower relapse rate than ATRA/IDA	2012 https://www.ncbi.nlm.nih.gov/pubmed/22715121
RCT	Arsenic trioxide and all-trans retinoic acid treatment for acute promyelocytic leukaemia in all risk groups (AML17): results of a randomised, controlled, phase 3 trial **Comment:** AML17; ATRA/ATO induction is safe and effective in high risk APL	2015 https://www.ncbi.nlm.nih.gov/pubmed/26384238

Images

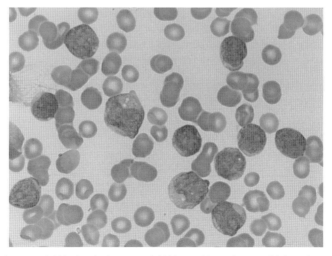

Figure 27.1 Acute myeloid leukemia. Large myeloid blasts with moderate to high nuclear to cytoplasmic ratio, fine chromatin, and prominent nucleoli. See color version on website.

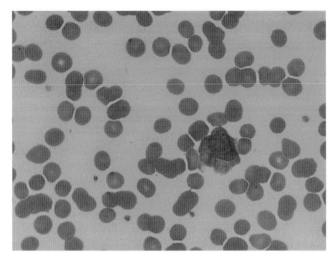

Figure 27.2 Acute promyelocytic leukemia. Promyelocytes with moderate nuclear to cytoplasmic ratio, slightly condensed nucleoli, prominent cytoplasmic granules, and prominent Auer rods. See color version on website.

Additional material for this chapter can be found online at:
www.wiley.com/go/oh/mountsinaioncology

This includes advice for patients, a case study, ICD codes, and multiple choice questions. The following images are available in color: Figures 27.1 and 27.2

CHAPTER 28

Acute Lymphoblastic Leukemia

Jaclyn C. Davis[1] and Birte Wistinghausen[2]
[1] Novartis Pharmaceuticals Corporation East Hanover, NJ, USA
[2] Children's National Health System, The George Washington University, Washington, DC, USA

OVERALL BOTTOM LINE

- Acute lymphoblastic leukemia (ALL) is the most common malignancy in the pediatric population but rare in adults with B-cell ALL accounting for ~80% of cases and T-cell ALL for ~20%.
- Presentations with vague systemic symptoms (including commonly fever, fatigue, bone pain), cytopenias and associated findings (pallor, petechiae, bruising) and, more often in T-ALL, lymphadenopathy, mediastinal masses, and hepatosplenomegaly.
- Tumor lysis syndrome, a medical emergency with hyperkalemia, hyperuricemia, and hyperphosphatemia, can occur spontaneously or with initiation of therapy.
- Steroids can achieve a temporary remission and should be avoided prior to diagnosis and risk stratification by immunophenotyping and cytogenetic/molecular analysis of blasts.
- Combination chemotherapy is standard of care and rapid early response to therapy and molecular markers correlate with prognosis.
- Age correlates with outcome with cure rates ranging from ~80–90% in children to 67.5% in adults.

Background
Definition of disease
Monoclonal malignant proliferation of lymphoid progenitor cells that disseminates throughout bone marrow and blood with potential organ infiltration.

Disease classification
- ALL was previously classified by morphology as L1 or L2 (FAB Classification).
- Current classifications include immunophenotype, molecular markers, WBC at diagnosis, testicular and/or CNS dissemination.

Incidence/prevalence
- ALL accounts for 0.4% of new adult cancer diagnoses with an incidence of 1.7 per 100000 per year but for 25% of pediatric cancers with >3000 newly diagnosed children each year.
- Incidence is highest in the 3–5 year age group.

Mount Sinai Expert Guides: Oncology, First Edition. Edited by William K. Oh and Ajai Chari.
© 2019 John Wiley & Sons Ltd. Published 2019 by John Wiley & Sons Ltd.
Companion Website: www.wiley.com/go/oh/mountsinaioncology

Etiology

- ALL arises from somatic genetic mutations in lymphoid progenitor cells including chromosomal translocations and intrachromosomal rearrangements with ~10–20 additional acquired mutations.
- Most cases are sporadic.

Pathology/pathogenesis

- Lymphoblasts are small to medium sized with scant cytoplasm and large nuclei with smooth chromatin, nucleoli, and expression of lymphoid progenitor markers:
  - B-cell ALL (B-ALL): CD19, cyCD79a, CD22, CD10, TdT, PAX5, +/− CD20, CD34
  - T-cell ALL (T-ALL): TdT, cyCD3, CD7, +/− CD1a, CD2, CD4, CD8.

Predictive/risk factors

- Concordance in identical twin: 20%.
- Prenatal X-ray exposure.
- Prior chemotherapy.
- Radiation exposure.
- Viral infections:
  - HTLV-1 (T- ALL in adults)
  - Epstein–Barr virus (EBV) (B-ALL).
- Certain genetic conditions.

Prevention and screening

- Screening is not recommended.
- There are no known preventive strategies.

Diagnosis (Algorithm 28.1)

Diagnosis is confirmed by morphologic, cytogenetic, and immunophenotypic analysis of blasts from bone marrow and/or peripheral blood.

Differential diagnosis

Differential diagnosis	Features
AML	Similar clinical presentation Morphologic evaluation of blasts show larger size, cytoplasmic granules, and/or Auer rods (M1–M7 morphology) Immunophenotyping is needed, with myeloblasts positive for myeloid markers such as CD13, CD33, and MPO
Reactive lymphocytosis – seen with EBV, cytomegalovirus (CMV), *Bordetella* pertussis, and parvovirus	EBV and CMV commonly cause fever, hepatosplenomegaly, lymphadenopathy (LAD), cytopenias *Bordetella* pertussis causes upper respiratory symptoms Parvovirus can cause anemia Bone marrow retains trilineage hematopoiesis without blasts Viral titers or cultures are necessary
Aplastic anemia	Pancytopenia No organomegaly or lymphadenopathy Hypocellular bone marrow without blasts
Idiopathic thrombocytopenic purpura (ITP), autoimmune hemolytic anemia (AIHA), or Evans syndrome	Positive direct antiglobulin test in AIHA Isolated thrombocytopenia in ITP Lack of systemic symptoms Trilineage hematopoiesis without blasts occasionally with hyperplasia of erythroid precursors (AIHA) or megakaryocytes (ITP)

(Continued)

Differential diagnosis	Features
Osteomyelitis	Focal bone pain Fever Absence of pancytopenia
Metastatic cancer, most commonly in childhood stage IV neuroblastoma	Widespread metastatic disease to the bone marrow in children can present with pancytopenia Localizing symptoms pointing to a primary site Imaging studies can aid in diagnosis Pathology may be needed to distinguish neuroblastoma Urine catecholamines
Stage IV lymphoma	Primary mass is usually present Bone marrow aspirate/biopsy <25% blasts
MDS	Similar clinical presentation with pancytopenia Hypercellular or dysplastic bone marrow, blasts <20%
Juvenile idiopathic arthritis	Pediatric patient with fever, rash, lymphadenopathy, and joint pain Leukocytosis, anemia, and thrombocytosis are common Bone pain, lymphocytosis, thrombocytopenia, and neutropenia are uncommon

Algorithm 28.1 Diagnosis of ALL

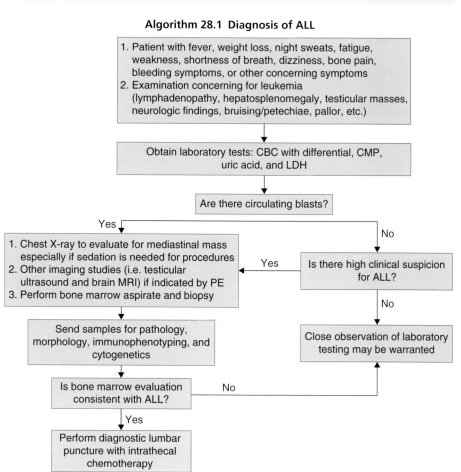

Typical presentation
- Vague symptoms including fever, fatigue, malaise, decreased appetite, weight loss, and bone pain.
- Pallor, increased bruising, or petechiae.
- Shortness of breath with mediastinal masses (Figure 28.1).

Clinical diagnosis
History
- Systemic symptoms:
  - Fever
  - Night sweats
  - Unintentional weight loss.
- Neurologic complaints with CNS involvement:
  - Headache
  - Vomiting
  - Changes in vision
  - Vertigo, ataxia
  - Cranial nerve palsies
  - Lethargy
  - Seizures.
- Easy bruising, epistaxis due to thrombocytopenia.
- Dizziness, fatigue, and weakness caused by anemia.
- Shortness of breath, wheezing, and chest pain caused by mediastinal mass.
- Bone pain leading to refusal to walk in young children.

Physical examination
- A comprehensive physical examination is required with attention to:
  - Lymphadenopathy, hepatosplenomegaly, and testicular enlargement
  - Thorough neurologic examination
  - Signs of superior vena cava (SVC) syndrome or respiratory compromise from mediastinal mass
  - Tachycardia, flow murmur, pallor, bruising, and petechiae from cytopenias.

Disease severity classification
Constantly evolving risk classifications determine risk of relapse and guide intensity of therapy:
- Immunophenotype
  - Favorable:
    - childhood: B-ALL
    - adults: T-ALL.
- Presenting WBC
  - Favorable:
    - childhood B-ALL: WBC <50 000/μL
    - adult B-ALL: WBC <30 000/μL
    - adult T-ALL: WBC <100 000/μL.
- Age
  - NCI criteria for childhood ALL:
    - standard risk:
      - age >1 year and <10 years *and* WBC <50 000/μL.

- high risk:
  - age ≥10 years
  - WBC >50 000/μL.
  - Age <1 year: infant ALL is associated with a poor prognosis.
- Disseminated disease
  - Unfavorable:
    - CNS involvement
    - testicular infiltration.
- Recurrent cytogenetic and/or genomic markers (B-ALL only)
  - Favorable:
    - *ETV-RUNX6* fusion (t(12;21)(p12;q22))
    - hyperdiploidy
    - trisomies of chromosomes 10 and 17.
  - Unfavorable:
    - t(9;22)(q34;q11)/*BCR-ABL1*
    - *MLL* rearrangements (chromosome 11q23)
    - *IKZFI* deletions/mutations
    - Ph-like ALL
    - hypodiploidy
    - t(17;19)(q22;p13)/TCF3(E2A)-HLF.
- Rapid early response is the most important predictor of outcome
  - Clearance of peripheral blood blasts within one week of therapy
  - Negative minimal residual disease by flow cytometry or polymerase chain reaction at the end of induction and/or consolidation.

Laboratory diagnosis

List of diagnostic tests

- CBC with differential (Figure 28.2).
- CMP, LDH, uric acid.
- PT/PTT, fibrinogen, D-dimer.
- Bone marrow aspirate (Figure 28.3) and biopsy:
  - Immunophenotyping
  - Cytogenetic and FISH analysis
  - If available genomic profiling for Ph-like ALL.
- Cerebrospinal fluid cytology.

Lists of imaging techniques

- Chest X-ray.
- Testicular ultrasound as needed.
- MRI of the brain as needed.

Potential pitfalls/common errors made regarding diagnosis of disease

- The diagnosis can be delayed in patients without circulating lymphoblasts because symptoms are nonspecific.
- If ALL is suspected, corticosteroids are *contraindicated*, because they can induce a temporary remission and delay diagnosis.

Treatment (Algorithms 28.2 and 28.3)
Treatment rationale
- The primary goal of induction chemotherapy is to achieve remission. The rationale of continuation chemotherapy is to deepen and maintain remission leading to cure.
- Adolescent and young adult (AYA) patients (aged 15–40 years) have improved survival when treated with "pediatric" protocols.
- Most pediatric patients are cured with combination chemotherapy.
- Age, performance status, and organ function at diagnosis influence therapy in adults.
- Bone marrow transplantation (BMT) in first remission is reserved for very high risk groups in children and for some adults.
- Patients with early relapse have a poor prognosis and are candidates for experimental strategies such as chimeric antigen receptor T cells as well as BMT in second remission.

Algorithm 28.2 Management of ALL

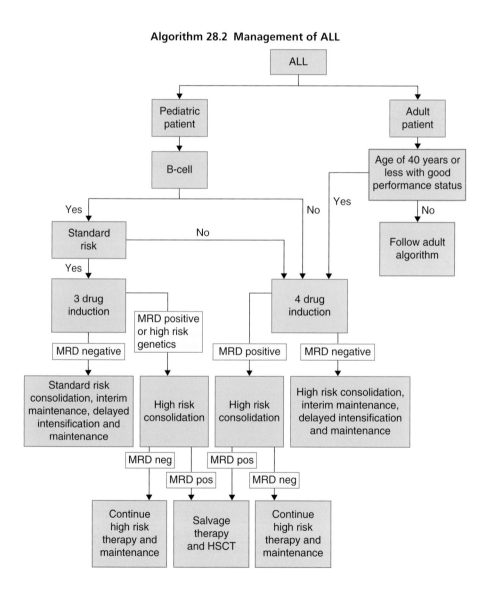

Algorithm 28.3 Management of T-cell ALL

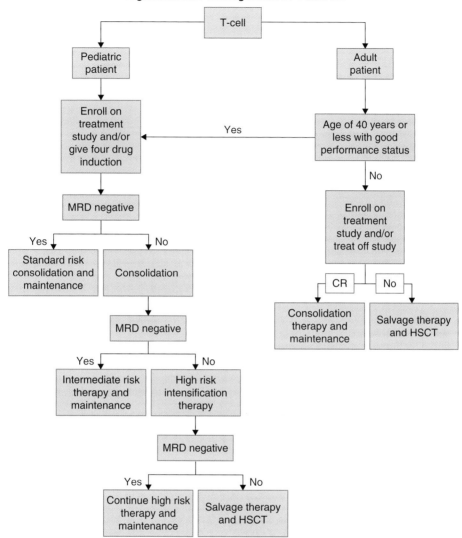

- Please note risk stratifications, definitions of remission, and minimal residual disease are constantly evolving with newer molecular methods. As such treatment algorithms require continuous updating.

When to hospitalize
- Patients undergoing evaluation for leukemia and starting induction chemotherapy because of risk for tumor lysis syndrome (TLS), infections, and other complications from pancytopenia or hyperleukocytosis.
- Most febrile neutropenic patients because of the high risk of bacterial and/or fungal sepsis.
- Some chemotherapy regimens.

Managing the hospitalized patient
This requires the oversight of experienced oncologists.

Table of treatment

Treatment	Comments
Childhood ALL	
Induction (28 days): • Goal: remission induction • Medications: vincristine, prednisone/dexamethasone, peg-asparaginase, +/− daunorubicin (for all T-ALL and high risk B-ALL) Risk stratification after completion of induction chemotherapy guides further therapy consolidation (Cons), interim maintenance (IM), and delayed intensification (DI) (5–8 months): • Goal: deepening of remission • Cons: vincristine, mercaptopurine +/− cytarabine, +/− cyclophosphamide, +/− peg-asparaginase • IM: methotrexate (high dose in high risk B-ALL), vincristine, +/− mercaptopurine, +/− peg-asparaginase • DI: vincristine, dexamethasone, doxorubicin, cytarabine, cyclophosphamide, peg-asparaginase, thioguanine Maintenance chemotherapy: • Goal: maintenance of remission • Medications: dexamethasone/prednisone, vincristine, mercaptopurine and methotrexate • Length varies by sex in the USA (2 years from the start of IM1 for females, 3 years from the start of IM1 for males) Select very high risk groups (hypodiploid or induction failures) are offered BMT following consolidation therapy Intrathecal methotrexate and/or cytarabine and/or hydrocortisone is given throughout therapy Depending on protocol, patients with CNS involvement at diagnosis and some other high risk groups receive cranial radiation (12–18 Gy). If testicular disease persists through induction, testicular radiation is given during consolidation Ph+ ALL and some Ph-like patients may benefit from a TKIs and are treated with different chemotherapy protocols	Fatigue, nausea, vomiting, hair loss, increased risk of infection due to leukopenia, anemia, and/or increased risk of bleeding due to thrombocytopenia are common and require close monitoring Side effects by drug: • Vincristine: peripheral neuropathy, constipation, jaw pain • Prednisone/dexamethasone: weight gain, hyperglycemia, cushingoid appearance, bone pain, muscle weakness, hypertension • Peg- or L-asparaginase: anaphylaxis, pancreatitis, hyper- and/or hypocoaguability/monitor DIC labs • Daunorubicin: discolored secretions, cardiomyopathy, mucositis • Methotrexate: hepatic dysfunction, acute renal failure, mucositis • Mercaptopurine: bone marrow suppression • Cyclophosphamide: hematuria or hemorrhagic cystitis • Cytarabine: at high doses causes fevers, conjunctivitis, mucositis • Intrathecal chemotherapy: leukoencephalopathy, seizures • In the 1970s the BFM group introduced delayed intensification or re-induction which increased cure rates in childhood ALL from 50% to >70%. Cure rates now exceed 80%
Adult ALL	

Various regimens are used including CALGB 8811 and hyper-CVAD/methotrexate-cytarabine CALGB 8811:
 • Induction:
   • If <60 years: cyclophosphamide, daunorubicin, vincristine, prednisone, and L-asparaginase
   • If 60 years or older: cyclophosphamide, daunorubicin, and prednisone
 • Followed by four courses of intensive chemotherapy
 • Maintenance chemotherapy lasts for up to 2 years from diagnosis
 • Cranial radiation is given during IM to all patients
 Hyper-CVAD/methotrexate-cytarabine: eight cycles of alternating courses is given followed by up to 2 years of maintenance chemotherapy	

(Continued)

Treatment	Comments
• Course A: cyclophosphamide, vincristine, doxorubicin, and dexamethasone • Course B: methotrexate and cytarabine • Maintenance: prednisone, vincristine, mercaptopurine, and methotrexate	
Relapse therapy	
Cure after relapse requires allo-BMT in most patients Late relapse and/or isolated CNS relapse can be cured with chemotherapy alone Allo-BMT is reserved for patients achieving a second CR Salvage therapy often includes experimental therapies given on research protocols Agents in development/clinical research include: • Nelarabine in T-ALL • Bortezomib • Bi-specific T-cell engagers (BiTEs) • Chimeric antigen receptor T-cells (CARTs) • TKIs for patients with targetable expression of tyrosine kinases • mTOR inhibitors	

Prevention/management of complications

- Risk of TLS at diagnosis and initiation of therapy:
  - Aggressive IV hydration
  - Allopurinol and/or rasburicase
  - Monitoring of electrolytes, uric acid, and renal function every 6–8 hours.
- Hyperleukocytosis:
  - Leukapheresis to temporarily lower the WBC before initiation of chemotherapy.
- Neutropenic fever
  - Broad spectrum antibiotics.
- Mediastinal mass, airway compromise, SVC syndrome:
  - Methylprednisolone (20 mg/m^2/day)
  - Mediastinal irradiation.
- Intracranial hemorrhage and/or ischemic brain injury:
  - Leukapheresis for hyperleukocytosis
  - Multidisciplinary management
  - Replacement of coagulation factors and platelets.
- Symptomatic anemia and thrombocytopenia:
  - Filtered and irradiated blood products
  - For potential BMT candidates, avoidance of related blood donors.

> **CLINICAL PEARLS**
> - Treatment of ALL includes several phases of combination chemotherapy with the goal of achieving, deepening, and maintaining remission.
> - The majority of children with ALL are cured. Age is an adverse prognostic factor.
> - AYA patients have superior outcomes on pediatric regimens.
> - Rapid early response is the best predictor of outcome.

- Novel therapies undergoing investigation include mTOR inhibitors, bidirectional T-cell engagers, cellular therapies, and TKIs in subgroups of ALL with targetable lesions.
- Retrieval of patients with relapsed ALL is ~50%.

Special populations
Pregnancy
- Limited data exist.
- The risk of fetal anomalies in early pregnancy is significant with chemotherapy. If feasible, conservative management with prednisone alone may be warranted before the third trimester.

Elderly
- Elderly patients are at higher risk of complications.

Others
- **Infants:** children <1 year at diagnosis have poor prognosis and are treated with more intensive regimens. BMT does not improve the outcome.
- **Down syndrome:** patients with Down syndrome have a higher incidence of ALL, a poorer prognosis, and higher risk of infectious complications, requiring very close monitoring during periods of intensive chemotherapy and/or neutropenia.
- HTLV1 ATLL.

Prognosis

BOTTOM LINE/CLINICAL PEARLS
- Untreated ALL is universally fatal.
- Cure rates are excellent in childhood.

Prognosis for treated patients
- 5-year survival rates for pediatric patients are 80–90%.
- Cure rates in AYA patients are approaching 70%.
- 5-year survival rates in adult patients are poor with only 30–40% of those <60 years and only 5–15% >60 years surviving.
- Increasing options for relapsed ALL: BITE, CART.

Follow-up tests and monitoring
- CBCs to monitor for relapse and/or treatment-related myelodysplastic syndrome/secondary AML.
- Testicular examinations in males to screen for relapse.
- Monitoring for treatment-related liver and/or renal dysfunction.
- Echocardiograms to assess for anthracycline-induced cardiomyopathy.

Reading list
Curran E, Stock W. How I treat acute lymphoblastic leukemia in older adolescents and young adults. Blood 2015;125:3702–3710.
Gökguget N. How I treat older patients with ALL. Blood 2013;122:1366–1375.

Guzaukas GF, Villa KF, Vanhove TF, et al. Risk–benefit trade-off of pediatric-inspired versus hyper-CVAD protocols for Philadelphia negative acute lymphocytic leukemia (ALL) in adolescents and young adults: a modeling
analysis. Blood 2014;124:1281.

Hunger SP, Mullighan CG. Acute lymphoblastic leukemia in children. N Engl J Med 2015;373:154–152.

Litzow, MR, Ferrando, AA. How I treat T-cell acute lymphoblastic leukemia in adults. Blood 2015;126:
833–841.

Milojkovic D, Apperley JF. How I treat leukemia during pregnancy. Blood 2014;123:974–984.

Nakano TA, Hunger SP. Blood consult: Therapeutic strategy and complications in the adolescent and young
adult with acute lymphoblastic leukemia. Blood 2012;119:4372–4374.

Guidelines

No guidelines exist for treatment of adults or pediatric patients with ALL as the field is constantly
envolving. For this reason, it is important for patients, especially those with unfavorable disease,
to be enrolled in clinical trials.

Evidence

Type of evidence	Title and comment	Date and weblink
Phase III study	Dexamethasone and high-dose methotrexate improve outcome for children and young adults with high risk B-acute lymphoblastic leukemia: a report from Children's Oncology Group Study AALL0232 **Comment:** Pediatric and young adult patients with high risk B-ALL had improved survival when they received high-dose methotrexate as compared with Capizzi methotrexate during the IM-1 phase of therapy. Dexamethasone given during induction benefited younger children but provided no benefit and was associated with a higher risk of osteonecrosis among participants 10 years and older	2016 https://www.ncbi.nlm.nih.gov/pubmed/27114587
Phase III study	Improved survival for children and young adults with T-lineage acute lymphoblastic leukemia: results from the Children's Oncology Group AALL0434 Methotrexate Randomization **Comment:** Pediatric and young adult patients with T-ALL have improved survival when receiving Capizzi methotrexate and nelarabine	2018 https://www.ncbi.nlm.nih.gov/pubmed/30138085
Phase III study	Improved early event free survival (EFS) with tolerable toxicity in children with Philadelphia chromosome positive (Ph+) acute lymphoblastic leukemia (ALL) with intensive imatinib mesylate with dose-intensive multiagent chemotherapy: Children's Oncology Group (COG) Study AALL0031 **Comment:** The addition of imatinib to chemotherapy doubled the survival rates for pediatric patients with Ph+ ALL. Survival rates were similar for those treated with imatinib and chemotherapy vs. BMT	2014 http://www.ncbi.nlm.nih.gov/pmc/articles/PMC4282929/
Phase II study	A pediatric regimen for older adolescents and young adults with acute lymphoblastic leukemia: results of CALGB 10403 **Comment:** Using a pediatric treatment regimen in adults <40 is feasible and leads to improved outcome	2019 https://www.ncbi.nlm.nih.gov/pubmed/30658992

Images

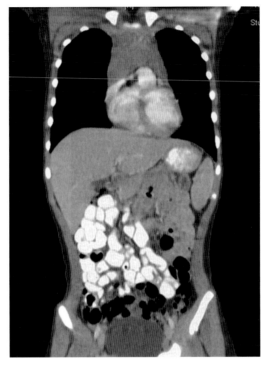

Figure 28.1 Mediastinal mass in T-ALL.

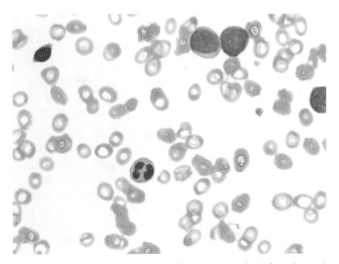

Figure 28.2 Peripheral blood smear from a patient with B-ALL. See website for color version.

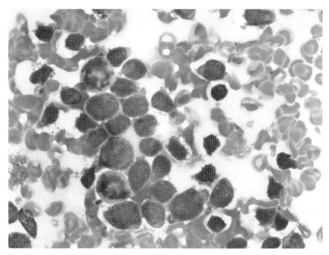

Figure 28.3 Bone marrow aspirate from a patient with B-ALL. See website for color version.

Additional material for this chapter can be found online at:
www.wiley.com/go/oh/mountsinaioncology

This includes advice for patients, a case study, ICD codes, and multiple choice questions. The following images are available in color: Figures 28.2 and 28.3.

CHAPTER 29

Chronic Lymphocytic Leukemia

Adam F. Binder and Janice L. Gabrilove
Icahn School of Medicine at Mount Sinai, New York, NY, USA

OVERALL BOTTOM LINE

- Chronic lymphocytic leukemia (CLL) is a lymphoproliferative disorder defined by the presence of an absolute clonal B-cell lymphocytosis greater than 5000/μL for a duration of at least 3 months.
- CLL is primarily a disease of the elderly. The median age of diagnosis is approximately 70 years.
- The clinical course varies from an indolent course and active surveillance (median life expectancy greater than 10 years) to an aggressive course requiring treatment (median life expectancy of less than 3 years).
- The clinical course of the disease is largely dependent on immunohistologic variation, IGVH chain mutation status, genetic variation, and B-cell receptor (BCR) stereotyping.
- Novel therapies such as BCR inhibitors and BCL-2 antagonists are prolonging the life expectancy of the high risk/poor prognostic group.
- Treatment options for CLL are rapidly changing, particularly for those patients with high risk disease.

Background
Definition of disease

- CLL is a lymphoproliferative disorder defined by the presence of an absolute clonal B-cell lymphocytosis greater than 5000/μL for a duration of at least 3 months.
- CLL can be preceded by monoclonal B-lymphocytosis (MBL), defined as fewer than 5000 clonal B cells/μL, with progression to frank CLL at a rate of 1–2% per year.
- CLL can also be defined by cytopenias with bone marrow biopsy revealing a typical marrow infiltrate even in the absence of an absolute lymphocytosis.
- Small lymphocytic lymphoma (SLL) has an identical histopathologic appearance, but requires the presence of lymphadenopathy and/or splenomegaly and a circulating absolute lymphocytosis of less than 5000/μL.

Disease classification

The WHO classifies CLL as a mature B-cell neoplasm, only distinguishable from SLL by its leukemic appearance.

Incidence/prevalence

The estimated incidence of CLL in 2015 was 14 620 (0.9% of all new cancer diagnoses). The estimated number of deaths in 2015 was 4650.

Mount Sinai Expert Guides: Oncology, First Edition. Edited by William K. Oh and Ajai Chari.
© 2019 John Wiley & Sons Ltd. Published 2019 by John Wiley & Sons Ltd.
Companion Website: www.wiley.com/go/oh/mountsinaioncology

Economic impact
- The estimated cost of treating CLL is expected to rise as novel agents come to market.
- Current estimates suggest that the 10-year cost for 100 CLL patients will rise from $4 565 929 to $6 309 162–19 037 495.

Etiology
- The inciting event leading to mutational change is unknown, but CLL is the result of multiple changes within a specific B-cell phenotype and its environment.
- There is evidence that a subset of CLL is "stereotyped," or containing a nearly identical BCR immunoglobulin (BCR immunoglobulin, along with associated proteins, is necessary for specific antigen recognition).
  - There are over 200 distinct stereotypes, but eight subsets account for about 30% of all stereotyped CLL cases.
  - Subset identification may be prognostic of disease course (i.e. more aggressive or more indolent).
- These stereotyped subsets suggest that among patients, there may be common antigens that stimulate mutational change and development of a clonal lymphoproliferative process.
- Specific chromosomal alterations (11q, 17p, 13q, and trisomy 12) and the recent discovery of a number of specific mutations (*NOTCH*, *SF3B1*, and *BIRC3*) have also emerged as initial genetic alterations potentially contributing to disease pathogenesis and clearly to prognosis.

Pathology/pathogenesis
- The development of a mature B-cell clone is thought to be a complex association of cell autonomous antigenic independent stimulation, gene mutations, cytogenetic abnormalities, epigenetic modifications, and bone marrow microenvironment changes.
- Most CLL is preceded by an MBL, which has all the histopathologic changes of CLL, but the peripheral absolute B-cell lymphocyte count is less than 5000/μL.
- MBL progresses to CLL by proliferation of the B-cell clonal population at a rate of about 1–2% per year.

Predictive/risk factors

Risk factor	Odds ratio
Agent Orange exposure and other herbicides used in farming Family history (first degree relatives) Ethnicity (North American and European descent)	Twice the risk
Prior history of airway infection	
• Laryngitis	1.7
• Sinusitis	2.0
• Otitis/mastoiditis	1.5
• Influenza	1.3

Prevention
Secondary prevention
- CLL is generally incurable, unless the patient undergoes HSCT. When indicated, therapy is administered to control the disease and prevent symptomatic recurrence.

Diagnosis (Algorithm 29.1)

Algorithm 29.1 Diagnosis of chronic lymphocytic leukemia

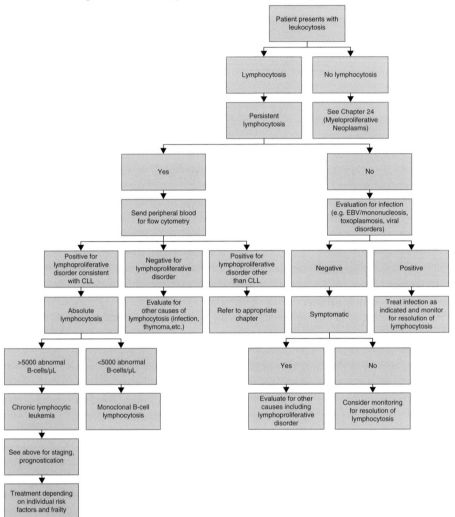

CLINICAL PEARLS
- The majority of patients are initially diagnosed incidentally when leukocytosis and absolute lymphocytosis are seen on routine CBC and differential.
- Some patients present with fatigue, splenomegaly, autoimmune hemolytic anemia or immune-mediated thrombocytopenia, or classic "B" symptoms of fevers, night sweats, and weight loss (>10% of body weight).
- Physical examination should focus on lymph node examination including Waldeyer's ring as well as abdominal examination to evaluate for hepatosplenomegaly.
- Initial laboratory investigations should include CBC with differential, CMP, and flow cytometry of peripheral blood.

- CT scanning of the chest/abdomen/pelvis with contrast is helpful to evaluate the extent of lymphadenopathy, but not necessary in asymptomatic low risk disease. In patients with classical "B symptoms," PET/CT may be of utility in an effort to evaluate for evidence of Richter transformation of CLL.

Differential diagnosis

Differential diagnosis	Features
Infectious causes of lymphocytosis (e.g. EBV/mononucleosis, toxoplasmosis, viral disorders, pertussis, *Bartonella henselae*)	Patient will present with symptoms concerning for infection, lymphocytosis will be transient. (EBV infects B cells, but reactive lymphocytosis is T cell in origin)
Other malignant causes of lymphocytosis (prolymphocytic leukemia, mantle cell lymphoma, hairy cell leukemia, splenic marginal zone lymphoma, lymphoplasmacytic lymphoma, large granular lymphocyte disorder, lymphoblastic lymphoma	Clonal population of cells will express different immune-histopathologic features from CLL. In the case of hairy cell leukemia, patients commonly present with pancytopenia including leukopenia
Drug hypersensitivity reactions	Can present with eosinophilia or lymphocytosis
Post-splenectomy patients	Lymphocytosis will develop after splenectomy
Thymoma	Can have circulating T-cell lymphocytosis

Typical presentation
- Most patients are asymptomatic at presentation. Some patients present with adenopathy – often cervical adenopathy. Other patients present with splenomegaly, cytopenias (related to bone marrow infiltration, autoimmune phenomena, or immune-mediated such as pure red cell aplasia), and symptoms related to cytopenias (fatigue, dyspnea, and easy bruising).
- 5–10% of patients present with fevers, drenching night sweats, and weight loss (>10% of body weight).
- Patients can also have a history of frequent infections (encapsulated organisms) related to hypogammaglobulinemia.

Clinical diagnosis
History
It is important to ask about:
- Fevers
- Night sweats
- Weight loss
- Fatigue
- Early satiety, abdominal pain, or fullness related to splenomegaly
- Respiratory symptoms
- Easy bruising or bleeding
- Any "lumps or bumps" they have noticed that could be palpable lymph nodes
- Recent infections
- History of HIV, hepatitis B or C
- Rashes or cutaneous nodules.

Physical examination
- A thorough lymph node examination including Waldeyer's ring is important. Over 50% of patients present with lymphadenopathy.
- Physicians should perform a comprehensive abdominal examination.
- Examination for cutaneous findings.

Useful clinical decision rules and calculators
- The Binet and Rai classification systems have traditionally been used to risk stratify patients (see section on Disease severity classification for Rai classification).
- The NCCN guidelines use Ann Arbor staging as well as Rai staging to determine who should be treated.
- In general, patients are eligible for treatment if:
  - There is a clinical trial
  - Significant symptoms related to CLL: fevers, night sweats, weight loss, fatigue, symptomatic splenomegaly or adenopathy
  - Autoimmune hemolytic anemia or thrombocytopenia
  - Progressive cytopenias
  - Progressive, bulky lymphadenopathy
  - Threatened end organ damage.
- A new International Prognostic Index Score (CLL IPI) was presented at the ASCO conference in 2015, but has not been widely disseminated into practice.

Disease severity classification
See Tables 29.1 and 29.2.

Table 29.1 Rai Stage Classification.

Clinical presentation	Modified stage	Historic stage
Lymphocytosis >5000 abnormal B-cells/µL in blood or lymphoid cells >30% in bone marrow	Low risk	0
Lymphocytosis, lymphadenopathy, enlarged liver or spleen	Intermediate	1
		2
Disease-related anemia; Hgb <11 g/dL	High risk	3
Disease-related thrombocytopenia; Platelets <100 000		4

Table 29.2 Proposed CLL International Prognostic Index (5 independent risk factors: age; clinical stage; del(17p) and/or TP53 mutation; IGHV mutation status; and B2-microglobulin level).

Stage	Risk
0–1	Low risk
2–3	Intermediate risk
4–6	High risk
7–10	Very high risk

Laboratory diagnosis

List of diagnostic tests

- CBC with differential.
- Evaluation of the peripheral blood smear (evaluate for presence of mature lymphocytosis).
- Peripheral blood for flow cytometry (must ask to evaluate for lymphoproliferative disorder). If peripheral blood is nondiagnostic, may require bone marrow biopsy or, if lymphadenopathy is present, excisional biopsy of a lymph node.
- LDH.
- For prognostic/therapeutic implications:
  - B2-microglobulin
  - FISH for trisomy 12, del(11q), del(13q), del(17p)
  - Molecular analysis to detect IGHV mutation status
  - *TP53* sequencing for point mutation
  - Zap-70, CD38 evaluation by immunohistochemistry
  - Next generation sequencing for *BICc-3, SF3B1, ATM, NOTCH1* mutation.

Lists of imaging techniques

- The American Society of Hematology "Choosing Wisely" campaign recommends against baseline or surveillance CT scans for asymptomatic, early stage CLL.
- CT scan of the chest/abdomen/pelvis with contrast for late stage or symptomatic patients.
- PET scans are not recommended unless there is concern for transformation to an aggressive lymphoma.

Potential pitfalls/common errors made regarding diagnosis of disease

It is important to remember that CLL can be an aggressive disease and every patient must be appropriately staged and risk stratified.

Treatment (Algorithm 29.2)

- Treatment recommendations can vary, will be patient dependent, and are rapidly evolving, given the emergence of new agents being used in the newly diagnosed setting.
- It is important to remember that patients with del(17p) respond poorly to cytotoxic chemotherapy.

Treatment rationale

- Initiation of treatment and choice of therapy for CLL depends on various factors: age, comorbidities, symptoms, risk stratification, del(17p) status, TP53 mutational status, additional detected mutations by next generation sequencing, and associated disease processes (i.e. autoimmune hemolytic anemia).
- The goal of treatment is to control the disease.
- For high risk patients (refractory to purine analogs [e.g. fludarabine], relapse within 24 months of initial treatment), novel therapeutics such as BCR inhibitors or BCL-2 antagonists should be considered.
- Patients with high risk disease and del(17p) or TP53 point mutations should be treated with BCR inhibitors (BTK or PI3K inhibitors) as first line therapy.
- HSCT remains the only potentially curative therapy and is an option for high risk otherwise healthy patients with an appropriate stem cell donor.

Algorithm 29.2 Treatment of chronic lymphocytic leukemia

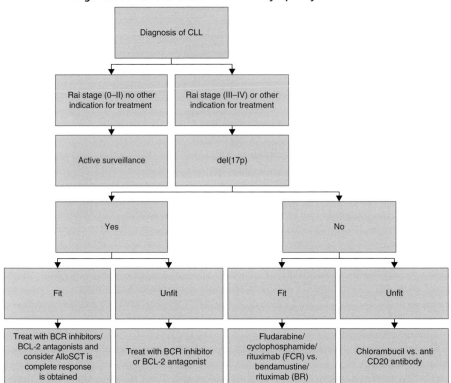

When to hospitalize
- Patients with CLL rarely require hospitalization.
- If they experience complications from their chemotherapy they may require hospitalization.
- If they experience autoimmune-related complications, they may require hospital admission.
- If patients with CLL develop Richter transformation, they may need hospitalization for additional therapy.

Managing the hospitalized patient
- If patients are on ibrutinib or idelalisib, these medications should not be stopped abruptly as they are at risk for a flare of their CLL.
- If the patient is on ibrutinib, it is important to be aware that ibrutinib can increase risk of bleeding and the patient should not be on anticoagulation medication while on ibrutinib.

Table of treatment

Treatment	Comments
Conservative	Active surveillance is appropriate for low risk, asymptomatic patients
Medical	See Algorithm 29.2

Prevention/management of complications

- Rituximab can result in a rate-related infusion reaction with the first dose. It is important to distinguish this from anaphylaxis. Once symptoms resolve, infusion can be restarted at a lower rate.
- Obinutuzumab, a second generation anti-CD20 monoclonal antibody, can result in infusion reactions.
- Ibrutinib, an oral Bruton's tyrosine kinase (BTK) inhibitor, can give rise to fatigue, diarrhea, stomatitis, arthralgias, and, rarely, atrial fibrillation which can require interruption of treatment.
- Idelalisib, an oral inhibitor of phosphatidylinositol-3 kinase (PI3K), can result in hepatitis, pneumonitis, and colitis that can result in treatment interruptions and initiation of corticosteroids.

CLINICAL PEARLS
- When considering treatment, one must consider histopathologic, immune, and cytogenetic risk factors in addition to the patient's fitness status.
- Patients who are otherwise asymptomatic may be monitored except for those with del(17p) for whom you may consider therapy earlier.
- The goal of treatment is to maintain durable remission.
- The only curative treatment option is HSCT and this treatment should only be considered in high risk, fit patients with an adequate stem cell donor.

Special populations
Pregnancy
- Chemotherapy can be administered in the third trimester.
- **Ibrutinib:** women should avoid pregnancy during treatment and for at least 3 months after cessation of treatment.
- **Idelalisib:** women should avoid pregnancy during treatment and for at least 1 month after cessation of treatment.

Elderly
- Treatment options vary based on frailty rather than age.

Prognosis

BOTTOM LINE/CLINICAL PEARLS
- Patients with indolent, low risk disease have a median life expectancy of over 10 years.
- Patients with high risk disease (del(17p), refractory to purine analog, relapse within 24 months), have a median life expectancy of 2–3 years.
- Life expectancy in high risk disease is changing as newer therapies are emerging that better target this high risk population.

Natural history of untreated disease
The natural history of the disease varies widely based on risk stratification.
- Patients can live for years without complications or treatment.
- Other patients will experience complications from autoimmune processes (e.g. autoimmune hemolytic anemia), cytopenias, splenomegaly, or bulky adenopathy.

Prognosis for treated patients

Based on the CLL prognostication index (see the section on Diagnosis) four prognostic groups have emerged:

Risk stratification	5-year OS (% alive)
Low (score 0–1)	93
Intermediate (score 2–3)	79
High (score 4–6)	64
Very high risk (score 7–10)	23

Follow-up tests and monitoring

- CBC with differential should be monitored every 3–6 months for recurrence of disease.
- Clinical symptoms such as fevers, night sweats, weight loss, or progressive bulky adenopathy should be monitored.
- CT scans every 3–6 months to evaluate nonpalpable adenopathy, except in low risk asymptomatic patients.
- If patients have rapid recurrence/progression, development of fevers, night sweats, weight loss, or appear very clinically ill, then you should consider transformation to an aggressive lymphoma such as diffuse large B-cell lymphoma (Richter transformation).

Reading list

Byrd JC, Furman RR, Coutre SE, et al. Targeting BTK with ibrutinib in relapsed chronic lymphocytic leukemia. N Engl J Med 2013;369:32–42.

Dreger P, Scheletig J, Andersen N, et al. Managing high-risk CLL during transition to a new treatment era: stem cell transplantation or novel agents? Blood 2014;124:3841–3849.

Furman RR, Sharman JP, Coutre SE, et al. Idelalisib and rituximab in relapsed chronic lymphocytic leukemia. N Engl J Med 2014;370:997–1007.

Hallek M. CME Information: chronic lymphocytic leukemia: 2015 Update on diagnosis, risk stratification, and treatment. Am J Hematol 2015;90:446–460.

Hallek M, Cheson BD, Catovsky D, et al. Guidelines for the diagnosis and treatment of chronic lymphocytic leukemia: a report from the International Workshop on Chronic Lymphocytic Leukemia updating the National Cancer Institute–Working Group 1996 guidelines. Blood 2008;111:5446–5456.

Rossi D, Spina V, Bomben R, et al. Association between molecular lesions and specific B-cell receptor subsets in chronic lymphocytic leukemia. Blood 2013;121:4902–4905.

Zenz T, Gribben JG, Hallek M, et al. Risk categories and refractory CLL in the era of chemoimmunotherapy. Blood 2012;119:4101–4107.

Suggested website

http://www.lls.org/

Guidelines
National society guidelines

Title	Source	Date and weblink
NCCN Diagnostic/Treatment Guidelines	NCCN	2019 https://www.nccn.org/store/login/login.aspx?ReturnURL=https://www.nccn.org/professionals/physician_gls/pdf/cll.pdf

International society guidelines

Title	Source	Date and weblink
Chronic Lymphocytic Leukaemia: ESMO Clinical Practice Guidelines	European Society for Medical Oncology (ESMO)	2019 https://www.esmo.org/Guidelines/ Haematological-Malignancies/Chronic-Lymphocytic-Leukaemia

Additional material for this chapter can be found online at:
www.wiley.com/go/oh/mountsinaioncology

This includes advice for patients, a case study, ICD codes, and multiple choice questions.

CHAPTER 30

Non-Hodgkin Lymphoma

Adam F. Binder and Joshua D. Brody
Icahn School of Medicine at Mount Sinai, New York, NY, USA

OVERALL BOTTOM LINE
- Non-Hodgkin lymphomas (NHLs) are neoplasms of mature B cells, T cells, or natural killer (NK) cells. In 2012 it was the seventh most common cancer in both men and women.
- There is a broad differential diagnosis for lymphadenopathy, both regional and systemic, and it is important to consider causes other than lymphoma.
- Excisional biopsy is key for the diagnostic investigation of lymphoma.
- In general, indolent lymphomas are incurable and treatment is focused on controlling symptoms or complications from the disease; aggressive lymphomas are acutely life threatening but potentially curable and the goal of treatment is cure.
- Treatment modalities primarily include chemo-immunotherapy, at times radiotherapy, and, rarely, surgery.

Background
Definition of disease
- NHLs are a group of diseases involving clonal lymphoproliferative disorder of B cells (most commonly), T cells, or NK cells; however, not all clonal populations are malignant.
- Clonality is established by certain characteristics seen on flow cytometry, such as light chain restriction, presence of translocations seen on FISH, gene sequencing demonstrating clonal rearrangement of B-cell or T-cell receptor, or gene expression profiling.

Disease classification
- The disease is classified according to morphologic, immunophenotypic, genotypic, and clinical characteristics.
- The most important classification distinction is between indolent lymphomas and aggressive or highly aggressive lymphomas as this affects prognosis and treatment considerations.

Incidence/prevalence
- In 2015, the incidence of NHL was expected to be 71 850, approximately 4.3% of all new cancer diagnoses, and to account for 19 790 or 3.4% of all cancer-related deaths.
- Based on the SEER database for 2005–2011, the OS rate from NHL at 5 years is 70%.

Mount Sinai Expert Guides: Oncology, First Edition. Edited by William K. Oh and Ajai Chari.
© 2019 John Wiley & Sons Ltd. Published 2019 by John Wiley & Sons Ltd.
Companion Website: www.wiley.com/go/oh/mountsinaioncology

Economic impact
- In 2010, the overall cost of lymphoma care (both Hodgkin lymphoma and NHL) was $12.14 billion. This is about 10% of the US national expenditure for cancer care of $124.57 billion. The total US national healthcare expenditure in 2010 was 2.604×10^3 billion dollars.
- This cost is expected to rise with a growing population, increased cost of pharmaceutical agents, and longer life expectancy for patients with NHL.

Etiology
- The etiology of most cases of NHL is unknown, although significant evidence indicates the accumulation of somatic mutations combined with growth signals provided by surrounding nontumor cells (i.e. the tumor microenvironment).
- Possible causative agents include pesticides, agricultural chemicals, hair dyes, radiation, as well as certain pathogens (e.g. *Helicobacter pylori* or human T-cell lymphotropic virus 1 [HTLV1]).
- Patients who are immunosuppressed, either as a result of medications (e.g. cyclosporine, TNF-α inhibitors), infections (e.g. HIV), inherited immunodeficiency, or autoimmune disease are at increased risk for developing lymphoma.

Pathology/pathogenesis
Various mechanisms account for the pathogenesis of NHL. It varies between B-cell and T-cell lymphomas.
- B-cell lymphoma:
  - The malignant B-cell clone can occur at various stages of maturation
  - Translocation events can occur in which the oncogene is constitutively activated by the immunoglobulin (Ig) locus (e.g. t(8:14) results in up-regulation of myc (8) by Ig locus (14) in Burkitt lymphoma). These translocation events can occur during V(D)J recombination, somatic hypermutation, or class switching
  - BCR signaling provides important survival signals to B-cell lymphoma cells. This can be caused either by stimulation from an exogenous source (i.e. *H. pylori*) or autoantibodies
  - Lymphoma microenvironment such as T-helper cells, tumor infiltrating T cells, or follicular dendritic cells can play an integral part in the development of certain lymphomas.
- NK/T-cell lymphoma:
  - Virally driven chronic T-cell proliferation alters cellular pathways driving accumulation of genetic abnormalities and clonal expansion of a subset of T cells.

Prevention

> **BOTTOM LINE/CLINICAL PEARLS**
> - No interventions have been shown to prevent the development of the disease except potentially in Epstein–Barr virus (EBV) driven post-transplant lymphoproliferative disorders.

Screening
- There are no screening recommendations for most patients with NHL. For the rare lymphoma subtypes occurring as a result of post-transplant EBV-driven lymphoproliferation, recommended screening exists for renal transplant and allogeneic HSCT recipients:
  - **For renal transplant:** EBV nucleic acid testing should occur within the first week, monthly for 3–6 months, then every 3 months for the first year. Retesting should occur after treatment

for acute rejection, although this may be based on risk stratification and can be center dependent.
- **For HSCT:** EBV nucleic acid testing should occur on the day of transplant, then weekly for 3 months. Screening should be longer if the patient has graft vs. host disease, a haploidentical graft, or history of EBV viremia.

Primary prevention
- In the rare instances described, it has been hypothesized that early treatment of EBV-driven lymphoproliferation with anti-CD20 antibodies might prevent progression to lymphoma. No preventions have otherwise been validated.

Secondary prevention
- For most lymphomas there are no strategies of secondary prevention. There have been some data to suggest maintenance therapy in certain NHL subtypes will prevent relapse.
- For lymphomas caused by chronic antigen stimulation (i.e. gastric mucosa-associated lymphoid tissue [MALT] lymphoma secondary to *H. pylori*), treatment of the underlying inflammatory process can result in eradication of the lymphoma and prevent recurrence.

Diagnosis

CLINICAL PEARLS
- Patients present with various symptoms depending on the location of the lymphoma, but a history of painless lymphadenopathy, fevers, night sweats, weight loss, erythroderma, abdominal fullness, or constitutional symptoms is suggestive of a malignant process.
- Providers should perform a thorough lymph node examination (including an examination of the oropharyngeal canal to assess for Waldeyer's ring), as well as an abdominal examination to evaluate for hepatosplenomegaly, a dermatologic examination for rashes or lesions that could suggest cutaneous involvement, and a neurologic examination to assess for CNS disease in aggressive lymphomas.
- Diagnostic evaluation should include excisional lymph node biopsy, CT of the chest/abdomen/pelvis or PET/CT, HIV, hepatitis B and C serologies, CMP, LDH, β2-microglobulin, and CBC with differential as well ancillary testing such as bone marrow aspiration or biopsy and peripheral blood flow cytometry in some patients.
- Lumbar puncture should be performed in patients with suspected CNS involvement (neurologic symptoms, more than two extranodal sites of disease, double hit lymphoma, Burkitt lymphoma).

Differential diagnosis

Differential diagnosis	Features
Sarcoidosis	Can be asymptomatic or symptomatic Tends to be hilar adenopathy
Infection	Adenopathy tends to be more regional and tender, but can have systemic adenopathy as well

(*Continued*)

Differential diagnosis	Features
Autoimmune disorders (lupus)	Adenopathy occurs in 50% of patients with systemic lupus erythematosus Other clinical symptoms of lupus present
Mycobacterial infections	Adenopathy can be localized or systemic, tends to enlarge over weeks to months without systemic symptoms
Metastatic malignancy	Enlarged lymph node could be presenting symptom of metastatic solid malignancy (e.g. Virchow node)
HIV lymphadenopathy	Nontender adenopathy occurs during acute infection (arises in week 2), but can persist
Castleman disease	Lymphoproliferative disorder characterized by fevers, hepatosplenomegaly, polyclonal hypergammaglobulinemia, lymphadenopathy Associated with HHV-8 infection Can be localized or multicentric adenopathy
Benign necrotizing lymphadenitis (Kikuchi disease)	Characterized by fevers and cervical adenopathy Tends to occur in young women
Medications	Certain medications can cause serum sickness reactions (fever, rash, arthralgias, lymphadenopathy); phenytoin can cause generalized lymphadenopathy without serum sickness symptom
Dermatopathologic lymphadenopathy	Can occur with diffuse benign skin lesions, pathologic diagnosis
Kimura disease	Inflammatory condition involving subcutaneous tissue and lymph nodes of head and neck Often with elevated IgE and eosinophilia
Rosai–Dorfman syndrome (sinus histiocytosis with massive lymphadenopathy)	Lymphadenopathy tends to be in the cervical region

Typical presentation

- The typical presentation of NHL varies given the diverse subtypes.
- Many patients with indolent lymphoma present with asymptomatic lymphadenopathy.
- Patients with more aggressive lymphomas or advanced indolent lymphomas can have pain symptoms related to the location and size of lymphadenopathy, symptoms related to anemia or thrombocytopenia if there is extensive bone marrow involvement, abdominal fullness/pain if there is profound splenomegaly, or classic B symptoms (fevers, night sweats, unintentional weight loss).
- Patients with cutaneous NHL will present with plaque lesions (mycosis fungoides; MF), papular lesions (acute T-cell leukemia/lymphoma), ulcerating/fungating lesions (MF, anaplastic large cell lymphoma), or erythroderma (MF, Sézary syndrome); one must always rule out systemic disease in patients presenting with cutaneous lymphoma.

Clinical diagnosis

History

- Ask about past medical history (e.g. autoimmune diseases).
- Ask about localizing symptoms to suggest either infectious etiology or malignancy.

- Ask about possible exposures to infectious agent (i.e. mononucleosis, mycobacterial, cat scratch disease, HIV).
- Ask about duration of adenopathy, growth rate, and whether nodes are tender or nontender.
- Ask about other symptoms (fever, night sweats, weight loss, rashes, pain, fatigue), medications, and recent travel.

Physical examination

- The clinician should conduct a thorough lymph node examination. It is important to evaluate Waldeyer's ring, epitrochlear nodes, cervical (anterior, posterior), clavicular (supra, infra), axillary, and inguinal lymph nodes.
  - Note whether the lymph nodes are tender or nontender
  - Measure diameter if possible; greater than 1 cm is typically considered enlarged
  - Note the consistency of the lymph nodes and whether they are fixed or mobile.
- Detailed abdominal examination with close attention to splenomegaly in the absence or presence of hepatomegaly (isolated splenomegaly is seen in various lymphoproliferative disorders).
- Dermatologic examination to evaluate for skin lesions.
- Full clinical examination to evaluate for systemic symptoms that will help in narrowing the differential diagnosis.

Useful clinical decision rules and calculators

For NHL, the Ann Arbor Staging system is used.

Ann Arbor Stage	Involvement
Stage I (A/B)[a]	Involvement of a single lymph node region or single extranodal site
Stage II (A/B)[a]	Involvement of two or more lymph node regions or lymphatic structures on the same side of the diaphragm or with involvement of limited, contiguous, extralymphatic organ or tissue
Stage III (A/B)[a]	Involvement of lymph nodes above and below the diaphragm, which may involve the spleen
Stage IV (A/B)[a]	Diffuse involvement including one or more extralymphatic organ (liver, bone marrow, or nodular involvement of the lungs)

[a]A/B used to denote absence (A) or presence (B) of constitutional symptoms: fevers (>38.5°C), drenching night sweats, weight loss (>10% unintentional weight loss over 6 months prior to diagnosis).

- Staging is important for overall prognosis, but in lymphoma it is not as powerfully prognostic as in solid malignancies. As a result, prognostic calculators exist for various NHLs. The International Prognostic Index (IPI) is used for diffuse large B-cell lymphoma. Variations on this prognostic scoring system are also used in other lymphomas such as follicular lymphoma (FLIPI). Prognostic calculators are available online.
- We also take into account the aggressive nature of the NHL, which is determined by disease type as well as immunohistochemical, transcriptional, and molecular markers to determine an appropriate treatment plan.

Disease severity classification

See Algorithm 30.1.

Algorithm 30.1 Disease severity classification of NHL

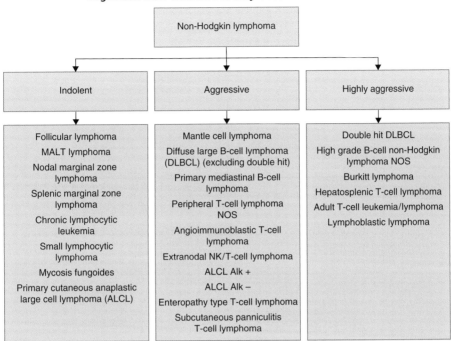

Laboratory diagnosis
List of diagnostic tests (Algorithm 30.2)
- Excisional lymph node biopsy is critical to preserve architectural integrity when evaluating for lymphoma. In some cases, core needle biopsy is sufficient to allow for architectural assessment. Fine needle aspirate is generally not sufficient to diagnose NHL.
- CBC with differential (pay attention to lymphocyte count, cytopenias to suggest bone marrow involvement).
- CMP.
- LDH.
- Phosphorous.
- β2-microglobulin (can be elevated in chronic kidney disease given its renal clearance).
- HIV, hepatitis B and C serologies.
- Uric acid (elevated in aggresive lymphomas with tumor lysis).
  In a subset of cases:
- Bone marrow biopsy (in most, but not all cases).
- *H. pylori* (e.g. in gastric MALT).
- Quantitative immunoglobulin assessment (in CLL patients with recurrent infections).
- Coombs test, reticulocyte count, and haptoglobin (e.g. in CLL patients with evidence of hemolysis or unexplained anemia).
- Serum viscosity (e.g. in patients with Waldenström macroglobulinemia).
- Serum EBV quantitative PCR (e.g. in patients with NK/T-cell lymphoma, post-transplant lymphoproliferative disorder).
- HTLV1 serology (e.g. in patients with adult T-cell leukemia/lymphoma).
- FISH of peripheral blood or tumor.

Algorithm 30.2 Diagnosis of NHL taking into account immunohistochemistry findings.
Some cytogenetic abnormalities are listed here that can also be helpful for diagnostic purposes.
One must also consider cytogenetic abnormalities for prognostication of certain disease
subtypes (i.e. double hit DLBCL)

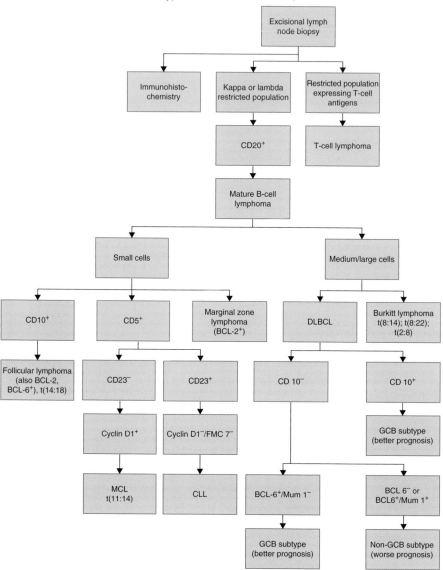

- Targeted gene sequencing (e.g. *p53*, *Myd88*, and *BRAF* in CLL, Waldenström macroglobulinemia, and hairy cell leukemia, respectively).

Lists of imaging techniques
- If indolent lymphoma is suspected, a CT scan of the chest, abdomen, and pelvis (sometimes
  neck) is indicated for staging purposes.

- If an aggressive lymphoma is suspected, often a CT scan is the first test performed to evaluate for the extent of lymphadenopathy. However, a PET/CT scan is ultimately required for staging and monitoring response to treatment once a diagnosis is made. If possible, a PET/CT scan should be part of the initial evaluation. A PET/CT scan can also guide which lymph node to biopsy.
- MRI of the brain, spine, or other regions is reserved for selected cases (e.g. suspected CNS involvement, spinal cord compression, or nasal NK/T-cell lymphoma).

Potential pitfalls/common errors made regarding diagnosis of disease

- Patients are frequently sent for a FNA of a lymph node. This commonly leads to indeterminate results causing a delay in diagnosis.
- If lymphoma is suspected, it is best for the patient to have an excisional lymph node biopsy as the initial diagnostic evaluation. In rare cases, core needle biopsy might be acceptable, though not preferred.
- An experienced hematopathologist should examine the biopsy to make an accurate diagnosis that will guide treatment decisions.

Treatment (Algorithm 30.3)

Algorithm 30.3 Treatment of NHL

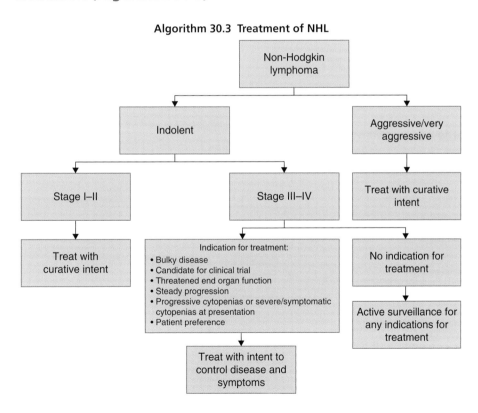

Treatment rationale

- Given the diverse disease classifications within the larger category of NHL, the treatment varies greatly according to diagnosis.

- In general, patients with B-cell lymphomas or B-cell rich T-cell lymphomas where CD20$^+$ cells are strongly expressed, rituximab (an anti CD20 monoclonal antibody) should be used in the treatment regimen.
- For patients with the, generally incurable, indolent lymphomas, the goal of treatment is to control the disease. If the patient is asymptomatic, one can actively monitor the disease and only treat when symptomatic or in case of impending end-organ effect (e.g. compression of vasculature, ureters, or bowel).
- For aggressive lymphomas, the goal of treatment is to cure the patient of the disease and first line therapy varies depending on disease type. However, for most lymphomas, the backbone of first line therapy involves some combination of steroids, anthracyclines, vinca alkaloids, and an alkylating agent + /– rituximab (see second point in this section for comment on rituximab use).

When to hospitalize
- Most patients with NHL can be treated as outpatients.
- If patients have an aggressive lymphoma and they appear acutely ill, they may need inpatient management for evaluation and treatment.
- Patients with spontaneous tumor lysis syndrome or at high risk for treatment-induced tumor lysis syndrome should be admitted to hospital.
- Some chemotherapy regimens need to be delivered as an inpatient because of a high risk of acute adverse effects or because of frequent or continuous dosing.
- Some patients need to be hospitalized for complications from chemotherapy such as acute infections, particularly while neutropenic.

Managing the hospitalized patient
Managing a hospitalized lymphoma patient is similar to managing other acutely ill patients.

Table of treatment

Treatment	Comments
Conservative	Suitable for stage III–IV indolent lymphomas. Active surveillance is an option for many asymptomatic patients in this setting
Medical Rituximab R-CHOP R-EPOCH Bendamustine Chlorambucil Ibrutinib Idelalisib Bortezomib Brentuximab Vaccine therapy BEAM/autologous stem cell transplant (salvage therapy after initial relapse)	Idelalisib: monitor closely for colitis, pneumonitis Ibrutinib: do not use if the patient requires anticoagulation for any indication; can cause atrial fibrillation in about 12% of patients
Radiologic	Radiation therapy is often used for bulky disease sites after chemotherapy, for palliative treatment in refractory symptomatic disease, or for stage I, contiguous stage II disease
Complementary	Acupuncture can be used for control of nausea

Prevention/management of complications

- Rituximab can result in a rate-related infusion reaction with the first dose. It is important to distinguish this from anaphylaxis. Once symptoms resolve, the infusion can be restarted at a lower rate.
- Neuropathy from vincristine can result in it being omitted from R-CHOP.
- Ibrutinib, an oral inhibitor of Bruton's tyrosine kinase, can result in hepatitis, pneumonitis, and colitis that can result in treatment interruptions.

CLINICAL PEARLS
- Patients tend to have rapid responses to initial therapy and can see complete responses after the first 2–4 cycles. Early response has improved prognostic implications in aggressive lymphomas.
- It is important to stay on schedule for chemotherapy cycles and to avoid complications with supportive medications.

Special populations

Pregnancy

- Certain chemotherapy can be safely administered in the second and third trimesters for aggressive disease requiring urgent therapy.

Elderly

- For many of the various treatment options, dose modifications can be made to minimize toxicity from chemotherapy in the elderly. For example, a dose modified R-CHOP regimen is effective in patients over the age of 80.
- A geriatric assessment scale should be used when deciding on treatment regimens. Certain regimens may not be appropriate for elderly or frail patients.

Others

- In the HIV population, depending on the type of NHL, treatment can differ from that for the general population. For example, in Burkitt lymphoma, a dose adjusted R-EPOCH regimen takes into account CD4 count.

Prognosis

BOTTOM LINE/CLINICAL PEARLS
- Prognoses for patients with advanced stage NHL are generally better than those for patients with solid malignancies.
- Many subtypes of aggressive NHL are curable in the majority of patients. Patients with common indolent subtypes frequently have a median OS greater than 10 years.
- Prognosis varies widely based upon given the diversity of NHL subtypes.
- Prognosis is determined by calculating prognostic index scores as well as taking into account immunophenotypic and genetic variations of the disease.
- In general, systemic T-cell lymphomas have a poorer prognosis. ALK + anaplastic large cell lymphoma is an exception.

Natural history of untreated disease

This varies dramatically based on aggressiveness of the lymphoma.

- For certain indolent lymphomas (e.g. follicular lymphoma), patients can live for years without indication for treatment.
- For highly aggressive lymphomas (e.g. Burkitt lymphoma), patients need to be treated urgently as the disease is life threatening.

Prognosis for treated patients

- Diffuse large B-cell lymphoma:
  - **Germinal center B-cell (GCB) subtype:** defined on immunohistochemistry by ($CD10^+$, or $CD10^-/BCL-6^+/MUM1^-$)low IPI (0–2): OS about 70% at 10 years, high IPI (3–5): OS 20–30% at 10 years
  - **Non-GCB subtype:** defined on immunohistochemistry by ($CD10^-/MUM1^+$) low IPI (0–2): OS about 50% at 10 years, high IPI (3–5): OS 0–5% at 10 years.
- Chronic lymphocytic leukemia:
  - **17p deletion:** median OS 28–30 months (prior to development of ibrutinib, which has activity in this population)
  - **13q deletion as sole abnormality:** median OS 84 months
  - **Other abnormalities:** median OS 120–156 months.
- Follicular lymphoma (based on FLIPI, 5-year OS): low risk ~90%, intermediate risk ~80%, high risk ~50–55%.

Follow-up tests and monitoring

- Follow-up monitoring has been under debate for various types of NHL and the recommendations are currently changing. For aggressive NHL, if the patient obtained a complete response on post-treatment imaging, then the current recommendation is to follow the patient clinically every 3–6 months and only repeat imaging if clinically indicated (i.e. development of symptoms or worsening cytopenias). For indolent lymphomas, following clinically is also recommended except in certain conditions such as gastric MALT lymphoma, for which it is recommended to perform an EGD 3 months after therapy.

Reading list

Al-Hamadani M, Habermann TM, Cerhan JR, et al. Non-Hodgkin lymphoma subtype distribution, geodemographic patterns, and survival in the US: a longitudinal analysis of the National Cancer Data Base from 1998 to 2011. Am J Hematol 2015;90:790–795.

Ansell SM. Non-Hodgkin lymphoma: diagnosis and treatment. Mayo Clin Proc 2015;90(8):1152–1163.

Gloghini A, Dolcetti R, Carbone A. Lymphomas occurring specifically in HIV-infected patients: from pathogenesis to pathology. Semin Cancer Biol 2013;23:457–467.

Kuppers R. Mechanisms of B-cell lymphoma pathogenesis. Nature Rev 2005;5:251–263.

Lenz G, Staudt LM. Aggressive lymphomas. N Engl J Med 2010;362:1417–1429.

Olsen EA. Evaluation, diagnosis, and staging of cutaneous lymphoma. Dermatol Clin 2015;33(4):643–654.

Suggested websites

http://www.cancer.gov/types/lymphoma
http://www.lls.org/
http://www.cancer.org/cancer/non-hodgkinlymphoma/
http://www.mdanderson.org/patient-and-cancer-information/cancer-information/cancer-types/non-hodgkins-lymphoma/nhl-full.jpg
http://media.oncologynurseadvisor.com/images/2011/06/08/ona_ce0611_tb1_171613.gif

Guidelines
National society guidelines

Title	Source	Date and weblink
Diagnostic/Treatment Guidelines	NCCN	2019 www.NCCN.org

International society guidelines

Title	Source	Date and weblink
Non-Hodgkin Lymphoma Guidelines	European Society for Medical Oncology (ESMO)	2019 http://www.esmo.org/Guidelines

Additional material for this chapter can be found online at:
www.wiley.com/go/oh/mountsinaioncology

This includes advice for patients, a case study, ICD codes, and multiple choice questions.

CHAPTER 31

Hodgkin Lymphoma

Jonah Shulman[1], Parth R. Rao[2], and Akshay Sudhindra[1]
[1] Icahn School of Medicine at Mount Sinai, New York, NY, USA
[2] Geisinger Medical Center, Danville, PA, USA

OVERALL BOTTOM LINE
- Hodgkin lymphoma (HL) is a highly curable disease even when patients present with late stage disease.
- FDG-PET has a central role in staging, assessing response as well as prognostication of disease.
- Brentuximab vedotin, an anti-CD30 antibody drug conjugate, is highly active against HL and is currently indicated in relapsed and/or refractory HL and also as a consolidation treatment post autologous SCT. It is now also approved for upfront use in advanced disease.
- Patients who receive radiation therapy as part of their treatment regimen are at a higher risk of developing secondary malignancies as well as cardiovascular disease.

Background
- HL is a lymphoid neoplasm characterized by the presence of atypical lymphoblasts surrounded by a heterogeneous infiltrate of inflammatory cells.

Disease classification
- HL is divided into two types that differ in morphology, clinical presentation, and management strategies: classic HL (cHL) and nodular lymphocyte predominant HL (NLPHL).
- cHL is further classified into four categories: nodular sclerosis, mixed cellularity, lymphocyte-rich, and lymphocyte-depleted HL. Histologies with the most and least lymphocyte infiltration have the best and worst outcomes, respectively.

Incidence/prevalence
- Incidence of HL is approximately 2.5–3 per 100 000 men and women per year and there are 0.3 deaths per 100 000 men and women per year.
- In 2016, there were an estimated 210 974 people living with HL in the USA.

Economic impact
- Recent studies show that the cost of first line therapy for HL is approximately $23 000; however, it increases seven to eightfold when patients relapse and undergo transplantation. The addition of Brentuximab vedotin has increased cost significantly.

Etiology
- The exact etiology is unknown.
- An association with exposure to EBV infection is well reported in up to 30% of cases; however, no causal relationship has been established.

Mount Sinai Expert Guides: Oncology, First Edition. Edited by William K. Oh and Ajai Chari.
© 2019 John Wiley & Sons Ltd. Published 2019 by John Wiley & Sons Ltd.
Companion Website: www.wiley.com/go/oh/mountsinaioncology

- There is increased incidence and severity of HL in patients with HIV/AIDS.
- According to the Swedish Family Cancer database, relatives of HL patients have a fourfold elevated risk of developing HL.
- There is an increased incidence of HL in carpenters, farmers, and meat processors.

Pathology

- cHL is characterized by the presence of typical large mononuclear or binucleated Reed–Sternberg cells on a background of inflammatory cells.
- Cells typically stain positive for CD30 and CD15, and are weakly positive for Pax5. They do not express CD20, CD79a, or CD45.
- NLPHL consists of numerous large, tightly packed nodules which are filled with scattered large "popcorn" cells or lymphocyte predominant cells that are CD20 and CD79a positive, but rarely CD15 or CD30 positive.

Prevention

> **BOTTOM LINE**
> - No interventions have been demonstrated to prevent the development of the disease.

Secondary prevention

- Brentuximab is approved for post ASCT consolidation therapy in patients with HL with risk factors for relapse or progression after transplantation.
- The AETHERA trial was a randomized, double-blinded, placebo-controlled trial which showed that early consolidation with brentuximab improved PFS for these patients.

Diagnosis

> **BOTTOM LINE**
> - Clinical findings include painless or sometimes painful cervical or axillary lymphadenopathy, night sweats, fevers, unintended weight loss, and splenomegaly.
> - The presence of atypical lymphoblasts, Reed–Sternberg cells, or lymphocyte predominant cells surrounded by heterogeneous infiltration of inflammatory cells on an excisional biopsy is diagnostic.
> - FDG-PET is considered standard of care to determine the extent of disease.

Differential diagnosis

Differential diagnosis	Features
Infectious mononucleosis	Bilateral and symmetrical adenopathy Involvement of posterior oropharynx Atypical lymphocytes in peripheral blood
Primary mediastinal B-cell lymphoma	Cells with clear and abundant cytoplasm B-cell lineage always positive, BCL-6 100% CD15/CD30 50–70%
Phenytoin-associated lymphadenopathy	History of exposure to Dilantin

Typical presentation

The most common presentation is nontender lymphadenopathy in the neck, supraclavicular region, or axillae. Mediastinal lymphadenopathy may cause chest pain, dyspnea, or cough, or may be found incidentally on chest X-ray. Up to one-third of patients with HL present with night sweats and unexplained weight loss defined as >10% of baseline weight. Pel–Ebstein fever, an unexplained fever that remits and relapses over weeks, is characteristic.

Clinical diagnosis (Algorithm 31.1)

Algorithm 31.1 Diagnosis of Hodgkin lymphoma

Lymphadenopathy
+/−
Presence of B symptoms

↓

Palpable lymphadenopathy
Assess for splenomegaly

↓

Excisional biopsy of most
readily accessible lesion

Large mononucleated or binucleated cells
CD15/CD30+ve,
CD20/CD79−ve, Pax5+/−
Classic Hodgkin lymphoma
(cHL)

Large tightly packed nodules of cells
CD20/CD79+ve, Pax5 +ve
CD15/CD30 −ve
Nodular lymphocyte predominant
Hodgkin lymphoma
(NLPHL)

PET-FDG
scan for staging

Early stage disease
(IA–IIA)

Advanced stage disease
(IIB–IVB)

Favorable

Unfavorable

History
- Unusual presentations include severe and unexplained itching, and pain at enlarged lymph node after consumption of alcohol. Patients with HIV and AIDS have increased frequency of HL, in whom it tends to involve extranodal sites and has an aggressive clinical course with poorer prognosis.

Table 31.1 Ann Arbor Staging System.

Stage	Extent of disease
I	Involvement of a single lymph node region or lymphoid structure
II	Involvement of two or more lymph node regions on one side of the diaphragm
III	Involvement of two or more lymph node regions on both sides of the diaphragm
IV	Disseminated involvement of a deep, visceral organ

Physical examination
- Physical examination should focus on assessment of hepatosplenomegaly in addition to lymph nodes.
- Palor and tachycardia are nonspecific findings that can occur in patients with advanced stage disease because of involvement of bone marrow.

Useful clinical decision rules and calculators (Table 31.1)
- Each stage is subdivided into A and B substages depending on whether constitutional symptoms ("B" symptoms) are absent (A) or present (B).
- Localized involvement of an extranodal site by direct extension from an involved lymph node is designated by the subscript E and does not qualify as stage IV.

Disease severity classification
- Poor prognostic factors for early stage HL (stage IA–IIA) include:
  - Bulky disease (greater than 10 cm in diameter or greater than one-third the mediastinal diameter)
  - Elevated ESR
  - More than two to three sites of nodal disease
  - Presence of extranodal sites.

International Prognostic Score for advanced stage HL (stage IIB–IV); 1 point for each condition:
- Age older than 45 years
- Male sex
- Stage IV disease
- Serum albumin less than 4.0 g/dL
- Hemoglobin levels less than 10.5 mg/dL
- White blood count higher than 15 000/μL
- Lymphocytes less than 600/μL and/or a lymphocyte count less than 8% of the white cell count.

Laboratory diagnosis
List of diagnostic tests
- CBC, CMP, LDH, and ESR.
- HIV and hepatitis serology.
- Excisional lymph node biopsy is the gold standard for definitive diagnosis. FNA biopsy is not recommended.
- Fertility counseling, egg/sperm collection and preservation.
- Bone marrow biopsy is not indicated in early stage disease and may not be necessary in patients who have FDG avid bone lesions on PET scan. Bone marrow biopsy can often be omitted as it usually does not affect management.

Table 31.2 PET 5-point scale by Deauville criteria.

Score	PET/CT result
1	No uptake
2	Uptake ≤ mediastinum
3	Uptake > mediastinum but ≤ liver
4	Uptake moderately higher than liver
5	Uptake markedly higher than liver or new lesions
X	New areas of uptake unlikely related to lymphoma

- If bleomycin is used, pulmonary function test at baseline, the end of the second cycle of treatment, and when bleomycin-related lung toxicity is clinically or radiographically suspected.

Lists of imaging techniques
- FDG-PET at baseline for staging of disease and at the end of the second cycle as well as at the end of treatment for prognostication (Table 31.2).
- Echo or MUGA scan to obtain baseline cardiac function before starting anthracycline therapy.

Potential pitfalls/common errors made regarding diagnosis of disease
- HL should be considered in young patients who present with persistent lymphadenopathy and constitutional symptoms.
- Diagnosis can be missed if fine needle biopsy was obtained instead of excisional biopsy.

Treatment (Algorithm 31.2)
Treatment principles
- Patients with early stage favorable cHL and without bulky adenopathy are treated with ABVD (adriamycin-bleomycin-vinblastine-dacarbazine) with or without involved field radiation therapy (IFRT).
- There is growing evidence that 4–6 cycles of ABVD alone results in similar OS, modestly inferior PFS, and less long-term toxicity compared with combination of chemotherapy and radiation therapy.
- Interim PET (i.e. PET after 2–3 cycles of ABVD) is highly predictive of treatment response and has a strong prognostic significance. Freedom from progression (FFP) is significantly higher in patients who are interim PET negative than patients who are positive after two cycles of ABVD.
- Patients with early stage cHL with unfavorable risk factors benefit from six cycles of ABVD.
- Patients with early stage cHL with bulky disease are treated with combined modality therapy – 4–6 cycles of chemotherapy plus IFRT.
- Patients with advanced stage (IIB–IV) are treated with six cycles of chemotherapy.
- Brentuximab vedotin has excellent response rates in relapsed/refractory HL and is often used as a bridge to ASCT.
- Salvage chemotherapy followed by ASCT is the standard approach for relapsed disease with around 50–60% of patients achieving long-term remission.
- Nivolumab is indicated for patients who relapse after transplant or are transplant-ineligible.
- For patients receiving 6 cycles of chemotherapy, if interim PET after 2 cycles of ABVD shows complete response, bleomycin can be omitted from subsequent cycles.

Algorithm 31.2 Treatment of Hodgkin lymphoma

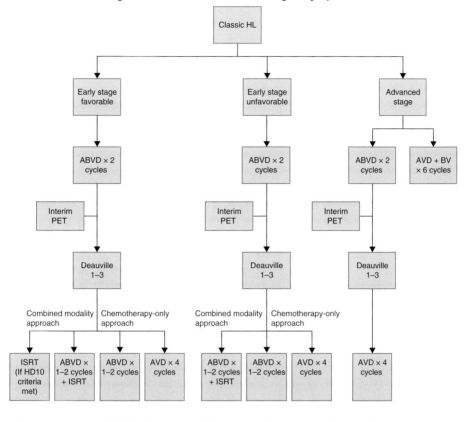

- Based on results of ECHELON-1 study, AVD + Brentuximab can also be considered for advanced stage HL.
- Early stage NLPHL is often treated with IFRT alone.
- Advanced stage NLPHL is treated with either R-CHOP or R-ABVD.

Table of treatment

Treatment	Comments
Conservative	During first trimester of pregnancy. ABVD during second trimester is generally safe
Medical • ABVD • Stanford V • BEACOPP	ABVD is standard of care BEACOPP is contraindicated specifically in elderly patients (i.e. > 60 years)
Radiologic	20–30 Gy in patients with bulky adenopathy outside chest region
Complementary	Treating underlying immunodeficiency in HIV-positive patients

Prevention/management of complications
- **Myelosuppression:** there is a high incidence of grade III and IV neutropenia with ABVD; however, patients rarely have neutropenic fever and sepsis. Patients should be counselled regarding increased risk of infections during this period.

- **Bleomycin-related pulmonary toxicity:** risk factors include older age, bleomycin dose, pulmonary irradiation, and history of smoking or lung disease. Use of growth factors has been shown to increase the incidence of pulmonary toxicity and hence NCCN guidelines do not recommend the use of growth factors. Pulmonary function tests should be repeated if clinical or radiologic evidence of pulmonary toxicity is present. Bleomycin should be discontinued if the patient's diffusing capacity of the lungs for carbon monoxide (DLCO) drops more than 50% from baseline. They should not be rechallenged with bleomycin.
- **Cardiovascular toxicity:** mediastinal irradiation and anthracycline-based chemotherapy are the two major risk factors. It is usually observed 5–10 years after completion of treatment. Aggressive management of cardiovascular risk factors (i.e. better control of BP, diabetes, hypercholesterolemia, etc.) is strongly recommended.
- **Secondary malignancies:** lung and breast cancer are the two most common secondary solid tumors (overall cumulative risk of 2%). Low dose chest CT should be considered for patients at increased risk (i.e. history of chest irradiation, and smoking). Annual breast screening with mammography and MRI beginning no later than 8–10 years after completion or at age 40 (whichever occurs earlier) is recommended for women who received chest or axillary radiation.
- Patients are also at an increased risk of developing NHL (1.5% at 15 years) and leukemia (1% at 15 years).
- **Hypothyroidism:** reported in about 50% of long-term survivors. Thyroid function tests should be carried out at least annually, especially in patients treated with radiotherapy to the neck.
- **Fertility:** cryoconservation should be offered to all patients undergoing chemotherapy. Gonadal dysfunction is significantly less common with ABVD compared to the BEACOPP regimen which leads to permanent infertility in most cases.
- Annual influenza vaccination.

CLINICAL PEARLS
- Most patients require 2–6 cycles of ABVD chemotherapy +/- ISRT depending on their stage.
- Interim PET is helpful in making further treatment decisions and provides prognostic information.
- Support with growth factors is not routinely recommended with ABVD given the increased incidence of bleomycin-induced pulmonary toxicity.

Special populations
Pregnancy
- HL is the fourth most common type of malignancy occurring during pregnancy.
- Treatment is avoided during the first trimester. ABVD is generally considered safe in the second and third trimesters. Treatment is delayed until after delivery when possible.
- Full-term delivery in all patients should be the goal. Premature delivery is more common in patients who received chemotherapy during pregnancy.

Elderly
- 15–20% of all HL occurs in patients older than 60 years of age. These patients have a worse prognosis and often have comorbid conditions and impaired performance status.
- Bleomycin should be used with caution and is sometimes omitted in older patients due to higher incidence of pulmonary toxicity.
- ABVD is the standard therapy for patients who can tolerate all four drugs.

Other

- Patients with HIV-associated HL should be treated with an ABVD-based regimen along with HAART.
- They have slightly lower complete remission rates and 5-year OS and PFS rates are lower (76% and 71% than the general population based on Phase II Spanish Trial).
- The immunologic response to antiretroviral therapy has a positive impact on OS and PFS.
- If the patient is on a ritonavir-based HAART regimen, monitor for increased chemotherapy toxicity due to drug–drug interactions.

Prognosis

BOTTOM LINE/CLINICAL PEARLS

- Patients with HL disease have a very good prognosis: >90% in early stage disease and >75% in patients presenting with advanced disease achieve long term remission.
- Interim PET (i.e. PET at the end of two cycles of ABVD) has been shown to be a good prognostic marker. Patients with PET positivity at the end of two cycles have higher chances of relapse and decreased PFS over the next 2 years.
- Brentuximab vedotin consolidation after ASCT in patients with relapsed or refractory disease has been shown to improve PFS and OS.

Natural history of untreated disease

- Initial spread of disease is through the lymphatic tissue network, involving adjacent lymph nodes first.
- In the advanced stage, it can extend to the adjacent organs and disseminate to spleen, bone marrow, and other organs.
- If the disease is left untreated, the life expectancy is approximately 1-2 years with less than 5% of patients alive at 5 years.
- NLPHL usually develops with solitary lymph node involvement. It spreads slowly and responds well to radiation therapy. Relapses are common but the disease is rarely fatal.

Prognosis for treated patients

- Patients with HL generally respond well to treatment, with patients presenting with stage IV disease having OS of approximately 70% at 5 years.
- Prognostic factors have been mentioned earlier. In addition, patients who received chest radiation or mediastinal radiation as part of initial therapy have an increased incidence of secondary solid tumors as well as cardiopulmonary toxicities.

Follow-up tests and monitoring

- General consensus guidelines recommend follow-up with history and physical examination every 3–6 months for the first 1–2 years, every 6–12 months for next 3 years, and then annually.
- It is acceptable to obtain a CT scan once during the first 12 months and then as clinically indicated.
- Patients should be counselled regarding long-term side effects.

Guidelines
National society guidelines

Title	Source	Date and weblink
Hodgkin Lymphoma	National Comprehensive Cancer Network	2019 http://www.nccn.org/professionals/physician_gls/ f_guidelines.asp#hodgkin
Adult Hodgkin Lymphoma Treatment	National Cancer Institute	2019 https://www.cancer.gov/types/lymphoma/hp/adult-hodgkin-treatment-pdq#section/all

International society guidelines

Title	Source and comments	Date and weblink
German Hodgkin Study Group	Prefer BEACOPP vs. ABVD as upfront therapy in patients <60 years of age	2019 https://en.ghsg.org/
European Organization for Research and Treatment of Cancer	Age ≤50 is considered an unfavorable factor in early stage disease Preference to BEACOPP in younger patients over ABVD	2015 http://www.eortc.org/research-groups/ lymphoma-group/

Evidence

Type of evidence	Comment	Date and weblink
RCT	GHSG HD 10 trial **Comment:** Concluded that two cycles of ABVD + 20cGy ISRT is effective treatment for patients with a very favorable presentation of early stage disease with no risk factors	2010 http://www.nejm.org/doi/full/10.1056/ NEJMoa1000067
RCT	NCIC HD 6 trial **Comment:** ABVD alone is a reasonable treatment option in early stage patients with favorable disease who are PET negative after 2–3 cycles of ABVD	2005 http://jco.ascopubs.org/content/23/21/4634.long
RCT	UK RAPID Trial/ EORTC H10 trial **Comment:** Evaluated the importance of interim PET in early stage favorable disease	2012 http://abstracts.hematologylibrary.org/cgi/content-embargo/abstract/ashmtg;120/21/547 http://jco.ascopubs.org/content/32/12/1188.long
RCT	GHSG HD 11 **Comment:** Four cycles of ABVD with IFRT is standard treatment for early stage unfavorable disease	2010 http://jco.ascopubs.org/content/28/27/4199.long

Additional material for this chapter can be found online at:
www.wiley.com/go/oh/mountsinaioncology

This includes advice for patients, a case study, ICD codes, and
multiple choice question.

CHAPTER 32

Primary Central Nervous System Lymphoma

Rebecca M. Brown and Adília Hormigo
Icahn School of Medicine at Mount Sinai, New York, NY, USA

OVERALL BOTTOM LINE
- Primary central nervous system lymphoma (PCNSL) is an aggressive infiltrative high grade neoplasm of the brain, spinal cord, eyes, and/or leptomeninges formed of extranodal non-Hodgkin lymphoma cells.
- PCNSL can occur in immunocompetent patients, but is more commonly associated with AIDS, congenital immunodeficiencies, or in post-transplant patients on immunosuppression.
- PCNSL appears as a homogenously enhancing lesion on MRI of the brain in immunocompetent patients, but definitive diagnosis is through stereotactically guided needle biopsy. Additional studies are necessary to rule out an alternate primary source.
- Gold standard treatment is high dose methotrexate-based chemotherapy ± radiotherapy.

Background
Definition of disease
PCNSL is a non-Hodgkin extranodal lymphoma located exclusively within the brain, leptomeninges, spinal cord, and/or intraocular compartment (vitreous and/or retina) (Figure 32.1).

Disease classification
- Two demographics are associated with PCNSL: immunocompetent patients and immunocompromised patients (congenital immunodeficiency, AIDS, or immunosuppressive therapy).
- HIV-infected patients and those on immunosuppressive therapy after organ transplant are most likely to have EBV associated PCNSL of the DLBCL type.
- Approximately 90% of all PCNSL is DLBCL-type, while the remaining 10% is classified as Burkitt lymphoma, T-cell lymphoma, or poorly characterized lymphoma with features of DLBCL and Burkitt lymphoma.

Incidence/prevalence
- Annual incidence is 0.44 per 100 000 people, with an estimated 1272 new cases in the USA per year.
- Overall incidence peaked in 1996, corresponding roughly to the highest incidence of AIDS. PCNSL occurs in 2–6% of AIDS patients and HIV infection confers a 3600-fold increased risk.

Mount Sinai Expert Guides: Oncology, First Edition. Edited by William K. Oh and Ajai Chari.

- Incidence in the >64 year age group has continued to rise, potentially as a result of improved diagnostic techniques.
- Immunocompetent patients are most commonly affected between 50 and 70 years of age.

Etiology
- Precise oncogenic mechanisms have yet to be described.
- There is an association with CD4+ T-cell leukopenia, or immunodeficiency with concurrent EBV infection.

Pathology/pathogenesis
- The origin is unknown. Possibilities include: (i) it develops *de novo* in the brain from normal lymphoid cells that have migrated in; (ii) neoplasm forms in the periphery but has a particular tropism for the brain; or (iii) neoplasm forms in the periphery but only persists in the brain where it is protected from antineoplastic defenses.
- The route of entry is also unknown. A lymphatic-like system (glymphatic system) has recently been identified in the CNS, but its role in PCNSL is unclear.

Predictive/risk factors

Risk factor	Risk
Age	Risk increases with age, with a peak at 75–84 years (incidence 2.08 per 100 000 individuals)
AIDS	>3000× increased risk of PCNSL
Congenital immunodeficiency • Ataxia telangiectasia • Wiskott–Aldrich syndrome • Common variable immunodeficiency • Severe combined immunodeficiency	~4% increased risk of PCNSL
Post-transplant patients or patients undergoing immunosuppressive therapy • Renal patients are at greater risk than lung, heart, or gastrointestinal transplant patients	Occurs in 1–2% renal transplant recipients, and 2–7% cardiac, lung, and liver recipients. Possible association with mycophenolate mofetil

Prevention

BOTTOM LINE/CLINICAL PEARLS
- Maintenance of normal CD4 levels >350 k has been demonstrated to prevent PCNSL in HIV+ individuals.
- No interventions are known to prevent PCNSL for patients with genetic immunodeficiencies.

Diagnosis (Algorithm 32.1)

BOTTOM LINE/CLINICAL PEARLS
- Neurologic signs and symptoms depend on tumor site, and typically progress over weeks to months.
- Lesions are hypointense in T1, hyperintense in T2, and show homogenous contrast enhancement and restricted diffusion on brain MRI in immunocompetent patients (Figure 32.2).

- In AIDS/organ transplant patients, tumors are frequently ring-enhancing.
- PCNSL tumors are usually supratentorial and periventricular, and can cross the corpus callosum.
- After brain imaging suggestive of PCNSL, lumbar puncture and ocular slit lamp examination are performed. Results of these ancillary studies can confirm the diagnosis (a positive cerebrospinal fluid [CSF] cytology or vitreous biopsy), avoiding brain biopsy. CT chest/abdomen/pelvis or PET imaging and bone marrow biopsy are required to exclude the possibility of a systemic lymphoma with secondary brain involvement.

Algorithm 32.1 Diagnosis of primary CNS lymphoma (PCNSL). Investigation and diagnosis are similar for immunocompromised and immunocompetent patients. It is important to exclude toxoplasmosis in the AIDS patient. If ocular pathology or CSF is positive for monoclonal lymphomatous cells, a brain biopsy can be avoided

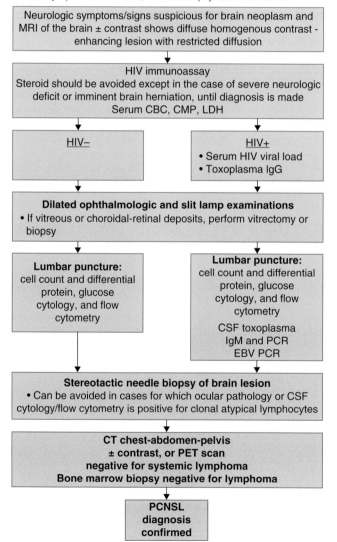

Neurologic symptoms/signs suspicious for brain neoplasm and MRI of the brain ± contrast shows diffuse homogenous contrast - enhancing lesion with restricted diffusion

↓

HIV immunoassay
Steroid should be avoided except in the case of severe neurologic deficit or imminent brain herniation, until diagnosis is made
Serum CBC, CMP, LDH

HIV–

HIV+
- Serum HIV viral load
- Toxoplasma IgG

Dilated ophthalmologic and slit lamp examinations
- If vitreous or choroidal-retinal deposits, perform vitrectomy or biopsy

Lumbar puncture:
cell count and differential
protein, glucose
cytology, and flow
cytometry

Lumbar puncture:
cell count and differential
protein, glucose
cytology, and flow
cytometry

CSF toxoplasma
IgM and PCR
EBV PCR

Stereotactic needle biopsy of brain lesion
- Can be avoided in cases for which ocular pathology or CSF cytology/flow cytometry is positive for clonal atypical lymphocytes

**CT chest-abdomen-pelvis
± contrast, or PET scan
negative for systemic lymphoma
Bone marrow biopsy negative for lymphoma**

**PCNSL
diagnosis
confirmed**

Differential diagnosis

Differential diagnosis	Features
Brain abscess	Ring-enhancing lesion with central T2 flair hypointensity. Core is bright on DWI and dark on ADC. MR spectroscopy may show a high succinate peak. Headache occurs in ~70% of patients and fever in <50%
Cerebral tuberculomas	Round, homogenously enhancing or ring-enhancing lesions
Chronic lymphocytic inflammation with pontine perivascular enhancement responsive to steroids (CLIPPERS)	Subacute progressive brainstem signs. Pontine + cerebellar punctate and curvilinear T2 hyperintense contrast-enhancing lesions
Glioma	Glioblastoma is usually heterogeneously contrast-enhancing on MRI
Metastases	Well circumscribed, contrast-enhancing lesions, often multiple, extensive surrounding edema
Multiple sclerosis (MS) and acute demyelinating encephalomyelitis (ADEM)	Tumefactive MS lesions are classically incomplete/horseshoe-shaped and ring-enhancing on MRI. CSF oligoclonal bands are <50% sensitive in tumefactive MS
Sarcoidosis	Numerous <5 mm contrast-enhancing lesions on MRI in the basal meninges involving apposing brain parenchyma ± cranial nerves
Toxoplasmosis	Common in AIDS. Ring-enhancing lesions on MRI. Uptake is decreased in SPECT, versus increased uptake in PCNSL

Typical presentation
- Weeks to months of headache, cognitive and personality changes, and/or decreased level of alertness.
- Seizures are uncommon (10%).
- Patients with ocular lymphoma may complain of "floaters."

Clinical diagnosis
History
- Headache, personality changes, and/or focal signs such as progressive lateralized weakness.
- History of HIV/AIDS or congenital immunodeficiency.
- Use of immunosuppressant agents.
- Painless blurry vision and/or floaters in patients with ocular lymphoma.

Physical examination
- A careful neurologic examination may reveal cognitive or focal neurologic deficits.
- Lymph node and testicular examinations to search for signs of systemic lymphoma.

Useful clinical decision rules and calculators
- On presentation, 30–40% of immunocompetent patients present with a solitary lesion whereas 90–100% of AIDS patients have multiple lesions.
- Supratentorial lesions are nine times more common than brainstem lesions, with the most common location being periventricular.

- Two-thirds of patients have detectable tumor cells in their CSF.
- 15% of patients with brain PCNSL have concurrent or preceding ocular lymphoma, whereas 60–90% of patients with intraocular lymphoma subsequently develop brain PCNSL.

Disease severity classification
- Indicators of worse prognosis are age >60 years, immunocompromise, and comorbid health conditions at diagnosis.

Laboratory diagnosis
List of diagnostic tests
- **Serum:** CBC, basic metabolic panel (BMP), LDH, CD4 count, HIV 1 and 2 screening, and HIV viral load if HIV test is positive.
- **Bone marrow biopsy:** to rule out systemic disease.
- **Lumbar puncture:** CSF protein >50 mg/dL, normal to low-normal glucose, 50% pleiocytosis (atypical/reactive lymphocytes), toxoplasma serology and EBV PCR+ in immunocompromised patients. Cytology and flow cytometry are informative in only 15–20% of studies. Therefore, lumbar puncture may be repeated two more times. Heavy-chain gene rearrangement analysis can be informative. Elevated CSF LDH and β2-microglobulin support the diagnosis.
- **For intraocular PCNSL:** vitrectomy/chorioretinal biopsy demonstrating IL10+ lymphomatous cells (or IL10 : IL6 ratio >1).
- **For brain PCNSL:** stereotactic needle biopsy with pathology showing highly mitotic, angiocentric, densely cellular, atypical lymphocytes.

Lists of imaging techniques
- MRI +/− contrast: demonstrates an infiltrative, homogenously enhancing (immunocompetent) versus ring-enhancing (immunocompromised) lesion, typically periventricular. Lesions are bright on DWI. Rare necrosis/hemorrhage.
- Brain SPECT or PET can distinguish between AIDS-associated toxoplasmosis and lymphoma.
- Slit lamp ophthalmologic examination may show vitreous or subretinal lymphoma cell infiltration.
- CT chest/abdomen/pelvis or whole body PET scan to rule out systemic disease.

Potential pitfalls/common errors made regarding diagnosis of disease
- Do not administer steroids prior to biopsy, except in life-threatening brain herniation. Tumors are exquisitely responsive to even low doses, which can severely compromise diagnosis.
- Always perform a slit lamp examination to investigate for ocular lymphoma, whether or not visual complaints are present.

Treatment (Algorithm 32.2)
Treatment rationale
- **DLBCL, Burkitt lymphoma, T-cell lymphoma subtypes:**
  - First line: high dose methotrexate (HD-MTX) ≥3.5 g/m^2 polychemotherapy regimen. Rituximab is added to the regimen for DLBCL.
  - Second line: consider whole brain radiation therapy (WBRT) and/or non-MTX-based chemotherapy.
- **AIDS-associated PCNSL:** HAART in addition to HD-MTX based regimen +/− WBRT.

Algorithm 32.2 Management of PCNSL. HD-MTX-based chemotherapy is the primary treatment modality. Dose adjustment may be made for patients with CKD stage 2–3 (GFR 30–90). For patients with CKD stage 4–5 (GFR <30), MTX may need to be omitted in favor of an alternate agent. Patients with poor functional status should receive MTX monotherapy because of the risk of chemotoxicity. WBRT and ASCT are alternatives that can be reserved for refractory or recurrent tumors, or in young, otherwise healthy patients. Ocular involvement is treated with intraocular MTX or rituximab, or ocular radiation

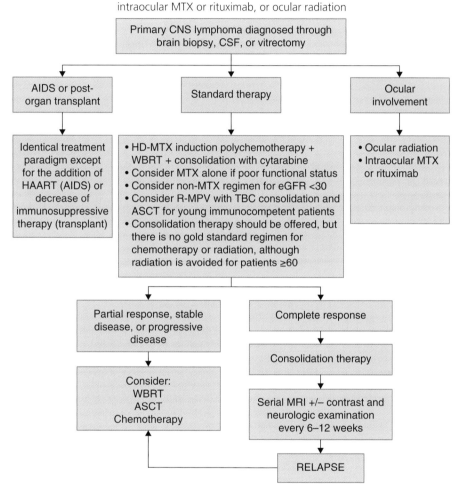

When to hospitalize
- Administration of the MTX-based chemotherapy regimen.
- Neutropenic fever.
- Suspected infection of the Ommaya reservoir.

Managing the hospitalized patient
- Daily CBC, BMP, and serum MTX levels.
- Monitor fluid balance, urine pH, and more intensive hydration and leucovorin rescue 24 hours after MTX.

Table of treatment (see also Figure 32.3)

Treatment	Comments
Medical	
Brain PCNSL: • HD-MTX-based regimen is gold standard R-MPV induction (rituximab, HD-MTX, procarbazine, vincristine) → TBC regimen (thiotepa, busulfan, and cyclophosphamide), ASCT Intraocular lymphoma: • Intravitreal MTX or rituximab Relapse/refractory PCNSL: no gold standard therapy. Consider RT AIDS-PCNSL: start HAART in addition to standard chemotherapy Primary leptomeningeal lymphomatosis: intrathecal MTX-based chemotherapy in addition to systemic chemotherapy	HD-MTX regimen can be followed by consolidation with cytarabine or sequential induction with thiotepa, cyclophosphamide, and busulfan and ASCT instead of WBRT High dose steroid monotherapy alone causes a striking clinical and radiographic improvement over weeks to months followed by tumor recurrence A phase II trial of R-MPV induction, TBC consolidation, and ASCT resulted in improved survival (see section on Evidence). BTK inhibitors and IMiDs can be used
Surgical	
	Consider for large life-threatening lesions associated with brain herniation
Radiologic	
Whole brain radiation therapy (WBRT): 30 doses of 1.5 Gy	High risk of dementia and ataxia in patients >60 years old Sometimes included in consolidation after HD-MTX-based chemotherapy
Psychologic	
	Neuropsychiatric testing before and after chemotherapy can identify neurotoxic sequelae
Other	
ASCT	See Medical treatment

Prevention/management of complications
- In patients with serosal fluid collections (e.g. pericardial effusion, pleural effusion, ascites), there is an increase in the volume of distribution but no change in clearance of MTX, which can cause toxicity.
- During HD-MTX, avoid drugs that delay MTX clearance (e.g. NSAIDs, co-trimoxazole, pencillins).
- Screen for nephrotoxicity, myelosuppression, mucositis, and deep venous thrombosis.
- MTX can cause pneumonitis and leukoencephalopathy.
- Dexamethasone should be tapered as tolerated.
- Chemotherapy-associated delayed neurotoxicity including leukoencephalopathy with progressive memory loss, ataxia, and incontinence can sometimes be improved by placing a ventriculoperitoneal shunt.

> **CLINICAL PEARLS**
> - The mainstay of treatment for PCNSL is a polychemotherapy regimen based on HD-MTX.
> - Surgery is rarely indicated unless the lesion causes brain herniation and imminent death.
> - WBRT has the potential to improve survival in young adults but is highly associated with neurocognitive impairment.
> - Intrathecal chemotherapy using an Ommaya reservoir should be reserved for patients with proven leptomeningeal lymphomatosis defined as characteristic MRI findings or neoplastic cells identified in CSF.
> - ASCT can be considered for patients in the <60 year age range.

Special populations

Pregnancy
- Treatment is determined on an individualized basis. Patients diagnosed during pregnancy with significant neurologic impairments may opt for early delivery or elective termination of pregnancy (based on gestational age and patient preference) so that cytotoxic chemotherapy can be administered.

Children
- PCNSL is exceedingly rare in children. Chemotherapy-based regimens are recommended.

Elderly
- Elderly patients are at higher risk of neurocognitive sequelae of treatment and omission of WBRT is indicated.

Others
- AIDS patients:
  - Start HAART to reconstitute the immune system.
  - Immune reconstitution syndrome is rare but can occur.
  - HD-MTX-based regimens can improve response rates.
- Patients with post-transplant lymphoproliferative disorder with PCNSL can be treated similarly to immunocompetent patients with the additional recommendation of decreasing the dosage of immunosuppressive therapies.

Prognosis

> **BOTTOM LINE/CLINICAL PEARLS**
> - Prognosis is best for patients <60 years old with a high Karnofsky Performance Score (KPS) score at diagnosis.
> - Rapid response to chemotherapy correlates with longer survival.
> - AIDS-associated PCNSL has a poorer prognosis.

Natural history of untreated disease
- Untreated patients, whether immunocompromised or immunocompetent, have a median survival of ~2.5 months.

Prognosis for treated patients

- Average 1-year and 5-year survival in immunocompetent individuals receiving standard therapy was 76% and 37% in a retrospective study.
- Prognosis is poorer for AIDS-associated PCNSL: 25% 2-year survival.
- 2-year PFS is dependent on treatment regimen, but ranges between 30% and 75%, with 2-year OS of 40–81%.
- The most reliable predictors of poor survival include increasing age and low KPS.
- All patients with intraocular lymphoma eventually develop brain lesions.

Follow-up tests and monitoring

- Patients should be screened with a neurologic examination and MRI +/– contrast 1 month after completing therapy and then every 2 months for the first year. Further screening decisions should be made on an individual basis.

Reading list

Abrey LE, Ben-Porat L, Panageas KS, et al. Primary central nervous system lymphoma: the Memorial Sloan-Kettering Cancer Center prognostic model. J Clin Oncol 2006;24:5711–5715.

Abrey LE, Yahalom J, DeAngelis LM. Treatment for primary CNS lymphoma: the next step. J Clin Oncol 2000;18:3144–3150.

Campo E, Swerdlow SH, Harris NL, et al. The 2008 WHO classification of lymphoid neoplasms and beyond: evolving concepts and practical applications. Blood 2011;117:5019–5032.

Chan CC, Rubenstein JL, Coupland SE, et al. Primary vitreoretinal lymphoma: a report from an International Primary Central Nervous System Lymphoma Collaborative Group symposium. Oncologist 2011;16:1589–1599.

Gavrilovic IT, Hormigo A, Yahalom J, et al. Long-term follow-up of high-dose methotrexate-based therapy with and without whole brain irradiation for newly diagnosed primary CNS lymphoma. J Clin Oncol 2006;24:4570–4574.

González-Aguilar A, Soto-Hernández JL. The management of primary central nervous system lymphoma related to AIDS in the HAART era. Curr Opin Oncol 2011;23:648–653.

Korfel A, Schlegel U. Diagnosis and treatment of primary CNS lymphoma. Nature Rev Neurol 2013;9:317–327.

Hottinger AF1, Alentorn A, Hoang-Xuan K. Recent developments and controversies in primary central nervous system lymphoma. Curr Opin Oncol 2015;27:496–501.

Pels H, Schmidt-Wolf I, Glasmacher A, et al. Primary central nervous system lymphoma: results of a pilot and phase II study of systemic and intraventricular chemotherapy with deferred radiotherapy. J Clin Oncol 2003;21:4489–4495.

Suggested websites

National Cancer Institute, AIDS related lymphoma: http://www.cancer.gov/types/lymphoma/patient/aids-related-treatment-pdq

National Clinical Trials Database: https://clinicaltrials.gov/

Society for Neuro-Oncology: https://www.soc-neuro-onc.org/

PCNSL treatments: http://www.cancer.gov/types/lymphoma/hp/primary-cns-lymphoma-treatment-pdq

Guidelines
National society guidelines

Title	Source	Date and weblink
Central Nervous System Cancers Version 1.2015	National Comprehensive Cancer Network	2015 http://www.nccn.org/professionals/physician_gls/PDF/cns.pdf

International society guidelines

Title	Source	Date and weblink
Diagnosis and treatment of primary CNS lymphoma in immunocompetent patients: guidelines from the European Association for Neuro-Oncology	European Association for Neuro-Oncology	2015 https://www.ncbi.nlm.nih.gov/pubmed/26149884
Guidelines on the diagnosis and management of adult patients with primary CNS lymphoma (PCNSL) and primary intra-ocular lymphoma (PIOL)	British Society for Haematology British Committee for Standards in Haematology	2009 https://b-s-h.org.uk/media/16266/pcnsl_-bcsh-2007.pdf
Primary diffuse large B-cell lymphoma of the CNS	World Health Organization	2008 World Health Organization classification of tumours pathology and genetics of tumours of the haematopoietic and lymphoid tissues. IARC Press, Lyon: 2008, pp. 240–241

Evidence

Type of evidence	Title and comment	Date and weblink
RCT	Randomized phase III study of whole-brain radiotherapy for primary CNS lymphoma **Comment:** WBRT increased PFS but not OS, compared with chemotherapy alone	2015 https://www.ncbi.nlm.nih.gov/pubmed/25716362
RCT	R-MPV followed by high-dose chemotherapy with TBC and autologous stem-cell transplant for newly diagnosed primary CNS lymphoma **Comment:** Phase II study of 32 PCNSL patients treated with R-MPV followed by TBC and ASCT resulted in 81% 5-year PFS and OS	2015 https://www.ncbi.nlm.nih.gov/pmc/articles/PMC4342354
Retrospective review	Intensive chemotherapy with thiotepa, busulfan and cyclophosphamide and hematopoietic stem cell rescue in relapsed or refractory primary central nervous system lymphoma and intraocular lymphoma: a retrospective study of 79 cases **Comment:** R-MPV induction, BTC consolidation, and autologous stem cell transplant benefits some patients with refractory PCNSL	2012 https://www.ncbi.nlm.nih.gov/pmc/articles/PMC3487451

Images

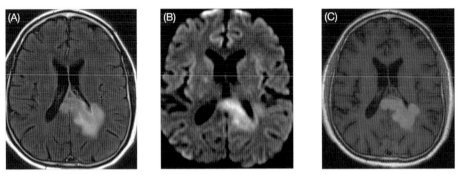

Figure 32.1 Primary central nervous system lymphoma (PCNSL) imaging. (A) T2 flair: left posterior infiltrative occipito-parietal hyperintensity. (B) Diffusion weighted imaging (DWI): the lesion demonstrates restricted diffusion. (C) PCNSL is homogenously enhancing on T1+ contrast.

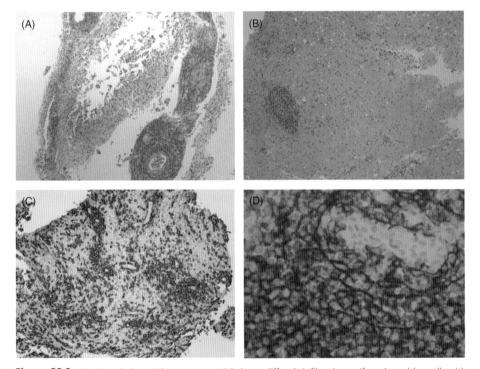

Figure 32.2 PCNSL pathology. (A) Low power H&E shows diffusely infiltrating uniform large blue cells with vascular cuffing that is typical of PCNSL. (B) Low power H&E with angiocentric clustering. (C) Low power CD20 stain. Positivity indicates diffuse large B-cell lymphoma (DLBCL) type. (D) High power CD20 stain. (Courtesy of Drs. Marco Hefti and Mary Fowkes, Mount Sinai Hospital, Icahn School of Medicine.) See color version on website.

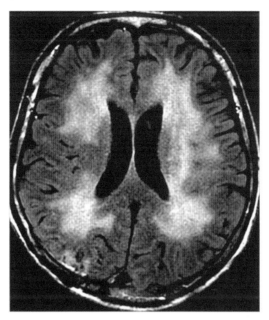

Figure 32.3 Methotrexate-induced leukoencephalopathy bilateral T2 hyperintensities involving primarily the white matter without mass effect.

Additional material for this chapter can be found online at:
www.wiley.com/go/oh/mountsinaioncology

This includes advice for patients, a case study, ICD codes, and multiple choice questions. The following image is available in color: Figure 32.2.

PART 3

Bone Marrow Transplant

Autologous Stem Cell Transplantation for Plasma Cell Disorders

Keren Osman

Mount Sinai Medical Center, New York, NY, USA

OVERALL BOTTOM LINE
- Autologous stem cell transplantation (ASCT) is a safe and effective treatment modality for both multiple myeloma and AL amyloidosis.
- Careful selection of patients for transplant results in the best outcomes for patients with these diseases.
- Both PFS and OS are enhanced for patients with plasma cell disorders who undergo ASCT.

Background
Definition of disease
Plasma cell disorders are diseases that result from an abnormal proliferation of a monoclonal population of plasma cells that may or may not secrete detectable levels of a monoclonal immunoglobulin or immunoglobulin fragment (paraprotein or M protein). The plasma cell disorders for which ASCT is a common treatment modality include multiple myeloma and AL amyloidosis.

Disease classification
- **Multiple myeloma:** a disease characterized by a clonal proliferation of plasma cells in the bone marrow which results in a wide variety of symptoms and clinical presentations. Destruction of bone can lead to bone pain from lytic lesions, hypercalcemia, and the replacement of normal marrow function can lead to anemia. Patients can also present with renal dysfunction from protein deposition in the kidneys.
- **AL amyloidosis:** a disease that results from the extracellular tissue deposition of fibrils composed of fragments of monoclonal light chains. Patients can have AL amyloidosis alone or in association with other plasma cell disorders such as multiple myeloma, MGUS, or Waldenström macroglobulinemia. Patients can present with a variety of symptoms such as, but not limited to, nephrotic range proteinuria, edema, hepatosplenomegaly, heart failure, and carpal tunnel syndrome.

Etiology
The etiology of both multiple myeloma and amyloidosis is not well known. Genetic factors, viral infections, exposure to radiation, organic chemicals such as benzene, herbicides, and insecticides have all been implicated but not definitively proven.

Mount Sinai Expert Guides: Oncology, First Edition. Edited by William K. Oh and Ajai Chari.
© 2019 John Wiley & Sons Ltd. Published 2019 by John Wiley & Sons Ltd.
Companion Website: www.wiley.com/go/oh/mountsinaioncology

Background

The landscape of treatment for plasma cell disorders has changed dramatically over the last few years with numerous new therapies and improved patient outcomes. As a result, the paradigm for therapy and the use of ASCT has evolved and continues to change with new discoveries. In addition, as the utilization of ASCT has increased, the demographics of this therapy have shifted. As a result, there are several considerations when deciding whether ASCT is suitable for a patient with plasma cell disease: timing, status of disease, optimal preparatory regimen, role of single versus double transplant, and recommendations for post-transplant follow-up.

Indications in AL amyloidosis

Patients should be assessed by a multidisciplinary team and use of risk stratification is employed to select patients for ASCT.

Eligibility criteria include:
- Histologic proof of amyloidosis
- Clonal plasma cell dyscrasia
- Performance status 0–2
- Left ventricular ejection fraction over 40%
- Oxygen saturations over 95% on air
- Supine blood pressure over 90 mmHg
- Troponin T <0.06 ng/mL
- N-terminal pro-brain natriuretic peptide (NT-proBP) <5000.

Indications in multiple myeloma

- Clonal plasma cell dyscrasia with symptomatic disease requiring treatment.
- Post induction chemotherapy usually incorporating a novel agent.
- Age up to 70 years (frailty index which takes into account cardiac, renal, hepatic, and pulmonary comorbidities is preferred to an absolute age cutoff).
- No major restrictions for renal function.
- No requirement for response to induction.

Procedures
Stem cell mobilization

Chemotherapy mobilization:
- Cyclophosphamide 1.5 g/m^2 on days 1 and 2.
- G-CSF 5 µg/kg daily on day +3 after initiation of cyclophosphamide and daily thereafter until mobilization procedure is complete.
  When white blood cell count is ≥10/µL, check blood CD34 levels:
- If CD34 is ≥10/µL, begin apheresis.
- If CD34 is <10/µL, continue G-CSF and measure CD34 daily. When CD34 is >10/µL, begin apheresis.
- If CD34 <10/µL and white blood cells are >1/µL for 3 days, start plerixafor. When CD34 is >10/µL, begin apheresis.
  Growth factor-only mobilization:
- G-CSF 10 µg/kg every day (day +1) and daily thereafter until mobilization procedure is complete. On day 4, measure CD34 levels.
  - If the goal is to collect for 1 transplant and day 4 CD34 is <10/µL, begin plerixafor and collect cells the next morning.
  - If the goal is to collect for >1 transplant and day 4 CD34 is <20/µL, begin plerixafor and collect cells the next morning.

Plerixafor dosing
- Renal clearance ≥50 mL/min: 0.24 mg/kg
- Renal clearance <50 mL/min: 0.16 mg/kg.

Dose never to exceed 24 mg.

Transplant procedure

Conditioning:
- Standard nonprotocol remains melphalan 200 mg/m^2 for fit patients.
- Melphalan 140 mg/m^2 if the patient is frail or serum creatinine ≥2.0 mg/dL.
  Procedural:
- Infusion of stem cells 18–24 hours post conditioning
  - Oral antibiotic prophylaxis: penicillin, levofloxacin, acyclovir, and fluconazole
  - Manage breakthrough fever of >38.5°C with vancomycin and cefepime until culture results are negative for 3 days or engraftment.

Timing

Multiple myeloma

Patients with newly diagnosed symptomatic multiple myeloma are treated with several cycles of induction chemotherapy, traditionally a triplet regimen with three active drugs. The goal is to achieve at least a partial remission prior to stem cell collection and ASCT. There has been much controversy over whether to proceed to ASCT immediately after collection of stem cells or wait until first relapse. Recent data from several different multicenter studies has confirmed that patients have a PFS advantage if they undergo ASCT immediately after induction chemotherapy and stem cell collection is complete. Thus, the current recommendation is to proceed to ASCT right after completion of induction chemotherapy and stem cell collection and not to wait for relapse of the disease.

Amyloidosis

Over the last 10 years, the OS of patients with AL amyloidosis has improved significantly, largely because of improvement in supportive care, access to novel chemotherapies, and better selection criteria for transplantation. A recent review was conducted comparing early with deferred ASCT for patients with AL amyloidosis who are transplant eligible. Transplantation was considered "early" if it took place within the first 90 days of stem cell collection. When comparing PFS and OS, early transplant improved PFS but OS was equivalent in both early and late transplant. Thus, the current recommendation is that patients may proceed to transplant at either time point.

Single or double transplant

- Tandem transplant was first demonstrated to improve OS in patients with multiple myeloma in 2003. Survival benefit was seen after extended follow-up in patients who did not achieve a very good partial response (VGPR) after the first transplant.
- A second transplant need not always be performed in tandem. The second transplant can be delayed until progression and becomes a useful salvage strategy. Thus, the recommendation is to collect stem cells for two or more transplants, therefore making a second mobilization procedure unnecessary. Second stem cell transplantation in relapsed myeloma can also be associated with superior OS and PFS compared with conventional chemotherapy if the response duration from the first transplant exceeds 18 months.
- Single and tandem transplants are both appropriate options for the management of myeloma. Collecting stem cells for a future salvage transplant is justifiable.

Complications

At time of infusion:
- Fever
- Chills
- Chest tightness
- Hypotension
- Cough.
  Early post infusion (weeks 1–4):
- Bacterial, viral, or fungal infections
- Nausea/vomiting
- Mucositis
- Need for blood and platelet transfusions
- Diffuse alveolar hemorrhage (rare)
- Veno-occlusive disease of the liver (exceedingly rare).
  Late complications (months to years):
- Recurrence of the plasma cell disease (common)
- Myelodysplastic syndrome
- Secondary leukemia.

Maintenance therapy

Multiple myeloma
- Lenalidomide
- Bortezomib
- Lenalidomide/bortezomib for high risk patients.

Amyloidosis
- Patients not achieving a VGPR or CR after ASCT could be considered for further chemotherapy with bortezomib or immunomodulatory imide drugs (ImiDs) to improve response.
- Results of ongoing trials addressing bortezomib in induction and maintenance or consolidation are awaited.

Follow-up

Multiple myeloma, every 2–3 months
- Quantitative immunoglobulins plus quantitation of M protein (serum protein electrophoresis, free light chains (FLCs) +/– urine protein electrophoresis) at least every 3 months.
- CBC, differential, platelets.
- Blood, urea, nitrogen (BUN) test, creatinine, calcium.
- Immunofixation (serum/urine) to confirm complete response 2 or in select situations (relapse, MGUS associated with complete 2 response particularly after SCT, etc.).
- Bone survey annually or if symptomatic.
- Bone marrow biopsy as clinically indicated to confirm a complete remission, with testing for minimal residual disease an area of active research.
- Consider MRI as clinically indicated.
- Consider a PET/CT scan as clinically indicated.

Amyloidosis
Hematologic response: every 1–3 months:
- Monitoring of response with FLC or M-protein should be carried out every 1–3 months.

- Difference between the involved and uninvolved light chain (dFLC) should be used to monitor hematologic response as long as dFLC is >50 mg/L at diagnosis. The M protein can be used if >5 g/L.
Organ response: every 3–6 months:
- Electrocardiography (ECG)/echocardiography/NT-proBNP.
- Routine measurements of renal function, including creatinine clearance and 24-hour urine protein excretion and/or urine protein–creatinine ratio.
- Liver function tests or assessment of other organ function as indicated.

Special populations
Elderly
- In patients aged >70 years selected for transplant, the toxicity and outcomes are comparable to those found for younger patients.
- A frailty index should be applied which measures activities of daily living plus cardiac, renal, and hepatic comorbidities to identify a population with low risk of transplant-related complications. This is a more realistic approach to patient eligibility than age alone.

Renal dysfunction
- Maintain hydration to avoid renal failure.
- Avoid use of NSAIDs.
- Avoid gadolinium if creatinine ≥ 2 mg/dL.
- Avoid iodine IV contrast.
- Not a contraindication to transplant.
- Monitor for renal dysfunction with chronic use of bisphosphonates.

Dialysis
- Patients on dialysis are eligible for ASCT.
- Dialysis patients require a reduction in their conditioning dose of melphalan to 140 mg/m^2.
- Special attention should be paid to the increased risk of mucositis.
- Other medications should be adjusted accordingly.

Reading list
Suggested websites
Amyloidosis Foundation: http://www.amyloidosis.org/
Amyloidosis Support Groups: http://www.amyloidosissupport.org/
International Myeloma Foundation: https://myeloma.org/Main.action
Multiple Myeloma Research Foundation: https://www.themmrf.org/

Guidelines
National society guidelines

Title	Source	Date and weblink
Hematopoietic stem cell transplantation for multiple myeloma	American Society for Blood and Marrow Transplantation (ASBMT)	2015 http://tgapp.asbmt.org/#/article-content-hematopoietic-stem-cell-page

International society guidelines

Title	Source	Date and weblink
Diagnosis and investigation of AL amyloidosis	British Society for Haematology	2014 http://www.bcshguidelines.com/documents/Amyloid_2014.pdf

Evidence

Type of evidence	Title	Date and weblink
	Update on treatment of light chain amyloidosis	2014 https://www.ncbi.nlm.nih.gov/pmc/articles/PMC3912950/
	How we manage autologous stem cell transplantation for patients with multiple myeloma	2014 http://www.bloodjournal.org/content/124/6/882.long?sso-checked=true

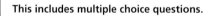

Additional material for this chapter can be found online at:
www.wiley.com/go/oh/mountsinaioncology

This includes multiple choice questions.

CHAPTER 34

Allogeneic Stem Cell Transplantation Overview

Parth R. Rao[1], Amir Steinberg[2], and Luis Isola[2]

[1] Geisinger Medical Center, Danville, PA, USA
[2] Icahn School of Medicine at Mount Sinai, New York, NY, USA

OVERALL BOTTOM LINE

- Allogeneic stem cell transplantation (AlloSCT) is a potentially curative treatment for leukemias, high risk and relapsed lymphomas, and certain benign hematologic conditions. This treatment transplants healthy hematopoietic stem cells from a matched donor after the elimination of diseased stem cells with the help of high dose consolidation chemotherapy.
- Development of large donor registries and advances in molecular methods to more accurately type donors, along with use of umbilical cord blood banks, have had a major role in the wider application of AlloSCT.
- Graft versus host disease (GVHD) is the leading cause of AlloSCT-related mortality.
- Patient survivorship is crucial as life expectancy post AlloSCT continues to improve as a result of accurately matched donors and better strategies in management of GVHD.

Background

- The first successful matched AlloSCT was performed in 1968 in an infant with X-linked immunodeficiency.
- The International Bone Marrow Transplant Registry (IBMTR) was formed in 1972 in Europe and then moved to the USA in 1980.
- Initially, only matched unrelated donor transplants were required to be reported to the Center for International Blood and Marrow Transplant Research (CIBMTR); however, the Stem Cell Transplant Outcomes Database was formed in 2007 after which all AlloSCTs were required to register through CIBMTR.
- The incidence of AlloSCTs is increasing in the USA, exceeding 8000 patients every year.
- The number of AlloSCTs continues to increase in elderly patients (>60 years), with around 15–20% of recipients in this age group, as a result of increased ability to use nonmyeloablative conditioning regimens in AlloSCT recipients.

Indications
Hematologic malignancies

- Acute myelogenous leukemia
  - Intermediate and high risk group in first complete remission (CR1)
    - All patients in CR2.

Mount Sinai Expert Guides: Oncology, First Edition. Edited by William K. Oh and Ajai Chari.
© 2019 John Wiley & Sons Ltd. Published 2019 by John Wiley & Sons Ltd.
Companion Website: www.wiley.com/go/oh/mountsinaioncology

- Chronic myelogenous leukemia
  - TKI intolerant/refractory in chronic phase
  - Accelerated as well as blast phase.
- Acute lymphoblastic leukemia
  - Standard as well as high risk group in CR1
  - All patients in CR2.
- Myelodysplastic syndromes (MDS)
  - High risk group and therapy-related MDS.
- Multiple myeloma
  - Refractory patients
  - Plasma cell leukemia
  - Relapse after autologous transplant.
- Myelofibrosis and myeloproliferative disorders.
- Relapsed/refractory Hodgkin lymphoma.
- Relapsed/refractory non-Hodgkin lymphoma.

Non-malignant conditions
- Aplastic anemia
- Sickle cell disease
- Beta-thalassemia
- Severe combined immune deficiency
- Paroxysmal nocturnal hemoglobinuria
- Refractory hemophagocytic syndrome
- Mast cell disorders
- Chronic granulomatous disease
- Wiskott–Aldrich syndrome.

Procedure
Donor selection
- Selection of donor is largely dependent on the matching of major histocompatibility complex (MHC) which mainly includes the HLA.
- The ideal donor is a matched sibling. Patients have better clinical outcomes as they have less incidence of acute and chronic graft versus host reaction.
- If a matched sibling cannot be found, a search would occur for a matched unrelated donor in the National Marrow Donor Program (NMDP) registry.
- Haploidentical transplants are increasing in number and involve the use of family members who share half-matched compatibility to the recipients.
- Children, parents, and half siblings are considered potential haploidentical donors.
- All potential donors undergo detailed history and physical assessment, basic blood testing as well as testing for HIV, hepatitis viruses, and cytomegalovirus infection.
- They must have normal liver, kidney, and cardiopulmonary function and should have the ability to tolerate general anesthesia if bone marrow is considered for stem collection.

Patient selection
- Patients who are considered for transplantation require in depth counseling regarding their current disease process, preparation for transplant including conditioning regimens, as well as a psychosocial assessment.

- Recipients undergo similar assessment to donors and in addition require disease-specific restaging, discussion regarding the potential impact on fertility, and options for fertility preservation.
- Some of the important factors that have consistently impacted the outcomes post-transplant are disease status at transplantation, donor type, patient's age, and comorbid conditions.

Donor cell procurement

- Collection of stem cells from bone marrow via aspiration is generally performed under regional or general anesthesia.
- Complications from bone marrow stem cell collection are rare and involve problems related to periprocedural anesthesia, bleeding, or infection.
- Donors may receive G-CSF prior to bone marrow collection to increase the yield.
- Historically, bone marrow was the source of stem cell procurement; however, with use of G-CSF and other mobilizing drugs like plerixafor, peripheral blood has become the most common source of stem cell procurement in the current era.
- Potential complications from G-CSF exposure include bone pain and, extremely rarely, splenic rupture.
- Cord blood is a source of stem cells that is obtained by collecting blood from umbilical cord and placenta after delivery of an infant.
- Usually, two umbilical cord units are used for most adult recipients, as the stem cell dose is relatively low in cord blood.

Conditioning regimens

- Types of conditioning regimen include myeloablative, reduced intensity, and nonablative.
- Myeloablative regimens aim to kill malignant cells and achieve adequate immunosuppression to prevent rejection of donor stem cells by the recipient.
- Examples of myeloablative regimens include total body irradiation (TBI) of 1200–1320 cGY plus cyclophosphamide/etoposide or a combination of cyclophosphamide and busulfan.
- Reduced intensity conditioning regimens that use lower doses of chemotherapy drugs and radiation have decreased the incidence of acute and chronic toxicity, and hence are typically used in patients with comorbid conditions or in elderly patients. Examples include combining fludarabine with melphalan or busulfan.
- Nonablative regimens are primarily used in indolent malignancies and nonmalignant conditions. Examples include fludarabine with TBI of 200 cGY.

Engraftment

- Engraftment of stem cells depends on a number of factors including use of conditioning regimen, underlying indication for AlloSCT, and source of stem cells.
- ANC recovery is defined as an ANC of $\geq 0.5 \times 10^9$/L for three consecutive laboratory values obtained on different days.
- Platelet recovery is defined as when the recipient's platelet count is $\geq 20 \times 10^9$/L seven days after platelet transfusion and is maintained for three consecutive laboratory values obtained on different days.
- Bone marrow stem cells usually engraft by 17–21 days, whereas peripheral blood stem cells (PBSCs) take the shortest time to engraft – around 7–14 days, likely because of higher stem cell dose.
- Cord blood stem cells may take up to 6 weeks to engraft.
- Patients receive G-CSF support until neutrophil recovery occurs.

Complications

Mucositis

- Mucositis is the most common complication of AlloSCT.
- Involvement of the gastrointestinal system can cause nausea, cramping, and diarrhea requiring parenteral nutrition.

Hepatic veno-occlusive disease

- Veno-occlusive disease (VOD) often occurs within the first 3 weeks of transplantation.
- Endothelial damage to hepatic sinusoids is the inciting event.
- Risk factors include underlying liver disease, elevated transaminases, and myeloablative regimens like busulfan, cyclophosphamide, and TBI.
- Patients usually present with painful hepatomegaly, fluid retention, and hyperbilirubinemia.
- Treatment is largely supportive.
- Preliminary trials using defibrotide, a polydeoxyribonucleotide with adenosine receptor agonist activity, have shown favorable results in patients with established VOD.
- Heparin and ursodiol have been shown to have a role in treatment; however, strong evidence to support their use is lacking.

Infection

- AlloSCT recipients are highly susceptible to infections given the deficiency of humoral as well as cell-mediated immunity.
- All AlloSCT recipients receive prophylaxis against bacterial, viral, fungal, and parasitic infections as standard of care.
- The incidence of bacterial infections is highest during the pre-engraftment period (i.e. within 1–2 months), when neutropenia and mucositis are common.
- Fungal and *Pneumocystis* pneumonia infections occur during the post engraftment period (i.e. from the third to fifth month).
- After the first 6 months, the frequency of invasive *Aspergillus* infection increases as a result of use of steroids for GVHD. See Chapter 37 for further details.

Graft versus host disease

- Acute GVHD (aGVHD) usually occurs within the first 100 days post-transplant.
- It can take place in up to 30% of AlloSCT.
- Incidence and severity of aGVHD correlates with extent of HLA disparity between donor and recipient.
- It is the most important cause of transplant-related mortality, morbidity, and diminished quality of life.
- Other risk factors include older age, alloimmunized donor, and less intense immunosuppression.
- Primary organs involved are skin, gastrointestinal system, or liver.
- The mainstay of treatment is steroids, which in turn can cause profound immunodeficiency, making the patient highly susceptible to life-threatening infections.
- Steroid refractory aGVHD responds poorly to second line therapy and is associated with high mortality.
- Chronic GVHD (cGVHD) can occur in up to 50% of patients.
- It usually occurs in patients with history of aGVHD; however, it can also take place *de novo*.
- Limited disease usually involves skin with no or minimal liver involvement whereas extensive disease, which includes other organ involvement, is associated with poor long-term survival.

- Treatment options include calcineurin inhibitors, and biologic agents like TNF-α inhibitors and photopheresis.
- Patients with cGVHD on long-term immunosuppressive treatment require penicillin prophylaxis to prevent infections from encapsulated organisms.

Transplantation-related lung injury

- The most common pulmonary complication is interstitial pneumonitis.
- Risk factors include prior lung injury from conditioning regimens and prior exposure to radiation therapy.
- Prompt treatment with steroids, after ruling out infectious causes, is indicated.
- Diffuse alveolar hemorrhage is a rare but potentially fatal post AlloSCT complication. Patients usually present with progressive dyspnea, significant hypoxia, and diffuse alveolar infiltrates.

Graft failure

- Graft failure is defined as failure to recover hematologic function or loss of bone marrow function after initial reconstitution.
- Factors known to increase risk include inadequate stem cell dose, degree of mismatch, inadequate immunosuppression, prior history of alloimmunization, and certain infections.
- It can take place within first 2 months of transplantation; however, late graft failure has been known to occur.
- Marrow and peripheral stem cells have a 1–2% rate of engraftment failure whereas the engraftment failure rate of cord blood approaches 10%.
- Initial treatment includes continuing support with G-CSF; however, infusion of additional stem cells, depending on the availability, may be required.

Patient survivorship post-transplant

Cardiovascular disease

- AlloSCT recipients are at higher risk of developing cardiovascular disease as well as worsening of known cardiovascular risk compared with an age-matched controlled general population.
- Risk factors include exposure to chemotherapy drugs like anthracyclines, high dose cyclophosphamide, exposure to TBI, and use of calcineurin inhibitors and steroids.
- Clinicians should have a high degree of suspicion for the development of heart failure in these patients.
- Close surveillance with ECG should be carried out as clinically indicated.

Respiratory disease

- cGVHD of lung can occur in up to 10% of patients and chronic lung disease accounts for 5% of nonrelapse mortality in AlloSCT recipients.
- Potential causes include exposure to TBI, chemotherapy drugs like bleomycin, and interstitial pneumonitis.
- Pulmonary function testing should be performed 6 months after AlloSCT as it is an important predictor of long-term lung impairment and mortality after allogeneic transplant.
- In addition to additional diagnostic investigation to search for definitive causes, patients with abnormal post-transplant pulmonary function testing should continue to be tested annually.

Liver disease

- AlloSCT patients can have an increased incidence of liver damage because of cGVHD, reactivation of hepatitis B or C, and iron overload from multiple blood transfusions.

- Patients with history of exposure of hepatitis B/C should have regular PCR levels checked as well as consideration for liver biopsy 8–10 years after AlloSCT to assess for cirrhosis, especially in patients with chronic hepatitis C.
- Plasma ferritin is used as a screening test for iron overload when clinically suspected.

Endocrine disorders

- AlloSCT recipients are at an increased risk for developing a number of endocrine disorders including diabetes mellitus, hypothyroidism, metabolic syndrome, osteoporosis, hypogonadism, and infertility.
- Recipient conditioning regimens like TBI increase the risk of hypothyroidism as well as hypogonadism.
- All AlloSCT recipients should have thyroid-stimulating hormone (TSH) checked 6–12 months after transplant and then on an annual basis.
- Steroids and calcineurin inhibitors used for treatment of cGVHD significantly increase the risk of diabetes mellitus in these patients.
- Bone density screening is recommended at 1 year post-transplant and repeated based on clinical condition.
- Most women remain infertile post-transplant; however, men can regain fertility and should be counseled regarding contraception and safe sexual practices.
- Sex hormone levels may be checked in clinically indicated cases and replacement therapy can be given 1 year after transplant.

Secondary malignancies

- The incidence of secondary malignancies is as high as 10–13% in AlloSCT patients.
- The most common secondary malignancies include skin neoplasms, head and neck cancer, non-Hodgkin lymphoma, and other solid tumor malignancies.
- The cumulative incidence of solid tumors in all transplant patients is 1–2% in the first 10 years and 3–4% in the next 10 years post-transplant.
- Risk factors include exposure to TBI, use of alkylating chemotherapeutic agents, and cGVHD.
- Incidence of breast cancer is increased especially in women who are young and had TBI as part of a conditioning regimen.
- Early mammography is recommended for women with a history of TBI, starting at age 25 or 8 years after radiation, whichever occurs later, but no later than age 40.
- Regular examination of oral cavity and thyroid should be performed. All patients should be educated on importance of sunscreen protection and regular skin examination.
- Post-transplant lymphoproliferative disorder (PTLD) occurs in approximately 1% of AlloSCT patients. It is driven by EBV infection and risk factors include having a HLA mismatched donor, use of antithymocyte globulin, and cGVHD. It requires reducing immunosuppression and treatment with rituximab.

Vaccinations

- All AlloSCT patients should be routinely vaccinated and revaccinated until they regain complete function of their immune system.
- Patients, especially those with history of cGVHD, are immunocompromised for a longer time and are highly susceptible to infections.
- Pneumococcal and influenza vaccine should be administered 3 months post AlloSCT, followed by international consensus guidelines for vaccinations for the general population.

- All other vaccines such as diphtheria, tetanus, and pertussis vaccine, *Hemophilus* influenza B, and hepatitis B vaccine can be given within 6–12 months post AlloSCT.
- Measles, mumps, and rubella (MMR) vaccine is not recommended in AlloSCT patients during first 24 months post AlloSCT, or those with cGVHD or with active immunosuppression. See Chapter 37 for further details.

Relapse after transplant

- Some patients may be eligible for donor lymphocyte infusions to elicit for graft versus tumor effect.
- A smaller proportion of the patients may be candidates for repeat or second transplantation.
- For patients who do not qualify for transplant, care must be individualized with strong consideration to enroll in clinical trials.
- Studies using chimeric antigen receptor-T cells show promise for their use as a potential adjunct or alternative, prior or post-transplant.

Reading list
Suggested websites
Bethematch.org
Cibmtr.org
Factwebsite.org

Additional material for this chapter can be found online at:
www.wiley.com/go/oh/mountsinaioncology

This includes advice for patients, a case study, ICD codes, and multiple choice questions.

CHAPTER 35

Allogeneic Stem Cell Transplantation for AML and MDS

Alla Keyzner

Icahn School of Medicine at Mount Sinai, New York, NY, USA

> **OVERALL BOTTOM LINE**
> - Allogeneic stem cell transplant (SCT) is the only curative treatment for myelodysplastic syndrome (MDS).
> - Patients with intermediate-2 and high risk MDS should undergo allogeneic SCT at the time of diagnosis.
> - Patients with high risk AML benefit from allogeneic SCT in the first remission.
> - Patients with relapsed favorable risk AML can be cured by undergoing allogeneic SCT in the second remission.

Background
Definition of disease
- The MDS is a malignant hematopoietic stem cell disorder characterized by ineffective hematopoiesis in the setting of multilineage dysplasia.
- AML is a group of myeloid hematopoietic neoplasms characterized by clonal proliferation and reduced differentiation into mature cell types.

Disease classification
- Both MDS and AML diseases are classified using the WHO classification system based on combination of morphologic features, immunophenotype, genetic abnormalities, and clinical presentation.
- Cytogenetic and molecular genetic data are used to risk stratify patients into favorable, intermediate, and adverse risk groups allowing tailoring of therapeutic options including allogeneic SCT.

Etiology
See Chapters 25 and 27.

Pathology/pathogenesis
See Chapters 25 and 27.

Prevention
Screening
- Patients treated with radiation and/or cytotoxic agents, especially alkylating agents and topoisomerase II inhibitors, should be monitored for development of cytopenias.

Mount Sinai Expert Guides: Oncology, First Edition. Edited by William K. Oh and Ajai Chari.
© 2019 John Wiley & Sons Ltd. Published 2019 by John Wiley & Sons Ltd.
Companion Website: www.wiley.com/go/oh/mountsinaioncology

Diagnosis
Indications
- High risk MDS (intermediate-2/high risk disease by the International Prognostic Scoring System, IPSS).
- Intermediate-1 risk disease by IPSS with evidence of disease progression.
- Therapy-related MDS.
- Very poor and poor risk groups of AML based on ELN modified classification in first remission.
- Intermediate risk AML with evidence of MRD in first complete remission (CR1).
- Core binding factor AML with c-kit mutation.
- Relapsed AML.

History
During evaluation for allogeneic SCT, the clinician should enquire about:
- Symptoms of heart, lung, liver, and kidney disease.
- History of psychiatric disease.
- Substance abuse.
- Available support system identified.
- Detailed family history.
- History and number of units of packed red blood cells and/or platelet transfusions.

Physical examination
- Comprehensive physical examination including liver and spleen size.

Useful clinical decision rules and calculators
- Revised IPSS score is used to risk stratify patients with MDS.
- Cytogenetic and molecular data are used to risk stratify patients with AML into favorable, intermediate-1, intermediate-2, and adverse risk groups of patients.
- Stem Cell Transplant Comorbidity Index is used to help predict nonrelapse mortality and OS following allogeneic SCT.

Disease severity classification
- Disease Risk Index (DRI) is a useful tool to help assign patients into four OS groups (low, intermediate, high, and very high risk) based on disease type and status of the disease at the time of transplantation (Table 35.1).

Laboratory diagnosis
List of diagnostic tests
- Bone marrow aspirate and biopsy.
- CBC with differential, CMP, and coagulation studies.
- Infectious disease testing.
- HLA typing.
- Anti-HLA antibodies.

Lists of imaging techniques
- Echocardiography.
- Pulmonary function tests.

Table 35.1 Disease Risk Index (DRI).

Disease	Stage	DRI group	2-year OS (%)	95% CI
AML favorable cytogenetics CR		Low	66	63–68
AML intermediate cytogenetics CR		Intermediate	51	50–52
Low risk MDS adverse cytogenetics	Early	Intermediate		
Low risk MDS intermediate cytogenetics	Advanced	Intermediate		
High risk MDS intermediate cytogenetics	Early	Intermediate		
AML favorable cytogenetics	Advanced	High	33	31–35
High risk MDS intermediate cytogenetics	Advanced	High		
AML adverse cytogenetics CR		High		
High risk MDS adverse cytogenetics	Advanced	High		
Low risk MDS adverse cytogenetics	Advanced	High		
AML adverse cytogenetics	Advanced	Very high	23	20–27

Advanced stage refers to induction failure or active relapse.
(Source: Adapted from Armand et al. 2014.)

Potential pitfalls/common errors made regarding diagnosis of disease

Referral to transplant center is delayed until the patient is in remission.

Treatment

- All patients should be offered participation in a clinical trial when available.
- All willing and eligible siblings should undergo HLA typing to identify an HLA-matched donor.
- An unrelated donor search is performed for patients who lack an HLA-matched donor.
- Patients who do not have an HLA-matched related or unrelated donor should be evaluated for an alternative source of stem cells such as umbilical cord blood or haploidentical donor.
- Patients under the age of 55 years with no significant comorbidities should be offered myeloablative allogeneic SCT.
- Older patients over the age of 55 or patients with significant comorbidities should be offered reduced intensity allogeneic SCT.
- Maintenance therapy with sorafenib should be considered in FLT3 positive patients.
- Use of hypomethylating agents as maintenance therapy in the post-transplant setting is an area of ongoing clinical investigation.

When to hospitalize

- Patients are hospitalized during the early part of transplantation during the conditioning preparative regimen through engraftment of donor cells.
- Patients can be discharged upon resolution of neutropenia, lack of active infection or active GVHD, with close follow-up for assessment of symptoms and signs of GVHD, infectious symptoms, transfusion needs, and transplant-related toxicities.
- Patients may require re-hospitalization if they developed transplant-related complications, such as GVHD or infection, or relapsed disease.

Table of treatment

Treatment	Comments
Conservative	
Antimicrobial prophylaxis: • Acyclovir 800 mg twice daily to prevent herpes zoster • Levofloxacin 500 mg/day • Posaconazole 300 mg daily to prevent invasive fungal infection • Bactrim 1 DS MWF or atovaquone 1500 mg/day should be started on day +30 to prevent PCP infection	Prophylactic antimicrobials start on Day 0 • Renally dosed • During neutropenic period

Growth factor support:
• Filgrastim 5 µg/kg/day
Transfusion:
• All products should be leukoreduced and irradiated
• Patients who are CMV negative should receive CMV negative blood products
• Transfusion parameters:
  ◦ Hemoglobin <7.0 g/dL
  ◦ Platelets <10 K, or <20 K if febrile
  ◦ If patient is bleeding transfuse for platelets <50 K
	• Starts on day + 7

Medical	

Myeloablative preparative regimens:
• Bu/Cy: busulfan IV 12.8 mg/kg administered over 4 days with cyclophosphamide 120 mg/kg administered over 2 days
• Flu/Bu: fludarabine 120–180 mg/m^2 and busulfan IV 12.8 mg/kg each administered over 4 days
• Cy/TBI: cyclophosphamide 120 mg/kg total dose administered over 2 days with total body irradiation (TBI 12 Gy) administered over 4 days
 	
Reduced intensity regimens:
• Flu/Mel: fludarabine (125–150 mg/m^2 total dose) administered over 5 days with melphalan (140 mg/m^2) administered over 2 days
• Flu/Bu: fludarabine (150–160 mg/m^2 total dose) administered over 4–5 days with busulfan IV (6.4–8 mg/kg) administered over 2–3 days
Immunosuppression (IS):Combination of calcineurin inhibitor (CI) (tacrolimus or cyclosporine) with methotrexate:
• Tacrolimus CIV 0.02 mg/kg/24 hours– goal trough level 5–10
	• Cytoxan administered prior to busulfan is associated with decreased risk of hepatic sinusoidal obstruction syndrome.
	• Busulfan can be given IV or PO. IV administration is associated with more predictable pharmacokinetics and improved tolerance
	• All hepatotoxic drugs should be discontinued during busulfan administration and for 48 hours after completion
	• Hold acetaminophen on days of busulfan administration
	• Antiseizure prophylaxis with levetiracetam is administered 24 hours prior to start of busulfan and continues for 72 hours following its completion
	
	• IS drugs are dosed based on ideal body weight unless stated otherwise
	• Methotrexate is dosed based on actual body weight
	• IV to PO conversion:
	  ◦ cyclosporine – 1 : 4
	  ◦ tacrolimus – 1 : 3
	• CIs interact with CYP450 inducers/inhibitors – requiring dose adjustment.
	• Tacrolimus adsorbs to IV tubing – level must be drawn from periphery or non-tacrolimus-containing line

(Continued)

(*Continued*)

Treatment	Comments

• Cyclosporine IV 1.5 mg/kg every 12 hours – goal trough level 200–400
• Methotrexate:
  • Full dose: 15 mg/m^2 on day 1; 10 mg/m^2 on days +3, 6, 11
  • Mini: 5 mg/m^2 on days +1, 3, 6, 11
Other IS drugs used:
• Mycophenolate 15 mg/kg twice to three times daily
• Sirolimus 6–12 mg PO loading dose followed by 4 mg/kg/day – goal trough level 3–12
• Rabbit ATG 1–3 mg/kg/day given over 3 days prior to day 0
	
	• IV : PO conversion 1 : 1
	• Not available as IV
	• Interacts with CYP450 inducers/inhibitors
	• Dosed based on actual body weight

Surgical	
Placement of triple lumen Hickman catheter	
Psychologic	
Allogeneic SCT is very stressful both for patients and their significant others. Social workers are an integral part of the transplant team and work very closely with patients and family members in addressing their needs	

Prevention/management of complications
- Transplant-associated thrombotic microangiopathy is associated with the use of calcineurin inhibitors (CI). First line therapy is discontinuation of CI and starting alternative non-CI immunosuppressive therapy. Rituxan, eculuzimab, and plasma exchange can be used in some cases.
- Hepatic sinusoidal obstruction syndrome, also known as VOD, is characterized by painful hepatomegaly, jaundice, and ascites. Risk factors include myeloablative preparatory regiments TBI and busulfan. Supportive measures that address fluid balance and pain management are used. In severe cases, defibrotide has been shown to be effective in reversing sinusoidal obstruction syndrome.
- Sirolimus is associated with pneumonitis necessitating discontinuation of the medication.
- Mycophenolate can cause colitis that at times can be confused with gastrointestinal GVHD.
- Fludarabine has been associated with irreversible neurotoxicity.
- High dose cyclophosphamide is associated with hemorrhagic cystitis. Aggressive hydration during drug administration is required to prevent it.
- Acute GVHD – see Chapter 39 for further details
- Chronic GVHD occurring months to years following allogeneic SCT can affect multiple organs and require ongoing immunosuppression.
- Infectious complications are very frequent during the post-transplant period requiring prophylaxis as well as active surveillance:
  - Invasive fungal infections
  - Viral reactivation – CMV, BK virus, EBV

- Bacterial infection
- Pneumocystis pneumonia.
- Long-term survivors of allogeneic SCT are at risk for cardiac, pulmonary, and endocrine toxicities as well as secondary malignancies.

Special populations
Elderly
- Reduced intensity preparative regimens are associated with decreased treatment-related morbidity and mortality allowing older patients to undergo allogeneic SCT. Age alone is not a significant prognostic factor for nonrelapse mortality, disease-free survival, or OS and should not be a limiting factor.

Others
- Finding HLA-matched donors for non-Caucasian patients can be challenging, leading to use of alternative sources of donor cells, such as umbilical cord blood and haploidentical donors.

Prognosis

> **BOTTOM LINE/CLINICAL PEARLS**
> - Allogeneic SCT is the only curative therapeutic option for patients with MDS with long-term disease-free survival of 25–60% depending on prognostic features.
> - Allogeneic SCT improves survival of AML patients with high risk cytogenetic or molecular abnormalities.
> - Combination of the Hematopoietic Cell Transplantation Comorbidity Index (SCT-CI) and Disease Index Score determines long-term outcomes.

Reading list
Armand P, Kim HT, Cutler CS, et al. A prognostic score for patients with acute leukemia or myelodysplastic syndromes undergoing allogeneic stem cell transplantation. Biol Blood Marrow Transplant 2008;14:28–35.

Cornelissen JJ, Gratwohl A, Schlenk RF, et al. The European LeukemiaNet AML Working Party consensus statement on allogeneic HSCT for patients with AML in remission: an integrated-risk adapted approach. Nat Rev Clin Oncol 2012;9:579–590.

Cutler CS, Lee SJ, Greenberg P, et al. A decision analysis of allogeneic bone marrow transplantation for the myelodysplastic syndromes: delayed transplantation for low-risk myelodysplasia is associated with improved outcome. Blood 2004;104:579–585.

Koreth J, Pidala J, Perez WS, et al. Role of reduced-intensity conditioning allogeneic hematopoietic stem-cell transplantation in older patients with de novo myelodysplastic syndromes: an International Collaborative Decision Analysis. J Clin Oncol 2013;31:2662–2670.

Sekeres MA, Cutler C. How we treat higher-risk myelodysplastic syndromes. Blood 2014;123(6):829–836.

Schlenk RF, Döhner K, Krauter J, et al. Mutations and treatment outcome in cytogenetically normal acute myeloid leukemia. N Engl J Med 2008;358:1909–1918.

Vyas P, Appelbaum FR, Craddock C. Allogeneic hematopoietic cell transplantation for acute myeloid leukemia. Biol Blood Marrow Transplant 2015;21:8–15.

Suggested websites
http://c.ymcdn.com/sites/www.asbmt.org/resource/resmgr/Docs/AdultAML_PositionStatement.pdf
http://c.ymcdn.com/sites/www.asbmt.org/resource/resmgr/Docs/PediatricAML_PositionStateme.pdf
http://c.ymcdn.com/sites/www.asbmt.org/resource/resmgr/Docs/MDS_PositionStatement.pdf

Guidelines
National society guidelines

Title	Source	Date and weblink
	NCCN	2019 http://www.nccn.org/professionals/physician_gls/pdf/aml.pdf
	NCCN	2019 http://www.nccn.org/professionals/physician_gls/pdf/mds.pdf

International society guidelines

Title	Source	Date and weblink
The European LeukemiaNet AML Working Party consensus statement on allogeneic HSCT for patients with AML in remission: an integrated-risk adapted approach	European LeukemiaNet AML Working Party	2012 http://www.ncbi.nlm.nih.gov/pubmed/22949046

Evidence

Type of evidence	Title and comment	Date and weblink
Systematic review	Allogeneic SCT for acute myeloid leukemia in first complete remission: systematic review and meta-analysis of prospective clinical trials **Comment:** This analysis confirmed survival benefit of allogeneic SCT over chemotherapy for patients with intermediate-risk to high-risk AML	2009 https://www.ncbi.nlm.nih.gov/pmc/articles/PMC3163846/
Retrospective analysis	Comparative analysis of the value of allogeneic HSCT in acute myeloid leukemia with monosomal karyotype versus other cytogenetic risk categories **Comment:** This analysis shows that allogeneic SCT improves outcomes in AML with monosomal karyotype that otherwise carries a particularly poor outcome	2012 https://www.ncbi.nlm.nih.gov/pubmed/22564995
Decision analysis	A decision analysis of allogeneic bone marrow transplantation for the myelodysplastic syndromes: delayed transplantation for low risk myelodysplasia is associated with improved outcome **Comment:** This analysis showed that allogeneic SCT should be offered to patients with intermediate-2 and high-risk MDS at the time of diagnosis	2004 https://www.ncbi.nlm.nih.gov/pubmed/15039286

Additional material for this chapter can be found online at:
www.wiley.com/go/oh/mountsinaioncology

This includes advice for patients, a case study, ICD codes, and
multiple choice questions.

CHAPTER 36

Stem Cell Transplantation for Lymphoproliferative Disorders

Doyun Park[1], Eileen Scigliano[2], and Amir Steinberg[2]
[1] NYU School of Medicine, New York, NY, USA
[2] Icahn School of Medicine at Mount Sinai, New York, NY, USA

OVERALL BOTTOM LINE
- ASCT can be used for salvage or consolidative therapy for aggressive and low grade B- and T-cell lymphomas.
- ASCT is a standard of care for relapsed or chemo-sensitive refractory Hodgkin lymphoma and diffuse large B-cell lymphoma.
- Maintenance therapy given following ASCT can improve PFS in some lymphomas, such as brentuximab (anti-CD30 antibody) for Hodgkin lymphoma and rituximab (anti-CD20 antibody) for mantle cell lymphoma.
- Allogeneic stem cell transplant (AlloSCT) is sometimes an option for patients who relapse after multiple lines of therapy and/or ASCT.

Background
Description of transplant
- **ASCT:** stem cells have the potential to differentiate into white blood cells, red blood cells, or platelets. Stem cells are collected from the patient and frozen prior to high dose chemotherapy. High dose chemotherapy is then given to the patient to destroy malignant cells, but will also eradicate normal hematopoietic cells. Infusion of the previously collected autologous stem cells, after the high dose chemotherapy has been cleared, will enable recovery of the patient's blood counts within approximately 3 weeks.
- **AlloSCT:** uses a donor's immune system to attack the lymphoma ("graft versus lymphoma"). The conditioning regimen of chemotherapy and/or radiation, given prior to infusion of the donor stem cells, functions to eradicate any residual lymphoma in the patient and to eliminate the patient's immune system to prevent rejection of the donor graft. More myeloablative conditioning regimens are more effective in eradicating residual tumor and result in lower relapse rates, but are associated with greater toxicity. Reduced intensity or nonmyeloablative regimens have less toxicity and rely more on the graft versus tumor effect of the donor immune system and are used more often in indolent, or slower growing, lymphomas and in patients who are older or who have comorbidities that preclude more toxic myeloablative regimens.

Background
- Successful AlloSCT was first performed in the 1960s and successful ASCT for lymphomas followed in the 1970s.

Mount Sinai Expert Guides: Oncology, First Edition. Edited by William K. Oh and Ajai Chari.
© 2019 John Wiley & Sons Ltd. Published 2019 by John Wiley & Sons Ltd.
Companion Website: www.wiley.com/go/oh/mountsinaioncology

- Purpose of ASCT is to overcome the marrow toxicity of high dose therapy by infusing stem cells and allowing them to repopulate, and "rescue" the marrow.
- In AlloSCT, donor cells not only repopulate the marrow, but a graft versus tumor effect can have a significant role in this type of transplant.
- The incidence of lymphomas is increasing annually and as a result transplants have increased in number with approximately 3000 ASCT in the USA for non-Hodgkin lymphoma, 1000 AlloSCT, and approximately 1200 transplants (mostly ASCT) for Hodgkin lymphoma according to the Center for International Blood and Marrow Transplant Research (CIBMTR) 2013 data.
- ASCT are in the range $100 000–150 000 and AlloSCT $200 000–250 000 in insurance reimbursement costs.

Indications
- Diffuse large B-cell lymphoma (DLBCL)
- Hodgkin lymphoma
- CNS lymphoma
- Follicular lymphoma
- Small lymphocytic lymphoma (SLL)/CLL
- MCL
- Peripheral T-cell lymphoma.

Diffuse large B-cell lymphoma
- The PARMA trial demonstrated a 5-year survival advantage of 53% vs. 32% for ASCT vs. conventional salvage chemotherapy, in patients with relapsed or chemo-sensitive refractory DLBCL, and established ASCT as standard of care for patients with relapsed/refractory DLBCL.
- Although not universal standard of care, some institutions consider consolidation ASCT in first remission for patients with high International Prognostic Index (IPI), c-myc expression, and double hit lymphomas (this is what refractory disease is, so not first remission).
- AlloSCT can be considered in patients with stem cell mobilization failure or relapse following an ASCT.
- Most studies show no benefit for maintenance rituximab following ASCT for DLBCL.

Hodgkin lymphoma
- ASCT has been shown to improve PFS (40–50%) and, in some studies, OS, in patients with relapsed or refractory Hodgkin lymphoma.
- In the Athera trial, brentuximab, given as maintenance following ASCT, has been shown to improve PFS in high risk patients (those with primary refractory disease, relapse <12 months, or relapse with extranodal disease).
- AlloSCT may be indicated for patients whose disease relapses after ASCT with 50% 2-year OS and 25% PFS rates.

CNS lymphoma
- Treatment of primary CNS lymphoma includes induction chemotherapy with methotrexate-based regimens followed by consolidation therapy with WBRT, which has been associated with neurotoxicity.
- High dose chemotherapy with thiotepa-based regimens and ASCT in nonrandomized studies has shown excellent results and may replace WBRT as consolidation even in younger patients. Most recently, Memorial Sloan Kettering Cancer Center reported 2-year PFS and OS of 79% and 81%, respectively, in their single center phase 2 study (Omuro et al. 2015).

- Cancer and Leukemia Group B (CALGB) is currently conducting a phase 3 trial comparing ASCT with chemotherapy alone for patients in first complete remission.
- Limited data exist for AlloSCT in the form of case reports.

Follicular lymphoma

- The indications and timing of ASCT and AlloSCT for follicular lymphoma are based on patient (age, performance status, comorbidities) and disease characteristics and are evolving in the era of many new biologic agents used to treat follicular lymphoma.
- ASCT is associated with low transplant-related mortality and can result in prolonged remissions in patients with chemo-sensitive disease transplanted in first or second remission, but does not usually result in cure.
- AlloSCT is associated with higher transplant-related mortality and long-term complications such as chronic graft versus host disease, but is associated with lower relapse rates. Most studies comparing ASCT with AlloSCT for relapsed follicular lymphoma show equivalent OS rates.
- AlloSCT might be considered for patients who only have a partial response to salvage therapy, bone marrow involvement with lymphoma, inadequate stem cell collection, or relapse after ASCT.

Small lymphocytic lymphoma/chronic lymphocytic leukemia

- The role of ASCT and AlloSCT for SLL/CLL is evolving with the advent of novel agents and indications and timing of transplant should take into account patient risk factors (age, comorbidities) and disease-related factors (prognostic markers, chemo-sensitivity).
- There are no randomized studies comparing outcomes for chemo-immunotherapy, ASCT, and alloSCT in patients with SLL/CLL.
- AlloSCT is the only potentially curative therapy in CLL because of a potent graft versus leukemia effect.
- Reduced intensity conditioning is associated with lower transplant-related mortality and improved PFS and OS than myeloablative conditioning.
- AlloSCT should be considered in young(er) patients with high risk clinical and biologic features including 17p or 11q deletions, disease refractory to fludarabine, relapse within 24 months of induction, and transformation to a more aggressive disease (Richter transformation).

Mantle cell lymphoma

- Recent emerging novel therapies have put in question the use of ASCT in MCL.
- ASCT should be an option as part of frontline therapy for young and fit patients, as thus far it has been shown to result in the most durable PFS.
- Consolidation with ASCT in first complete remission should be considered for patients with very poor risk features including high Ki67+ (proliferation index), blastic subtype, SOX11-positive, and high MCL International Prognostic Index (MIPI) score.
- ASCT can also be considered for patients with only a partial response to induction or those who require multiple regimens to achieve a clinical complete remission.
- For selected patients, AlloSCT can offer the best chance for long-term remission with 3-year OS rates of about 50% (CIBMTR data).

T-cell lymphoma

- T-cell lymphomas comprise a heterogeneous group of diseases with a poorer prognosis than the B-cell lymphomas.

- ASCT should be considered as consolidation in first remission in all subtypes, except for ALK-positive anaplastic large cell lymphoma in patients with low IPSS scores, and is associated with improved PFS and OS compared with ASCT in patients with partial response to induction or subsequent remission (CR2).
- AlloSCT for patients with relapsed or refractory T-cell lymphomas results in 3-year PFS rates of about 35–50% in nonrandomized trials including CIBMTR data, and provides cure for some patients.

References and reading list

Gribben JG, Zahrieh D, Stephans K, et al. Autologous and allogeneic stem cell transplantations for poor-risk chronic lymphocytic leukemia. Blood 2005;106:4389–4396.

Metzner B, Pott C, Müller TH, et al. Long-term clinical and molecular remissions in patients with follicular lymphoma following high-dose therapy and autologous stem cell transplantation. Ann Oncol 2013;24:1609–1615.

Omuro A, Correa DD, DeAngelis LM, et al. R-MPV followed by high-dose chemotherapy with TBC and autologous stem-cell transplant for newly diagnosed primary CNS lymphoma. Blood 2015;125:1403–1410.

Philip T, Guglielmi C, Hagenbeek A, et al. Autologous bone marrow transplantation as compared with salvage chemotherapy in relapses of chemotherapy-sensitive non-Hodgkin's lymphoma. N Engl J Med 1995;333:1540–1545.

Rashidi A, Ebadi M, Cashen AF. Allogeneic hematopoietic stem cell transplantation in Hodgkin lymphoma: a systematic review and meta-analysis. Bone Marrow Transplant 2016;51:521–528.

Reimer P, Rüdiger T, Geissinger E, et al. Autologous stem-cell transplantation as first-line therapy in peripheral T-cell lymphomas: results of a prospective multicenter study. J Clin Oncol 2009;27:106–113.

Tam CS, Bassett R, Ledesma C, et al. Mature results of the M. D. Anderson Cancer Center risk-adapted transplantation strategy in mantle cell lymphoma. Blood 2009;113:4144–4152.

Additional material for this chapter can be found online at:
www.wiley.com/go/oh/mountsinaioncology

This includes advice for patients, a case study, ICD codes, and multiple choice questions.

CHAPTER 37

Infectious Complications of Stem Cell Transplantation

Meenakshi M. Rana and Amir Steinberg
Icahn School of Medicine at Mount Sinai, New York, NY, USA

OVERALL BOTTOM LINE
- Stem cell transplantation affects the body's immune response to infection brought about by neutropenia, mucous membrane inflammation, alterations in cell-mediated and humoral immunity, and via the various effects of immunosuppressants in allogeneic recipients.
- The neutropenic phase increases the risk for bacterial and fungal infections which may necessitate the use of prophylaxis.
- *Pneumocystis jiroveci* pneumonia prophylaxis and prophylaxis against herpetic viruses are necessary measures to prevent complications.
- In allogeneic recipients, viral infections, especially cytomegalovirus, significantly factor into post-transplant complications and pre-emptive monitoring is recommended.
- Active graft versus host disease can increase infectious risk through the use of immunosuppressants but also through its effects.
- Vaccines should be administered starting 6–12 months post-transplantation in both autologous and allogeneic transplant patients.

Background
- SCT is a method of treating several hematologic malignancies, testicular cancer, autoimmune disorders, and hemoglobinopathies.
- Transplantation can affect the body's immune response through a period of neutropenia, alterations in cell-mediated and humoral immunity, and the various effects of immunosuppressants in allogeneic recipients.
- Bacterial, fungal, and viral infections are the main categories of infections that occur in transplant patients and methods have evolved over the past four decades to prevent, sometimes pre-emptively monitor, and treat such pathogens.

Prevention
- Prophylactic medications are discussed within each category of bacterial, fungal, and viral infections.
- Foundation for the Accreditation of Cellular Therapy (FACT) standards require the use of high efficiency particulate air (HEPA) filtration rooms to be available for transplant patients.
- Hand hygiene should be universally practiced and other precautions (contact, droplet, airborne) may be needed to prevent transmission in the setting of certain infections.

Mount Sinai Expert Guides: Oncology, First Edition. Edited by William K. Oh and Ajai Chari.
© 2019 John Wiley & Sons Ltd. Published 2019 by John Wiley & Sons Ltd.
Companion Website: www.wiley.com/go/oh/mountsinaioncology

Bacterial infections

- Bacterial infections are one of the leading causes of morbidity and mortality in transplant patients.
- There are three periods of risk that dictate the type of bacterial infections patients are at risk for and when specific prophylaxis is indicated (Figure 37.1).

Immediate post-transplant neutropenic period

- The first period of infection risk is immediately after SCT when patients become neutropenic for, on average, 1–4 weeks.
- Risk of infection is from decreased protection from neutropenia but also from inflammation of the mucous lining which leads to translocation of bacteria.
- Bacterial infections are the most common infection in the immediate post-transplant period.
- Gram-positive bacterial infections:
  - Gram-positive infections, particularly *Staphylococcus aureus* and coagulase-negative staphylococci, are the most common bacterial infections.
  - The Gram-positive infections can often be seen with central line infections.
- Gram-negative bacterial infections:
  - Common Gram-negative bacteria, which make up 40% of bacterial infections, include *Klebsiella* and *Pseudomonas aueruginosa*, though routine use of bacterial prophylaxis has decreased the incidence of these particular infections.
  - Fluoroquinolones, such as levofloxacin, are typically used as prophylaxis for these Gram-negative bacteria and streptococcus.
  - The addition of an anti-Gram-positive agent to the prophylaxis is not indicated and fluoroquinolone resistance is increasing.
  - For those patients allergic to fluoroquinolones, macrolides such as azithromycin can be considered. Augmentin may also be considered as an alternative.
- *Clostridium difficile:*
  - Routine prophylaxis has led to an increase in *Clostridium difficile* infection because of alterations in normal gut flora.
  - Therapy for *Clostridium difficile* involves a course of metronidazole, with oral vancomycin reserved for refractory and recurrent cases.
  - Once a patient is no longer neutropenic, antibiotics can be discontinued.
- Febrile neutropenia:
  - If a patient develops febrile neutropenia during the early post-transplant period, broad spectrum antibiotics covering both Gram-positive and Gram-negative infections are prescribed.
  - A common combination is vancomycin with cefepime. Aztreonam can be given as an alternative to cefepime if the patient has a penicillin allergy.
  - Coverage can be narrowed if a source of infection or fever is identified.
  - Once neutropenia resolves and the patient is afebrile, the antibiotics can be stopped provided there is no further source of infection.

Post-engraftment period

- Cell-mediated and humoral immunity have important roles during this period and dysfunction in such immunity increases the risk for parasitic infections and viral infections.
- Transplant recipients are at high risk for *Pneumocystis jiroveci* pneumonia (formerly known as *Pneumocystis carinii* pneumonia), commonly known as PCP.

- Nonmyeloma autologous transplant recipients (primarily patients with lymphoma) typically begin receiving PCP prophylaxis 1 month after transplant and continue prophylaxis until 3–6 months after the date of transplant to coincide with the period of highest infectivity so as not to affect engraftment.
- Allogeneic transplant recipients generally follow the same guidelines as patients receiving autologous transplantations. However, prophylaxis for PCP should continue for as long as patients are on immunosuppressants which often occurs for longer than the 3–6 month period.
- Co-trimoxazole is considered the standard for PCP prophylaxis. If there is a strong contraindication to co-trimoxazole or co-trimoxazole allergy, alternative agents include atovaquone, dapsone, and pentamidine.

Late phase/chronic graft versus host disease
- GVHD affects the immune system through the need for immunosuppressants as well as modulations in cell-mediated and humoral immunity.
- Increased risk against encapsulated organisms is particularly concerning in chronic GVHD.
- For patients with chronic GVHD, prophylaxis against *Streptococcus pneumonia* should be administered. The suggested prophylaxis is penicillin.
- For patients allergic to penicillin, macrolides such as azithromycin are an alternative.

Viral infections
Common viral infections in SCT recipients include CMV, HSV, and respiratory viral infections (RVI), on which further detail is provided here. Other viral infections seen in SCT recipients include BK virus which can cause hemorrhagic cystitis, or human herpesvirus 6 (HHV-6) which can cause CNS syndromes. Please refer to the reading list for further information on these topics.

Cytomegalovirus infection
- CMV is a herpesvirus that remains latent in the human body after initial primary infection then reactivates to cause infection after allogenic HSCT.
- The majority of CMV infections occur post engraftment before day 100 after HSCT. However, the prevalence of late onset CMV disease (>100 days) has increased in the past few years.
- Reconstitution of CMV-specific CD8+ T-cell response after SCT correlates with protection from CMV and improved outcomes after CMV disease.

Risk factors/prevention
- In allogeneic HSCT recipients, the most important risk factor relates to the serologic status of donor and recipient. CMV serology should be assessed pretransplant to determine a recipient's risk for CMV infection.
- Recipients who are seronegative for CMV (R–) have a low risk of primary infection if cells from a CMV seronegative donor (D–) are used, as long as they do not acquire primary infection and CMV safe blood products are used.
- About 30% of CMV seronegative recipients with a seropositive donor (D+R–) will develop CMV infection.
- The risk is highest in those who are seropositive, and about 80% of CMV seropositive patients will develop CMV infection after HSCT.
- Other risk factors include the use of corticosteroids, T-cell depletion, acute and chronic GVHD, and the use of mismatched or unrelated donors.

- Letermovir has been FDA approved for prevention of CMV reactivation in CMV seropositive recipients.

Diagnosis/clinical manifestations

- After allogeneic HSCT, a pre-emptive strategy is used, in which weekly CMV PCR tests are monitored and antiviral treatment is initiated upon diagnosis of CMV infection. This includes either a positive PCR and/or signs and symptoms consistent with CMV.
- Fever is a common manifestation as is thrombocytopenia and leukopenia.
- CMV can affect any portion of the gastrointestinal tract, and typically ulcers are seen on endoscopy, often macroscopically very similar to GVHD. Other manifestations of CMV disease include pneumonia, retinitis, hepatitis, and encephalitis.
- On pathologic specimens, the presence of CMV inclusions is diagnostic of invasive CMV disease, and can be present even in the absence of ongoing CMV viremia in the blood.

Treatment

- Ganciclovir remains the first line agent for CMV infection and is available in intravenous formulation. The most common side effect is myelosuppression.
- Valganciclovir is the orally available pro-drug of ganciclovir.
- Foscarnet is considered second line therapy, because of side effects including nephrotoxicity and neurotoxicity.
- CMV immunoglobulin or pooled immunoglobulin can be used in the setting of severe CMV disease, specifically CMV pneumonia.

Herpes simplex virus

- HSV establishes latency in the neuronal cells of sensory nerve ganglia after primary infection and can then reactivate after transplantation in the setting of immunosuppression.
- Up to 80% of adult patients are HSV seropositive and reactivation occurs in seropositive patients after HSCT. Primary infection with HSV is unusual.

Prevention

- Acyclovir prophylaxis should be given to HSV seropositive recipients to prevent HSV infection after HSCT. This is based on clinical trials in which recipients of acyclovir were significantly less likely to develop HSV reactivation than those who received placebo.

Clinical manifestations

- While mucocutaneous disease is most common, other manifestions include HSV esophagitis, pneumonia, and meningitis or meningoencephalitis.

Treatment

- Intravenous acyclovir remains first line therapy for severe mucocutaneous disease. Randomized control trials have shown acyclovir treatment decreases viral shedding and lesion pain, reducing the time to lesion healing.
- Oral acyclovir can also be used, as can valacyclovir which is more bioavailable and can thereby be given in less frequent regimens.
- Acyclovir requires dose modification for patients with renal insufficiency.

Respiratory viral infections
- Respiratory viruses commonly recognized include influenza A and B, parainfluenza 1–4, respiratory syncytial virus, and adenovirus; recently, human metapneumovirus, enterovirus, and rhinovirus have gained importance.
- The prevalence of RVI varies and is often based on circulation of seasonal viruses, exposure, and detection methods used.

Prevention
- General infection control measures vary for each RVI, but typically include droplet or/and contact precautions. Staff and visitors who may be ill with an RVI should refrain from working or interacting with patients.

Diagnosis/clinical presentation
- RVIs can cause upper and/or lower respiratory tract illness.
- Upper respiratory tract infection is usually limited to cough, sore throat, fever, and malaise.
- In lower respiratory tract infection, these symptoms can be accompanied by shortness of breath, rales or crackles on examination, with evidence of interstitial infiltrates or reticular noduar infiltrates on imaging.
- Direct fluorescent antibody is limited to certain viruses and has poor sensitivity. PCR testing for respiratory viruses has increased sensitivity with rapid turnaround time and should be considered in critically ill patients or in patients where diagnosis will alter management.

Treatment
- Influenza A or B should be treated with neuraminidase inhibitors, such as oseltamivir.
- The use of ribavirin (aerosolized or oral) and/or palivizumab (RSV-specific monoclonal antibody) is controversial given its limited data for efficacy; randomized clinical trials are needed.
- Otherwise, supportive care and ventilator support, if needed, remain the mainstay of therapy.

Invasive fungal infections
- Invasive fungal infections (IFIs) remain a cause of significant morbidity and mortality in patients receiving HSCT.
- Based on Transplant Associated Infections Surveillance Program (TRANSNET) data collected from 23 transplant centers between 2001 and 2006, the overall incidence of IFIs in allogeneic and autologous HSCT was around 3.4%. In addition, invasive aspergillosis surpassed *Candida* as the most common IFI in HSCT recipients (43% vs. 28%), given the increased use of fluconazole prophylaxis. This was followed by other mold infections such as *Fusarium* and *Scedosporium* (16%) and zygomycetes (8%).
- Risk factors for IFIs in HSCT recipients includes prolonged duration of neutropenia, CMV infection, GVHD, and allogeneic or cord transplant.

Prevention
- Autologous SCT recipients should receive prophylaxis against *Candida* infection with fluconazole.
- Allogeneic and cord transplant recipients should receive mold-active prophylaxis with either voriconazole or posaconazole.

- Side effects of azoles should be monitored for in this setting, including liver function test elevations and QTc prolongation. Drug interactions in the setting of azole therapy should be carefully considered and typically a 50–60% dose reduction in calcineruin inhibitors is required in the setting of voriconazole or posaconazole therapy.

Diagnosis/clinical presentation

Candida:
- *Candida* infection should be suspected early after SCT, in the first 40 days.
- Typically, patients present with neutropenic fever and have mucositis or a central venous catheter.
- More recently, non-*albicans Candida* is being increasingly diagnosed, especially in the era of routine azole prophylaxis.
- Rarely, *Candida* infections can occur late after SCT in the setting of GVHD.

Invasive aspergillosis:
- Invasive aspergillosis and other mold infections can occur early pre-engraftment, in the setting of prolonged neutropenia as seen with allogeneic or cord blood transplant.
- They can also be diagnosed late after HSCT, in the setting of GVHD and cell-mediated immunodeficiency.
- Typically, patients present with cough, fever, hemoptysis, pleuritic chest pain, or dyspnea but occasionally clinical signs can be subtle in the setting of heavy immunosuppression.
- Diagnosis of invasive aspergillosis can be challenging given the poor sensitivity of sputum and bronchoalveolar lavage cultures; however, when positive, they have a high positive predictive value for invasive disease.
- While histopathologic diagnosis is required for proven disease, lung biopsies may be difficult to obtain in the setting of leukopenia and thrombocytopenia. Therefore, other noninvasive methods of diagnosis are often used to evaluate for possible or probable invasive aspergillosis, including chest imaging and the use of fungal antigen testing.
- Chest imaging can vary from diffuse nodular infiltrates to cavitary lesions; CT findings may show a "halo" sign of low attenuation surrounding a nodular lesion.
- A serum test for galactomannan, a cell wall component of *Aspergillus*, is often used for diagnosis although may not be useful in the setting of azole prophylaxis. False positive galactomannans have been reported, especially in the setting of ampicillin/sulbactam and piperacillin/tazobactam use.
- A cell wall polysaccharide, $(1-3)$-β-D-glucan, found in most fungi, with the exception of *Cryptococcus* and zygomycetes, can also be used as a screening tool for IFIs and pneumocystis. False positive tests can be seen in the setting of hemodialysis filters and immunoglobulins.

Treatment

- Typically, echinocandins or azoles can be used for *Candida* infections, depending on whether identified as *albicans* or non-*albicans* species.
- For invasive aspergillosis, the drug of choice is voriconazole, based on a randomized clinical trial comparing voriconazole with amphotericin which showed significantly improved survival in the voriconazole arm.
- However, voriconazole has no activity against the zygomycetes, so without microbiologic or histopathologic confirmation of invasive aspergillosis, liposomal amphotericin or posaconazole should be considered.

Vaccinations

Stem cell transplantation can lead to loss of prior vaccine immunity to several infections.

Revaccination of patients after both autologous and allogeneic transplantation is recommended. Consider at least 1 month intervals between doses.

- **Pneumococcus:** three doses of pneumococcal conjugate (PCV, also known as PCV13 or Prevnar 13) starting 3–6 months after transplant. A fourth dose of PCV may be given if chronic GVHD is present. Otherwise, a dose of 23-valent polysaccharide pneumococcal vaccine (PPSV23) is suggested after completion of the three doses of PCV.
- **Tetanus, diphtheria, acellular pertussis:** DTaP preferred. Tdap may be an alternative if DTaP unavailable to healthcare provider. Three doses starting 6–12 months after transplantation. Acellular pertussis vaccine is preferred. Whole-cell pertussis may be an alternative if unavailable to healthcare provider.
- *Haemophilus* **influenza:** three doses starting 6–12 months after transplant.
- **Polio:** inactivated vaccine. Three doses starting 6–12 months after transplant.
- **Hepatitis B:** three doses starting 6–12 months after transplant.
- **Hepatitis A:** considered optional.
- **Influenza:** inactivated. Yearly beginning 4–6 months after transplant. Additional dose if patient is under 9 years old.
- **Measles–mumps–rubella:** usually given as 1–2 doses of combined MMR vaccine if patient is at least 24 months after transplant, has no active GVHD, and is not on immunosuppression.
- **Varicella:** optional. Like MMR, Varivax is a live vaccine so should be given only if the patient is at least 24 months after transplant, has no active GVHD, and is not on immunosuppression.

Supportive care

- For allogeneic patients with severe gammaglobulinemia (i.e. IgG <400 mg/dL), intravenous immunoglobulin can be considered at a dosage of 500 mg/kg/week.

Reading list

Kumar D, Humar A. Respiratory viral infections in transplant and oncology patients. Infect Dis Clin N Am 2010;24:395–412.

Ljungman P, Hakki M, Boeckh M. Cytomegalovirus in hematopoietic stem cell transplant recipients. Infect Dis Clin N Am 2010;24:319–337.

Person A, Kontoyiannis DP, Alexander BD. Fungal infections in transplant and oncology patients. Infect Dis Clin N Am 2010;24:439–459.

Singh N, Paterson DL. Aspergillus infections in transplant recipients. Clin Microbiol Rev 2005;18:44–69.

Styczynski J, Reusser P, Einsele H, et al. Management of HSV, VZV and EBV infections in patients with hematological malignancies and after SCT: guidelines from the Second European Conference on Infections in Leukemia. Bone Marrow Transplant 2009;43:757–770.

Tomblyn M, Chiller T, Einsele H, et al. Guidelines for preventing infectious complications among hematopoietic cell transplantation recipients: a global perspective. Biol Blood Marrow Transplant 2009;15;1143–1238 and Bone Marrow Transplant 2009;44:453–455.

Suggested websites

American Society for Blood and Marrow Transplantation: www.asbmt.org
Foundation for the Accreditation of Cellular Therapy: www.factwebsite.org
Infectious Disease Society of America: www.idsociety.org
National Comprehensive Cancer Network: www.nccn.org

Image

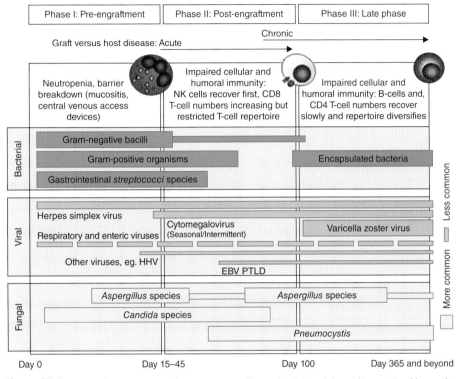

Figure 37.1 Phases of opportunistic infections among allogeneic HSCT recipients. (Source: Tomblyn et al. 2009. Reproduced with permission from Elsevier.)

Additional material for this chapter can be found online at:
www.wiley.com/go/oh/mountsinaioncology

This includes advice for patients, a case study, ICD codes, and multiple choice questions.

CHAPTER 38

Acute Graft Versus Host Disease

Anne S. Renteria, James L.M. Ferrara, and John E. Levine
Icahn School of Medicine at Mount Sinai, New York, NY, USA

OVERALL BOTTOM LINE
- Acute graft versus host disease (GVHD) develops in ~50% allogeneic HSCT recipients, targets the skin, gastrointestinal tract, and liver, and is the major cause of nonrelapse mortality.
- Diagnosis is based on clinical symptoms but other post-HSCT complications can present similarly and should be evaluated.
- The standard first line therapy is high dose steroids but 50% of cases, primarily gastrointestinal GVHD, are steroid refractory.
- The loss of diversity in the gastrointestinal microbiota is associated with increased GVHD mortality and is related to several factors, including exposure to antibiotics.

Background
Definition of disease
- Acute GVHD is an immune-mediated phenomenon and occurs when activated *donor* T cells from the graft attack normal *recipient* tissues (skin, liver, gastrointestinal tract).
- It can occur up to 6 months after hematopoietic stem cell transplantation (HSCT) and time of onset is influenced by multiple factors (intensity of conditioning, donor type, prevention strategies).

Incidence/prevalence
- Acute GVHD develops in 40–60% of HSCT recipients.
- Major factors that increase risk are unrelated donors, human leukocyte antigen (HLA) mismatch, and high dose radiation conditioning.

Etiology
- Donor conventional T cells (Tcons) respond to genetically defined protein antigens expressed on antigen-presenting cells (APCs) and then proliferate and target host tissues.

Pathology/pathogenesis
- The development of GVHD involves three distinct phases:
  - **First:** tissue damage (especially in the gastrointestinal tract) from the conditioning initiates an inflammatory immunologic cascade starting with the release of danger signals from the gastrointestinal lumen (LPS, PAMPs, DAMPs) and proinflammatory cytokines (TNFα, IL-1, IL-6) that promote the activation of host APCs.

Mount Sinai Expert Guides: Oncology, First Edition. Edited by William K. Oh and Ajai Chari.
© 2019 John Wiley & Sons Ltd. Published 2019 by John Wiley & Sons Ltd.
Companion Website: www.wiley.com/go/oh/mountsinaioncology

- **Second:** host APCs drive Tcon proliferation which then traffic to the target organs (skin, gastrointestinal tract, liver).
- **Third:** Tcons cause tissue destruction through cytotoxic activity and through cytokines (e.g. TNFα). Regulatory T cells (Tregs) can dampen GVHD.

Predictive/risk factors
- HLA matching: better matching between the donor and recipient lessens the risk of acute GVHD.
- Unrelated adult donors confer increased risk compared with sibling donors.
- Umbilical cord transplant: less risk for same degree of HLA match.
- Children are at lower risk.
- Older donor age increases risk.
- Conditioning regimen: high dose radiation during conditioning increases risk.

Prevention

> **CLINICAL PEARLS**
> - Younger male donors are preferred.
> - *In vivo* or *ex vivo* donor T-cell removal or inhibition decreases the incidence of acute GVHD.
> - Prevention of acute GVHD with immunosuppression starts prior to stem cell infusion.
> - Post-HSCT cyclophosphamide has emerged as an alternative prophylaxis regimen.

Screening
- There are no validated screening tests for acute GVHD.
- Validated serum GVHD biomarkers are closest in terms of clinical development.

Primary prevention
- Calcineurin inhibitors (cyclosporine, tacrolimus) are the most widely used drugs for GVHD prevention:
  - Always given in combination with either methotrexate (MTX) or mycophenolate mofetil.
  - *In vivo* T-cell depletion (with antibodies such as antithymocyte globulin or alemtuzumab) further reduces GVHD risk.
- *Ex vivo* T-cell depletion is an alternative prevention strategy to calcineurin inhibitors.
- High-dose cyclophosphamide given on days +3 and +4 post-HSCT depletes activated and proliferating T cells while relatively sparing quiescent T cells, stem cells, and Tregs.
  - Commonly used for HLA-haploidentical HSCT.
- T-cell depletion strategies delay immune reconstitution and increase risk for infections and relapse.

Diagnosis (Algorithm 38.1)

> **CLINICAL PEARLS**
> - Acute GVHD should always be considered in a patient post-HSCT presenting with a skin rash, diarrhea, nausea, vomiting, or elevation of bilirubin.
> - The diagnosis of acute GVHD is primarily based on clinical manifestations but histopathologic confirmation should be pursued whenever possible.
> - Its clinical spectrum ranges from mild disease that can be managed in the outpatient setting to severe life-threatening disease requiring hospitalization.

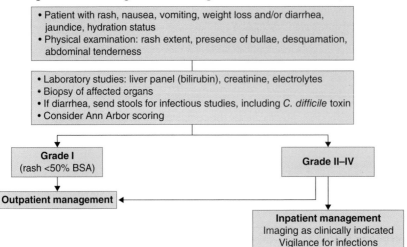

Algorithm 38.1 Diagnosis of acute graft versus host disease (GVHD)

Differential diagnosis

Symptoms	Features
Skin rash	
Engraftment syndrome	Fever, capillary leak syndrome, weight gain
Acral erythema (palmoplantar erythrodysesthesia)	Chemotherapy complication, blistering, and desquamation may develop
Drug rash	Difficult to distinguish from GVHD; cessation of offending agent often helpful
Viral exanthems (e.g. HHV-6, CMV)	Biopsy shows sparse perivascular lymphocytic infiltrates
Nausea, vomiting, diarrhea	
Conditioning regimen-induced enteritis	Improves over time without treatment
Clostridium difficile colitis	Presence of toxin in stool
Viral infection (e.g. CMV)	Detectable on biopsy or stool study
Drug toxicity	Improves with cessation of offending agent
Typhlitis (neutropenic enterocolitis)	Severe neutropenia, abdominal distension
Jaundice	
Veno-occlusive disease	Weight gain, painful hepatomegaly, increased abdominal girth
Iron overload	Elevated ferritin
Viral infection	Hepatitis A, B, C; CMV
Toxic drug effect	Contraceptives, TPN
Gallstones	Ultrasound usually diagnostic
Sepsis	Transaminases also elevated

Table 38.1 GVHD target organ staging.

Stage	Skin (active erythema only)	Liver (bilirubin)	Upper gastrointestinal tract	Lower gastrointestinal tract (stool output/day)
0	No active (erythematous) GVHD rash	<2 mg/dL	No or intermittent nausea, vomiting, or anorexia	Adult: <500 mL/day Child: <10 mL/kg/day
1	Maculopapular rash <25% body surface area (BSA)	2–3 mg/dL	Persistent nausea, vomiting, or anorexia	Adult: 500–999 mL/day Child: 10–19.9 mL/kg/day
2	Maculopapular rash 25–50% BSA	3.1–6 mg/dL	–	Adult: 1000–1500 mL/day Child: 20–30 mL/kg/day
3	Maculopapular rash > 50% BSA	6.1–15 mg/dL	–	Adult: > 1500 mL/day Child: > 30 mL/kg/day
4	Generalized erythroderma (> 50% BSA) plus bullous formation and desquamation > 5% BSA	>15 mg/dL	–	Severe abdominal pain with or without ileus, or grossly bloody stool (regardless of stool volume)

Typical presentation
- GVHD develops at a median of 25 days post HSCT but may occur up to 6 months after HSCT (influenced by conditioning intensity, donor type, and prevention strategies).
- GVHD can develop in any target organ, but skin and /or gastrointestinal presentations are most common. Severity staging is based on symptoms and provided in Table 38.1.

Clinical diagnosis
History
- Patients should be questioned about the presence of the symptoms listed in Table 38.1. Pruritus is often associated with *skin GVHD*. Abdominal cramping and tenesmus often accompany the diarrhea associated with *gastrointestinal GVHD (GI GVHD)*.

Physical examination
- Erythematous maculopapular rash in *skin GVHD* (Figure 38.1).
- Weight loss is often seen in *upper GI GVHD*.
- Pain on abdominal palpation can be occasionally elicited in *lower GI GVHD*.
- Icterus suggests *liver GVHD*.

Disease severity classification
Maximal severity correlates with OS.
Overall clinical grade (based upon most severe target organ involvement):
- **Grade 0:** no stage 1–4 of any organ.
- **Grade I:** stage 1–2 skin without liver, upper, or lower gastrointestinal tract involvement.
- **Grade II:** stage 3 rash and/or stage 1 liver and/or stage 1 upper gastrointestinal tract and/or stage 1 lower gastrointestinal tract.
- **Grade III:** stage 2–3 liver and/or stage 2–3 lower gastrointestinal tract, with stage 0–3 skin and/or stage 0–1 upper gastrointestinal tract.
- **Grade IV:** stage 4 skin, liver, or lower gastrointestinal tract involvement, with stage 0–1 upper gastrointestinal tract.

Laboratory diagnosis

List of diagnostic tests

- **Liver GVHD:** elevated conjugated bilirubin and alkaline phosphatase. Transaminitis is not a diagnostic component but is seen in severe disease. Disease is staged according to the total bilirubin only, but the clinical picture is one of cholestasis resulting from loss of bile ducts.
- **GI GVHD:** frequently complicated by enteric losses of electrolytes and bicarbonate. With severe diarrhea there is a significant risk of acute renal insufficiency.
- **Stool analysis** for infectious enteritis (e.g. rotavirus, adenovirus, *C. difficile*) as these can be present at the same time as GI GVHD.
- **GVHD biomarkers** (ST2 and REG3α) at diagnosis can be used to stratify patients for nonrelapse mortality (NRM) and treatment failure according to the Ann Arbor scoring system (Ann Arbor 1 <10% 6-month NRM; Ann Arbor 2 = ~25% NRM; Ann Arbor 3 > 40% NRM).

Pathology features on biopsy

- **Skin:** interface dermatitis and apoptosis at the base of the crypts are the most common findings.
- **Gastrointestinal:** crypt cell apoptosis is the histologic hallmark. The patchy nature of GI GVHD histology sometimes leads to false negative biopsies. In severe disease whole areas may be denuded, with total loss of epithelium.
- **Liver:** transjugular biopsies are safer than percutaneous access. Histologic examination reveals extensive damage to the bile canaliculi.

List of imaging techniques

Ultrasound, CT, or MRI are not specific for acute GVHD and are used primarily to exclude other diseases.

Potential pitfalls/common errors in diagnosis

- Harmful delays in initiating treatment when attempting to obtain a biopsy specimen.
- A negative tissue biopsy does not exclude the diagnosis of GVHD.
- Failure to evaluate a patient with watery diarrhea for *C. difficile* colitis.
- Invasive CMV disease (e.g. CMV colitis) may not be associated with a detectable serum CMV DNA PCR.

Treatment (Algorithm 38.2)

Treatment rationale

- The primary goal of treatment is to suppress donor T-cell-driven tissue destruction, and to allow tissue repair.
- Standard practice for grade II–IV acute GVHD is intravenous methylprednisolone 2 mg/kg/day or the oral equivalent if tolerating oral intake.
- Infectious risk increases with increased immunosuppression. Antibacterial, antiviral, and anti-fungal drugs prophylaxis are optimized and immunoglobulin infusions are provided to the patients with low IgG levels (<400 mg/dL) and/or recurrent infections.

When to hospitalize

- GVHD can worsen rapidly and patients who require systemic steroids are usually admitted until responding to treatment and, for those with GI GVHD, until oral intake can be resumed.
- If the diarrhea is voluminous, if intractable vomiting, and/or if the patient is showing signs of volume depletion and electrolyte imbalance.
- Skin GVHD with bullous formation and desquamation to start "burn-like" treatment.

Algorithm 38.2 Management of acute GVHD

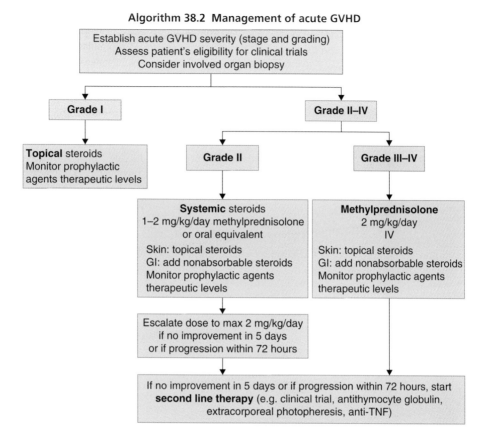

Table of treatment

Treatment	Comment
Always consider obtaining a biopsy of the involved organ	
Grade I	
Topical steroids + optimization of prophylactic agents	Carefully assess response to treatment
Grade II–IV	
Gastrointestinal: systemic steroids ± nonabsorbable oral steroids	Evaluate for infectious causes of diarrhea: CMV, *C. difficile* toxin Bowel rest and if diarrhea persists > 3 days consider starting TPN
Skin: systemic steroids + optimization of prophylactic agents	Monitor response to treatment and secondary skin infections
Liver: systemic steroids	Monitor for coagulopathy

Prevention/management of complications

- Vigilance for infections, myopathy, osteoporosis, avascular necrosis of bones, and cataracts.
- Maintain good nutrition and physical activity.
- Treat hypogammaglobulinemia with IVIg.
- About half of patients will not respond to systemic steroid treatment and no standard agent is defined for steroid-refractory GVHD. In this setting, enrollment on a clinical trial is preferred. In the absence of a clinical trial, antithymocyte globulin, extracorporeal photopheresis, and anti-TNF inhibitors are commonly used but responses are variable.

CLINICAL PEARLS

- The diagnosis of acute GVHD is primarily based on clinical manifestations but histopathologic confirmation should be pursued whenever possible.
- Grade I acute GVHD is usually managed in the outpatient setting, and selected patients with grade II GVHD (diarrhea <500 mL, no intractable vomiting, and no evidence of dehydration) can often be managed as outpatients.
- Most patients with grade II–IV GVHD require initial management in the inpatient setting as their disease can rapidly progress.
- Initial therapy for GI GVHD typically includes bowel rest and intravenous medications until symptoms respond to treatment.

Prognosis

CLINICAL PEARLS

- Acute GVHD accounts for 20% of deaths post HSCT.
- GI GVHD carries a higher risk of steroid-refractory disease and is associated with a low survival rate.
- Survival for grade IV disease is very low (5% at 5 years).

Reading list

Deeg HJ. How I treat refractory acute GVHD. Blood 2007;109:4119–4126.

Ferrara JL, Levine JE, Reddy P, et al. Graft-versus-host disease. Lancet 2009;373:1550–1561.

Jagasia M, Arora M, Flowers ME, et al. Risk factors for acute GVHD and survival after hematopoietic cell transplantation. Blood 2012;119:296–307.

Hartwell MJ, Özbek U, Holler E, et al. An early-biomarker algorithm predicts lethal graft-versus-host disease and survival. JCI Insight 2017;2:e89798.

Teshima T, Reddy P, Zeiser R. Acute graft-versus-host disease: novel biological insights. Biol Blood Marrow Transplant 2016;22:11–16.

Suggested websites

Pasquini MC. Current use and outcomes of hematopoietic stem cell transplantation, CIBMTR Summary slides, 2014: http://www.cibmtr.org.

Guidelines
National society guidelines

Title	Source	Date and weblink
EBMT-NIH-CIBMTR Task Force position statement on standardized terminology & guidance for graft-versus-host disease assessment	EBMT-NIH-CIBMTR	2018 https://www.ncbi.nlm.nih.gov/pubmed/29872128
First- and second-line systemic treatment of acute graft-versus-host disease: recommendations of the American Society of Blood and Marrow Transplantation	ASBMT	2012 https://www.ncbi.nlm.nih.gov/pubmed/22510384

Image

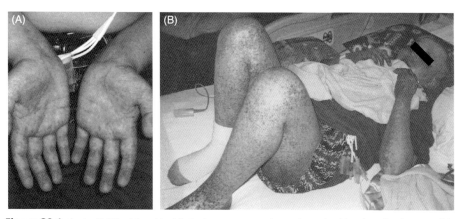

Figure 38.1 Acute GVHD of the skin. (A) Erythematous maculopapular rash with palmar involvement. (B) Stage 3 disease: >50% BSA with no bullous formation or desquamation. See color version on website.

Additional material for this chapter can be found online at: www.wiley.com/go/oh/mountsinaioncology

This includes advice for patients, a case study, ICD code, and multiple choice questions. The following image is available in color: Figure 38.1.

PART 4

Multidisciplinary Care of Cancer Patients

CHAPTER 39

Oncologic Emergencies

Scot A. Niglio and Adriana K. Malone
Icahn School of Medicine at Mount Sinai, New York, NY, USA

OVERALL BOTTOM LINE

Efficient diagnosis and proper management of life-threatening oncologic emergencies is crucial. In this chapter we review four of the most common emergencies:
- Malignancy-associated hypercalcemia
- Tumor lysis syndrome
- Neutropenic fever
- Malignant spinal cord compression.

Malignancy-Associated Hypercalcemia

Background

Malignancy-associated hypercalcemia (MAH) is a frequent occurrence which carries a poor prognosis.

Incidence/prevalence

- Up to 23% of all cancer patients have been reported to develop hypercalcemia.
- Over 33% of the total cases of hypercalcemia presenting to the emergency department are associated with cancer.

Etiology/pathology/pathogenesis

See Table 39.1.

Prevention
Primary prevention

- Denosumab, a RANK ligand inhibitor, has been shown to be more efficacious than treatment with zoledronic acid in delaying or preventing MAH in breast, other solid tumors, and multiple myeloma.

Secondary prevention

- Worsening hypercalcemia will inevitably develop with tumor progression and many patients with metastatic bone disease will receive IV pamidronate every 3–4 weeks to prevent skeletal complications and, as a result, recurrent hypercalcemia.

Diagnosis
Clinical diagnosis

- Signs and symptoms of hypercalcemia include lethargy, confusion, constipation, hypovolemia, and cardiac dysrhythmias.

Mount Sinai Expert Guides: Oncology, First Edition. Edited by William K. Oh and Ajai Chari.
© 2019 John Wiley & Sons Ltd. Published 2019 by John Wiley & Sons Ltd.
Companion Website: www.wiley.com/go/oh/mountsinaioncology

Table 39.1 Classifications of hypercalcemia associated with malignancy.

Etiology	Mechanism	Malignancy
Humeral hypercalcemia	Parathyroid hormone–related hormone (PTHrP)	Breast, ovarian, endometrial, squamous (head and neck, esophagus, cervix, lung), renal; human T-lymphotrophic virus-associated lymphoma
Local osteolysis	Cytokines (IL-1, IL-6, IL-8), chemokines, PTHrP	Breast, multiple myeloma, lymphoma
Calcitriol secreting tumors	1,25(OH)$_2$-dihydroxyvitamin D	Hodgkin, non-Hodgkin lymphomas
Ectopic parathyroid hormone secretion	Parathyroid hormone	Parathyroid, ovary, lung primitive neuroectoderm

Laboratory diagnosis
- Severity of hypercalcemia is divided into three categories:
  - Mild: 10.5–11.9 mg/dL
  - Moderate: 12.0–13.9 mg/dL
  - Severe: ≥14.0 mg/dL.
- Clinical outcomes of hypercalcemia are affected more by the rate of rise of serum calcium and by the underlying volume depletion from osmotic diuresis than by the absolute serum concentration.
- Half of serum calcium is protein bound. Formulas to correct for hypoalbuminemia are imprecise and ionized calcium more accurately represents true serum calcium levels.

Treatment
Hydration, calciuresis, and supportive measures
- Restoring intravascular volume is important in improving glomerular filtration rate and decreasing passive sodium–calcium absorption from the proximal tubule. IV saline should be started at 200–500 mL/hour and adjusted for a urine output of 100–150 mL/hour. However, less than 30% of patients will achieve a normal calcium level with IV hydration alone.
- Furosemide can be administered at 20–40 mg IV after rehydration to elicit calciuresis.
- Removal of calcium from parenteral feeding solutions and discontinuation of calcium supplements is recommended.
- Discontinuation of therapies that can cause hypercalcemia including lithium, calcitriol, vitamin D, and thiazides.
- Hypophosphatemia typically develops in patients with MAH regardless of the underlying etiology secondary to decreased food intake, saline diuresis, and use of loop diuretics.

First line pharmacologic therapies: bisphosphonates
- Bisphosphonates (pamidronate and zolendronic acid) are pyrophosphate analogs that bind hydroxyapatite, and inhibit bone crystal dissolution and osteoclastic reabsorption.
- Calcium levels decrease 2–4 days after administration, reach a nadir at 4–7 days, and usually normalize for 1–4 weeks.
- Dosing of pamidronate is 60–90 mg intravenously over a 2-hour period in a solution of 50–200 mL of normal saline (NS) or dextrose 5% in water (D5W).

- Dosing of zolendronic acid is 4 mg IV over a 15-minute period in 50 mL of NS or D5W.
- Bisphosphonates carry the risk of renal failure, osteonecrosis, and flu-like symptoms (aches, chills, and fever).

Second line pharmacologic therapies

- Calcitonin can be administered at 4–8 IU/kg SC or IM every 12 hours, and may result in a more rapid decrease in serum calcium. However, its short duration of action and potential tachyphylaxis has left it second line compared with newer agents.
- Glucocorticoids can decrease extrarenal calcitriol production in lymphoma and myeloma, increase renal calcium excretion, and inhibit osteoclastic bone reabsorption (prednisone 40–100 mg/day orally, or hydrocortisone 200–400 mg/day IV for 3–5 days). However, glucocorticoids can trigger tumor lysis syndrome.
- Denosumab is a nuclear factor-kappa ligand monoclonal antibody that can be used in patients with severe symptomatic MAH that is refractory to bisphosphonates. Unlike bisphosphonates, denosumab is not cleared although the kidneys and can be used in patients with chronic kidney disease, for whom bisphosphonates are used with caution or contraindicated. Initial dose is 60 mg SC, with repeat dosing based upon response. Patients should be monitored post denosumab for profound hypocalcemia.
- Mithramycin can be administered at single dose 25 µg/kg over 4–6 hours in NS. Use is limited because of adverse events including thrombocytopenia, platelet-aggregation defect, anemia, leukopenia, hepatitis, and renal failure.
- Gallium nitrate (100–200 mg/m^2 IV administered over 24 hours for 5 days) lowers serum calcium. Its use is also limited because of potential renal failure.

Dialysis

- Hemodialysis is indicated in patients with congestive heart failure, severe kidney injury (glomerular filtration rate <10–20 mL/min), clinically significant neurologic findings, or calcium concentration >18 mg/dL.

Prognosis

- Hypercalcemia in malignancy carries a poor prognosis, with approximately 50% of patients dying within 30 days.

Reading list

Bech A, de Boer H. Denosumab for tumor-induced hypercalcemia complicated by renal failure. Ann Intern Med 2012;156(12):906–907.

Cicci JD, Buie L, Bates J, et al. Denosumab for the management of hypercalcemia of malignancy in patients with multiple myeloma and renal dysfunction. Clin Lymphoma Myeloma Leuk 2014;14:e207–211.

Diel IJ, Body JJ, Stopeck AT, et al. The role of denosumab in the prevention of hypercalcaemia of malignancy in cancer patients with metastatic bone disease. Eur J Cancer 2015;51:1467–1475.

Dietzek A, Connelly K, Cotugno M, et al. Denosumab in hypercalcemia of malignancy: a case series. J Oncol Pharm Pract 2015;21:143–147.

McCurdy MT, Shanholtz CB. Oncologic emergencies. Crit Care Med 2012;40:2212–2222.

Stewart AF. Clinical practice. Hypercalcemia associated with cancer. N Engl J Med 2005;352:373–379.

Tumor Lysis Syndrome

Background

Definition of disease

Acute tumor lysis syndrome (TLS) results from the release of intracellular contents leading to potentially life-threatening metabolic abnormalities including hyperkalemia, hyperphosphatemia, hypocalcemia, and hyperuricemia. The metabolic shifts can lead to cardiac dysrhythmias, acute kidney injury, seizures, tetany, and even sudden death. TLS is either classified as laboratory TLS (LTLS) or clinical TLS (CTLS), which is further described in this section.

Incidence/prevalence
- TLS most frequently occurs in hematologic malignancies, including high grade lymphomas and leukemias.
- Increasingly reported in malignancies that it had previously rarely been associated with including endometrial carcinoma, hepatocellular carcinoma, chronic lymphocytic leukemia, and chronic myelogenous leukemia.

Etiology
Risk factors for TLS:
- Bulky tumor or extensive metastasis
- Organ infiltration by cancer cells
- Bone marrow involvement
- Renal infiltration or outflow tract obstruction
- High proliferation of cancer cells
- Cancer cell sensitivity to anticancer therapy
- High intensity of initial chemotherapy
- Nephropathy prior to cancer diagnosis
- Dehydration or volume depletion
- Acidic urine
- Hypotension
- Exposure to nephrotoxins
- Exogenous potassium
- Exogenous phosphate
- Delayed uric acid removal.

Pathology/pathogenesis
- TLS occurs in malignancies with a high proliferative rate, large tumor burden, and high sensitivity to chemotherapy.
- The initiation of cytotoxic chemotherapy, steroids, cytolytic antibody therapy, and/or radiation therapy leads to rapid lysis of tumor cells resulting in a large release of potassium, phosphorus, and nucleic acids into the bloodstream.
- Hyperkalemia can lead to fatal dysrhythmias.
- Hypocalcemia results secondarily from hyperphosphatemia and can cause tetany, dysrhythmia, and seizure.
- Calcium phosphate can deposit in various organs including the kidneys leading to injury.
- Nucleic acids are metabolized into hypoxanthine, xanthine, and eventually uric acid, which can crystallize, leading to acute kidney injury.

Prevention
- IV fluids are administered to prevent TLS in at-risk patients:
  - **Adults:** roughly double maintenance rate, 2.5 mL/kg/hour (200 mL/hour in an 80-kg patient)
  - **Children:** 200 mL/kg per day (~8 mL/kg/hour) in children weighing ≤10 kg
  - **Target urine output:** 2 mL/kg/hour for children and adults, 4–6 mL/kg/hour if ≤10 kg.
- Allopurinol alone can be used in patients whose uric acid level is <7.5–8 mg/dL and are not high risk for developing TLS.
  - 100 mg/m^2 by mouth every 8 hours (maximum 800 mg/day)
  - In acute kidney injury, reduce dose by 50%

- 200 mg/day for creatinine clearance 10–20 mL/minute
- ≤100 mg/day for creatinine clearance 3–10 mL/minute
- ≤100 mg/dose at extended intervals for creatinine clearance <3 mL/minute in adults.
- Intermediate to high risk individuals whose uric acid is ≥7.5 mg/dL can receive 0.15 mg/kg rasburicase for prevention.
- Exogenous potassium and phosphate should be limited unless a deficiency is seen.

Diagnosis

TLS is classified either as laboratory TLS (LTLS) or clinical TLS (CTLS).

Diagnosis of LTLS

Two or more of the following laboratory changes within 3 days prior to initiation OR by day 7 of cytotoxic therapy.

Diagnosis of CTLS

Requires the presence of LTLS in addition to one or more of the following clinical complications: renal insufficiency, cardiac arrhythmias, seizure, neuromuscular irritability, or sudden death (see Table 39.2).

Table 39.2 Diagnosis of laboratory tumor lysis syndrome.

Metabolic item	Laboratory values
Potassium	≥6.0 mmol/L or 6 mEq/dL or 25% increase from baseline
Phosphorus	≥2.1 mmol/L for children or ≥1.45 mmol/L for adults or 25% increase from baseline
Calcium	≤1.75 mmol/L or 25% decrease from baseline
Uric acid	≥476 mmol/L or 8 mg/dL or 25% increase from baseline

Treatment (Table 39.3)

- Aggressive hydration and diuresis are fundamental not only for the prevention but also the management of TLS.
- Rasburicase is a recombinant urate oxidase that works by catabolizing uric acid to the more soluble allantoin. Whether given therapeutically or prophylactically, the agent is highly effective at rapidly normalizing uric acid levels.
- Rasburicase is contraindicated in patients with glucose 6-phosphate deficiency because hydrogen peroxide is a by-product of uric acid catabolism to allantoin, which can cause hemolytic anemia or methemoglobinemia in this subgroup of patients.
- Dialysis for TLS is indicated in significant AKI, poor response to medical management, or symptomatic life-threatening metabolic derangements.

Prognosis

- TLS is associated with increased mortality.
- AKI in TLS is associated with higher morbidity and mortality, making prevention and treatment critical.

Table 39.3 Treatment of laboratory tumor lysis syndrome.

Metabolic abnormality	Potential clinical outcome	Treatment
Hyperkalemia	Muscle cramps, paresthesias, peaked T waves on ECG, dysrhythmias, ventricular fibrillation, cardiac arrest	• Polystyrene sulfonate 1 g/kg • Insulin 0.1 unit/kg with 25% dextrose 2 mL/kg • Sodium bicarbonate 1-2 mEq/kg IV push • Calcium gluconate 100-200 mg/kg slow IV infusion for cardiac membrane stabilization
Hyperphosphatemia	Nausea, vomiting, diarrhea, lethargy, acute kidney injury	• IV fluids • Removal of phosphate from IV fluids • Oral (non-calcium containing) phosphate binders • Hemodialysis
Hypocalcemia	Hypotension, dysrhythmias, neuromuscular irritability (tetany, muscle twitching, carpopedal spasm, Trousseau sign, Chvostek sign, laryngospasm, or bronchospasm)	• Calcium gluconate 50–100 mg/kg slow IV infusion with electrocardiogram monitoring. • Give only if symptomatic
Hyperuricemia	Acute kidney injury	• IV fluids • Rasburicase (0.2 mg/kg IV once or twice daily given for 5–7 days) • Allopurinol by mouth or IV (dosing listed in Prevention section)

Reading list

Coiffier B, Altman A, Pui CH, et al. Guidelines for the management of pediatric and adult tumor lysis syndrome: an evidence-based review. J Clin Oncol 2008;26:2767–2778.

Howard SC, Jones DP, Pui CH. The tumor lysis syndrome. N Engl J Med 2011;364:1844–1854.

McCurdy MT, Shanholtz CB. Oncologic emergencies. Crit Care Med 2012;40:2212–2222.

Guidelines

Title	Source	Date and weblink
Guidelines for the management of pediatric and adult tumor lysis syndrome: an evidence-based review	Coiffier B, Altman A, Pui CH, et al.	2008 https://www.ncbi.nlm.nih.gov/pubmed/18509186

Neutropenic Fever
Background
Definition of disease

- Neutropenia is defined as an absolute neutrophil count (ANC) of <500 cells/mm^3 or an ANC that is expected to decrease to <500 cells/mm^3 during the following 48 hours.
- Neutropenic fever is defined by the Infectious Diseases Society of America (IDSA) as a single oral temperature >38.3°C (100.4°F) or a temperature of 100.4°F sustained over a 1-hour period in a neutropenic patient.

Etiology

- Causal risk factors include indwelling Foley catheters, exposure to hospital-acquired pathogens, and chemotherapy-induced mucositis.

Pathology/pathogenesis

- Bacteria are the most common cause of neutropenic fever.
- Fungal pathogens are common in high risk patients with neutropenic fever, with *Candida* and *Aspergillus* accounting for the majority of infections.
  Most common bacterial organisms found in neutropenic fever:
- Gram-positive pathogens:
  - Coagulase-negative staphylococci
  - *Staphylococcus aureus,* including methicillin-resistant strains
  - *Enterococcus* species, including vancomycin-resistant strains
  - Viridans group streptococci
  - *Streptococcus pneumonia*
  - *Streptococcus pyogenes.*
- Gram-negative pathogens:
  - *Escherichia coli*
  - *Klebsiella* species
  - *Enterobacter* species
  - *Pseudomonas aeruginosa*
  - *Citrobacter* species
  - *Stenotrophomonas maltophilia.*

Prevention

- Fluoroquinolone prophylaxis should be considered in high risk patients with expected duration of an ANC $\leq$100 cells/mm^3 for >7 days.
- The National Comprehensive Cancer Network (NCCN) also recommends considering prophylaxis for intermediate risk groups including autologous hematopoietic cell transplantation, lymphoma, chronic myelogenous leukemia, multiple myeloma, and patients receiving purine analog therapy.
- Levofloxacin (500 mg once daily) and ciprofloxacin (500 mg twice daily) are considered to be equivalent.
- Addition of an empiric Gram-positive active agent to fluoroquinolone prophylaxis is generally not recommended.
- IDSA does not recommend a specific antifungal agent for prophylaxis. Fluconazole (400 mg/day orally), which covers most *Candida* species, is typically used. Fluconazole does not have *Aspergillus* coverage, so voriconazole (200 mg twice daily orally) and posaconazole (300 mg/day orally) are used.
- *Pneumocystis jiroveci* pneumonia (PCP) prophylaxis (either trimethoprim-sulfamethoxazole 160–800 mg/day orally or atovaquone 1500 mg/day orally) is recommended for patients with acute lymphoblastic leukemia, those undergoing hematopoietic stem cell transplantation, patients receiving a glucocorticoid dose equivalent to $\geq$20 mg/day of prednisone for 1 month or longer, and for patients receiving temozolomide and radiotherapy until recovery of lymphopenia.
- Herpes simplex virus seropositive patients undergoing allogeneic HSCT or leukemia induction therapy should receive acyclovir prophylaxis 800 mg twice daily orally (off label).

Diagnosis
Clinical diagnosis
History
- Oral, pharyngeal, or esophageal pain can be a result of mucositis.
- Headache or sinus pain could represent sinusitis.
- Respiratory symptoms may be secondary to pneumonia.
- Abdominal pain may be secondary to typhlitis.

Physical examination
- A thorough physical examination is of the upmost importance.
- Oral examination is used to evaluate for mucositis.
- Palpate sinuses to evaluate for sinusitis.
- Decreased breath sounds or crackles can be signs of pneumonia.
- Abdominal examination is important to evaluate for typhlitis.
- The perirectal region should be evaluated to rule out abscess.
- Digital rectal examination or rectal temperature should be avoided to prevent colonizing gastrointestinal organisms from entering the surrounding mucosa and soft tissues.

Diagnostic tests and imaging techniques
- Blood cultures should be obtained on the onset of fever prior to administration of antibiotics.
- CBC with differential can be used to further guide the ANC.
- Patients with respiratory symptoms should have a chest X-ray to evaluate for pneumonia.
- CT of the head, sinuses, chest, abdomen, and pelvis should be performed as clinically indicated (Figure 39.1).

Treatment
- Empiric antibiotic therapy should be given as early as possible, with some evidence showing decreased mortality if given as early as within 30 minutes of fever onset.
- High risk patients require hospitalization for IV empiric antibiotic therapy with an antipseudomonal β-lactam, such as cefepime, a carbapenem (meropenem or imipenem-cilastatin), or piperacillin-tazobactam.
- Vancomycin is not recommended as an initial standard empiric therapy, but indications are as follows:
  - Hemodynamic instability or other evidence of severe sepsis
  - Clinically suspected catheter-related infection
  - Pneumonia or skin/soft tissue infection at any site
  - Positive blood culture for Gram-positive bacteria, prior to final identification and availability of susceptibility data
  - Colonization with methicillin-resistant *Staphylococcus aureus* (MRSA)
  - Severe mucositis, if fluoroquinolone prophylaxis has been given and ceftazidime is used as empiric therapy.
- In patients with clinically or microbiologically documented infections, the particular organism and site determine the duration of therapy. The appropriate antibiotics should be continued for at least the duration of neutropenia or longer if clinically necessary.
- Empiric antifungal coverage should be considered in high risk patients who have a persistent fever after 4–7 days of broad spectrum antibiotics and no identified fever source. Antifungal therapy should be instituted if there are any indications of a possible invasive fungal infection.

- In patients with unexplained fever, it is recommended that the initial regimen be continued until there is a clear sign of marrow recovery with an ANC >500 cells/mm^3.
- If the appropriate treatment course has been completed and all signs and symptoms of the documented infection have resolved, the patient may be transitioned back to fluoroquinolone prophylaxis until no longer needed.

Prognosis
Neutropenic fever is associated with a high mortality; early recognition and antibiotic therapy is critical.

Reading list
Coiffier B, Altman A, Pui CH, et al. Guidelines for the management of pediatric and adult tumor lysis syndrome: an evidence-based review. J Clin Oncol 2008;26:2767–2778.

Flowers CR, Seidenfeld J, Bow EJ, et al. Antimicrobial prophylaxis and outpatient management of fever and neutropenia in adults treated for malignancy: American Society of Clinical Oncology clinical practice guideline. J Clin Oncol 2013;31:794–810.

Freifeld AG, Bow EJ, Sepkowitz KA, et al. Clinical practice guideline for the use of antimicrobial agents in neutropenic patients with cancer: 2010 update by the Infectious Diseases Society of America. Clin Infect Dis 2011;52:e56–93.

Rosa RG, Goldani LZ. Cohort study of the impact of time to antibiotic administration on mortality in patients with febrile neutropenia. Antimicrob Agents Chemother 2014;58:3799–3803.

Suggested website
NCCN Guidelines Prevention and Treatment of Cancer-Related Infections, Version 1.2018. 2017: http://www.nccn.org.

Guidelines

Title	Source	Date and weblink
Clinical practice guideline for the use of antimicrobial agents in neutropenic patients with cancer	Infectious Diseases Society of America	2010 https://www.ncbi.nlm.nih.gov/pubmed/21205990
Clinical Practice Guidelines in Oncology: Prevention and treatment of cancer-related infections	National Comprehensive Cancer Network (NCCN)	2017 http://www.nccn.org
Antimicrobial prophylaxis and outpatient management of fever and neutropenia in adults treated for malignancy	American Society of Clinical Oncology	2013 https://www.ncbi.nlm.nih.gov/pubmed/23319691

Image

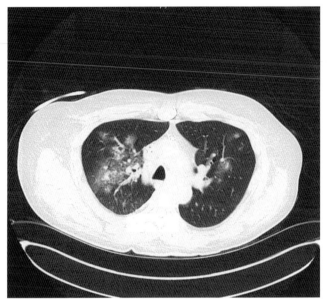

Figure 39.1 Chest CT with multifocal pneumonia.

Malignant Spinal Cord Compression
Background
Malignant spinal cord compression (MSCC) occurs when a primary or metastatic lesion encroaches on the spinal cord.

Incidence/prevalence
- MSCC occurs in 5% of incurable cancer patients within the last 2 years of life.
- Median survival after diagnosis is less than 6 months.

Etiology/pathology/pathogenesis
Tumors that are most commonly responsible for MSCC include lymphoma, myeloma, breast, prostate, lung cancer, melanoma, sarcoma, and renal cell carcinoma.

Diagnosis
History
- Back pain is the first symptom in 95% of patients presenting with MSCC.
- Approximately 50% of patients have bowel or bladder dysfunction.

Physical examination
- Sensory abnormalities are seen in 40–90% of patients.
- Weakness is present in 60–85% of patients with MSCC at the time of diagnosis.
- Post-void residual function aids in the diagnosis of cauda equina syndrome with 90% sensitivity and 95% specificity.

List of imaging techniques

- MRI is the gold standard for diagnosing MSCC with a sensitivity of 93% and a 97% positive predictive value.
- The entire spine should be evaluated with T1- and T2-weighted imaging in axial, sagittal, and coronal planes as one-third of patients have multiple sites of metastasis (Figure 39.2).
- Gadolinium enhanced images enhance the ability to improve both identification of leptomeningeal and intramedullary metastasis and underlying nearby anatomy, but are not necessary to evaluate epidural spinal cord compression.
- CT with myelography can be used as an alternative when MRI is unavailable or contraindicated.
- Noncontrast CT without myelography can still be of use if contrast cannot be administered.
- If MRI or CT myelography is not available, bone scintigraphy combined with plain films has a sensitivity of 98% but a poor specificity.

Treatment

- Rapid treatment improves short-term prognosis.
- Corticosteroids mitigate vasogenic edema and are a standard of treatment; however, dosing remains somewhat controversial. High dose dexamethasone (96 mg IV bolus, then 24 mg orally every 6 hours for 3 days, followed by a 10-day taper) had significant preservation of ambulation at 3 months in a randomized controlled clinical trial, but can have severe side effects.
- Several studies have suggested that lower doses can be effective but they have not been assessed in randomized trials.
- High dose steroids are recommended for patients with an abnormal neurologic examination and moderate dose steroids (dexamethasone 10 mg IV bolus, then 4 mg orally four times daily with a 2-week taper) for all others because of the detrimental side effects of high dose steroids. Multiple studies have suggested that lower doses can be effective and are most commonly used.
- Patients with radiosensitive tumors should undergo radiotherapy; nearly half of survivors that receive radiation are ambulatory at 1 year (Table 39.4).

Table 39.4 Radiosensitivity of tumors.

Radiosensitive	Radioresistant
Lymphoma	Melanoma
Myeloma	Sarcoma
Breast	Renal cell carcinoma
Prostate	
Small-cell lung cancers	

- Indications for surgery include: spinal instability, previous radiation to the area, radioresistant tumors, unknown primary tumor, paraplegia <48 hours, or a single area of cord compression.
- Longer median duration of ambulation (122 vs. 13 days), maintenance of continence (156 vs. 17 days), and median survival (126 vs. 100 days) is seen with selective surgical decompression followed by postoperative radiotherapy vs. radiation alone.

Prognosis

Longer median duration of ambulation, maintenance of continence, and survival is seen with selective surgical decompression followed by postoperative radiotherapy vs. radiation alone.

Reading list

George R, Jeba J, Ramkumar G, et al. Interventions for the treatment of metastatic extradural spinal cord compression in adults. Cochrane Database Syst Rev 2015;9:CD006716.

Heimdal K, Hirschberg H, Slettebo H, et al. High incidence of serious side effects of high-dose dexamethasone treatment in patients with epidural spinal cord compression. J Neurooncol 1992;12:141–144.

Helweg-Larsen S, Sorensen PS. Symptoms and signs in metastatic spinal cord compression: a study of progression from first symptom until diagnosis in 153 patients. Eur J Cancer 1994;30A:396–398.

McCurdy MT, Shanholtz CB. Oncologic emergencies. Crit Care Med 2012;40:2212–2222.

Sorensen S, Helweg-Larsen S, Mouridsen H, et al. Effect of high-dose dexamethasone in carcinomatous metastatic spinal cord compression treated with radiotherapy: a randomised trial. Eur J Cancer 1994;30A: 22–27.

Image

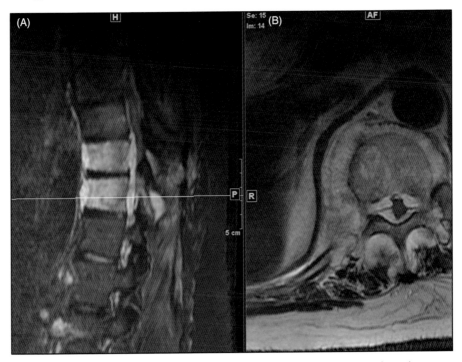

Figure 39.2 CT/MRI images of cord compression. A 50-year-old male with metastatic colorectal cancer presented with 1 week of new onset severe lower thoracic bandlike pain that wraps around the umbilicus bilaterally. He also had bilateral leg weakness, urinary retention, as well as reduced sensory on examination from T12–L1. MRI showed severe canal compression due to metastatic soft tissue deposits involving the thoracic spine from T9–T11 seen in (A) in a T2 sequence sagittal view. Epidural cord compression at T11 can be further seen in (B) on axial view T2 sequence. (Courtesy of Amy M. Chan, MD, Neuroscience and Medicine, Icahn School of Medicine at Mount Sinai.)

Additional material for this chapter can be found online at:
www.wiley.com/go/oh/mountsinaioncology

This includes advice for patients, a case study, ICD codes, and multiple choice questions.

CHAPTER 40

Thrombosis in Cancer Patients

Doyun Park[1], Caroline Cromwell[2], Mala Varma[2], and Ilan Shapira[2]

[1] NYU School of Medicine, New York, NY, USA
[2] Icahn School of Medicine at Mount Sinai, New York, NY, USA

OVERALL BOTTOM LINE
- Twenty percent of all venous thromboembolism (VTE) is associated with cancer.
- Cancer-associated VTE is the second leading cause of death in cancer patients and negatively impacts both short- and long-term survivals.
- Low molecular weight heparin has been shown to be more efficacious than vitamin K antagonist therapy in cancer-associated VTE.
- Further research is needed to determine the efficacy of novel oral anticoagulants in cancer-related VTEs.

Background
Definition of the disease
Types of cancer-associated thromboembolisms include deep venous thrombosis (DVT) and pulmonary embolism (PE), as well as visceral or splanchnic venous thrombosis (SVT). They also include arterial occlusion such as stroke and myocardial infarction.

Disease classification
Frequent imaging has led to an increase in diagnoses of unsuspected or incidental venous thrombosis (IVT). The latest American College of Chest Physicians guidelines for the treatment of VTEs recommend treating IVTs in the same way as symptomatic DVTs, although there are no randomized studies to support this approach.

Incidence/prevalence
- Annual incidence of VTE is estimated to be 1 in 200.
- The cancers most strongly associated with VTE are those of pancreas, ovary, and brain.
- Myeloproliferative neoplasms constitute the most common cause of SVTs.
- Of cancer-related VTEs, 78–80% are estimated to occur on an outpatient basis, with the 2-year incidence of VTE in the range of 0.6–7.8% per year.
- Up to 10% of patients diagnosed with idiopathic VTE are found to have cancer within 1 year of their thromboembolic event.

Economic impact
- A retrospective analysis showed that the difference in annual medical costs for solid cancer patients was about $32 378 for patients with VTE compared with those without VTE.

Mount Sinai Expert Guides: Oncology, First Edition. Edited by William K. Oh and Ajai Chari.
© 2019 John Wiley & Sons Ltd. Published 2019 by John Wiley & Sons Ltd.
Companion Website: www.wiley.com/go/oh/mountsinaioncology

- A retrospective analysis of lung cancer patients showed that medical cost was 40% greater in those who developed VTE than in those who did not.
- In a 2005 study, the mean cost per patient with cancer treated with dalteparin for 6 months was Can$4162 compared with Can$2003 per patient treated with warfarin.

Etiology
Historically, Virchow's triad (hypercoagulability, vascular wall injury, and circulatory stasis) has represented the three main factors that predispose patients to thrombosis. Cancer patients often demonstrate abnormalities in each component of Virchow's triad.

Pathology/pathogenesis
Tumor cells stimulate blood coagulation by:
- Increased production of procoagulant factors (e.g. tissue factor), which also promotes angiogenesis and vascular permeability.
- Release of cytokines (TNFα, IL-1β) and vascular endothelial growth factor (VEGF).
- Direct cell–cell interaction via cell adhesion molecules expressed on tumor cells with patient endothelial cells, leukocytes, and platelets. The result is the promotion of fibrin formation, the final step in the coagulation pathway.

Predictive/risk factors

Risk factor	Relative risk
First 3 months after diagnosis	53.5
Advanced/metastatic cancer stage	19.8
3–10 months after diagnosis	14.3
Chemotherapy administration	6.5
1–3 years after diagnosis	3.6
Body mass index (BMI) >35	2.5
Hemoglobin <10	2.4
White blood cells >11 000/mL	2.2
Platelets >350 000/mL	1.8
Red blood cell transfusion	1.60
Platelet transfusion	1.20

Prevention

CLINICAL PEARL
- There is good evidence supporting the use of postoperative thromboprophylaxis in patients undergoing surgery for cancer.
- Based on post hoc subgroup analyses, routine thromboprophylaxis in hospitalized patients with cancer is also supported.
- Routine thromboprophylaxis is not recommended for ambulatory cancer patients.

Screening
- Routine screening for thromboembolism beyond history taking and physical examination is not recommended.
- Conversely, CT of the chest of patients with idiopathic VTE is not recommended because it has not been shown to reduce time to diagnosis or mortality.
- Despite the assumption that the validity of D-dimer may be compromised in cancer, several studies have reported high negative predictive value and sensitivity of D-dimer testing for diagnosing PE among oncology patients. Although many cancer patients have elevated D-dimer levels, there is no consensus on the cutoff levels predictive of cancer-associated thrombosis.

Primary prevention
- Thromboprophylaxis is currently recommended for hospitalized medical and surgical cancer patients without contraindications by American Society of Clinical Oncology (ASCO) and National Comprehensive Cancer Network (NCCN) guidelines.
- Most guidelines do not recommend routine prophylaxis in ambulatory settings except for myeloma patients treated with thalidomide or lenalidomide who are receiving treatment with these agents in combination with chemotherapy or dexamethasone.
- Extended prophylaxis with low molecular weight heparin (LMWH) for up to 4 weeks should be considered for postoperative patients who have undergone major abdominal or pelvic surgery for cancer and have high risk features such as immobilization, obesity, and history of VTE.
- Although its use is not recommended by the NCCN guidelines, patients' Khorona risk score (site of tumor, CBC parameters, BMI) can be calculated and used to determine the use of thromboprophylaxis.

Secondary prevention
- Secondary prevention after initial VTE with LMWH for a minimum of 6 months is recommended by most guidelines. However, in clinical practice, indefinite anticoagulation beyond 6 months is frequently adopted for patients with active or metastatic cancer. Clinicians can also use the recently validated Ottawa prognostic score, which takes into account sex, primary tumor site, tumor state, and history of VTE to determine risk of recurrence.

Diagnosis (Algorithm 40.1)

CLINICAL PEARLS
- Thromboembolism should always be considered in a cancer patient not in remission who presents with swelling in the lower extremity or shortness of breath.
- DVT affecting the lower extremity is the most common type of thrombosis in cancer patients.
- The incidence of upper extremity thrombosis has markedly increased, estimated to be up to 25% of all venous thrombotic episodes among cancer patients.
- Examination findings of the involved extremity include: increased warmth, edema, and erythema. Phlegmasia cerulea dolens, an extreme manifestation of proximal venous thrombosis caused by compartment syndrome, occurs most often in the setting of malignancy and should not be missed.

Algorithm 40.1 Diagnosis of deep venous thromboembolism (DVT)

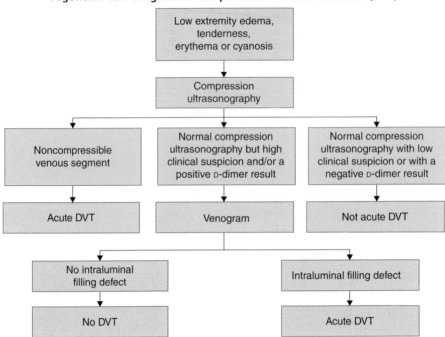

Differential diagnosis

Differential diagnosis	Features
Lymphedema	Can arise from prior radiotherapy or surgical cancer treatment
Post-thrombotic syndrome	Must be ruled out from new thrombosis if new symptoms occur; marked by reduced vein diameter caused by fibrotic thickening of the recanalized vein walls, and an irregular appearing multichanneled lumen
Enlarged lymph nodes or metastases compressing the veins	Enlarged lymph nodes can compress inferior vena cava (IVC) and iliac nodes causing lower extremity edema
Pulmonary metastasis, symptomatic anemia, angina	Symptoms may be similar to those of PE
Tumor thrombus	Extension of tumor itself rather than bland thrombosis caused by hypercoagulability, most often encountered in hepatocellular carcinoma, renal cell carcinoma, and retroperitoneal sarcoma

Typical presentation

- VTE in the form of PE and DVT is the most frequent clinical presentation of cancer-associated thrombosis.
- Catheter-related VTE is another common occurrence. Cancer patients are three times more likely to develop catheter-associated DVTs than noncancer patients.

- Incidentally encountered, asymptomatic VTE is a common entity in cancer patients caused by frequent radiographic restaging, with similar mortality as to symptomatic VTE.
- As discussed in the section on Predictive/risk factors, VTE most often occurs in the initial phase of diagnosis (first 3 months), at an advanced stage of the cancer, or during the active treatment phase.

Clinical diagnosis
History
- Inquire routinely about swelling, pain, and erythema of any extremity (calf, thigh, upper arm), as well as exertional dyspnea, pleuritic chest pain, cough, and hemoptysis.
- Abdominal pain (for SVT), headaches (for sagittal sinus thrombosis), and symptoms of myocardial infarction and stroke should be further investigated when more common causes have been ruled out.

Physical examination
Evaluate patients for:
- Signs of swelling, erythema of lower extremity
- Tachycardia, tachypnea, hypoxia, concerning for pulmonary embolus
- Neurologic/cardiovascular symptoms suspicious for arterial ischemia
- Right upper quadrant tenderness, hepatomegaly, and ascites concerning for SVT.

Useful clinical decision rules and calculators
The Khorona risk score can be used to predict risk of primary VTE occurrence and decide upon thromboprophylaxis. The Ottawa prognostic score can be used to determine the risk of VTE recurrence and duration of secondary prophylaxis. A number of risk prediction tools have been developed to quantify individual risk of hemorrhage for patients receiving anticoagulation, though none are specific to oncology.

Disease severity classification
Treatment guidelines for PE have not differed based on the location, size, or number of filling defects. However, one exception is subsegmental PE (SSPE). There is evidence that treating SSPE without presence of DVT may not reduce the risk of thromboembolic recurrence, suggesting that SSPE may not be clinically relevant. However, consensus remains that, in the absence of contraindications, cancer patients with SSPE should receive anticoagulants.

Laboratory diagnosis
- Laboratory biomarkers predictive of cancer-related thrombosis are thrombocytosis >350 000/μL or leukocytosis >11 000/μL, hemoglobin less than 10 g/dL, tissue factor, soluble P-selectin, and D-dimer.
- Thrombophilia investigation is not recommended in cancer-related thrombosis as the role of hereditary thrombophilia in cancer remains unclear.

List of imaging techniques
- Although standard catheter-based venography is considered the gold standard for diagnosing thrombosis, it is generally not needed to establish a diagnosis of DVT.
- Compression ultrasonography is the noninvasive standard for diagnosis of patients with suspected DVT.

- CT or MRI can be useful for patients with high clinical suspicion for DVT despite negative or equivocal ultrasound results and for evaluation of iliocaval veins.
- CTPA is the first choice diagnostic imaging modality for PE in most situations. Ventilation–perfusion (V/Q) scanning is usually reserved for patients with suspected PE in whom CTPA is contraindicated (i.e. pregnancy, renal failure, multiple myeloma especially if not in remission).

Potential pitfalls/common errors made regarding diagnosis of disease

- PE may not be immediately recognized in patients with symptomatic anemia, primary and metastatic burden in lung, radiation injuries, or chronic obstructive pulmonary disease (COPD) from longstanding smoking history.
- Nonthrombotic pulmonary embolism (i.e. fat embolism in the setting of trauma and orthopedic procedures and amniotic fluid embolism) should be distinguished, as treatment for these entities is mainly supportive.
- Chronic DVT must be distinguished from acute DVT, as anticoagulation remains ineffective in preventing post-thrombotic syndrome.
- Tumor thrombus should be distinguished from bland thrombus as tumor-directed therapy rather than anticoagulation would be indicated in the former.

Treatment (Algorithms 40.2 and 40.3)

Algorithm 40.2 Diagnosis of PE

Algorithm 40.3 Management of DVT and PE

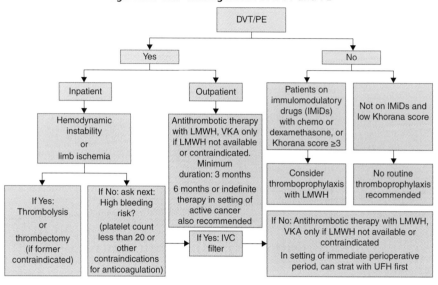

Treatment rationale
- The primary goal of treatment is to reduce mortality from PE and to prevent recurrence of future clots while minimizing bleeding risk.
- In the CLOT trial, dalteparin was found to be more effective than warfarin in reducing risk of recurrent DVT at 6 months, as well as improving survival with LMWH in a subgroup of patients who did not have metastatic disease. Based on available evidence, LMWH is supported by multiple consensus guidelines as the initial therapy of choice for cancer patients.
- However, multiple phase 2 and 3 prospective randomized trials specifically evaluating LMWHs for survival in cancer patients found no survival benefit with use of LMWH in advanced cancer patients.
- Unfractionated heparin can be used in patients with severe renal impairment and fondaparinux is a reasonable replacement for those with a history of heparin-induced thrombocytopenia (HIT).
- Extended, indefinite anticoagulation is generally practiced in clinical settings, especially for those with metastatic or progressive disease.

When to hospitalize
We recommend hospitalizing patients with massive thrombus (swelling of proximal and distal limbs, acrocyanosis, limb ischemia, extension of thrombus into proximal veins and into the IVC), symptomatic pulmonary embolism (hypoxia, hemodynamic instability), as well as those at high risk for anticoagulation-induced bleeding complications (recent bleeding episode, thrombocytopenia, metastases, coagulopathy), and with multiple significant comorbidities (immobility, cognitive impairment, severe pain from the thrombus requiring analgesia).

Managing the hospitalized patient
- Patients with signs of venous gangrene (i.e. phlegmasia cerulea dolens) should receive local thrombolysis, surgical thrombectomy, or percutaneous mechanical thrombectomy.
- Pulmonary emboli patients who have hemodynamic instability should be considered for thrombolysis or embolectomy if thrombolytic therapy is contraindicated.

Table of treatment

Treatment	Comments
Conservative	None (guidelines recommend treating entities that may be treated conservatively in patients without cancer, such as SSPE or isolated distal DVT, still warrant therapy in patients with cancer)
Medical	**Acute VTE** LMWH (recommended as first line for cancer patients): Dalteparin: 200 u/kg once daily Enoxaparin 1 mg/kg twice daily, or 1.5 mg/kg once daily (no consensus regarding frequency between the major guidelines; smaller retrospective studies suggested recurrence of VTE was higher in the once daily regimen. Ultimately, the decision is driven by patient preference) Tinzaparin 175 u/kg once daily or Fondaparinux (minimal risk of HIT) 5 mg (<5 kg), 7.5 mg (50–100 kg) or 10 mg (>100 kg) once daily Partial thromboplastin time (PTT) adjusted unfractionated heparin infusion in initial acute inpatient setting LMWH still preferred but vitamin K antagonist (VKA) with International Normalized Ratio (INR) 2–3 (if LMWH not available, cost prohibitive, or severe renal insufficiency) Can reduce LMWH treatment to 75% after first month. ≥3 months' duration recommended (except for ASCO 2013 guidelines which recommend ≥6 months' duration) **Recurrent VTE** If after VKA, switch to LMWH. If recurrent while on LMWH, increase dosage by 20–25%. If recurrent again, anti-factor Xa levels can be used to tailor LMWH escalation **Thrombocytopenia** Anticoagulation can be given if platelet count >50 000/mL Dose reduction by 50% if platelet count 20–50 000/mL Hold anticoagulation if platelet count <20 000/mL **Novel oral anticoagulants (NOACs)** Given the lack of prospective evidence supporting use of NOACs for VTEs in cancer patients, consensus guidelines do not recommend use of NOACs. Of note, however, pooled analyses of the two major NOAC trials, EINSTEIN and RECOVER, showed that while higher recurrence and bleeding were observed in cancer patients compared with patients without cancer, efficacy was no different between cancer patients treated with NOACS or warfarin. Also important to note is that many "active" cancer patients were not included in these trials whereas those with past history of cancer were entered **Catheter-related thrombosis** Can be treated with LMWH × 3–5 days followed by long-term anticoagulation for ≥3 months while catheter remains in place. Catheter should be removed only if venous access is no longer required, device is nonfunctional, or if line-related sepsis occurs
Surgical	IVC filter, for those with absolute contraindications to anticoagulation Thrombectomy should be considered for severe iliofemoral DVT at high risk for post-thrombotic syndrome, and in whom thrombolysis is contraindicated. For similar reasons, embolectomy in patients with PE should be considered

(*Continued*)

Treatment	Comments
Radiologic (interventional)	IVC filter: see Surgical recommendation
Complementary	Ambulation, compression stockings IVC filter can be used as adjunct therapy in patients with recurrent embolism despite adequate anticoagulation, and in patients in whom an additional embolic event would be near fatal (i.e. those with poor cardiopulmonary reserve from massive PE or pre-existing cardiopulmonary comorbidities, or those with hemodynamic instability)

Prevention/management of complications

Emergent bleeding complications:

- **On LMWH (enoxaparin):** patient should be given 1 mg protamine sulfate for every 1 mg enoxaparin given in previous 8 hours. Fresh frozen plasma should not be given in LMWH-related bleeding.
- **On warfarin:** vitamin K 10 mg (repeat dosing every 12 hours as needed), fresh frozen plasma (2–4 units), and prothrombin complex concentrates (per institutional protocol) are used.

CLINICAL PEARLS
- LMWHs are preferred over VKAs for their superior efficacy in preventing recurrent VTEs as well as survival benefit as suggested in multiple studies.
- Minimum therapy duration of 3–6 months is recommended. Extended/indefinite anticoagulation in the setting of active cancer is supported by consensus guidelines.
- IVC filters should be used only in patients with absolute contraindications for anticoagulation.
- Use of NOACs for treatment of VTE in cancer patients is not supported by expert guidelines because of insufficient evidence.

Special populations
Pregnancy
- Warfarin is generally avoided during pregnancy because of well-documented negative effects on the developing fetus. NOACs are not used during pregnancy because of lack of information on fetal safety and efficacy.

Elderly
- Low dietary vitamin K intake and polypharmacy prevalence in the elderly mean that initial doses of warfarin should start at 3–4 mg/day and be lowered to 2.5 mg in the setting of severe malnourishment, frailty, or liver disease.

Renal insufficiency
- If LMWH is administered at therapeutic dosage in patients with renal insufficiency, dosage reduction should be considered. When creatinine clearance is found to be <30 mL/min, dose reduction of enoxaparin from 1 mg/kg every 12 hours to 1 mg/kg once daily is recommended. Alternatively, anti-factor Xa monitoring and/or dose reduction should be considered. The usually accepted target range for anti-factor Xa activity (measured 4 hours post injection) is 0.6–1.0 IU/mL for twice daily dosing and 1.0–2.0 IU/mL for once daily dosing.

Heparin-induced thrombocytopenia

- Fondaparinux can be used in patients with history of HIT; however, when calculating a HIT score, it is important to keep in mind that myelosuppression from cancer chemotherapy provides a very likely alternative explanation to HIT.

Multiple myeloma patients on IMiDs

- Twenty percent of patients with multiple myeloma being treated with immunomodulatory imide drugs (ImiDs) and dexamethasone will develop a VTE (even higher rates if given with concurrent erythropoiesis stimulating agents). While low dose warfarin has been shown to be ineffective, aspirin 81 mg/day or LMWH for those at higher risk of thrombotic events reduces the risk of VTE to <5%.

Disseminated intravascular coagulation

- Disseminated intravascular coagulation (DIC) can be associated with bleeding or clotting. The risk of DIC is particularly increased in patients with adenocarcinomas, acute promyelocytic leukemia, or with the use of L-asparaginase in acute lymphocytic leukemia regimens. The management of DIC requires balancing the risk of thrombosis with the risk of bleeding in the setting of possible hypofibrinogenemia and thrombocytopenia. If the latter concurrent conditions are present with a thrombotic event, consideration can be given to using low dose unfractionated heparin as the underlying condition is being treated.

Prognosis

CLINICAL PEARLS
- Cancer patients who develop VTE have reduced life expectancy.
- Patients with cancer and thrombosis have a lower survival rate than those with cancer alone, reflecting VTE-related deaths and the more aggressive course of malignancies associated with VTE.

Prognosis for untreated patients

- Untreated PE is associated with a mortality of 30%, usually from recurrent embolism. If left untreated, symptomatic DVT results in a 50% chance of PE.

Prognosis for treated patients

- VTE recurrence is three times more common in cancer patients than in patients without cancer. Risk of recurrence varies depending on location and stage of primary tumor, mode of anticoagulation, and histology.

Follow-up tests and monitoring

CBC should be checked on a regular basis to monitor platelet count while the patient remains on anticoagulation. Follow-up imaging is not routinely carried out.

Reading list

Kearon C, Akl EA, Comerota AJ, et al. Antithrombotic therapy for VTE disease: Antithrombotic Therapy and Prevention of Thrombosis, 9th ed. American College of Chest Physicians Evidence-Based Clinical Practice Guidelines. Chest 2012;141(2 Suppl):e419S–494S.

Khorana A. Cancer-associated thrombosis: updates and controversies. Hematology Am Soc Hematol Educ Program 2012;2012:626–630.

Lee AY, Peterson EA. Treatment of cancer associated thrombosis. Blood 2013;122:2310–2317.

Lyman GH, Khorana AA, Kuderer NM, et al. Venous thromboembolism prophylaxis and treatment in patients with cancer: American Society of Clinical Oncology Clinical Practice Guideline Update. J Clin Oncol 2013;31:2189–2204.

Suggested website
National Comprehensive Cancer Network. Clinical Practice Guidelines in Oncology Venous Thromboembolic Disease version 2.2013: http://www.nccn.org/professionals/physician_gls/pdf/vte.pdf.

Guidelines
National society guidelines

	American College of Chest Physicians (2012)	National Comprehensive Cancer Network (2011)	American Society of Clinical Oncology (2013)
Initial therapy	Not specifically addressed in cancer patients	LMWH (dalteparin, enoxaparin, tinzaparin), fondaparinux or PTT-adjusted UFH infusion	LMWH preferred in initial 5–10 days
Long-term therapy	LMWH to VKA to NOACs	LMWH preferred as monotherapy in patients with proximal DVT or PE in metastatic/advanced cancer	LMWH preferred but VKA acceptable if LMWH not available
Duration of therapy	At least 3 months	Minimum 3 months but indefinite for active cancer or persistent risk factors	≥ 6 months but consider indefinite AC for patients with metastatic cancer and those receiving chemotherapy

Evidence

Type of evidence	Title and comment	Date and weblink
RCT	Low-molecular-weight heparin versus coumarin for the prevention of recurrent venous thromboembolism in patients with cancer: CLOT **Comment:** Demonstrated that dalteparin is more effective than warfarin in reducing risk of recurrent thromboembolism in cancer patients	2003 https://www.ncbi.nlm.nih.gov/pubmed/ 12853587.
RCT	Nadroparin for the prevention of thromboembolic events in ambulatory patients with metastatic or locally advanced solid cancer receiving chemotherapy: a randomised, placebo-controlled, double-blind study: PROTECHT **Comment:** Demonstrated that nadroparin, a LMWH, reduces incidence of thromboembolic events in ambulatory patients with metastatic/locally advanced cancer receiving chemotherapy	2009 https://www.ncbi.nlm.nih.gov/pubmed/ 19726226

Additional material for this chapter can be found online at:
www.wiley.com/go/oh/mountsinaioncology

This includes advice for patients, a case study, ICD code, and
multiple choice questions.

CHAPTER 41

Imaging of Cancer Patients

Idoia Corcuera-Solano, Mathilde Wagner, and Bachir Taouli

Icahn School of Medicine at Mount Sinai, New York, NY, USA

OVERALL BOTTOM LINE
- Medical imaging is an essential component of the care of cancer patients in all phases of cancer management: screening, diagnosis, staging of cancer, assessment of treatment response, and monitoring cancer recurrence.
- Cancer imaging is mandatory to allow optimal patient management and increase the chances of patients' survival.
- The main focus of this chapter is to overview the different imaging technologies available for diagnosing cancer and to review the current role of imaging in cancer management.

Medical imaging technologies
Ultrasound
- Ultrasound uses high frequency sound waves to bounce off tissues and internal organs.
- Because sound waves are highly scattered at bone and air interfaces, many parts of the body are inaccessible, and effective imaging depth is limited in most organs to approximately 10 cm.
- Especially good at imaging soft tissues and distinguishing between solid tumors and fluid-filled cysts.
- It is one of the most common diagnostic imaging methods used in the initial diagnosis of tumors in the liver, pancreas, kidney, thyroid, breast, prostate, ovaries, and uterus.
- Useful in determining blood vessels' involvement, especially in the assessment of liver cancer.
- Frequently used to guide biopsies for thyroid, breast, liver, and prostate and to guide minimally invasive therapies in cancers such as in the liver.
- Advantages of ultrasound include the absence of radiation exposure, widespread availability of the technique, and low cost. The principal disadvantage of ultrasound is that it is operator dependent and not reproducible.
- Used as the initial modality in children because of the lack of radiation.

Computed tomography (CT)
- CT is a cross-sectional imaging technique using X-rays. In most cases, CT needs intravenous contrast injection although this is contraindicated in patients with a history of allergy to iodine and for those with renal insufficiency, and relatively contraindicated in patients with multiple myeloma.
- Images can be reconstructed in any plane requested and use any slice thickness to help build a more definitive diagnosis of the patient's disease.

Mount Sinai Expert Guides: Oncology, First Edition. Edited by William K. Oh and Ajai Chari.
© 2019 John Wiley & Sons Ltd. Published 2019 by John Wiley & Sons Ltd.
Companion Website: www.wiley.com/go/oh/mountsinaioncology

- CT scans are among the most common imaging technologies used in diagnosing cancer, as well as in planning and monitoring cancer treatment.
- CT scans are useful in detecting cancer of the liver, pancreas, lungs, and bones. CT is also important in providing information on cancer in the stomach, intestines, and brain.
- CT has also been very important in allowing the development of image-guided procedures and radiotherapy.
- Advantages of CT include excellent spatial resolution, rapid image acquisition, and examination reproducibility. The principal disadvantage of CT is the radiation dose involved and the risk of adverse reaction from the iodine contrast material.
- Modern imaging devices are constantly being improved to generate higher resolution images while significantly decreasing the amount of radiation and exposure time.

Magnetic resonance imaging (MRI)

- MRI uses radio frequency waves in the presence of a strong magnetic field. These radio frequency waves are used to get tissues to emit radio waves of their own. Different tissues (including tumors) emit a more or less intense signal based on their chemical composition.
- MRI can be used to produce two- or three-dimensional images of sections of the body. MRI has a better contrast resolution than CT and is often better than CT scanning in distinguishing soft tissues.
- MRI is used in the same way as CT in cancer detection, staging, therapy response monitoring, biopsy guidance, and minimally invasive therapy guidance.
- MRI is especially useful for imaging of the central nervous system, particularly for brain tumors. It is often the best method for detecting and characterizing cancer in the head, neck, prostate, bones, and muscles. There has also been considerable interest in MRI as a whole-body imaging technique.
- Advances in MRI techniques go beyond morphologic study to obtain functional and structural information about different physiologic processes of tumor microenvironment, such as oxygenation levels, cellular proliferation, or tumor vascularization through MRI analysis of some characteristics: angiogenesis (perfusion MRI), metabolism (MR spectroscopy), cellularity (diffusion-weighted MRI), or hypoxia (blood-oxygen-level-dependent [BOLD] MRI).
- Advantages of MRI include the absence of radiation exposure, very good contrast resolution, and the ability to provide multiplanar imaging.
- Limitations of MRI include the fact that patients with metallic prostheses may not be suitable for scanning, limited availability, cost, and contraindications (such as severe claustrophobia, pacemaker devices, and so on).

Nuclear medicine

- Nuclear medicine employs radiopharmaceuticals: radiolabeled ligands that have the ability to interact with molecular targets involved in the causes or treatment of cancer. These exogenous agents using radionuclides are injected intravenously and are relatively noninvasive.
- Radioactive substances can be traced to evaluate where and when they concentrate. By targeting to a disease-specific biomarker it is possible to get accumulation in diseased tissue that can be imaged.
- Cancer cells can be identified in tissue and bone, thus assisting with more precise diagnosis and effective treatment.
- Nuclear medicine is very sensitive in determining the presence or spread of cancer.

Positron emission tomography computed tomography (PET-CT)

- PET-CT is a technique that combines a PET and a CT examination.
- PET-CT improves cancer staging and the assessment of early therapy response showing metabolic changes in tumor and tissue.
- The most commonly used tracer is fludeoxyglucose (FDG) but many other specific tracers are available (e.g. gallium 68, C11 choline).
  - The sensitivity of FDG-glucose is poor in uncontrolled diabetes; recommended blood glucose level prior to FDG-PET is less than 250; it is also recommended that patients fast prior to FDG-PET.
- PET-CT is mainly indicated in head and neck, esophageal, lung, colorectal, and cervical cancers, lymphoma, and melanoma.
- Limitations include that FDG is not accurate across all tumor types and that tissue changes such as inflammation/infection will also take up FDG, so it is not a truly tumor-specific ligand. The other key disadvantages of PET are that it involves radiation dose and high cost.

Current role of imaging in cancer management

Screening

- The purpose of a cancer screening test is to identify the presence of a specific cancer in an asymptomatic individual at risk.
- Early detection has been the major factor in the reduction of mortality and cancer management costs.
- Current screening imaging tests recommended by the American Cancer Society (ACS) include:
  - Annual mammography in patients older than 40 years for breast cancer screening.
  - Annual low dose CT scan (LDCT) of the chest for lung cancer screening in high risk patients.
  - CT colonography has been proposed as screening for the detection of colorectal neoplasia in patients older than 50 years; however, strong need exists to clinically validate its widespread use.
- Liver screening with ultrasound in high risk patients is also recommended by the American Association for the Study of Liver Disease (AASLD) for early hepatocellular carcinoma (HCC).

Diagnosis and staging

- Imaging has a major role in the detection of cancer as it provides a detailed insight into the exact location and extent of the disease (local extent and presence of metastases).
- Imaging is by far the most effective method to stage cancer accurately.
- Staging can have a critical impact on treatment outcome by facilitating appropriate patient selection for specific therapeutic interventions.
- Cancer clinical staging systems are useful to select the appropriate primary and adjuvant therapy and can provide a more accurate prognostic assessment before and after treatment intervention by providing risk stratification information.
- Local extent is assessed in most cancers with CT, except for uterine, cervix, prostate, and rectum, in which MRI has shown better accuracy.
- CT, PET-CT, and, increasingly, MRI, are the most commonly used methods employed in metastatic staging, particularly where a whole body examination is required. While complete staging relies on a combination of clinical findings, including blood tests, radiology provides the central and pivotal staging process.

Treatment and monitoring

- Imaging techniques can be used to monitor therapy. Information about treatment response is crucial, as it is used to plan the next steps.

- Tumor responses to treatment are still largely assessed from imaging measurements of reductions in tumor size.
- Various response criteria models have been developed for this purpose, of which the most commonly used is the Response Evaluation Criteria In Solid Tumors (RECIST) model.
- RECIST is a standardized procedure that has been widely adopted by academic institutions, medical research groups, and pharmaceutical companies and has been applied in clinical practice and trials where the main endpoints were the "objective response to therapy" or the "time to progression" of the disease. Various imaging techniques, mostly CT, PET-CT, and MRI, can be used for treatment monitoring but for consistency the same modality should be used at baseline and during follow-up.
- To assess RECIST, an initial scan is taken before the treatment starts, against which later scans will be compared. When the course of treatment ends, a final examination is performed to assess the response of the cancer to treatment.
- RECIST guidelines are based on the assessment of the size changes of neoplastic lesions, in order to evaluate objectively the degree of response to therapy. The estimation of the overall response to therapy is based on the change of all neoplastic lesions (target, measurable, and nonmeasurable) and on the appearance of new lesions comparing the baseline images with the follow-up examinations. Depending on the total tumor burden, the case will be categorized as complete response, partial response, or progressive disease (Figure 41.1).
- RECIST has showed some limitations since the development of targeted therapies. Those treatments can lead to a response and an increased survival without any tumor size decrease. New criteria have been developed (e.g. Choi in GIST, mRECIST in HCC).

Follow-up

- Because of the resilient and pervasive nature of cancer cells it is important that patients undergo regular follow-up after they have been declared to be in remission.
- Follow-up care involves a series of regular examinations in order to monitor cancer remission and pinpoint any possible recurrence.
- Patients should undergo follow-up checks to ensure their cancer remains in remission because the earlier recurrence is detected, the better the prognosis.
- The importance of imaging is that it can noninvasively detect the state of the disease or its recurrence before symptoms appear.

Cancer type and imaging modality indication

	Locoregional staging	Distant metastatic disease	Comments
Chest			
Lung cancer	CE-chest CT (include liver and adrenals): modality of choice	Chest-abdomen-pelvis CT	
	MRI chest: for superior sulcus tumors (Pancoast) to assess brachial plexus invasion	Brain MRI (if neurologic symptoms)	
Primary mediastinal neoplasm	CE-chest CT: modality of choice		Thymoma: octreotide scan or PET if chest CT inconclusive
	MRI chest: reserved for clarifying problems encountered on CT		

(Continued)

	Locoregional staging	Distant metastatic disease	Comments
Pleural tumors	CE-chest CT: modality of choice MRI: reserved for clarifying problems encountered on CT	Whole body FDG-PET/CT	
Liver, biliary tract, and pancreas			
Liver cancer: HCC and fibrolamellar HCC	Multiphasic CT/MRI: for lesion characterization and staging	Chest CT Bone scan	
Cholangiocarcinoma	Multiphasic CT/MRI: for lesion characterization and staging	FDG-PET/CT	
Pancreatic cancer	CE: abdominal CT Endoscopic ultrasound ERCP MRCP	Chest CT	Pancreatic neuroendocrine tumors: octreotide scans PET
Gastrointestinal tract			
Esophageal cancer	Chest-abdomen CT Neck CT if upper chest	PET	
Gastric and duodenal carcinoma	Chest with contrast, abdomen and pelvis CT with contrast or without	PET: if gastric cancer >T2 with no metastatic disease by CT or MRI	
Small bowel malignant tumors	CT abdomen and pelvis with contrast		
Colorectal cancer	CT abdomen and pelvis with contrast	CT chest, abdomen and pelvis with contrast or PET/CT	If liver lesion, consider MRI of the abdomen with contrast or without
Genitourinary			
Renal tumors	Abdomen/pelvis CT or Abdomen/pelvis MRI with contrast or without	Chest CT with contrast or without	
Bladder cancer and upper tracts	CT abdomen and pelvis with contrast or without or MRI abdomen and pelvis with contrast or without	CT chest with contrast or PET/CT	
Testicular germ cell tumors	Testicular ultrasound	Chest and abdomen and pelvis CT with contrast	
Primary adrenal malignancy	CT abdomen with contrast or without or MRI abdomen with contrast or without	PET/CT	
Prostate cancer	MRI pelvis contrast	Bone scan	

(Continued)

(*Continued*)

	Locoregional staging	Distant metastatic disease	Comments
Gynecologic and imaging of women			
Uterine tumors	Pelvic MRI with contrast	CT chest and abdomen/pelvis with contrast	
Cervical cancer	Pelvic MRI with contrast	CT chest and abdomen/pelvis with contrast	
Ovarian cancer	TV ultrasound: initial imaging modality Pelvic MRI with contrast	CT abdomen and pelvis with contrast	
Breast cancer	Mammography, supplemented with ultrasound, occasionally breast MRI	Chest and abdomen/pelvis CT: if stage III or IV Bone scan: if bone pain	PET if inconclusive CT or bone scan
Lymphomas and hematologic imaging			
Lymphoma	CT chest, abdomen/pelvis with contrast and/or PET/CT		
Myeloma	Whole body low dose CT, whole body MRI and/or PET/CT		Whole body low dose CT preferred over skeletal survey

Reading list

Eisenhauer EA, Therasse P, Bogaerts J, et al. New response evaluation criteria in solid tumours: revised RECIST guideline (version 1.1). Eur J Cancer 2009;45:228–247.

Fass L. Imaging and cancer: a review. Mol Oncol 2008;2:115–152.

Hricak H. Oncologic Imaging: Essentials of Reporting Common Cancers. Elsevier/Saunders, 2007.

Silverman PM. Oncologic Imaging: A Multidisciplinary Approach. Elsevier/Saunders, 2012.

Tirkes T, Hollar MA, Tann M, et al. Response criteria in oncologic imaging: review of traditional and new criteria. Radiographics 2013;33(5):1323–1341.

Guidelines

Title	Source	Date and weblink
Guidelines for the Early Detection of Cancer Oncology imaging guidelines. V 17.0	American Cancer Society (ACS)	2015 https://www.nccn.org/

Image

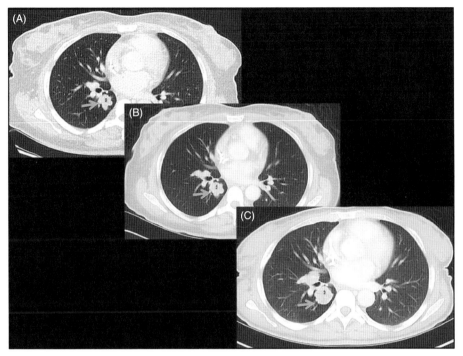

Figure 41.1 Lung cancer. (A) Baseline chest CT and follow-up scans after (B) 3 and (C) 6 months, with interval increase in size of the right pulmonary nodule (arrows) demonstrating progression of disease as per RECIST criteria.

Additional material for this chapter can be found online at:
www.wiley.com/go/oh/mountsinaioncology

This includes advice for patients, a case study (Figure 41.2 and Figure 41.3), and multiple choice questions. Additional figures for this chapter are also available Figure 41.2A,B and Figure 41.3A–E.

CHAPTER 42

Overview of Radiation Oncology

Ronald D. Ennis

Robert Wood Johnson Medical School and New Jersey Medical School of Rutgers University, New Brunswick, NJ, USA

OVERALL BOTTOM LINE
- Radiotherapy is used in half of all cancer patients as sole curative treatment, curative treatment in combination with surgery and/or chemotherapy, or palliative treatment.
- Radiotherapy is most commonly given externally via techniques such as intensity modulated radiotherapy with or without image guidance, stereotactic radiosurgery, and three-dimensional conformal radiotherapy.
- Radiotherapy is also delivered by brachytherapy – which is the implantation of radioactive source(s) directly into or adjacent to the tumor.
- Radiotherapy can also be delivered by oral or IV/intra-arterial injection of unsealed radioactive sources, sometimes termed radionuclide therapy.
- In all these settings, the radiation oncologist weighs the radiation dose–volume response relationships of the tumor and all the exposed normal tissues, in the context of the patient's disease, general health, and social milieu to choose whether and by which technique to treat each patient.

External beam radiation therapy (EBRT)
Indications
This treatment is used in nearly every malignancy in a curative, adjuvant, or palliative role.

Basic principles of EBRT
Linear accelerator
- EBRT is generally delivered from one of the most sophisticated machines in medicine – a 10-ton, multimillion dollar, linear accelerator (linac).

Generating the beams
- This machine converts electricity to high energy X-rays by accelerating electrons to high speed and then having the electrons pass through a high density material like tungsten.
- The interactions of electrons with the tungsten nuclei bend/slow the electrons and result in the generation of a beam of high energy X-rays (the Bremsstrahlung effect).
- Alternatively, the high energy electrons themselves, without interacting with tungsten nuclei, can be allowed to emanate as a beam from the linac.
- EBRT can also be delivered from a machine housing a radioactive material, almost always Cobalt-60, which generates continuous high energy gamma rays (physically the same as X-rays).

Mount Sinai Expert Guides: Oncology, First Edition. Edited by William K. Oh and Ajai Chari.
© 2019 John Wiley & Sons Ltd. Published 2019 by John Wiley & Sons Ltd.
Companion Website: www.wiley.com/go/oh/mountsinaioncology

Beam shaping

- Once the beam (X-rays/gamma rays or electrons) is generated, it is shaped to match the clinical needs (i.e. the shape of the tumor being treated).
- The beam shaping in modern linacs is achieved via dozens of software controlled, individually motor driven, 2–10 mm width, beam shapers known as leaves.
- Each leaf can remain stationary during treatment or can move to shape the beam dynamically.

Positioning

- Patient, tumor, and linac positioning and their interplay are crucial to optimizing the treatment of each patient.
- The treatment table on which the patient lies, part of the linac, is made of carbon fiber allowing X-ray beams to traverse it unperturbed on their way to the patient.
- The table can move to any angle relative to the linac.
- Immobilization devices, individually constructed to immobilize the patient and tumor, are locked into the table providing high accuracy and reproducibility.
- The precision of positioning the part of the linac from which the radiation beam emanates and the linac table are both 1° and 1 mm.

Clinically relevant characteristics of treatment beams

- Electrons treat superficially with minimal exposure to tissues deeper in the body and are therefore ideal for skin tumors and breast tumors.
- X-rays are used for deeper tumors and are therefore used much more often.
- The energy of the X-ray or electron beam determines its penetration depth.
- Linacs generally have the capability to generate beams of several X-ray and electron energies, thereby providing flexibility to optimize treatment.
- A Cobalt-60 treatment machine only provides the fixed natural energies that emanate as Cobalt-60 decays.

Treatment planning

- The radiation oncologist harnesses all these capabilities to meet the clinical needs of the patient through treatment planning.
- The first step in the planning process is a simulation.
- During the simulation, the optimal positioning of the patient is decided and the necessary immobilization device(s) are created and a CT (or MRI) scan is performed.
- The images are then loaded into sophisticated software that allows the radiation oncologist, assisted by dosimetrists and physicists, to develop a virtual treatment evaluating all of the possible treatment delivery options provided by the linac.

Types of EBRT
Three-dimensional conformal radiotherapy (3DCRT)

- Using the 3D representation of the tumor and normal tissues from the planning CT scan, the full spectrum of beam angles, patient angles, and static beam shapes is explored to optimize treatment to fit the clinical situation.
- This type of treatment is used extensively in modern radiotherapy, for example in breast and lung cancers.

Intensity modulated radiation therapy (IMRT)

- This type of EBRT exploits the capability of dynamically changing the beam shape while the beam is delivering treatment.

- This capability, achieved by having the leaves move dynamically while the beam is delivering treatment, adds an almost infinite number of ways to treat a patient as every shape is possible for any length of time.
- To fully exploit this, IMRT entails a change in how the planning process is performed by the radiation oncologist, termed inverse planning. Instead of deciding a priori on the shape of the beams from each treatment angle, the treatment planning software is provided by the radiation oncologist with a series of goals for treatment. The software algorithm then creates the optimal dynamic beam shaping.
- The goals given to the algorithm include a series of dose–volume relationships for the tumor(s) and surrounding normal tissues, in addition to a prioritization score for each organ (e.g. no more that 50% of the kidney can receive 18 Gy, all of the tumor must receive the full dose, etc.).

Image guidance: basic
- Prior to treatment, after reproducing the patient positioning from the simulation on the treatment table, the radiation technologist obtains a series of X-ray images (the linac also has the capability to image the patient with high quality X-rays) to verify that patient positioning, beam shaping, and beam angles are as devised in the treatment plan.
- Only after the radiation oncologist has approved these images can treatment commence.
- If any adjustments are needed they are made prior to actual treatment delivery.
- These images are repeated on a regular basis (e.g. weekly) to assure no changes have developed.

Image guidance: advanced
- When needed, more sophisticated and more frequent forms of image guidance (IG) are performed allowing visualization of more than can be seen on a plain X-ray.
- The radiation oncologist can place (or have a surgeon or interventional radiologist place) radio-opaque markers (fiducials) into the organ of interest. Then, when the X-ray is taken, the markers are visualized and thereby the location of the soft tissue organ of interest can be precisely known and its position adjusted so that it is precisely (~1 mm accuracy) in the correct location.
- Fiducial-based IG is commonly used in prostate, liver, pancreas, and lung cancers, especially in conjunction with stereotactic body radiotherapy (SBRT).
- Fiducial-based IG is most commonly performed before each treatment.
- The second form of advanced IG is accomplished by performing a CT scan of the patient, with the linac, on the treatment table prior to treatment.
- Known as cone beam CT (CBCT), this can be performed daily and allows the radiation oncologist to note positioning of the tumor in addition to significant variations in internal anatomy which if undetected could result in excessive dose to normal tissues. As with fiducial-based CBCT, the tumor's position can be adjusted to the correct location (~2 mm accuracy for soft tissues). Other changes can be made for changes seen in normal tissues.

IG-IMRT and IG-3DCRT
- When daily IG is combined with 3DCRT or IMRT, these are termed IG-3DCRT and IG-IMRT, respectively. It is common, but not essential or uniform, to combine these, especially with IMRT, in current radiation oncology practice. For example, IG-IMRT is commonly used in prostate and head and neck cancers and IG-3DCRT is used in lung cancer (Figure 42.1).

Stereotactic radiosurgery (SRS)/stereotactic body radiotherapy (SBRT) (a.k.a. stereotactic ablative body radiosurgery (SABR))
- This type of treatment incorporates all of the above advances together with precise tumor localization, not just at the beginning of each treatment, but throughout an entire treatment.

- This requires accounting for patient movement and internal organ motion via either rigid immobilization of patient and her/his internal organ of interest or dynamic tracking of the organ of interest.
- This level of precision obviates the usual need for a margin of tissue around the tumor be to included in the treatment volume. This allows the radiation oncologist to prescribe a much higher dose with a single treatment.
- Higher doses per treatment results in the need for fewer treatments, a significant convenience.
- Aside from the convenience of fewer treatment sessions, this method allows biologically significantly higher doses than can be achieved in non-SRS/SBRT settings yielding improved rates of tumor control.
- SRS is the term used for application of this technique in the brain.
- SRS is used routinely for brain metastases, and malignant and benign brain tumors.
- SRS can be delivered using a linac or a dedicated unit known as a Gamma Knife®.
- When applied in the body, this approach is termed SBRT or SABR.
- SBRT/SABR is commonly used in lung, prostate, and liver cancers, and selected metastases.
- For certain malignancies, the high dose per treatment used in these techniques has a biologic advantage yielding significantly improved tumor control rates above what would be expected for the given dose. This is most clearly seen in renal cell carcinoma, but may also be true in melanoma and prostate cancer.

Adaptive planning

- An additional benefit of CBCT-based IG is the ability to note dramatic decreases in tumor volume as a result of treatment when they occur.
- The consequence of a dramatic decrease in tumor volume during the treatment course is that the normal tissues now occupy the space previously occupied by the tumor thereby exposing these surrounding tissues to higher doses than intended.
- When noted, the radiation oncologist can adapt to this change by repeating the planning CT-simulation and re-planning the treatment to this smaller volume.
- This maneuver assuredly decreases the risk of toxicity from radiotherapy. The degree of benefit of adaptive planning in a variety of settings is a current area of research.

Charged particle EBRT – protons

- A proton beam has the appealing physical characteristic that no radiation is delivered to the tissues beyond a certain depth, that depth being determined by the beam energy.
- This differs from X-rays in which gradually decreasing doses are delivered to tissues beyond the tumor.
- The proton beam also delivers a lower entry dose prior to reaching the targeted depth compared to X-rays.
- When used clinically, the net result of this is that significantly lower doses are delivered to tissues not immediately adjacent to the tumor compared with X-rays.
- Due to a variety of uncertainties, this is not true, currently, in close proximity to the tumor.
- Because X-ray therapies can usually keep the dose to normal tissues below the threshold dose at which serious complications develop using the techniques described, it is unclear what the benefit of delivering an even lower dose to these tissues via proton EBRT will be.
- One of the leading rationales for using proton therapy is that it should lead to a lower risk of radiation-induced second malignancies.
- As a result, one of the leading uses of proton therapy is in pediatric radiation oncology.

- Treatment of skull-based tumors, eye tumors, and recurrent head and neck cancers are other common uses for proton therapy.
- All of the techniques discussed for X-rays already exist or are currently being developed for proton therapy.
- A proliferation of proton treatment centers worldwide has occurred over the last decade.
- Emerging data will likely clarify in what settings the superior characteristics of a proton beam can be translated into clinical benefit.

Heavy charged particle beam EBRT
- An innovation on the horizon is the use of beams of heavy charged particles such as carbon ions for therapy.
- The theoretical advantages of these beams is the particle is more damaging over short distances thereby providing greater lethality in a single "hit" of a cell.
- This appears to overcome the inherent relative resistance of hypoxic tumor tissue to X-ray and proton radiotherapy.
- Few particle beam facilities are in use clinically worldwide to date.

Brachytherapy
Indications
Brachytherapy plays an important curative role in prostate, cervical, and head and neck cancers, among others. It is used as an adjunct to surgery in soft tissue sarcomas, uterine cancers, and recurrent tumors in a variety of settings.

Basic principles of brachytherapy
- Implantation of radioactive materials, encapsulated in seeds, pellets, or wires, directly into or adjacent to a tumor is termed brachytherapy.
- This approach allows the delivery of exceptionally high doses of radiation to the tumor.
- The amount of radiation exposure decreases rapidly as distance from the radioactive source increases, thereby creating a favorable ratio of dose to tumor vs. dose to normal tissues.
- Key elements in the successful application of brachytherapy are: (i) a localized tumor/tumor bed that can be encompassed by the radiation emanating from the implanted radioactive materials; (ii) a method for reliably and safely placing the radioactive material into the tumor/tumor bed; and (iii) the normal tissues within or immediately adjacent to the implant volume can tolerate their expected doses.
- An example of a situation in which brachytherapy is not applicable is when treatment to a region of the body is needed (e.g. the pelvis, whole breast).

Types of brachytherapy
Brachytherapy can be divided into temporary and permanent implants.
- Permanent implants use radioactive materials with physical characteristics of low energy, which results in radiation being delivered within a short distance (~5–10 mm) of each source and a half-life that results in complete delivery of their therapeutic dose over a period of weeks–months.
  - This type of treatment allows the patient to go home immediately after outpatient placement of the sources has been performed.
  - The radioactive sources decay into a nonradiative element and remain inertly in the patient permanently.
  - The most common setting in which this is carried out is prostate cancer.

- Temporary implants are performed with materials that deliver their radiation over a relatively short period of time. (These materials also have high energies which mean that patients should not go out in public with such an implant in place.) Temporary implants are further subdivided into low dose and high dose rate implants.
  - A low dose rate (LDR) implant typically delivers its therapeutic dose over a 24–48 hour implant session with 1–2 sessions per patient. This means that these sessions require an inpatient stay.
  - A high dose rate (HDR) implant delivers a therapeutic dose very quickly (over a period of 5–45 minutes).
  - Such a rapid dose rate results in a higher biologic effect per dose to normal tissues.
  - Therefore, to be carried out safely, the treatment must be divided into several (2–6) treatments over a few (1–6) weeks.
  - An important advantage of this approach is that treatments are often performed on an outpatient basis.
  - The trend in recent years has been an increasing use of outpatient multifaction HDR brachytherapy in place of temporary LDR inpatient brachytherapy.

Unsealed source radiotherapy/radionuclide therapy
Indications
Unsealed source radiotherapy or radionuclide therapy has an important role in the treatment of thyroid cancer and liver tumors, can be used in lymphomas, and has an emerging role in bone metastases particularly from prostate cancer.

Basic principles of unsealed source radiotherapy/radionuclide therapy
- Delivery of radioactive material directly into the patient (intra-arterially, intravenously, or orally) which is not sealed inside a seed or wire is termed unsealed source radiotherapy.
- These are typically delivered by nuclear medicine physicians or radiation oncologists.
- The radioactivity is delivered to the tumor via: (i) inherent tumor or normal tissue biochemistry (iodine-131 for thyroid cancer, radium-223 for bone metastases); (ii) attachment to a monoclonal antibody targeted to a tumor-expressed antigen (yttrium 90-ibritumomab for CD20 positive lymphoma); or (iii) direct selective delivery into an artery feeding the tumor (yttrium-90-microspheres into a hepatic artery branch for liver tumors).
- The therapeutic radiation, which travels only a short distance from the radioactive molecule or compound, is delivered via beta particles (equivalent to electrons) (I-131, Y-90), or alpha-particles (Ra-223).
- Gamma rays are also delivered from I-131 allowing it to be imaged.

Intraoperative radiotherapy
Indications
This therapy is most commonly used to treat tumors in conjunction with complex surgical resections, particularly in regions difficult to treat with more conventional forms of radiotherapy, such as previously irradiated areas and retroperitoneal sarcomas. There is current interest in using this to treat breast cancer in conjunction with a lumpectomy.

Basic principles of intraoperative radiotherapy
- This treatment can be delivered via an external source of radiation beams such a mobile electron beam treatment machine, a mobile low energy X-ray machine sometimes referred to as an electronic brachytherapy machine, or a linac.
- It can also be delivered via brachytherapy using intraoperative HDR or intraoperative placement of catheters which are then loaded postoperatively with LDR sources.

Complications
Basic principles
- Every normal tissue has a different response to radiation. Some tissues tolerate high doses with minimal effect (vaginal mucosa) and other are exquisitely sensitive (bone marrow).
- The types of tissue damage induced by radiotherapy broadly include fibrosis, vascular injury, and depletion of normal cells, but the symptomatic consequences of these vary depending on the organ; from bowel urgency to dyspnea, from renal failure to infertility.
- The dose–complication relationships are complex; they are organ and/or tissue specific and highly influenced by the volume of the organ exposed to the dose. Increasing dose to increasing volume of an organ leads to increasing risk, but the shape of the dose volume–complication curve varies by organ.
- An important aspect of complications of radiotherapy is the importance of the dose delivered per unit time. For any given dose, the same dose given over a few minutes has a much greater deleterious effect than when given over hours. While the same can be said about the effect of the dose on the tumor, in general, the differential effect of time is much greater for normal tissues than tumor.
- Dose, volume and dose per unit time do not fully explain the complications that patients experience.
- Some complications are likely random events based on the stochastic nature of radiation's effect.
- Genetic predispositions likely have an important role.
- Research into genetic predispositions to radiation toxicity is beginning to emerge, but is not yet used routinely in clinical practice.
- The radiation oncologist must weigh the dose–response relationships of the tumor and all the exposed normal tissues in the region, in the context of the patient's disease, general health, and social milieu to optimize the care of each patient.

Special populations
Pregnancy
- Special care must be undertaken when treating the pregnant patient because a developing fetus is exquisitely sensitive to radiation. Treatment can only be considered if the treatment area is a considerable distance from the fetus. In addition, if treatment must be given, it is preferable to avoid the first trimester when the fetus is most sensitive. Decisions about whether to treat, how to treat, what to treat, and when need to be carefully considered on a case-by-case basis.

Children
- Children are particularly sensitive to the deleterious effects of radiation in several ways including effects on growth and intellectual development, and an increased risk of treatment-induced cancer. Nevertheless, the benefits of radiotherapy often outweigh these risks and radiotherapy has an important role in many pediatric malignancies. Fortunately, through the work of pediatric cancer cooperative groups, these issues have been and continue to be well studied.

Elderly
- There are no specific contraindications to using radiotherapy in the elderly other than, as for all other patients, taking into account the patient's overall functional and specific organ function status. It is worth noting that there is an increasing awareness that many studies in oncology have excluded the elderly, leaving oncologists uncertain about the risks–benefits of treatment in this population. Furthermore, in the extreme elderly, radiation appears to be tolerable even when chemotherapy is not.

Reading list

DeVita VT, Lawrence TS, Rosenberg SA, eds. DeVita, Hellman, and Rosenberg's Cancer: Principles and Practice of Oncology, 10th edition, 2015, pp. 136–157.
Hoppe R, Phillips T, Roach M, eds. Leibel and Phillips Textbook of Radiation Oncology, 3rd edition. Saunders: 2010, pp. 1–330.

Guidelines
National society guidelines

Title	Source	Weblink
Guidelines and White Papers from the American Radiation Oncology Society	American Society for Radiation Oncology	https://www.astro.org/Patient-Care-and-Research/Clinical-Practice-Statements
Guidance from the American Nuclear Medicine Society	Society of Nuclear Medicine and Molecular Imaging	http://www.snmmi.org/ClinicalPractice/content.aspx?ItemNumber=10817&navItemNumber=10786
Appropriateness Criteria and Practice Parameters from the American Radiology Society	American College of Radiology	https://www.acr.org/Clinical-Resources/Practice-Parameters-and-Technical-Standards/Practice-Parameters-by-Subspecialty

Image

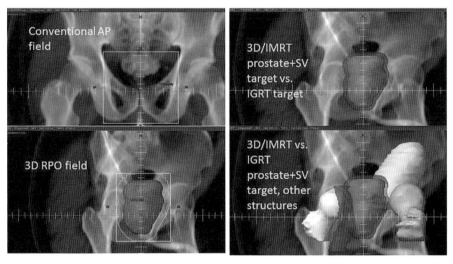

Figure 42.1 Evolution in RT techniques: prostate cancer. Comparison of treatment volume for conventional, 3D conformal/IMRT and IG-3DCRT/IG-IMRT treatment of prostate cancer. Upper left: a prostate cancer anteroposterior (AP) field prior to advent of 3DCRT. Lower left:right posterior oblique (RPO) 3DCRT field. Note field shape matches the red structure which is the prostate and seminal vesicles (SV) and a margin around them to account for set-up variability and organ motion from this oblique nonintuitive angle. Upper right: red is the same structure, green is the smaller structure (prostate and seminal vesicle with much smaller margin) treated when image guidance techniques are used. Lower right: same as upper right but showing relationship with all other adjacent structures. See color version on website.

Additional material for this chapter can be found online at:
www.wiley.com/go/oh/mountsinaioncology

This includes advice for patients and multiple choice questions.
The following image is available in color: Figure 42.1.

CHAPTER 43

Orthopedic Oncology

Meredith K. Bartelstein[1] and Ilya Iofin[2]
[1] Memorial Sloan Kettering Cancer Center, New York, NY, USA
[2] Icahn School of Medicine at Mount Sinai, New York, NY, USA

OVERALL BOTTOM LINE

- Musculoskeletal lesions of bone and soft tissue can be benign or malignant and also primary or metastatic. Cure is possible for primary bone and soft tissue sarcomas and involves wide resection of the tumor. Conversely, goals of care are palliative for metastatic disease and multiple myeloma, and treatment is usually intralesional.
- Key clinical findings include pain with activity, night pain, and expanding soft tissues masses.
- Thorough radiologic investigation is necessary and includes X-ray and cross-sectional imaging of the entire involved bone as well as staging studies.
- Early referral to an orthopedic oncologist is an important early step in the evaluation of a patient with a suspected musculoskeletal lesion.
- Treatment of bone and soft tissue sarcomas involves a multidisciplinary team and a combination of surgery, radiation, and chemotherapy.

Background

Definition of disease

- Musculoskeletal tumors include both benign and malignant conditions of the bone and soft tissues. These may be primary bone or soft tissue sarcomas, of which there are more than 30 varieties, metastatic lesions, multiple myeloma, or lymphoma.
- The carcinomas that most commonly metastasize to bone include: lung, breast, prostate, renal, and thyroid.
- Metastatic lesions and myeloma are more common than sarcoma in patients older than 40 years of age. The reverse is true of patients younger than 40 years of age.

Disease classification

- The World Health Organization (WHO) classifies bone and soft tissue sarcomas by their cell of origin, but molecular genetic techniques are having an increasingly important role (Table 43.1).

Incidence/prevalence

- Bone and soft tissue sarcomas comprise less than 1% of all adult malignant tumors.
- There are approximately 3000 new bone sarcomas diagnosed each year in the USA. The WHO estimates an incidence of 8 cases per million people. These are most common in patients under 40 years of age.

Mount Sinai Expert Guides: Oncology, First Edition. Edited by William K. Oh and Ajai Chari.
© 2019 John Wiley & Sons Ltd. Published 2019 by John Wiley & Sons Ltd.
Companion Website: www.wiley.com/go/oh/mountsinaioncology

Table 43.1 WHO classification of bone tumors (Doyle et al. 2014).

Chondrogenic	Notochordal
Osteogenic	Vascular
Fibrogenic	Myogenic
Fibrohistiocytic	Lipogenic
Ewing sarcoma	Epithelial Undifferentiated high grade pelpmorphic sarcoma
Osteoclastic giant cell rich	Tumors of undefined neoplastic nature

- There are approximately 12 000 new soft tissue sarcomas diagnosed each year in the USA. The WHO estimates an incidence of 30 cases per million people. These are seen in patients of all ages.

Etiology
- Primary malignant bone and soft tissue tumors are sarcomas, or cancers of mesenchymal origin.

Pathology/pathogenesis
- In regards to pathogenesis, sarcomas can be divided into two groups: those with known changes in the cell cycle, such a p53 or Rb mutation, and those with altered karyotypes leading to chromosomal translocations or aneuploidy.

Predictive/risk factors
Most bone and soft tissue sarcomas are idiopathic. However, known risk factors include:
- Genetic alterations: i.e. retinoblastoma (Rb), Li–Fraumeni syndrome (p53)
- Paget disease
- Radiation exposure
- Chronic osteomyelitis
- Chemical exposure: i.e. vinyl chloride.

Prevention

BOTTOM LINE/CLINICAL PEARLS
- No interventions have been demonstrated to prevent the development of primary bone and soft tissue tumors.
- Prevention measures for carcinoma, such as smoking cessation, will aid in prevention of bone and soft tissue metastases.

Screening
- Currently, no screening tests are used for primary bone and soft tissue tumors.
- However, screening tests can be performed for some carcinomas that commonly metastasize to bone. These include PSA for prostate cancer, mammography for breast cancer, and chest CT scan for lung cancer in high risk populations.
- Some genetic screening tests can be performed for those with a family history of cancer syndromes.

Diagnosis (Algorithm 43.1)

Algorithm 43.1 Diagnosis of bone and soft tissue lesions

- Important findings on patient history include pain with activity, night pain and rest pain, weight loss, and any personal or family history of cancer.
- Thorough examination includes assessment for palpable masses, areas of tenderness to palpation, swelling, decreased range of motion, and alteration of gait.
- Initial investigation of suspicious lesions should include X-ray of the entire involved bone. Findings will dictate the need for further imaging such as CT, MRI, or bone scan.
- Initial laboratory testing should include CBC, CMP, ESR, CRP, and serum protein electrophoresis/immunofixation, and serum free light chains.
- Bone and soft tissue sarcomas most often metastasize to the lungs. CT scan of the chest should be performed for staging.

Differential diagnosis

Differential diagnosis	Features
Metastatic disease	This is the most common bone malignancy in adults >40 years of age. Consider any personal history of carcinoma as well as risk factors. Lesions may be lytic, blastic, or mixed
Multiple myeloma	Patients present with hypercalcemia, renal dysfunction, anemia, and/or lytic lesions. Laboratory testing is critical to this diagnosis
Lymphoma	The most common lymphoma of bone in the USA is a diffuse large B-cell lymphoma
Infection	Infection is a common mimicker of tumor

Typical presentation
- Malignant bone tumors often occur as painful or growing masses in the extremities.
- Another presentation is that of an injury that does not resolve as expected.
- Any painless, enlarging, soft tissue mass deep to fascia should prompt suspicion of sarcoma.

Clinical diagnosis
History
As with all conditions, the clinician should take a thorough history, including:
- Location and quality of pain, if present
- Time course
- Presence of masses
- Need for assistive device, such as cane or walker
- History of cancer makes metastatic lesions more likely, but does not rule out a primary lesion or unrelated malignancy.

Physical examination
- Masses
- Skin changes
- Tenderness
- Neurovascular examination.

Useful clinical decision rules and calculators
- For patients under 40 years of age, primary sarcomas are more likely than other diagnoses such as metastatic disease and multiple myeloma. The opposite holds true for patients over 40 years of age. Exceptions occur.
- Infection can mimic tumor in some cases. A common adage is to "culture every tumor and biopsy every infection."

Disease severity classification
- Musculoskeletal lesions, both benign and malignant, are staged by the Enneking system (Enneking et al. 1980; Tables 43.2 and 43.3).
- The AJCC TNM system is also used and is similar to that for other cancers.

Laboratory diagnosis
List of diagnostic tests
- CBC
- CMP
- ESR and CRP.
- Serum protein electrophoresis/immunofixation, and serum free light chains.
- Serum alkaline phosphatase may be elevated at diagnosis, and acts as a tumor marker in some diseases.

Table 43.2 Enneking staging system for benign musculoskeletal tumors (Enneking et al. 1980).

Stage	Description
1	Latent
2	Active
3	Aggressive

Table 43.3 Enneking staging system for malignant musculoskeletal tumors (Enneking et al. 1980).

Stage	Grade	Site	Metastasis
Ia	Low	Intracompartmental	M0
Ib	Low	Extracompartmental	M0
IIa	High	Intracompartmental	M0
IIb	High	Extracompartmental	M0
III	Any	Any	M1

- Biopsy is the ultimate diagnostic tool for bone and soft tissue lesions that are concerning for malignancy. This can be performed via core needle biopsy or open incisional biopsy. Fine needle aspiration is less useful in sarcoma as it does not preserve tissue architecture. Biopsy should be performed as the final step of the diagnostic investigation, after all other staging examinations.

Lists of imaging techniques
- X-ray of lesion, including the entire involved bone, is the first step. In some circumstances, the diagnosis can be made with X-ray alone. X-rays may demonstrate calcifications, changes in bone matrix, and periosteal reaction (Figure 43.1).
- CT scan is useful in showing bony details.
- CT scan of the chest, abdomen, and pelvis is used for staging and to differentiate between primary and metastatic lesions.
- MRI with and without contrast is useful in delineating soft tissue details (Figure 43.2).
- Technetium 99 bone scan is useful for detecting areas of bone production and detects metastases. While bone scan is sensitive, it is not specific for malignancy, and will also be positive in cases of healing fracture and degenerative joint disease.
- The role of PET scan is emerging. FDG avidity can be sensitive for detecting metastatic lesions for many cancers. The CT portion of a PET scan may be useful, but is typically of lower resolution, so a dedicated CT may be needed for more detailed analysis.

Potential pitfalls/common errors made regarding diagnosis of disease
- Even with appropriate physical examination and imaging, diagnosis of bone and soft tissue tumors is challenging. Biopsy is usually required for definitive diagnosis.
- Biopsy should only be performed in coordination with the surgeon who will ultimately be performing the tumor resection. Inappropriately planned biopsy can lead to more complex resections, or even amputation.

Treatment (Algorithms 43.2 and 43.3)
Treatment rationale
- Each tumor requires its own treatment approach which is determined by tumor type, location, and involvement of any adjacent neurovascular structures. Surgical resection is the mainstay of treatment. Limb sparing surgery is usually possible with use of adjuvants such as chemotherapy and radiation therapy.
- Survival rates with limb sparing surgery are equal to those of amputation. However, amputation has a role for patients in whom excision of the tumor would leave a nonfunctional limb.
- Radiation is an important adjunct in treatment of soft tissue sarcomas, bone metastases, and myeloma.
- Chemotherapy has been shown to be an important adjunct in the treatment of high grade bone sarcomas; however, its role in soft tissue sarcoma is still unclear.

Algorithm 43.2 Treatment of bone lesions

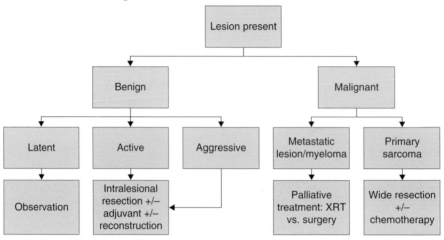

Algorithm 43.3 Treatment of soft tissue lesions

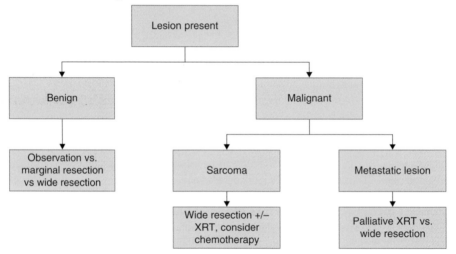

When to hospitalize

- Hospitalization should be considered for patients who present with pathologic fracture and those at high risk for pathologic fracture. One useful evaluation tool is the Mirels criteria (Mirels 1989; Table 43.4).
- To calculate this, scores from the four categories are added. Scores of 9 or more usually require surgical treatment, while scores of 7 or less do not. Treatment for a score of 8 depends on multiple other patient factors.

Table 43.4 Mirels criteria.

Score	1	2	3
Site	Upper extremity	Lower extremity	Peritrochanteric
Pain	Mild	Moderate	Functional
Nature of lesion	Blastic	Mixed	Lytic
Size of lesion	<1/3 bone diameter	1/3–2/3 bone diameter	>2/3 of cortex

Table of treatment

Treatment	Comments
Nonoperative	Appropriate for patients with benign lesions or metastatic ones without fracture risk, and for those whom goals of care are such that the risks of treatment outweigh the benefits. In these cases, the focus should be on comfort
Surgical • Intralesional resection • Wide resection • Amputation	• Intralesional resection violates the tumor capsule, leaving tumor cells behind. It is appropriate for benign lesions as well as metastases and myeloma • Wide resection involves removing the entire tumor with surrounding normal tissue. This is used in sarcoma • Amputation is reserved for cases where limb salvage is not possible. This occurs in cases where excision involves critical nerves and blood vessels such that complete excision would leave a nonfunctional limb
Chemotherapy	Chemotherapy is used with curative intent for sarcoma, usually both before and after surgery, and for palliation in metastatic disease and myeloma
Radiation	Used as an adjunct in most soft tissue sarcomas. Radiation therapy can be used either before or after surgical treatment. It can also be used as a primary treatment modality for metastatic disease and myeloma

Prevention/management of complications
• Thorough investigation to establish the correct diagnosis prior to surgery minimizes complications such an inappropriate intralesional resection of sarcomas, which may jeopardize life and limb.
• Early involvement of multiple specialties improves care.

CLINICAL PEARLS
• Surgical resection varies according to the aggressiveness of the lesion in question; more aggressive lesions require wide margins.
• Chemotherapy, in combination with surgical resection, is an integral part of treatment of high grade osteosarcoma and Ewing sarcoma. The utility of chemotherapy for soft tissue sarcoma is uncertain.
• Radiation therapy can be used for definitive treatment of Ewing sarcoma, although surgery is preferred whenever feasible. It is used as an adjunct therapy in soft tissue sarcoma. It provides palliation for metastatic lesions and myeloma, and improves local tumor control after surgery.

Special populations
Children
• Bone sarcomas are most common in the young and account for 4% of tumors in children, and 7% in adolescents.
• Soft tissue sarcomas make up 7% of tumors in pediatric patients, but are more prevalent in adults.
• The most common musculoskeletal malignancies in children are osteosarcoma, Ewing sarcoma, and rhabdomyosarcoma.
• Expandable prostheses are useful in making up for remaining growth in children as the growth plate is usually resected with sarcoma.

Elderly
- Bone sarcoma in older patients is rare. It is often secondary to radiation, Paget disease, or bone infarcts. Prognosis is worse than in the young.

Prognosis

BOTTOM LINE/CLINICAL PEARLS
- For most primary bone tumors, the 5-year relative survival is 60–70%.
- If metastatic disease is present, 5-year survival rates decrease to 15–30%.
- For metastases to bone and myeloma, prognosis depends on subtype, but the disease is not curable.

Follow-up tests and monitoring
- Patients should continue surveillance after treatment for bone or soft tissue sarcomas. Patients should be followed every 3–6 months for the first 2–3 years, and then yearly after that. Higher grade lesions tend to require more frequent initial follow-up. Patients should be followed with history and physical examination, and appropriate imaging studies.

References and reading list
Doyle LA. Sarcoma classification: an update based on the 2013 World Health Organization classification of tumors of soft tissue and bone. Cancer 2014;120:1763–1774.

Enneking WF, Spanier SS, Goodman MA. A system for the surgical staging of musculoskeletal sarcoma. Clin Orthop Relat Res 1980;153:106–120.

Gilbert NF, Cannon CP, Lin PP, et al. Soft-tissue sarcoma. J Am Acad Orthop Surg 2009;17:40–47.

Greenspan A, Jundt G, Remagen W, et al. Differential Diagnosis of Orthopaedic Oncology. Philadelphia, PA: Lippincott Williams & Wilkins, 2007.

Messerschmitt PJ, Garcia RM, Abdul-Karim FW, et al. Osteosarcoma. J Am Acad Orthop Surg 2009;17:515–527.

Mirels H. Metastatic disease in long bones: a proposed scoring system for diagnosing impending pathologic fractures. Clin Orthop Relat Res 1989;249:256–264.

Peabody TD, Attar S. Orthopaedic Oncology: Primary and Metastatic Tumors of the Skeletal System, 2014.

Scharschmidt TJ, Lindsey JD, Becker PS, et al. Multiple myeloma: diagnosis and orthopaedic implications. J Am Acad Orthop Surg 2011;19:410–419.

Weber KL. Evaluation of the adult patient (aged >40 years) with a destructive bone lesion. J Am Acad Orthop Surg 2010;18:169–179.

Suggested websites
Musculoskeletal Tumor Society: www.msts.org
National Comprehensive Cancer Network: www.nccn.org

Guidelines
National society guidelines

Title	Source	Date and weblink
NCCN Clinical Practice Guideline in Oncology: Bone Cancer	National Comprehensive Cancer Network	2015 http://www.nccn.org/professionals/ physician_gls/pdf/bone.pdf
NCCN Clinical Practice Guideline in Oncology: Soft Tissue Sarcoma	National Comprehensive Cancer Network	2015 http://www.nccn.org/professionals/ physician_gls/pdf/sarcoma.pdf

International society guidelines

Title	Source	Date and weblink
Bone Sarcomas: ESMO Clinical Practice Guidelines	European Society for Medical Oncology	2014 http://www.esmo.org/Guidelines/Sarcoma-and-GIST/Bone-Sarcomas
Soft Tissue and Visceral Sarcomas: ESMO Clinical Practice Guidelines	European Society for Medical Oncology	2014 http://www.esmo.org/Guidelines/Sarcoma-and-GIST/Soft-Tissue-and-Visceral-Sarcomas

Images

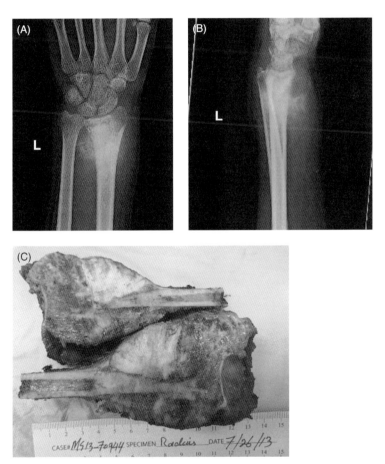

Figure 43.1 (A) Anteroposterior (AP) and (B) lateral X-ray images, and (C) clinical specimen of a distal radius osteosarcoma. See website for color version.

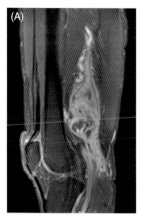
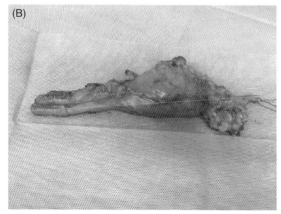

Figure 43.2 (A) Post-contrast sagittal MRI image showing heterogeneous enhancement and (B) clinical specimen of a malignant peripheral nerve sheath tumor arising from the tibial nerve. See website for color version.

Additional material for this chapter can be found online at:
www.wiley.com/go/oh/mountsinaioncology

This includes advice for patients, a case study, ICD codes, and multiple choice questions. The following images are available in color: Figures 43.1(B) and 43.2(B).

CHAPTER 44

Ophthalmologic Oncology

Albert Y. Wu[1] and Kalla A. Gervasio[2]

[1] Stanford University School of Medicine, Palo Alto, CA, USA
[2] Wills Eye Hospital, Philadelphia, PA, USA

OVERALL BOTTOM LINE

- Ophthalmologic tumors are rare in the overall population. The most common primary intraocular tumors are uveal melanoma in adults and retinoblastoma in children.
- Diagnosis of most intraocular tumors is made clinically by dilated fundus examination and confirmed with additional imaging such as fundus photography, A- and B-scan ultrasound, IV fluorescein angiography, optical coherence tomography, and CT/MRI.
- Uveal melanoma most commonly affects the choroid and is often asymptomatic at the time of diagnosis, with plaque brachytherapy being the first line treatment. Nearly half of all patients with uveal melanoma will eventually die from metastases, even with early treatment.
- Patients with retinoblastoma typically present with leukocoria or strabismus. Retinoblastoma has excellent overall prognosis in the USA, where systemic chemotherapy with focal adjuvant therapy and intra-arterial chemotherapy are the mainstays of treatment. There are both sporadic and familial forms of retinoblastoma.
- Systemic cancer and its treatment can cause ocular complications prompting immediate referral to an ophthalmologist including decreased vision, new onset diplopia or cranial nerve palsies, visual field defects, and proptosis.

Background
Definition of disease

- The field of ophthalmologic oncology encompasses primary and metastatic tumors of the eye and ocular adnexa. Given the breadth of anatomic structures included under this term, this chapter focuses primarily on the most common primary intraocular tumors – uveal melanoma and retinoblastoma (Figures 44.1 and 44.2). This chapter also reviews ocular complications of cancers and their treatments.

Disease classification

- Primary intraocular tumors arise from the globe itself, while adnexal tumors develop from the orbit, conjunctiva, or eyelids.
- Metastatic tumors to the eye tend to involve the choroid and most commonly arise from the breast or lungs.

Mount Sinai Expert Guides: Oncology, First Edition. Edited by William K. Oh and Ajai Chari.
© 2019 John Wiley & Sons Ltd. Published 2019 by John Wiley & Sons Ltd.
Companion Website: www.wiley.com/go/oh/mountsinaioncology

Incidence/prevalence
- The most common primary intraocular tumor in adults is uveal melanoma (iris, ciliary body, and choroid), which typically originates from the choroid and has an annual incidence of 4.3 new cases per million people in the USA.
- Retinoblastoma is the most common primary intraocular tumor in children, with 300 new cases diagnosed annually in the USA. In the USA survival rates are 95% but only 50% worldwide.
- Other intraocular tumors include primary intraocular lymphoma, leukemia, and metastatic tumors to the globe, which often target the choroid because of its rich vascular supply.

Etiology
- The etiology of most ophthalmologic tumors is unknown.
- Excessive UV light exposure is a potential cause of uveal melanoma, although the evidence is less than that for cutaneous melanoma.
- Retinoblastoma is either a sporadic/nonheritable (94%) or familial/heritable (6%) tumor that arises via Knudson's "two-hit" hypothesis through inactivation of the Rb tumor suppressor gene.

Pathology/pathogenesis
- Uveal melanoma develops through uncontrolled proliferation of uveal melanocytes, though the molecular pathogenesis of this tumor is still unknown. Proposed mechanisms include constitutive Bcl-2 expression leading to apoptosis resistance or inhibition of the Rb and p53 tumor suppressor pathways causing the development of dormant nevi that either remain as such or undergo malignant degeneration.
- Retinoblastoma develops from germline or somatic mutations that inactivate both alleles of the *RB1* retinoblastoma gene on chromosome 13q14 coding for the pRB tumor suppressor protein. Hereditary retinoblastoma is bilateral (one-third of cases), while sporadic retinoblastoma is usually unilateral (two-thirds of cases).

Predictive/risk factors
- Uveal melanoma risk factors: gender – male > female (OR: 4.9 to 3.7); UV light exposure (welding occupations OR 2.05; other occupations OR 1.37); fair skin color (OR 1.80), light eye color (blue or green OR 1.75), propensity to sunburn (OR 1.64); Caucasian race (98% of cases); atypical cutaneous nevi (OR 2.82), common cutaneous nevi (OR 1.74), cutaneous freckles (OR 1.22), or iris nevi (OR 1.53); genetic factors (chromosome 3 monosomy is a predictor of worse prognosis).
- Retinoblastoma: family history and genetic factors; inheritance of germline mutation in *RB1* gene on chromosome 13q14 – autosomal dominant transmission with 80% penetrance.

Prevention

> **BOTTOM LINE/CLINICAL PEARLS**
> - No interventions have been demonstrated to prevent initial development of either uveal melanoma or retinoblastoma.
> - Secondary prevention of retinoblastoma is best achieved with chemoreduction (systemic chemotherapy with focal adjuvant therapy) or intra-arterial chemotherapy with melphalan.

Screening
- Given the rarity of ophthalmologic tumors, there are currently no evidence-based standardized screening methods for uveal melanoma or other less common tumors. Annual ophthalmologic

examinations including slit lamp and dilated fundus examination can assist in detecting cancer of the eye and ocular adnexa.
- Family members (mainly offspring and siblings) of patients diagnosed with familial retinoblastoma can undergo screening dilated fundus examination and genetic screening and counseling for the *RB1* germline mutation, which indicates increased susceptibility.

Primary prevention
- While decreasing UV light exposure (both real and artificial from tanning salons) may decrease the risk of uveal melanoma, there are no proven interventions for primary prevention of most ophthalmologic tumors.

Secondary prevention
- Plaque brachytherapy has a role in preventing re-occurrence of uveal melanoma, although nearly half of all treated patients will still develop metastases.
- Chemoreduction with systemic chemotherapy and focal adjuvant therapy or intra-arterial chemotherapy with melphalan have been shown to prevent reoccurrence of retinoblastoma in children.

Diagnosis

CLINICAL PEARLS
- For uveal melanoma, clinicians should ask about a history of excessive UV light exposure, dysplastic nevus syndrome or cutaneous melanoma, and a history of other cancers such as breast or lung. Visual complaints such as flashes, floaters, or blurry vision as well as systemic symptoms such as anorexia or weight loss should also be inquired about. Retinal examination may reveal melanotic (brown) or amelanotic (yellow) masses in the choroid in uveal melanoma.
- Leukocoria and strabismus are the most common presenting signs of retinoblastoma, as well as a characteristic white–gray mass on dilated fundus examination. The differential should include other common causes of leukocoria in children such as congenital cataracts, persistent hyperplastic primary vitreous, Coats disease, and ocular toxocariasis.
- Fundus photography, A- or B-scan ultrasound, IV fluorescein angiography (IVFA), and CT/MRI can be used to confirm a diagnosis of retinoblastoma or uveal melanoma.

Differential diagnosis

Differential diagnosis	Features
Uveal melanoma differential: choroidal nevus	Pigmented or nonpigmented flat lesions of the choroid that are usually <2 mm thick and can gradually become elevated with age. Nevi may be associated with drusen, RPE atrophy, hyperplasia, and detachment
Congenital hypertrophy of the retinal pigmented epithelium (CHRPE)	Dilated fundus examination will show flat black lesions with well-delineated margins in the periphery surrounded by a depigmented and pigmented halo
Reactive hyperplasia of the retinal pigmented epithelium (RPE)	Arises secondary to prior trauma or inflammation. On examination, appears as flat black lesions with irregular margins and is often multifocal

(Continued)

(*Continued*)

Differential diagnosis	Features
Melanocytoma of the optic nerve	Black optic nerve lesion with fibrillated margins
Choroidal hemangioma	Red–orange choroidal mass but no mushroom shape
Metastatic tumors	Light brown flat or slightly elevated mass in a patient with a history of cancer (breast or lung)
Choroidal osteoma	Yellow–orange mass close to the optic disc with pseudopod projections

Typical presentation
- Most patients with uveal melanoma are asymptomatic at the time of diagnosis unless the tumor involves the macula by direct extension, secondary retinal detachment, or macular edema. If symptomatic, patients can present with decreased vision, visual field defects, floaters, light flashes, and, rarely, pain.
- Children with retinoblastoma typically present before age 3, with the most common signs being leukocoria (white pupillary reflex) and strabismus (misalignment of the eyes).

Clinical diagnosis
History
- When concerned about uveal melanoma, it is important to ask questions that help to differentiate primary ocular melanoma from metastatic disease. Inquiring about a past medical history of cancer, particularly breast, lung, and cutaneous melanoma, as well as systemic symptoms such as anorexia and weight loss, assists in the diagnosis.
- When concerned about retinoblastoma, clinicians should ask about the age at onset and a family history of the disease, especially in the patient's siblings and parents. It is also important to ask questions that help rule out other conditions that mimic retinoblastoma. Examples include inquiring about contact with puppies or ingesting dirt (ocular toxocariasis) and the patient's birth history (retinopathy of prematurity).

Physical examination
- For uveal melanoma, dilated fundus examination with indirect ophthalmoscopy may demonstrate an elevated brown choroidal mass, an amelanotic mass, orange lipofuscin at the retinal pigment epithelium, or a mushroom-shaped mass invading through Bruch's membrane with potential subretinal hemorrhage.
- For retinoblastoma, external ocular examination, slit lamp examination, and dilated fundus examination with indirect ophthalmoscopy under anesthesia will show a characteristic white mass.

Useful clinical decision rules and calculators
See Algorithms 44.1 and 44.2.

Disease severity classification
- Spindle-A cell melanomas have the best prognosis and epithelioid cell melanomas have the worst prognosis. Classification of uveal melanoma cell types is described by the ACS (http://www.cancer.gov/types/eye/hp/intraocular-melanoma-treatment-pdq/#section/_95).

Algorithm 44.1 Diagnosis of retinoblastoma

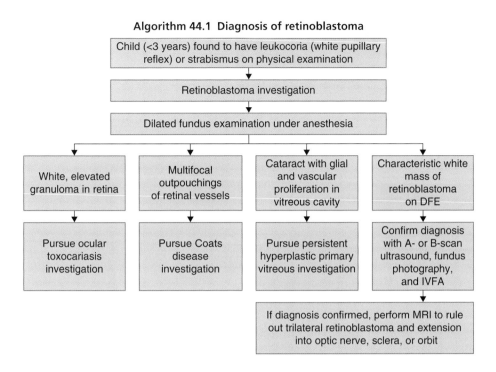

- Staging and prognosis of retinoblastoma was previously described by the Reese–Ellsworth classification and International Intraocular Retinoblastoma Classification (ABC classification). Both systems are described by the ACS (http://www.cancer.org/cancer/retinoblastoma/detailedguide/retinoblastoma-staging).

Laboratory diagnosis
List of diagnostic tests
- Laboratory tests are not used in the initial diagnosis of intraocular tumors. In patients with uveal melanoma, clinicians should rule out liver metastases biannually with lactate dehydrogenase (LDH), gamma-glutamyl transpeptidase (GGT), aspartate aminotransferase (AST), alanine aminotransferase (ALT), and alkaline phosphatase, followed by an MRI of the liver if any laboratory test levels are elevated.

Lists of imaging techniques
- IVFA, A- and B-scan ultrasound, and MRI can be used in the diagnosis of both uveal melanoma and retinoblastoma. MRI may demonstrate extension of uveal melanoma or retinoblastoma into the optic nerve, orbit, or brain.
- It is important to rule out trilateral Rb (bilateral retinoblastoma plus pineal primitive neuroectodermal tumor [PNET] tumors) in all retinoblastoma patients with ultrasound or MRI. CT is generally avoided because of the radiation exposure.
- In cases of confirmed uveal melanoma, annual chest X-ray or CT to rule out lung metastases, and MRI of the liver should be obtained.

Diagnosis of ocular complications of systemic cancer therapy
- Systemic cancers and their treatments can have adverse effects on the eye. It is important for medical oncologists to know when to refer patients to an ophthalmologist.

Algorithm 44.2 Diagnosis of uveal melanoma

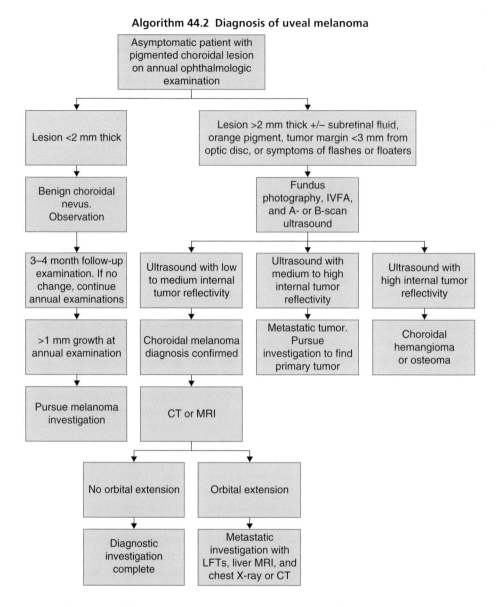

- It can be hard to differentiate symptoms of primary eye disease from those that are secondary to cancer therapies. A detailed history to determine the onset of ocular symptoms in relation to initiation of chemotherapy is important. A basic eye examination should be performed to assess pupils, near visual acuity, and visual fields before a more extensive investigation by an ophthalmologist.
- Ocular symptoms that require prompt referral to an ophthalmologist include significant vision loss (central and/or peripheral), binocular diplopia or misalignment of the eyes (both suggestive of new onset cranial nerve palsies), loss of the red reflex, eye and periocular pain, inflammation of the eyelids, conjunctiva, or sclera, and proptosis.
- Chemotherapies that have been associated with new onset cranial nerve palsies and/or diplopia include cytosine arabinoside, mitoxantrone, cisplatin, vinca alkaloids, chlorambucil,

5-fluorouracil (5-FU), carmustine, nitrosoureas, methotrexate, and interferon-alpha. Prompt referral to a neurologist or neuro-ophthalmologist is recommended.

- Certain ocular complications of chemotherapy are considered to be so common that specific preventative treatments are recommended. These include conjunctivitis secondary to 5-FU (treat with cool compresses), dry eye secondary to cyclophosphamide (treat with artificial tears), keratitis secondary to cytosine arabinoside (treat with topical corticosteroid drops and artificial tears or topical 2-deoxycytidine drops), canalicular fibrosis and resulting epiphora secondary to docetaxel (treat with temporary intubation of lacrimal puncta), and keratitis plus photophobia secondary to methotrexate (treat with artificial tears).

Diagnosis of ocular paraneoplastic syndromes

- Eye-related paraneoplastic syndromes include autoimmune phenomena in the retina such as cancer-associated retinopathy (CAR) and melanoma-associated retinopathy (MAR). CAR can progress rapidly over the course of 6–9 months and is most commonly associated with small cell lung cancer. MAR has a male sex predilection. Symptoms of both syndromes include ring scotomas, shimmering photopsias, and nyctalopia, which should prompt referral to an ophthalmologist, as diagnosis involves dilated fundus examination demonstrating very subtle retinal findings.
- Metastases to the eye most commonly affect the choroid but can also affect the retina and/or vitreous. Patients may be asymptomatic or experience nonspecific symptoms such as vision loss, floaters, photopsias, or peripheral field defects. In patients with a known cancer diagnosis, such symptoms should prompt referral to an ophthalmologist for further evaluation.
- Leukemia, lymphoma, multiple myeloma, and other lymphoproliferative disorders can result in retinal and/or vitreous hemorrhage secondary to thrombocytopenia, and retinal vein occlusion secondary to hyperviscosity syndrome, both of which result in visual loss. Hyperviscosity retinopathy can be reversed by plasmapheresis.

Potential pitfalls/common errors made regarding diagnosis of disease

- Significant delays in diagnosis of retinoblastoma are commonly reported in developing countries, where children are diagnosed at advanced stages of the disease and have a poorer prognosis.
- Patients with a prompt diagnosis of uveal melanoma are more likely to be eligible for eye-conserving treatments such as plaque brachytherapy. Those with a delay in diagnosis or misdiagnosis such as benign choroidal nevus or age-related macular degeneration are more likely to need enucleation if diagnosed at an advanced stage.

Treatment (Algorithms 44.3 and 44.4)
Treatment rationale

- The main goals of uveal melanoma treatment are prevention of tumor extension into the orbit or metastases, with the secondary goal being to salvage visual acuity.
- First line treatment for most uveal melanomas of medium or large size is immediate treatment with radiation with either plaque brachytherapy or proton beam radiation therapy (PBRT) as supported by the Collaborative Ocular Melanoma Study (COMS). If the initial tumor is too extensive for eye salvage therapy, patients undergo enucleation. Second line treatments include external eye wall resection surgery and transpupillary thermal therapy.
- The main goals of retinoblastoma treatment are patient survival and preservation of the globe, with the secondary goal being to salvage visual acuity. Treatment depends on ABC classification (see Algorithm 44.4).

Algorithm 44.3 Treatment of choroidal melanoma

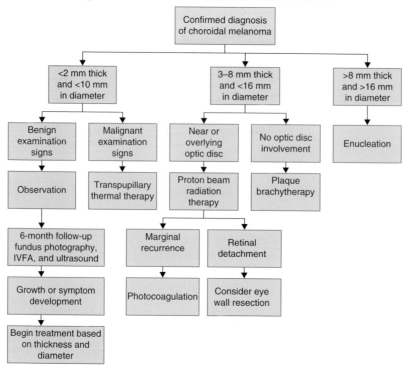

Algorithm 44.4 Treatment of retinoblastoma

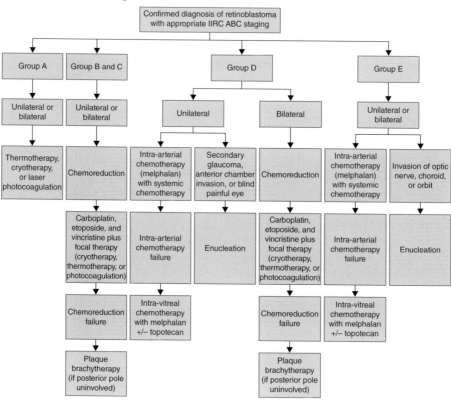

- Systemic chemotherapy with focal adjuvant therapy and intra-arterial chemotherapy are the mainstays of retinoblastoma treatment. Second line therapies include thermotherapy, cryotherapy, laser photocoagulation, plaque brachytherapy, external beam radiotherapy, and systemic chemotherapy for metastases.

When to hospitalize

- Adults with uveal melanoma metastatic to the liver may be hospitalized for 7–10 days for isolated hepatic perfusion therapy with high dose chemotherapy.
- Children treated for retinoblastoma should be hospitalized if they develop neutropenic fever and/or infection.

Uveal melanoma treatment	Comment
Conservative	
	Observation with 6-month follow-up imaging (fundus photography, IVFA, optical coherence tomography, and ultrasound) is recommended for choroidal lesions <2 mm in height and <10 mm in diameter and if the lesion is asymptomatic without signs of growth
Surgical	
Enucleation	May be necessary in patients with very large choroidal melanomas with extrascleral extensions or neovascular glaucoma in a painful eye. It is also used when the affected eye has no visual potential
Eye wall resection	Used in patients who develop extensive retinal detachment after radiation therapy or to preserve as much vision as possible when radiation therapy is unlikely to do so (poor plaque candidates). It can be performed when the tumor does not involve the posterior pole and is <15 mm in diameter
Radiologic	
Plaque brachytherapy - ^{125}I (most common) - ^{60}Co - ^{106}Ru/^{106}Rh - ^{103}Pd - ^{192}Ir	Used in tumors 3–8 mm in thickness or <16 mm in basal diameter
PBRT	Preferred in patients with tumors in close proximity to or overlying the optic disc where radioactive plaques cannot be placed. PBRT is also able to treat tumors with thickness >5 mm more effectively than plaque brachytherapy
Other	
Transpupillary thermal therapy	Can only be used in tumors with <3 mm thickness. It can be used as an adjunct to radiation to reduce tumor recurrence rates
Photocoagulation	Used in patients with marginal recurrences after proton therapy

Prevention/management of complications

- Nonproliferative and proliferative radiation retinopathy and optic neuropathy are complications of plaque brachytherapy, especially in diabetic patients. The choice of treatment and radioisotope for brachytherapy should be selected very carefully.
- Secondary malignancies can arise in patients treated with external beam radiation therapy (EBRT), particularly those with familial retinoblastoma who are already at increased risk for

osteosarcomas, soft tissue sarcomas, and lymphomas. EBRT has largely been replaced by systemic chemotherapy with focal adjuvant therapy.

CLINICAL PEARLS
- For most medium and large choroidal melanomas that do not involve the optic disc, plaque brachytherapy is the preferred method of treatment.
- Chemoreduction with focal adjuvant therapy and intra-arterial chemotherapy with melphalan are now the mainstays of vision-preserving treatment for retinoblastoma patients, especially those with group B–D classified tumors.
- Radiotherapy (plaque brachytherapy, EBRT, or PBRT) poses the risk of radiation retinopathy, particularly in diabetic patients, and the development of secondary malignancies, particularly in children with familial retinoblastoma.

Special populations
Pregnancy
- It has been suggested that uveal melanoma development may be accelerated by pregnancy because of increases in melanocyte-stimulating hormone. Treatment with plaque brachytherapy tends to be safer toward the end of pregnancy or after birth, with no reported complications or infant metastases.

Children
- Though rare (1% of all cases), uveal melanoma can develop in children, particularly at or after puberty, and has a better prognosis with lower risk of metastasis. Plaque brachytherapy is still first line therapy.

Prognosis

BOTTOM LINE/CLINICAL PEARLS
- Even with early diagnosis and treatment, nearly half of all patients with uveal melanoma will die from metastatic disease.
- Retinoblastoma patients with a germline mutation must undergo lifetime monitoring for the development of secondary malignancies.
- Both diseases are fatal if left untreated.

Natural history of untreated disease
- Untreated uveal melanoma has a mortality rate of 31% at 5 years.
- Untreated retinoblastoma is fatal within 2 years as a result of orbital extension and metastases.

Prognosis for treated patients
- The all-cause mortality rate for uveal melanoma patients treated with plaque brachytherapy is 18% at 5 years. Approximately 40–50% of patients treated for uveal melanoma will die from metastases. Liver metastases are most common (87% of patients) and carry the worst prognosis with a median survival time of 7 months. The overall median survival time of patients with metastatic uveal melanoma is less than 1 year.
- In the USA, the prognosis for treated retinoblastoma is excellent with a 5-year survival rate of >90%. If a child remains recurrence-free after 5 years post-treatment, they are considered cured of the disease.

Follow-up tests and monitoring

- After uveal melanoma treatment, patients are followed every 6 months with ophthalmologic examination, liver function tests (LFTs), liver MRI, and chest X-ray or CT to monitor for local recurrence and metastases to the liver and lung.
- After retinoblastoma treatment, ophthalmologic follow-up should occur every 3 months for 1 year, and then be tapered. Lifetime screening for secondary malignancies should take place in those with familial retinoblastoma.

Reading list

Aziz HA, LaSenna CE, Vigoda M, et al. Retinoblastoma treatment burden and economic cost: impact of age at diagnosis and selection of primary therapy. Clin Ophthalmol 2012;6:1601–1606.

Eagle RC Jr. Eye Pathology: An Atlas and Text, 2nd edition. Philadelphia, PA: Lippincott Williams and Wilkins, 2012.

Gerstenblith AT, Rabinowitz MP. The Wills Eye Manual: Office and Emergency Room Diagnosis and Treatment of Eye Disease. Philadelphia, PA: Lippincott Williams & Wilkins, 2012.

Harman LE. Ophthalmic complications related to chemotherapy in medically complex patients. Cancer Control 2016;23:150–156.

Karcioglu ZA, Haik BG. Eye, orbit, and adnexal structures. In: Niederhuber JE, Armitage JO, Doroshow JH, et al., eds. Abeloff's Clinical Oncology, 5th edition. Saunders, 2013.

Lin P, Mruthyunjaya P. Retinal manifestations of oncologic and hematologic conditions. Int Ophthalmol Clin 2012;52:67–91.

Rodriguez-Galindo C, Wilson MW. Retinoblastoma. New York: Springer, 2010.

Shah CP, Weis E, Lajous M, et al. Intermittent and chronic ultraviolet light exposure and uveal melanoma: a meta-analysis. Ophthalmology 2005;112:1599.

Shields CL, Shields JA. Diagnosis and management of retinoblastoma. Cancer Control 2004;11:317–327.

Singh AD, Bergman L, Seregard S. Uveal melanoma: epidemiologic aspects. Ophthalmol Clin North Am 2005;18:75–84.

Weis E, Shah CP, Lajous M, et al. The association between host susceptibility factors and uveal melanoma: a meta-analysis. Arch Ophthalmol 2006;124:54.

Weis E, Shah CP, Lajous M, et al. The association of cutaneous and iris nevi with uveal melanoma: a meta-analysis. Ophthalmology 2009;116:536.

Wilson MW, Haik BG, Rodriguez-Galindo C. Socioeconomic impact of modern multidisciplinary management of retinoblastoma. Pediatrics 2006;118:e331–e336.

Zanaty M, Barros G, Chalouhi N, et al. Update on intra-arterial chemotherapy for retinoblastoma. Sci World J 2014;2014:1–6.

Guidelines
National society guidelines

Title	Source and comment	Date and weblink
Physician Data Query (PDQ) Cancer Information Summaries	National Cancer Institute (NCI) **Comment:** Evidence-based approach to diagnosis and treatment	2018 https://www.cancer.gov/types/retinoblastoma/ hp/retinoblastoma-treatment-pdq https://www.cancer.gov/types/eye/hp/ intraocular-melanoma-treatment-pdq
The American Brachytherapy Society consensus guidelines for plaque brachytherapy of uveal melanoma and retinoblastoma	ABS-OOTF Committee	2014 https://www.ncbi.nlm.nih.gov/pubmed/ 24373763

International society guidelines

Title	Source and comment	Date and weblink
National Retinoblastoma Strategy Canadian Guidelines for Care	Canadian Retinoblastoma Society **Comment:** Guidelines for diagnosis and management	2009 https://www.ncbi.nlm.nih.gov/pubmed/ 20237571
Clinical Practice Guidelines for Ocular and Periocular Melanoma	Australian Cancer Network **Comment:** Guidelines for diagnosis and management	2008 https://www.cancer.org.au/content/pdf/ HealthProfessionals/ClinicalGuidelines/ ManagementofOcularmelanomasupplementary document2008.pdf

Images

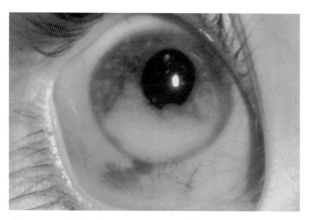

Figure 44.1 Pseudohypopyon. Although uncommon, pseudohypopyon can occasionally be the initial presenting sign of diffusely infiltrating retinoblastoma as in this patient. It represents cancer cell infiltration of the anterior chamber of the eye masquerading as a hypopyon or true pus collection. (Courtesy of Dr. Alan Friedman, Icahn School of Medicine at Mount Sinai, New York, NY, USA.) See color version on website.

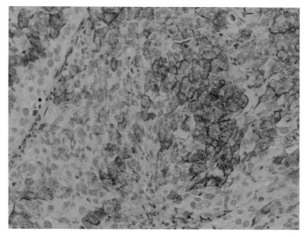

Figure 44.2 Uveal melanoma. If the diagnosis of uveal melanoma is unclear on examination, a biopsy with immunohistochemistry including HMB-45 staining can solidify the diagnosis. Uveal melanoma, just like cutaneous melanoma, stains positive for HMB-45, S-100, and Melan-A. (Courtesy of Dr. Alan Friedman, Icahn School of Medicine at Mount Sinai, New York, NY, USA.) See color version on website.

Additional material for this chapter can be found online at:
www.wiley.com/go/oh/mountsinaioncology

This includes advice for patients, a case study, ICD codes, and multiple choice questions. The following images are available in color: Figures 44.1 and 44.2.

CHAPTER 45

Cardio-Oncology

Gagan Sahni

Mount Sinai Cardiovascular Institute, New York, NY, USA

OVERALL BOTTOM LINE

- The combination of increased use of effective yet potentially cardiotoxic chemotherapy, overall increased cancer survival since the 1990s, and increased prevalence of traditional cardiovascular risk factors in this population have led to the emergence of chemotherapy induced cardiotoxicity as a major public health issue.
- Cardiologists dedicated to the care of either patients with chemotherapy induced cardiotoxicity or cancer patients with concomitant cardiovascular problems are a part of the emerging subspecialty of cardio-oncology or onco-cardiology.
- Cardiotoxicity related to cancer therapy is currently defined by a decrease in cardiac function and categorized into two types: irreversible injury (type 1) or reversible dysfunction (type 2).
- Early screening of cardiovascular diseases, risk stratification of patients, early detection of cardiotoxicity using tools such as global longitudinal strain imaging in echocardiography, and biomarkers such as troponin are valuable emerging tools to reduce the incidence of chemotherapy related cardiotoxicity.
- Preventive efforts should be considered for patients at estimated high risk for cancer therapy induced cardiotoxicity, with either pre-exposure drugs (e.g. angiotensin-converting enzyme inhibitors, angiotensin receptor blockers, and some beta blockers such as carvedilol) or post-exposure use of drugs (e.g. dexrazoxane to prevent anthracycline induced cardiotoxicity especially with the use of high doses or subsequent exposure).

Background
Definition of disease

- Cardiotoxicity encompasses a broad array of cardiovascular events of which heart failure or cancer therapeutics-related cardiac dysfunction (CTRCD) is most prominent.
- Although consensus is lacking, CTRCD as defined by the American Society of Echocardiography, is:
  - A decrease in left ventricular ejection fraction (LVEF) by 5% or more
  - Ejection fraction less than 53% in the presence of symptoms of heart failure, or
  - An asymptomatic decrease in LVEF by 10% or more to less than 53%.

  Other guidelines such as those by the European Society of Medical Oncology (ESMO), the European Society of Cardiology (ESC), and the Mayo Clinic suggest a normal baseline LVEF as 50% or more.

Mount Sinai Expert Guides: Oncology, First Edition. Edited by William K. Oh and Ajai Chari.

© 2019 John Wiley & Sons Ltd. Published 2019 by John Wiley & Sons Ltd.

Companion Website: www.wiley.com/go/oh/mountsinaioncology

Table 45.1 Classification of cancer therapy-induced heart failure.

	Type I	Type II
Chemotherapy agent	Doxorubicin	Trastuzumab
Clinical course and response to therapy	Appears to be irreversible	Likely to be reversible
Dose relation	Cumulative, dose related	Not dose related
Mechanism	Free radical formation, oxidative stress/ damage	Blocked ErbB2 signaling
Ultrastructure	Vacuoles; myofibrillar disarray and dropout; necrosis	No apparent ultrastructural abnormalities
Effect of re-challenge	High probability of recurrent dysfunction that is progressive	Increasing evidence for the relative safety of rechallenge

Disease classification
- Heart failure related to cancer therapy is currently defined by a decrease in cardiac function and categorized into two types: irreversible injury (type 1) or reversible dysfunction (type 2) (Table 45.1).

Incidence/prevalence
- For cancer survivors free of cardiovascular disease at 50 years of age, more than 50% of men and nearly 40% of women will develop cardiovascular disease during their remaining lifespan.

Economic impact
- The economic costs of cardiovascular disease and cancer in the USA in 2003 were estimated at $351.8 billion and $189.5 billion, respectively. The combined costs of these two diseases thus comprised almost 25% of the $2256.5 billion annual health expenditure.

Etiology
Heart failure in cancer patients has several causes.
   Pre-existing risk factors or underlying disease:
- Coronary artery disease and ischemia
- Hypertension
- Alcohol-related cardiomyopathy
- Diabetes
- Nutritional deficiencies
- Cardiac cachexia
- Thyrotoxicosis or hypothyroidism.
Related to cancer diagnosis:
- Amyloidosis
- Myocarditis
- Cardiotoxic chemotherapy
- Radiation
- Sepsis
- Capillary leak phenomenon
- Carcinoid syndrome
- Other

- Arterial venous fistula
- Endocarditis
- Pericardial disease, including constrictive pericarditis
- Pulmonary emboli
- Pulmonary hypertension
- Hemochromatosis and iron overload (frequent transfusions).

Pathology/pathogenesis

- The exact mechanism of cardiotoxicity is agent specific and not quite clear.
- Recent studies on anthracyclines showed that they target topoisomerase 2b in the cardiomyocytes to induce DNA double strand breaks and changes in the transcription of antioxidative and mitochondrial electron transport chain genes, leading to an increase in reactive oxygen species and mitochondrial dysfunction. Dexrazoxane, the only FDA approved drug for prevention of anthracycline cardiotoxicity, is a potent topoisomerase 2b inhibitor.

Risk factors for developing cardiotoxicity with anthracyclines

Risk factors	Odds ratio
Prior anthracycline use (increased cumulative dose)	NA
Cardiac radiation	NA
Other heart disease	1.53
Hypertension	1.58
Coronary artery disease	2.21
Age >65 years	2.25

Prevention

- Risk stratification of patients undergoing cardiotoxic chemotherapy to identify those at higher risk.
- Reducing cumulative dose for type 1 drugs such as doxorubicin which have dose related cardiotoxity.
- Use of alternative drugs (e.g. epirubicin and encapsulated doxorubicin) or alternative schedules (e.g. low dose continuous IV doxorubicin) that are less cardiotoxic than IV bolus conventional doxorubicin.
- Prevention of heart failure in patients at higher risk with drugs such as enalapril, candesartan, and carvedilol.
- Administration of cardioprotective drugs such as dexrazoxane in patients who will receive a high cumulative dose or a second lifetime exposure of anthracyclines.

Screening

- Cardiotoxicity risk score (CRS; see section on Useful clinical decision rules and calculators) assessment with comprehensive history and examination. This risk score includes age, hypertension, pre-existing coronary artery disease (CAD), pre-existing congestive heart failure (CHF), diabetes mellitus, prior or concurrent anthracycline therapy, prior or concurrent chest radiation.
- EKG.
- Echocardiogram with global longitudinal strain (GLS) imaging and 3D LVEF estimation (Figure 45.1).

Primary prevention

The following have been studied for primary prevention of cardiotoxicity in high risk individuals, those undergoing high dose chemotherapy, or stem cell transplant:

- Beta blockers such as carvedilol and nebivolol.
- Angiotensin-converting enzyme (ACE) inhibitors such as enalapril.
- Angiotensin receptor blockers (ARBs) such as valsartan and candesartan.
- Emerging role of statins.
- Use of lower doses of type 1 chemotherapeutic agents whose cardiotoxicity is dose related.

Secondary prevention

- Use of ACE-inhibitors/ARBs and beta blockers.
- Dexrazoxane for preventing anthracycline induced cardiomyopathy (currently approved in the USA only for patients with metastatic breast cancer who have already received a lifetime cumulative dose >300 mg/m^2 doxorubicin).
- Use of alternative drugs/schedules that are less cardiotoxic than doxorubicin.
- Avoiding combination cardiotoxic chemotherapy.

Diagnosis

BOTTOM LINE/CLINICAL PEARLS
- History of patients undergoing potentially cardiotoxic chemotherapy should include screening for CAD, CHF, prior irradiation or chemotherapy, cardiovascular risk factors such as diabetes and hypertension.
- Examination findings such as S3 gallop, tachycardia, unexplained weight gain, and edema should alert the physician to rule out new heart failure.
- Investigations should include a standard 12-lead EKG, biomarkers such as troponin I, and echocardiography.
- A decline in the GLS measurement during systole during echocardiography of >15% over baseline could predict early cardiotoxicity even prior to decline in the LVEF, and should be serially monitored during administration of anthracyclines and trastuzumab (Figure 45.2). Studies have suggested that as GLS is a marker of subclinical LV dysfunction and less affected by inter and intra-observer variability, it can help predict subclinical cardiac damage earlier than a measured ejection fraction.

Typical presentation

- Acute or subacute cardiotoxicity includes abnormalities prolongation of QT-interval on EKG, supraventricular and ventricular arrhythmias, acute coronary syndromes, pericarditis or myocarditis like syndromes, hypotension or hypertension, all of which can occur at the initiation of chemotherapy or up to 2 weeks after its termination.
- Chronic cardiotoxicity includes the entire spectrum from asymptomatic systolic or diastolic LV dysfunction to severe symptomatic CHF, accelerated CAD, chronic pericardial syndromes, and valvulopathy (Figure 45.3).

Clinical diagnosis

History

- Initial history should include screening for CAD, CHF, prior irradiation or chemotherapy, and cardiovascular risk factors such as diabetes and hypertension. Risk factor calculators such as the CRS (see section on Useful clinical decision rules and calculators) may be useful tools.

• Subsequent visits should include screening for symptoms such as new dyspnea, edema, palpitations, chest pain, and so on that could suggest new CHF, and ischemic or thromboembolic events.

Physical examination
• Tachycardia
• Elevated jugular venous pressure
• Presence of S3 gallop
• Rales on chest examination
• Lower extremity edema.

Useful clinical decision rules and calculators
Risk assessment by CRS. CRS risk categories by drug-related risk score plus number of patient-related risk factors: CRS >6, very high; 5–6, high; 3–4, intermediate; 1–2, low; 0, very low (Figure 45.4).

Medication-related risk	Patient-related risk factors
High (risk score 4) Anthracyclines, cyclophosphamide, ifosfamide, clofarabine, herceptin	Cardiomyopathy or heart failure CAD or equivalent (incl. peripheral artery disease) Hypertensive heart disease Diabetes mellitus
Intermediate (risk score 2) Docetaxel, pertuzumab, sunitinib, sorafinib	Prior or concurrent anthracycline Prior or concurrent chest radiation
Low (risk score 1) Bevacizumab, dasatinib, imatinib, lapatinib	Age <15 or >65 years Female gender
Rare (risk score 0) For example, etoposide, rituximab, thalidomide	

Other cardiotoxicities
Box 45.1 lists the entire spectrum of cardiotoxicity from chemotherapy and antibody-based regimens (Figure 45.5).

BOX 45.1 CARDIOTOXICITY OF CHEMOTHERAPY AND ANTIBODY-BASED THERAPY

Heart failure
   Anthracyclines
   Mitoxantrone (Novantrone)
   Alkylating agents
      Cyclophosphamide (Cytoxan)
      Ifosfamide (Ifex)
   Antimicrotubule agent
      Docetaxel (Taxotere)
   Monoclonal antibody-based TKI
      Bevacizumab (Avastin)
      Trastuzumab (Herceptin)
   Proteasome inhibitor
      Bortezomib (Velcade)
      Carfilzomib (Krypolis)

Small molecule TKIs
  Dasatinib (Sprycel)
  Lapatinib (Tykerb)
  Imatinib (Gleevec)
  Sunitinib (Sutent)
Antimetabolites
  Clofarabine (Clolar)
MEK inhibitors
  Trametinib (Mekinist)

Ischemia
  Bevacizumab (Avastin)
  Capecitabine (Xeloda)
  Docetaxel (Taxotere)
  Erlotinib (Tarceva)
  Fluorouracil (5-FU; Adrucil)
  Paclitaxel (Taxol)
  Sorafenib (Nexavar)
  Sunitinib (Sutent)
  Lapatinib (Tykerb)
  Pazopanib (Votrient)
  Cytarabine (Depocyt)
  Ifosfamide (Ifex)

Hypotension
  Alemtuzumab (Campath)
  All-*trans*-retinoic acid (Atra; Tretinoin)
  Decitabine (Dacogen)
  Denileukin (Ontak)
  Etoposide (Vepisid)
  Interferon-α
  Interleukin-2
  Paclitaxel (Taxol)
  Rituximab (Rituxan)

Hypertension
  Bevacizumab (Avastin)
  Sorafenib (Nexavar)
  Sunitinib (Sutent)
  Imatinib (Gleevec)
  Dasatinib (Sprycel)
  Mitoxantrone (Novantrone)
  Carfilzomib (Kyprolis)

Bradycardia
  Paclitaxel (Taxol)
  Thalidomide (Thalomid)
  Bortezomib (Velcade)
  Cisplatin (Platinol-AQ)

QT prolongation or torsade de pointes
  Arsenic trioxide (Trisenox)
  Dasatinib (Sprycel)
  Lapatinib (Tykerb)
  Nilotinib (Tasigna)

Vorinostat (Zolinza)
Pazopanib (Votrient)
Thromboembolism
Bevacizumab (Avastin)
Cisplatin (Platinol-AQ)
Erlotinib (Tarceva)
Lenalidomide (Revlimid)
Sunitinib (Sutent)
Thalidomide (Thalomid)
Vorinostat (Zolinza)
Pomalidomide (Pomalyst)
Pericarditis/pericardial effusion
Doxorubicin (Adriamycin)
Cyclophosphamide (Cytoxan)
Busulphan (Myleran)
Clofarabine (Clolar)
Dasatinib (Sprycel)
Imatinib (Gleevec)

List of laboratory diagnostic tests

- Biomarkers such as cardiac troponin I to predict cardiotoxicity have been well validated. Emerging data on myeloperoxidase need to be confirmed whereas the role of brain natriuretic peptides and C-reactive protein have not been established.
- Lipid panel to assess risk for vascular disease.
- Blood glucose monitoring to screen for diabetes.
- Anemia, especially common in cancer patients, has been directly correlated with outcomes in heart failure patients and should be part of a basic laboratory screen.

Lists of imaging techniques

- Standard 12-lead EKG should include evaluation for low voltage (which in the absence of artefact caused by obesity, raises concern for pericardial effusion or infiltrative cardiomyopathies particularly in an individual with longstanding hypertensive heart disease) and also calculation of the corrected QT interval. This should be monitored diligently for drugs that can potentially prolong the QT interval (e.g. arsenic, vorinostat, 5-HT$_3$ antagonists, macrolides).
- Comprehensive echocardiography as recommended by the American Society of Echocardiography for cardio-oncology including estimation of LVEF (ideally by 3D estimation) and GLS imaging. Based on numerous echo studies of strain rate imaging during cancer chemotherapy, which detects subclinical LV dysfunction, a >15% decline in GLS from baseline during and after completion of anthracycline-based chemotherapy or trastuzumab can be predictive of a future decrease in LVEF.
- Multiple gated acquisition scan can reduce inter-observer variability in LVEF but has the disadvantages of exposure to radioactivity and limited information about cardiac structure and diastolic function.
- Exercise or pharmacologic stress testing to diagnose CAD or risk stratification for non-cardiac surgery in cancer patients.
- Cardiac MRI can be used for assessment of LVEF in suboptimal echocardiography, to assess pericardial diseases, and to rule out infiltrative cardiomyopathies such as cardiac amyloid and hemochromatosis.

Potential pitfalls/common errors made regarding diagnosis of disease

- Calculation of GLS for early cardiotoxicity shows variability between different echo vendors and methods have not been completely validated.
- Estimation of LVEF by echo to detect cardiotoxicity has a significant inter- and intra-observer variability.
- Cardiotoxicity, especially in anthracyclines, can occur until 10 years after initial exposure. Therefore, if continued surveillance with serial echocardiograms is not carried out after completion of chemotherapy, cases of heart failure can be missed.

Treatment (Algorithms 45.1 and 45.2)
Treatment rationale

Algorithm 45.1 Treatment using anthracyclines (type 1 cardiotoxic agents) as used in clinical practice at Mount Sinai

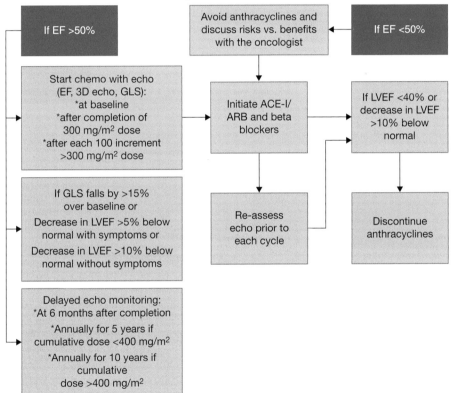

- ACE inhibitors/ARBs and beta-blockers remain the cornerstone of therapy for CHF caused by cardiotoxicity. Enalapril, carvedilol, nebivolol, valsartan, and candesartan have demonstrated the best outcomes when studied in this population.
- The precise role of aldosterone receptor antagonists (e.g. spironolactone) in the treatment of chemotherapy induced cardiomyopathy is currently unknown, but may be considered in those with New York Heart Association (NYHA) class >II symptoms.
- Loop diuretics can be used for volume overload.
- The combination of nitrates and hydralazine is of special benefit in African American patients, as well as in patients with renal insufficiency.

Algorithm 45.2 Treatment using trastuzumab (type 2 cardiotoxic agent) as used in clinical practice at Mount Sinai

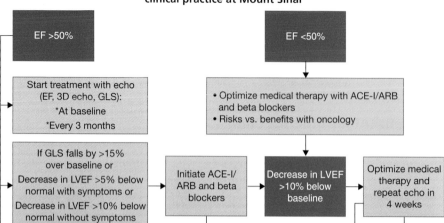

- In addition, risk factors for heart failure should also be aggressively treated such as hypertension and CAD.
- Device therapy including intracardiac defibrillator or biventricular pacemaker should be considered in patients whose LVEF remains <35% despite medical therapy and if their life expectancy from the oncologic perspective is >1 year.

When to hospitalize
- Decompensated CHF for intravenous diuretics, ultrafiltration, or ionotropic support with IV milrinone, dobutamine, and so on.
- For acute hemodynamic support with biventricular assist devices (e.g. in acute myopericarditis owing to cyclophosphamide).
- Alternatively, chronic left ventricular assist device support may become a bridge to transplant or destination therapy in End-stage heart failure.

Management of other cardiotoxicities

Cardiotoxicity	Management
Ischemia	Screening for CAD if cardiovascular risk factors present
	Anti-ischemic therapy with beta blockers, nitrates, calcium channel blockers, aspirin, and statins
	Revascularization with percutaneous coronary intervention (PCI) or coronary artery bypass graft (CABG) if medical therapy fails or high risk. Can consider bare metal stents during PCI if prolonged dual antiplatelet therapy is not possible because of surgery or bleeding risk (e.g. chemotherapy associated thrombocytopenia)
	Avoid higher dose regimens of drugs such as 5-fluorouracil

(*Continued*)

Cardiotoxicity	Management
Hypertension	Treatment with antihypertensives. ACE inhibitors, ARBs, and some beta blockers such as carvedilol and nebivolol have demonstrated the best cardioprotection against chemotherapy induced heart failure
Thromboembolism	Low molecular weight heparin is more effective than oral anticoagulant therapy with warfarin for the prevention of recurrent venous thromboembolism in patients with cancer who have had acute symptomatic proximal deep venous thrombosis (DVT), pulmonary embolism, or both IVC filter in cases of lower extremity DVT with high bleeding risk D-dimers can be falsely elevated in this population Prophylactic outpatient anticoagulation in high risk cancers such as multiple myeloma and pancreatic cancer if the thrombotic risk exceeds bleeding risk Newer oral antithrombotic agents such as dabigatran, rivaroxiban, edoxaban, and apixaban seem to be as effective and safe as conventional treatment in patients with cancer as suggested by smaller studies, but further clinical trials are required
Pericardial disease	Screening with echocardiogram. Suspect in case of metastatic disease, drugs such as cyclophosphamide, or prior radiation therapy Further assessment with a cardiac CT or MRI to rule out constrictive physiology, pericardial masses, or adhesions Pericardiocentesis of pericardial effusion if tamponade physiology or for diagnostic purposes Management of right heart failure caused by constriction Pericardial stripping in cases of constrictive pericarditis not amenable to medical therapy
Arrhythmias	Diligent monitoring of QT interval on EKG and electrolytes in case of QT prolonging drugs Dose adjustment of chemotherapy Use of prophylactic beta blockers and antiarrhythmics like amiodarone Avoid concomitant QT prolonging drugs Assess risk of bleeding vs. thromboprophylactic benefits of anticoagulation in atrial fibrillation

Prevention/management of complications

- Drugs such as dexrazoxane, although cardioprotective against anthracyclines, can reduce oncologic efficacy and increase the incidence of secondary malignancies and should be reserved only for anthracycline re-challenge in cumulative doses exceeding 300 mg/m^2.
- Anticoagulation for stroke prophylaxis in atrial fibrillation may have a higher bleeding risk than the normal population and devices such as the Watchman device (left atrial appendage closure device) can be considered as an alternative.
- Dual antiplatelet therapy (DAPT) for a year after coronary stents for CAD can pose a higher risk of bleeding and be prohibitive for any oncologic surgery. Bare metal stenting, which necessitates only a month of DAPT, can be considered as an alternative.

CLINICAL PEARLS

- A multidisciplinary approach with ongoing interaction between dedicated specialists comprising cardiologists, oncologists, and radiation oncologists in a cardio-oncology team is paving the way for standard of care in patients undergoing cardiotoxic chemotherapy.

- Early screening and risk stratification for developing cardiotoxicity should be performed routinely in all cancer patients.
- Institution-wide algorithms should be formulated based on current evidence-based medicine to guide use of cardiotoxic drugs like anthracyclines and trastuzumab.
- Evolving imaging techniques such as longitudinal strain in echo may establish themselves as a future modality for detection of early cardiotoxicity.

Special populations

Pregnancy

- ACE inhibitors and ARBs should not be used for treatment of heart failure from cardiotoxicity in pregnant patients because of its teratogenicity.
- Persistent LV dysfunction and presence of NYHA class III or IV symptoms of heart failure should be a contraindication for pregnancy because of the high rates of maternal and fetal morbidity and mortality.

Children

- Minimizing anthracycline dosage in pediatric cancer patients is a primary method of cardio-protection. Dexrazoxane and enalapril have also been studied as primary (pre-exposure) and secondary (post-exposure) cardioprotectant agents, respectively, in this population.

Elderly

- The incidence of cardiotoxicity increases with age >65 years with both anthracyclines and trastuzumab.

Prognosis

BOTTOM LINE/CLINICAL PEARLS
- As per the Cancer Trends Progress Report 2009/2010 Update, the length of cancer survival has increased for all cancers combined. The 5-year OS rate for all types of cancer has increased from 49% in 1977 to 68% in 2008. Today there are 14 million Americans alive with a history of cancer.
- Early detection and treatment of cardiovascular disease in these cancer survivors will provide improved prognosis and longevity.

Follow-up tests and monitoring

- Patients with history of anthracycline administration should have surveillance echocardiograms annually up to 5 years if their cumulative dose was <400 mg/m² and annually up to 10 years if dose was >400 mg/m².
- Those receiving mediastinal and chest radiation >30 Gy should be screened for latent CAD after 10 years and earlier in patients with multiple cardiovascular risk factors.

References and reading list

Bosch X, Rovira M. Enalapril and carvedilol for preventing chemotherapy-induced left ventricular systolic dys-function in patients with malignant hemopathies: the OVERCOME Trial. J Am Coll Cardiol 2013;61:2355–2362.

Ewer MS, Ewer SM. Cardiotoxicity of anticancer treatments. Nat Rev Cardiol 2010;7:564–575.

Gulati G, Heck SL, Ree AH. Prevention of cardiac dysfunction during an adjuvant Breast Cancer Therapy (PRADA) Trial: Late-Breaking Clinical Trials 4. Presented at: American Heart Association Scientific Sessions; Nov. 7–11, 2015; Orlando, FL, USA.

Heart Failure Clinics: Cardio-oncology Related to Heart Failure, Volume 7, Issue 3, Pages 299–440 (July 2011).

Iliescu CA, Grines CL, Marmagkiolis K. Evaluation, management, and special considerations of cardio-oncology patients in the cardiac catheterization laboratory. Catheter Cardiovasc Interv 2016;87:E202–E223.

Lyman GH, Bohlke K, Falanga A. Venous thromboembolism prophylaxis and treatment in patients with cancer: American Society of Clinical Oncology Clinical Practice Guideline Update. J Oncol Pract 2015;11:e442–e444.

Mackay B, Ewer M. Assessment of anthracycline cardiomyopathy by endomyocardial biopsy. Ultrastruct Pathol 1994;18:203–211.

Plana JC, Galderisi M, Barac A, et al. Expert consensus for multimodality imaging evaluation of adult patients during and after cancer therapy: a report from the American Society of Echocardiography and the European Association of Cardiovascular Imaging. Eur Heart J Cardiovasc Imaging 2014;15:1063–1093. doi: 10.1093/ehjci/jeu192

Sahni G, Scarabelli T, Yeh ETH. The diagnosis and management of cardiovascular disease in patients with cancer. In Fuster V, Harrington RA, Narula J, et al., eds. Hurst's The Heart, 14th edition. McGraw-Hill, 2017.

Vedovati MC, Germini F, Agnelli G, et al. Direct oral anticoagulants in patients with VTE and cancer: a systematic review and meta-analysis. Chest 2015;147:475–478.

Vejpongsa P, Yeh ET. Prevention of anthracycline-induced cardiotoxicity: challenges and opportunities. J Am Coll Cardiol 2014;64(9):938–945. doi: 10.1016/j.jacc.2014.06.1167

Yeh ET, Bickford C. Cardiovascular complications of cancer therapy: incidence, diagnosis, pathogenesis, and management. J Am Coll Cardiol 2009;53:2231–2247.

Guidelines
National society guidelines

Title	Source	Date and weblink
Expert consensus for multimodality imaging evaluation of adult patients during and after cancer therapy	American Society of Echocardiography (ASE) and the European Association of Cardiovascular Imaging	2014 https://www.ncbi.nlm.nih.gov/pubmed/25172399
Antithrombotic therapy and prevention of thrombosis, 9th edition	American College of Chest Physicians (ACCP)	2012 https://www.ncbi.nlm.nih.gov/pubmed/22315255
Expert consensus for multi-modality imaging evaluation of cardiovascular complications of radiotherapy in adults	European Association of Cardiovascular Imaging and the American Society of Echocardiography	2013 https://www.ncbi.nlm.nih.gov/pubmed/23998694

International society guidelines

Title	Source	Date and weblink
Cardiovascular toxicity induced by chemotherapy, targeted agents and radiotherapy	European Society of Medical Oncology (ESMO) Clinical Practice Guidelines	2012 https://www.ncbi.nlm.nih.gov/pubmed/22997448

Images

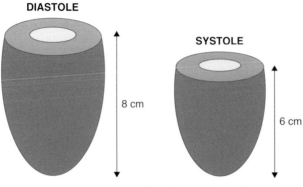

Longitudinal strain = $(8 - 6)/8 \times 100\% = -25\%$

Figure 45.1 Longitudinal strain: the shortening of ventricular length as the base moves towards the apex during systole. The figure on the left denotes end-diastole and the one on the right depicts end-systole. Note the downward descent of the mitral annulus toward the apex in systole. There is a reduction in length by 2 cm, which is a 25% decrease. As there is a decrease in the longitudinal length, it will be denoted by a negative (−) sign; hence the longitudinal strain will be −25%. (Source: Adapted from Echocardiography 2013;30(1):88–105. doi: 10.1111/echo.12079. Reproduced with permission from Wiley.)

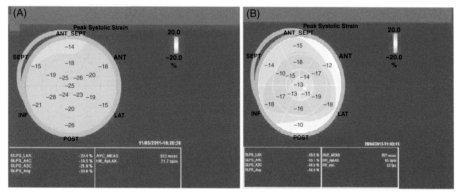

Figure 45.2 Bullseye plot showing global longitudinal strain (GLS) of a breast cancer patient. (A) GLS and regional longitudinal strain at baseline. (B) GLS and regional longitudinal strain 3 months during trastuzumab-based therapy after anthracylines. GLS has decreased from −22.6% to −14.4% (30% decrease). The decrease in GLS is therefore considered of clinical significance (>15% vs. baseline). (Source: Plana et al. 2014. Reproduced with permission from Oxford University Press.) See color version on website.

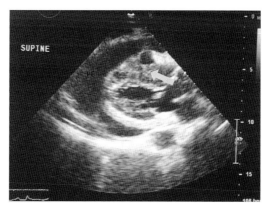

Figure 45.3 Parasternal long axis of a large circumferential pericardial effusion (PE) with involvement of the right ventricle with metastatic angiosarcoma (arrow) from the gluteal region. The RV cavity and free wall has been infiltrated with the metastatic tumor.

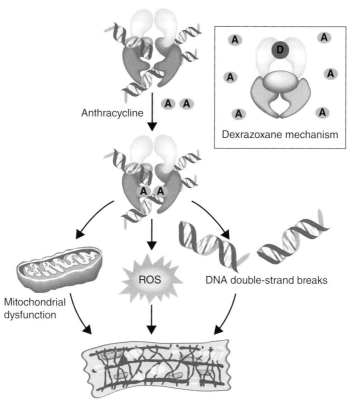

Figure 45.4 Mechanism of anthracycline-induced cardiotoxicity. Doxorubicin disrupts the normal catalytic cycle of topoisomerase (Top) 2β, causing DNA double-stranded breaks. It further changes the transcriptome, leading to defective mitochondrial biogenesis and an increase in reactive oxygen species (ROS). As a result, cardiomyocytes showed myofibrillar disarray and vacuolization. In the inset, dexrazoxane was shown to bind to Top2β to prevent anthracycline binding. (Source: Vejpongsa and Yeh 2014. Reproduced with permission from Elsevier.) See color version on website.

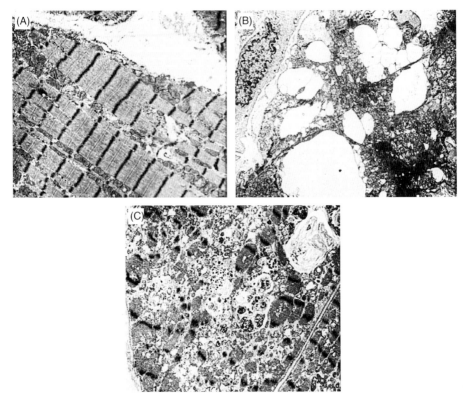

Figure 45.5 (A) Normal-appearing myocyte on cardiac biopsy. (B) Endomyocardial biopsy specimen showing a cell with vacuole formation following doxorubicin administration. (C) Endomyocardial specimen showing myocardial necrosis following doxorubicin administration. (Source: Mackay and Ewer 1994. Reproduced with permission from Taylor & Francis.)

Additional material for this chapter can be found online at: www.wiley.com/go/oh/mountsinaioncology

This includes advice for patients, a case study, ICD codes, and multiple choice questions. The following images is available in color: Figure 45.2 and 45.4.

CHAPTER 46

Psychiatric and Psychologic Dimensions of Cancer Care

Talia Wiesel

Icahn School of Medicine at Mount Sinai, New York, NY, USA

OVERALL BOTTOM LINE
- Beginning in 2015, the American College of Surgeons Commission on Cancer requires accredited cancer centers to have a program in place to identify and refer distressed patients for appropriate care.
- This chapter outlines the identification and management of psychological problems created or exacerbated by cancer, specifically, distress, anxiety depression, psychiatric emergencies, and delirium.

Indications

- The Institute of Medicine's 2008 report, Cancer Care for the Whole Patient: Meeting Psychosocial Health Needs, reviewed the scientific evidence demonstrating the effectiveness of services and interventions aimed at reducing psychologic problems created or exacerbated by cancer. It stressed the psychosocial domain must be integrated into routine cancer care.
- Beginning in 2015, the American College of Surgeons Commission on Cancer requires accredited cancer centers to have a program in place to identify and refer distressed patients for appropriate care.
- This places a burden on oncologists in busy practices to ensure patients with identified distress are appropriately treated, either by the primary oncology team or referred for specialized care.

Procedure

- The National Comprehensive Cancer Network (NCCN) has created Clinical Practice Guidelines in Oncology for Distress Management. Figure 46.1 (NCCN DIS-5) outlines the evaluation and treatment of distress.
- Figure 46.2 (NCCN DIS-A) shows the NCCN Distress Thermometer, a single question and problem checklist to identify the source of distress, recommended for screening patients. Validation studies have found that a score of 4 or greater should prompt a second evaluation by a team member to determine the nature of the distress and whether the patient should be referred to a psychiatrist, psychologist, social worker, or chaplain.

Clinical management
Distress

Patients who are most vulnerable to distress are those with:
- Prior psychiatric disorder (depression, substance abuse)
- Cognitive problems

Mount Sinai Expert Guides: Oncology, First Edition. Edited by William K. Oh and Ajai Chari.

© 2019 John Wiley & Sons Ltd. Published 2019 by John Wiley & Sons Ltd.

Companion Website: www.wiley.com/go/oh/mountsinaioncology

- Language or communication problems
- Comorbid medical illnesses
- Social problems (family, financial, living alone)
- Spiritual or religious concerns.

Anxiety disorders (Tables 46.1 and 46.2)

- Prevalence estimates of anxiety disorders vary, with rates approaching 30% in some studies
- The outline of the evaluation, treatment, and follow-up of anxiety disorders are outlined in Figure 46.3 (NCCN DIS-14).
- Treatment can be psychologic, particularly cognitive-behavioral approaches; relaxation and meditation are useful, as well as online interventions.
- If anxiety persists or is severe, several medications are useful. Table 46.3 outlines the most commonly used medications. However, olanzapine, an antipsychotic, is also often used off label to treat severe anxiety with good results.

Depressive disorders

- Sadness and grief are normal reactions to a cancer diagnosis and treatment. All patients will experience these reactions at times. Because sadness is common, it is important to distinguish between the normal continuum of sadness and depressive disorders.
- Prevalence estimates of depressive disorders range 15–25% of cancer patients.
- Depression often contributes to stopping or delaying treatment, and so contributes to a poorer outcome.
- DSM 5 Criteria for Major Depressive Episode:
  - Depressed mood
  - Diminished interest/pleasure in activities
  - Significant weight loss/gain or decrease/increase in appetite*
  - Insomnia or hypersomnia*
  - Fatigue or loss of energy*
  - Feelings of worthlessness or excessive guilt
  - Diminished ability to think or concentrate*, or indecisiveness
  - Recurrent thoughts of death or suicidal ideation.

*Careful history is needed to determine etiology of these symptoms. Because the etiology of vegetative/somatic symptoms can be difficult to determine, researchers recommend more emphasis be placed on psychologic symptoms.

Table 46.1 Signs and symptoms of anxiety.

Psychologic	Worry, apprehension, fear, sadness Often nonspecific and "free floating" Crying, rumination Difficulty in ability to "turn off" one's thoughts
Physical	Tachycardia, tachypnea Tremor, diaphoresis, nausea, dry mouth, insomnia, and anorexia May occur with panic attacks

(Source: Adapted from Psycho-Oncology: A Quick Reference on the Psychosocial Dimensions of Cancer Symptom Management. Reproduced with permission from Oxford University Press.)

Table 46.2 Etiology of anxiety.

Primary psychiatric disorders	During cancer diagnosis or recurrence exacerbation of prior anxiety disorders may be anticipated Primary mood disorders and dementia frequently experience symptoms of anxiety
Cancer related	Points of increased vulnerability to anxiety: • Finding a symptoms suspicious of cancer • Initial cancer diagnosis • Waiting for check-ups and testing • Awaiting initial treatment • Transitions in treatment • Finish of curative treatment • Transition from curative to palliative care • Advanced cancer and end of life Phobic reactions: • Needle phobia • Claustrophobic patients may have difficulty with MRI scans and enforced long-term confinement in hospital
Disease and treatment related	Congestive heart failure/pulmonary edema Pulmonary embolism Myocardial infarction Hormone-secreting tumors Seizure Untreated pain
Disease complications	Electrolyte abnormalities Delirium Early indication of sepsis Impending seizure Hypercalcemia Hyperthyroidism Hypoglycemia Hypoxia
Drugs	Anticholinergic Stimulants Sympathomimetics Steroids Drug withdrawal (from benzodiazepines, alcohol, narcotics, barbituates) Older antiemetics Antipsychotics

(Source: Psycho-Oncology: A Quick Reference on the Psychosocial Dimensions of Cancer Symptom Management. Reproduced with permission from Oxford University Press.)

- The evaluation, treatment, and follow-up of mood disorders are outlined in Figures 46.4 and 46.5 (NCCN DIS-10-11).
- Commonly used rating scales:
  - Patient Health Questionnaire (PHQ-9)
  - Hospital Anxiety and Depression Scale (HADS)
  - Psychopharmacolic treatment is outlined in Table 46.4).

Suicidal risk (Tables 46.5 and 46.6)

Passive suicidal thoughts are relatively common among cancer patients; many patients comment, "If the pain gets bad enough, I will kill myself." Studies indicate that the incidence of suicide

Table 46.3 Pharmacologic treatment of anxiety.

Drug	Starting dose (mg)	Maintenance dose
Selective serotonin reuptake inhibitors		
Escitalopram (Lexapro®)	10–20	10–20 mg/day PO
Fluoxetine (Prozac®)	10–20 every morning	20–60 mg/day PO
Citalopram (Celexa®)	10–20	10–20 mg/day PO
Benzodiazepines		
Alprazolam (Xanax®)	0.25–1.0	PO every 6–24 h
Clonazepam (Klonopin®)	0.5–2.0	PO every 6–24 h
Diazepam (Valium®)	2–10	PO/IV every 6–24 h
Lorazepam (Ativan®)	0.5–2.0	PO/IM/IVP/IVPB every 4–12 h

IM, intramuscular; IVP, IV push; IVPB, IV piggyback; PO, oral.
(Source: Psycho-Oncology: A Quick Reference on the Psychosocial Dimensions of Cancer
Symptom Management. Reproduced with permission from Oxford University Press.)

in cancer patients can be equal to the incidence in the general population or up to 2–10 times
as frequent. Overdosing with analgesics and sedatives is the most common method of suicide
among persons with cancer. Evaluation and risk assessment of any suicidal remarks is critical.

Patients at high risk for suicide:
- Active suicidal ideation with intent/plan to die.
- History of psychiatric disorders, especially those associated with impulsive behavior (e.g. bor-
  derline personality disorder).
- Family history of suicide.
- History of previous/prior suicide attempts.
- Patients with depression, hopelessness, or guilt for being a burden.
- Social isolation.
- Recent loss (death of a friend or spouse).
- Site of disease: lung cancer has the highest suicide rates followed by head and neck, stomach,
  pancreas, and colon.
- Severe uncontrolled pain.
- Physical and emotional exhaustion.
- Advanced stage of disease and poor prognosis.
- At initial diagnosis, especially within the first month and remains high for 6 months.
- Confusion/mild delirium.
- Alcohol/substance abuse.
- Male gender.
- Anticipation of debilitating or deforming surgery.

Delirium (Tables 46.7 and 46.8)
- Prevalence estimates of delirium are high, especially in hospitalized patients, with rates ranging
  from 28% to 48% in patients with advanced cancer.
- Delirium is a short-term cognitive impairment. It is usually reversible and occurs in cancer treatment related to any toxic state, and it often related to medication, particularly opioids.
- Delirium is often under-recognized and undertreated as it occurs commonly with fever, drugs,
  metabolic disturbances, central nervous system metastases, and paraneoplastic disorders.

Table 46.4 Selected antidepressants to treat depression in cancer patients.

Drug	Starting dose (mg/day)	Maintenance dose (mg/day)	Comments
Selective serotonin reuptake inhibitors			
Citalopram (Celexa®)	10	20–40	Soltabs available
Escitalopram (Lexapro®)	5–10	10–20	Possible nausea, sexual dysfunction
Fluoxetine (Prozac®)	10–20	20–60	Long half-life; possible nausea, sexual dysfunction; strong CYP450-2 D6 inhibitor
Paroxetine (Paxil®)	20	20–60	Possible nausea, sedation, strong CYP450-2D6 inhibitor
Sertraline (Zoloft®)	25–50	50–150	Possible nausea
Tricyclic antidepressants			
Amitriptyline (Elavil®)	25–50 qhs	50–200	Maximal sedation; anticholinergic effects; useful for neuropathic pain
Desipramine (Norpramin®)	25–50	50–200	Modest sedation; anticholinergic
nortriptyline (Pamelor®)	25–50 qhs	50–200	Moderate sedation; useful for neuropathic pain
Other agents			
Ibupropion (Wellbutrin®)	100	100–400 450 XL; 400 SR	Activating; sexual dysfunction; seizure risk in predisposed patients
Duloxetine (Cymbalta®)	20–40	60	Possible nausea, dry mouth; may be useful for neuropathic pain
Mirtazapine (Remeron®)	15 qhs	15–45 qhs	Sedating, variable appetite-stimulant, antiemetic effects
Desvenlafaxine (Pristiq®)	50	50–100	Nausea
Venlafaxine (Effexor®)	18.75–37.5	75–225; XR once daily	Can be used for neuropathic pain, hot flashes, nausea
Psychostimulants			
Dextroamphetamine Dexedrine®	2.5 BID	5–30	Possible blood pressure/cardiac complications
Methyphenidate Ritalin®	5 BID	10–60	Agitation, anxiety, nausea
Modafinil Provigil®	50 BID	50–200	Activating, nausea, cardiac side effects; usually well tolerated
Armodafinil Nuvigil®	50	50–200	Morning only; headache, nausea, dizziness, dry mouth

(Source: Psycho-Oncology: A Quick Reference on the Psychosocial Dimensions of Cancer Symptom Management. Reproduced with permission from Oxford University Press.)

Table 46.5 Assessment of suicidal risk.

Normalize. A discussion about suicide does not increase risk	Most patients with cancer have passing thoughts about suicide like, "If it gets bad enough I might do something." Have you had any thoughts like this?
Assess level of risk	Do you have any thoughts about wanting to end your life? How? How often do you have these thoughts? When was the last time you had this thought? Do you have a plan? Do you have any strong social supports? Do you have pills stockpiled at home? Do you have access to a weapon?
Obtain prior history	Have you ever had a psychiatric disorder or suffered from depression? Have you ever attempted to take your own life? Is there a family history of attempted or completed suicide?
Assess substance abuse	Have you ever had a problem with alcohol or drugs?
Identify bereavement	Have you lost anyone close to you recently?
Assess medical predictors of risk	Do you have pain that is not being relieved? How has the disease affected your life? How is your memory and concentration? Do you feel hopeless about the future? What do you plan for the future?

(Source: Psycho-Oncology: A Quick Reference on the Psychosocial Dimensions of Cancer Symptom Management. Reproduced with permission from Oxford University Press.)

Table 46.6 Interventions for suicidal patients.

Be prepared	Develop a "psychiatric code" procedure for psychiatric emergencies
	Useful institutional phone numbers should be kept on hand and easily available
	    Hospital security, 911, or police
	    Psychiatrist on call
	    Emergency room
	    Chaplaincy
	    Social work
	    Psychiatric hospital admission

Secure the safety of the patient	Do not leave the patient alone until they can be evaluated and started in treatment In the **hospital**, call a security officer. Does the patient need 1 : 1 observation? Dangerous objects that could be used for self-harm should be removed from the hospital room In the **clinic,** is there enough staff/assistance to monitor and control the patient's behavior? If not, call 911 At **home**, can family bring the patient to clinic or the emergency room? If not, call 911 to take the patient to the nearest emergency room Dangerous objects (e.g. guns, intoxicants) should be removed from the home Medications in the home should be secured
For acutely suicidal outpatients	Psychiatric hospitalization is necessary (voluntary or involuntary) Very medically ill patients may not be an appropriate admission to psychiatric units – they may be better treated with 1 : 1 constant observation on a medical floor A psychiatrist can assist in making these arrangements

(Source: Psycho-Oncology: A Quick Reference on the Psychosocial Dimensions of Cancer Symptom Management. Reproduced with permission from Oxford University Press.)

Table 46.7 Common causes of or contributors to delirium.

Infection	Fever
Metabolic disturbance	Hypoxia Hypo- or hyperglycemia Electrolyte disturbance Impaired liver function Impaired kidney function
Drugs	Corticosteroids Sympathomimetics Anticholinergic medications Opioid analgesics Benzodiazepine sedative hypnotics Alcohol or drug intoxication
Drug withdrawal	Especially alcohol or benzodiazepines
Cancer therapies	Chemotherapy agents (ifosfamide, methotrexate, cytosine arabinoside) Biotherapy agents, e.g. interleukin-2 (IL-2), interferon-alpha Brain radiation (early, late-delayed syndromes)
Seizure related	Post-ictal Complex partial status epilepticus
Disease related	Unrelieved pain Direct and indirect effects of primary brain tumors Central nervous system metastasis Paraneoplastic syndromes (rarely) Terminal stages of disease – may herald end of the disease trajectory

(Source: Psycho-Oncology: A Quick Reference on the Psychosocial Dimensions of Cancer Symptom Management. Reproduced with permission from Oxford University Press.)

Table 46.8 Management of delirium.

Prevent accidental self-harm	Falls Pulled IVs Pulled catheters
Close observation	Family Nurse Aid Physical restraints if necessary
Physical environment	Adequate, but not excessive, sensory stimulation Minimize disruptions of sleep–wake cycle Light on during the day Avoid long periods of daytime sleep Frequent reorientation Address sensory deficits (eyeglasses, hearing aids) Night: low level background light and sound (music or TV) is maintained Family presence is comforting
Caregiver concerns	Communicate and educate about delirium and its management Family members should be encouraged to take breaks. May be better if distressed family members do not stay with the patient, especially overnight 1 : 1 monitoring by professional patient aides helps ensure patient safety and allows family members to get needed rest

(Source: Psycho-Oncology: A Quick Reference on the Psychosocial Dimensions of Cancer Symptom Management. Reproduced with permission from Oxford University Press.)

Table 46.9 Selected medications for management of delirium in cancer patients.

Drug	Dosage	Comments
Antipsychotics		
Haloperidol[a] (Haldol®)	0.5–5 mg every 30 min–12 h PO, IM, IV	
Chlorpromazine[a] (Thorazine®)	25–100 mg every 4–12 h PO, IM, IV	
Risperidone (Risperdol®)	0.5–2 mg every 12 h PO	
Olanzapine (Zyprexa®)	2.5–5 mg every 12–24 h PO, IM	
Quetiapine (Seroquel®)	12.5–50 mg every 12 h PO	
Benzodiazepines		
Lorazepam[a] (Ativan®)	0.5–2 mg every 1–4 h PO, IM, IV	Only in the setting of alcohol withdrawal delirium
Midazolam[a] (Versed®)	0.003 mg/kg/h titrate to effect IV (per anesthesiologist)	
Anesthetics		
Propofol[a] (Diprivan®)	0.5 mg/kg/h titrate to effect IV	Rapid onset of sedation and recovery
Alpha agonists		
Dexmedetomidine (Precedex®)	1 µg/kg over 10 min followed by continuous infusion 0.2–0.7 µg/kg/h	Rapid onset sedation and recovery; no effect on cognition
Intensive care setting		
Propofol and dexmedetomadine provide rapid onset of sedation and recovery		

[a] May be administered by continuous infusion usually in the intensive care setting.
(Source: Psycho-Oncology: A Quick Reference on the Psychosocial Dimensions of Cancer Symptom Management. Reproduced with permission from Oxford University Press.)

- The outline of the evaluation, treatment, and follow-up of delirium is outlined in Figure 46.6 (NCCN DIS-9).
- Medication management of delirium in patients with cancer is outlined in Table 46.9.

Clinical features
- Acute onset
- Confusion, disorientation, impaired reality testing
- Distractibility
- Psychomotor agitation or retardation
- Illusions or hallucinations
- Diurnal variation
- Sleep–wake cycle disruption
- Lucid intervals
- Autonomic dysfunction
- Fear and anxiety
- Delusions, especially paranoid in nature.

Risk factors
- Advanced age
- Acuity of illness
- History of cognitive impairment
- Medication exposure
- Sensory deprivation
- End organ damage
- History of alcoholism
- Untreated pain.

Psychotherapeutic interventions
Psychotherapies in cancer care
- **Supportive psychotherapy:** aids patients in coping with distress associated with cancer, reinforces pre-existing strengths, and promotes adaptive coping strategies.
- **Cognitive-behavioral therapy (CBT):** a short-term therapy that addresses the current issues of coping with illness and assists the patient to perceive fears and concerns in a more constructive and realistic way.
- **Problem solving therapy:** encourages seeing illness in a new way, being optimistic, planning with family and patient to address the challenges together.
- **Interpersonal psychotherapy:** concentrates on the changed relationships caused by illness and explores ways to relate to the altered roles.
- **Dignity therapy and meaning centered therapy:** addresses existential and psychosocial distress related to life-threatening illness and end of life issues.
- **Narrative therapy:** the aim is to help patients vocalize their values, skills, and knowledge to live purposefully so they can confront illness. A focus on how identity is shaped by narratives.
- **Written emotional disclosure:** helps patients process the cancer experience by expressing their emotions through writing.

Behavioral interventions
- Progressive muscle relaxation exercises (for insomnia and anxiety)
- Mindfulness-based stress reduction/meditation
- Guided imagery
- Physical exercise
- Behavioral activation (depression).

Group and online therapies
- Groups for psychosocial support have been shown to be helpful for patients. They are most effective when they bring together patients who are coping with the same cancer.

Family and couples therapy
Complementary therapies
- Art therapy
- Music and dance therapy
- Writing and guided reading
- Acupuncture
- Massage
- Nutritional advice.

Patient education/resources
CancerCare 1800-813-HOPE (4673): www.cancercare.org.
Cancer Support Community (CSC) 1-888-793-9355: www.cancersupportcommunity.org.

American Psychosocial Oncology Society (APOS): www.apos-society.org (APOS provides a toll-free help line [1-866-276-7443] to which patients and their caregivers can be referred to help them find psychologic resources in their community.)

The LIVESTRONG Foundation: LIVESTRONG.org

Reading list

Holland JC, Golant M, Greenberg DB, et al., eds. Psycho-Oncology: A Quick Reference on the Psychosocial Dimensions of Cancer Symptom Management, 2nd edition. Oxford University Press, 2015.

Nelson CJ, Roth AJ, Alici Y, et al., eds. Geriatric Psycho-Oncology: A Quick Reference on the Psychosocial Dimensions of Cancer Symptom Management. Oxford University Press, 2015.

Wiener LS, Pao M, Kazak AE, et al., eds. Pediatric Psycho-Oncology: A Quick Reference on the Psychosocial Dimensions of Cancer Symptom Management, 2nd edition. Oxford University Press, 2015.

Suggested websites

Clinicians should be aware of the evidence supported interventions available for the management of distress. The following clinical practice guidelines will be useful to clinicians:

American Cancer Society: www.cancer.org

American Institute for Cancer Research: www.aicr.org

Association of Community Cancer Centers Cancer Program Guidelines: www.accc-cancer.org

Cancer.net, sponsored by ASCO: www.cancer.net

National Cancer Institute: www.cancer.gov

NCCN Clinical Practice Guidelines in Oncology: Distress Management: www.NCCN.org

A website developed by the NCI and several partners that provides information about research-tested intervention programs: http://rtips.cancer.gov/rtips/index.do

Images

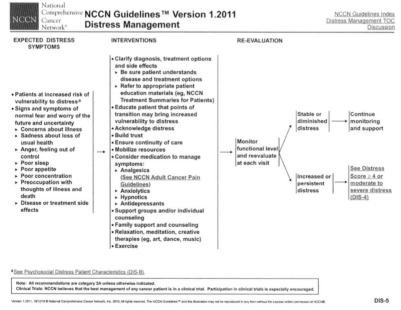

Figure 46.1 The evaluation and treatment of distress. (Source: Reproduced with permission from the NCCN Clinical Practice Guidelines in Oncology (NCCN Guidelines™) for Distress Management V.2.2014. © 2014 National Comprehensive Cancer Network, Inc. All rights reserved. The NCCN Guidelines and illustrations herein may not be reproduced in any form for any purpose without the express written permission of the NCCN. To view the most recent and complete version of the NCCN Guidelines, go online to NCCN.org. National Comprehensive Cancer Network, NCCN, NCCN Guidelines, and all other NCCN content are trademarks owned by the National Comprehensive Cancer Network, Inc.)

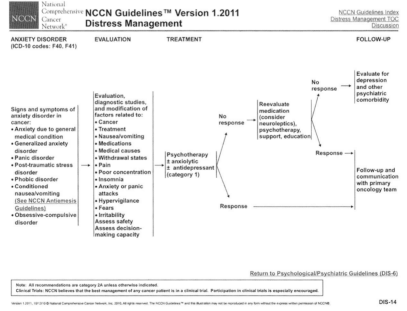

Figure 46.2 The NCCN Distress Thermometer. (Source: Reproduced with permission from the NCCN Clinical Practice Guidelines in Oncology (NCCN Guidelines™) for Distress Management V.2.2014. © 2014 National Comprehensive Cancer Network, Inc. All rights reserved. The NCCN Guidelines and illustrations herein may not be reproduced in any form for any purpose without the express written permission of the NCCN. To view the most recent and complete version of the NCCN Guidelines, go online to NCCN.org. National Comprehensive Cancer Network, NCCN, NCCN Guidelines, and all other NCCN Content are trademarks owned by the National Comprehensive Cancer Network, Inc.)

Figure 46.3 The evaluation, treatment, and follow-up of anxiety disorders. (Source: Reproduced with permission from the NCCN Clinical Practice Guidelines in Oncology (NCCN Guidelines™) for Distress Management V.2.2014. © 2014 National Comprehensive Cancer Network, Inc. All rights reserved. The NCCN Guidelines and illustrations herein may not be reproduced in any form for any purpose without the express written permission of the NCCN. To view the most recent and complete version of the NCCN Guidelines, go online to NCCN.org. National Comprehensive Cancer Network, NCCN, NCCN Guidelines, and all other NCCN Content are trademarks owned by the National Comprehensive Cancer Network, Inc.)

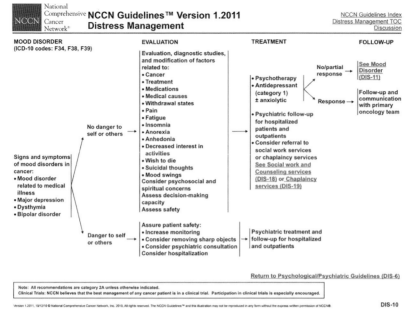

Figure 46.4 The evaluation, treatment, and follow-up of mood disorders. (Source: Reproduced with permission from the NCCN Clinical Practice Guidelines in Oncology (NCCN Guidelines™) for Distress Management V.2.2014. © 2014 National Comprehensive Cancer Network, Inc. All rights reserved. The NCCN Guidelines and illustrations herein may not be reproduced in any form for any purpose without the express written permission of the NCCN. To view the most recent and complete version of the NCCN Guidelines, go online to NCCN.org. National Comprehensive Cancer Network, NCCN, NCCN Guidelines, and all other NCCN Content are trademarks owned by the National Comprehensive Cancer Network, Inc.)

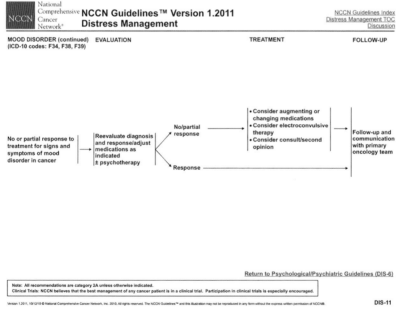

Figure 46.5 The evaluation, treatment, and follow-up of mood disorders. (Source: Reproduced with permission from the NCCN Clinical Practice Guidelines in Oncology (NCCN Guidelines™) for Distress Management V.2.2014. © 2014 National Comprehensive Cancer Network, Inc. All rights reserved. The NCCN Guidelines and illustrations herein may not be reproduced in any form for any purpose without the express written permission of the NCCN. To view the most recent and complete version of the NCCN Guidelines, go online to NCCN.org. National Comprehensive Cancer Network, NCCN, NCCN Guidelines, and all other NCCN Content are trademarks owned by the National Comprehensive Cancer Network, Inc.)

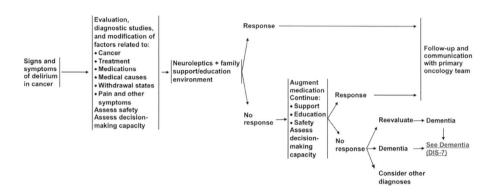

Figure 46.6 The evaluation, treatment, and follow-up of delirium. (Source: Reproduced with permission from the NCCN Clinical Practice Guidelines in Oncology (NCCN Guidelines™) for Distress Management V.2.2014. © 2014 National Comprehensive Cancer Network, Inc. All rights reserved. The NCCN Guidelines and illustrations herein may not be reproduced in any form for any purpose without the express written permission of the NCCN. To view the most recent and complete version of the NCCN Guidelines, go online to NCCN.org. National Comprehensive Cancer Network, NCCN, NCCN Guidelines and all other NCCN Content are trademarks owned by the National Comprehensive Cancer Network, Inc.)

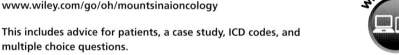

Additional material for this chapter can be found online at:
www.wiley.com/go/oh/mountsinaioncology

This includes advice for patients, a case study, ICD codes, and multiple choice questions.

CHAPTER 47

Geriatric Oncology

Ali John Zarrabi[1], Ran Huo[2], and Cardinale B. Smith[3]

[1] Emory University School of Medicine, Atlanta, GA, USA
[2] The Everett Clinic, Providence Regional Medical Center, Everett, WA, USA
[3] Icahn School of Medicine at Mount Sinai, New York, NY, USA

OVERALL BOTTOM LINE
- Geriatric oncology is a multidisciplinary field addressing the prevention, diagnosis, and treatment of cancer in older adults.
- Older adults are more likely to have medical comorbidities and functional decline than younger adults, and hence are at greater risk of chemotherapy related toxicity and worsening quality of life from standard cancer therapies.
- The Comprehensive Geriatric Assessment (CGA) is a multidimensional instrument used to collect data on medical, psychosocial, and functional capabilities of older adults.
- The CGA can be used to identify problems that may limit a patient's ability to tolerate standard cancer treatments, and thus provides actionable information to guide interventions that can improve the patient's ability to undergo treatment.
- Although most cancer diagnoses are among older adults, this population is highly underrepresented in clinical trials, and thus significant opportunities exist for further research in this emerging discipline.

Background
Definition of disease
- Geriatric oncology is an emerging discipline designed to identify and address the needs of the fastest growing segment of the population in the USA who are at increased risk for treatment related toxicities as a result of cancer treatment.

Incidence/prevalence
- Cancer is predominantly a disease of the elderly, comprising approximately 60% of new cancer cases (Ries et al. 2000).
- Seventy percent of cancer mortality occurs in patients over the age of 65 (Ries et al. 2000).
- Given the expected rise of cancer in the elderly, care of older adults with cancer will have an even larger role in the practice of oncologists.

Economic impact
- For elderly cancer patients, the net cost of care to Medicare aggregated over a 5-year timespan was estimated to be over $21 billion in 2004 (Yabroff et al. 2008).

Mount Sinai Expert Guides: Oncology, First Edition. Edited by William K. Oh and Ajai Chari.
© 2019 John Wiley & Sons Ltd. Published 2019 by John Wiley & Sons Ltd.
Companion Website: www.wiley.com/go/oh/mountsinaioncology

Etiology

- Older cancer patients are more likely to have decline in the function of organ systems as a result of age related loss of physiologic reserve.
- Patients with less physiologic reserve are at greater risk for decompensation from stressors such as systemic chemotherapy.
- *Chronologic age* does not always correlate with *physiologic age*; that is, not all older adults of the same age are at the same risk for decline with some adults having less functional reserve irrespective of their chronologic age.
- Given that some patients are more frail than others, there is a need to identify the frail older adult who may not tolerate standard cancer treatments and may need a more tailored treatment plan.

Pathology/pathogenesis

- Liver:
  - Older adults have decreased hepatic volume and hepatic blood flow, resulting in decreased drug metabolism and elimination, and consequently may have higher concentrations of drugs as they are less rapidly eliminated.
  - Given this baseline decrease in hepatic functioning, patients with liver metastases may have greater decompensation than younger patients.
- Kidney:
  - Older adults are expected to have a lower glomerular filtration rate.
  - Smaller decreases in intravascular volume can lead to more dramatic decreases in renal function.
  - Thus, patients with chemotherapy-induced vomiting or diarrhea are at increased risk for renal compromise.
- Bone marrow:
  - There is less bone marrow reserve among older adults.
  - This decreased reserve increases the risk of chemotherapy related cytopenias in older adults.
- Heart:
  - Older adults have an increased risk of coronary artery disease and valvular heart disease.
  - Older patients are at especially high risk of cardiotoxicity when certain toxic chemotherapies are used such as anthracycline-like agents.
- Muscle:
  - Older adults are at increased risk of sarcopenia.
  - Sarcopenic obesity, defined as muscle loss without loss or gain of fat, is found among patients with advanced cancer.

Prevention

Screening

The US Preventative Services Task Force (USPSTF) screening guidelines differ by cancer; see the following sections for a summary by cancer type. In general, elderly patients with comorbid illnesses and frailty may not derive as much benefit from screening for cancer. The decision to offer cancer screening should take into account the patient's estimated remaining life expectancy and current medical conditions. The decision should be made based on the patient's personal values and preferences (Smith et al. 2007).

Prostate

A discussion about prostate cancer screening is suggested between men and their healthcare providers beginning at age 50 in average-risk men. Healthcare providers should periodically discuss prostate cancer screening with men who are expected to live at least 10 years. Prostate-specific antigen (PSA) levels increase with age because of the higher prevalence of benign prostatic hyperplasia in older men. Raising the PSA biopsy threshold improves specificity and reduces the number of unnecessary biopsies (Qaseem et al. 2013).

Breast

Increasing age is the primary risk factor for breast cancer in most women. Of the approximately 230 000 new cases of female breast cancer arising annually in the USA, almost half are diagnosed in older women (age ≥65 years). Breast cancer screening with mammography should be continued as long as a woman has a life expectancy of at least 10 years or until age 75 (Walter and Schonberg 2014).

Colon

Randomized controlled trial (RCT) data for colorectal cancer screening shows that fecal occult blood testing (FOBT) is associated with a 15–20% reduction in cancer specific mortality. Screening for colon cancer should be continued as long as the life expectancy for an individual patient is at least 10 years or until age 75. One-time screening with colonoscopy or sigmoidoscopy is advised for adults who have never been screened for colorectal cancer, up to age 83 and 84, respectively (van Hees et al. 2014).

Lung

USPSTF recommends annual low dose chest CT scan screening for high risk individuals aged 55–80 years. Screening is appropriate until such time when a person has not smoked for 15 years or if life expectancy is limited. Many other organizations also support lung cancer screening for high risk older adults, and in 2015 Medicare began providing reimbursement for screening to age 77 (de Koning et al. 2014).

Cervical

Most major guidelines recommend stopping cervical cancer screening at age 65 for women who have had adequate recent screening and are not at increased risk for cervical cancer. Adequate screening is defined as three consecutive negative cytology tests or two consecutive negative HPV/Papanicolaou tests in the 10 years preceding, with the most recent test within 5 years. Older women who have never been screened have been shown to derive the most benefit from screening. Modeling studies suggest that screening older women who have never been screened could reduce mortality by 74%. Older women have the highest incidence of, and mortality from, cervical cancer and for these patients the recommendation by USPSTF is for screening until age 70–75 (Moyer 2012).

The USPSTF does not recommend routine screening for ovarian, pancreatic, oral, skin, bladder, or testicular cancers.

Diagnosis
Useful clinical decision rules and calculators

- Clinical decision-making tools to assess prognosis for elderly patients diagnosed with cancer without treatment can be found at http://eprognosis.ucsf.edu/.
- Several models have been developed to predict chemotherapy toxicity. These have been based upon the CGA. Some examples are summarized:
  - The Cancer and Aging Research Group (CARG) model is freely available online and can be useful in predicting risk for severe or fatal toxicity from chemotherapy. This assessment

requires laboratory test data and data about functional capacity, as well as type of cancer and proposed chemotherapy regimen in order to screen patients into risk categories. It was found to be significantly better than physician rated Karnofsky Performance Status for predicting toxicity from chemotherapy (Hurria et al. 2011).

- The Chemotherapy Risk Assessment Scale for High age (CRASH) score was developed to predict the risk of chemotherapy related toxicity in older adults. This assessment also utilizes laboratory data, functional capacity assessment, and proposed chemotherapy regimen, in order to predict the risk of toxicity (Extermann et al. 2012).

Treatment

Despite the high incidence of cancer in this group, older patients have been underrepresented in clinical trials that set the standards for care in oncology practice. Thus, the treatment for individual cancers is often extrapolated from data from younger patients.

Older patients should receive a screening geriatrics assessment. A full geriatrics assessment may be beyond the scope of an initial oncology clinic visit because of time and resource constraints. In these cases, it is recommended to refer the patients deemed at risk for treatment complications to a specialized geriatric medicine clinic. The issues revealed by the geriatrics assessment should be addressed using an interdisciplinary approach. For example, patients with complex pain could be seen by a pain or palliative specialist, patients with vision problems could see an ophthalmologist, and patients with cognitive impairment could be seen by geriatrician and/or neuropsychologist for evaluation (Sattar et al. 2014).

Prevention/management of complications

Based on the results of geriatric assessments conducted for elderly patients with cancer, consider dose reduction of standard dose chemotherapy for patients at risk of grade III–V toxicity (Hurria et al. 2011).

CLINICAL PEARLS
- Occult renal dysfunction is common and should guide decisions on chemotherapy dosage.
- Because of the high prevalence of polypharmacy, elderly patients are at increased risk from adverse drug events related to chemotherapy.
- Use caution when combining medications that affect hepatic P450 as they can vary the metabolism of chemotherapeutic agents.

Prognosis

In summary, geriatric oncology is a multidisciplinary field that can identify deficiencies that can limit a patient's ability to tolerate cancer treatment. Geriatric oncology provides a means to identify and intervene for at-risk patients prior to the development of therapy-related complications. By identifying frail patients who are the most vulnerable for treatment-related toxicity, geriatric oncology can guide decision making regarding appropriateness and aggressiveness of cancer-directed therapy.

References and reading list

de Koning HJ, Meza R, Plevritis SK, et al. Benefits and harms of computed tomography lung cancer screening strategies: a comparative modeling study for the US Preventive Services Task Force. Ann Intern Med 2014;160:311–320.

Extermann M, Boler I, Reich RR, et al. Predicting the risk of chemotherapy toxicity in older patients: the Chemotherapy Risk Assessment Scale for High-Age Patients (CRASH) score. Cancer 2012;118:3377–3386.

Hurria A, Togawa K, Tew WP, et al. Predicting chemotherapy toxicity in older adults with cancer: a prospective multicenter study. J Clin Oncol 2011;29:3457–3465.

Moyer VA. US Preventive Services Task Force. Screening for cervical cancer: US Preventive Services Task Force recommendation statement. Ann Intern Med 2012;156:880.

Qaseem A, Barry MJ, Denberg TD, et al. Clinical Guidelines Committee of the American College of Physicians. Screening for prostate cancer: a guidance statement from the Clinical Guidelines Committee of the American College of Physicians. Ann Intern Med 2013;158:761–769.

Ries EM, Kosary CL, Hankey BF, et al. SEER Cancer Statistics Review: 1975–2000. National Cancer Institute, Bethesda, MD.

Sattar S, Alibhai SMH, Wildiers H, et al. How to implement a geriatric assessment in your clinical practice. Oncologist 2014;19:1056–1068.

Smith RA, Cokkinides V, Eyre HJ. Cancer screening in the United States, 2007: a review of current guidelines, practices, and prospects. CA Cancer J Clin 2007;57:90–104.

van Hees F, Habbema JD, Meester RG, et al. Should colorectal cancer screening be considered in elderly persons without previous screening? A cost-effectiveness analysis. Ann Intern Med 2014;160:750–759.

Walter LC, Schonberg MA. Screening mammography in older women: a review. JAMA 2014;311:1336–1347.

Yabroff KR, Lamont EB, Mariotto A, et al. Cost of care for the elderly cancer patients in the United States. J Natl Cancer Inst 2008;100:630–641.

Suggested websites

https://eprognosis.ucsf.edu

www.mycarg.org/Chemo_Toxicity_Calculator

Additional material for this title can be found online at:
www.wiley.com/go/oh/mountsinaioncology

CHAPTER 48

Palliative Care

Lori Spoozak[1] and Bethann Scarborough[2]
[1] University of Kansas School of Medicine, Kansas City, KS, USA
[2] Icahn School of Medicine at Mount Sinai, New York, NY, USA

OVERALL BOTTOM LINE
- Palliative care improves the quality of life for patients with serious illness and their families by relieving suffering and providing an extra layer of support.
- Primary palliative care should be a clinical competency of all oncology care providers.
- Core palliative care skills include symptom management, prognostication, communication, transition planning, psychosocial support, and end of life care.

Background
Definition of palliative care
- Palliative care is specialized medical care focusing on management of physical symptoms and psychosocial distress for patients with serious illness. Palliative care can be provided throughout the continuum of illness and concurrently with disease-directed treatment.

Classification of palliative care
- **Primary palliative care:** skills and competencies required of all healthcare professionals.
- **Secondary palliative care:** specialist clinicians and organizations that provide consultation and specialty care.
- **Tertiary palliative care:** academic medical centers where specialist knowledge for the most complex cases is practiced, researched, and taught.
- Palliative care specialists are a limited resource. Oncologists, nurses, social workers, chaplains, and all members of the patient care team must be trained to address their patients' primary palliative care needs.

CLINICAL PEARLS
Components of primary palliative care:
- **Pain and symptom assessment:** Are there distressing physical or psychologic symptoms?
- **Social and spiritual assessment:** Are there significant social or spiritual concerns affecting daily life?
- **Understanding of illness/prognosis and treatment options:** Does the patient/surrogate understand the current illness, prognostic trajectory, and treatment options?

Mount Sinai Expert Guides: Oncology, First Edition. Edited by William K. Oh and Ajai Chari.
© 2019 John Wiley & Sons Ltd. Published 2019 by John Wiley & Sons Ltd.
Companion Website: www.wiley.com/go/oh/mountsinaioncology

> • **Identification of patient-centered goals of care:** What are the goals for care, as identified by the patient/surrogate? Are treatment options congruent with patient-centered goals? Has the patient participated in an advance care planning process?
> • **Transition of care post discharge:** What are the key considerations for a safe and sustainable transition from one setting to another?

Incidence/prevalence

• As of 2012, 61% of hospitals with 50 or more beds reported having a palliative care team (Figure 48.1). In addition, 87% of the National Cancer Institute's designated comprehensive cancer centers have a palliative care team.

Economic impact

• Healthcare value is the ratio of the quality of care to the cost of care. Palliative care raises the quality of care and lowers the cost of care. Palliative care improves symptom management and patient satisfaction. In addition, inpatient palliative care consultation teams have been shown to reduce direct hospital costs with savings of $1696–4908 per patient per admission.
• Two randomized controlled trials of early outpatient palliative care in advanced cancer revealed improved quality of life and survival for patients receiving the early intervention.

Criteria for palliative care assessment

CLINICAL PEARLS
Criteria for a palliative care assessment at the time of admission:
• The "surprise question": You would not be surprised if the patient died within 12 months.
• Frequent admissions (e.g. more than one admission for the same condition within several months).
• Admission prompted by difficult to control physical or psychologic symptoms.
• Complex care requirements (e.g. functional dependency, complex home support for ventilator/antibiotics/feedings).
• Decline in function, feeding intolerance, or unintended decline in weight (e.g. failure to thrive).

• In addition to patients with advanced or metastatic cancer, the expert consensus guidelines in the Clinical pearls box above identify patients in need of palliative care consultation during hospital admission. There are currently no consensus guidelines for outpatient palliative care consultation.

Core indicators for hospice eligibility

• Life expectancy of 6 months or less
• Multiple hospitalizations
• Physical decline
• Weight loss
• Serum albumin <2.5 g/dL
• Stage 3–4 pressure ulcers
• Multiple comorbidities

- Dependence on assistance for most activities of daily living (ADLs)
- Signs and symptoms such as increasing pain, dyspnea, nausea, edema, ascites
- Karnofsky or Palliative Performance Scale Score of ≤70%.

Symptom management

Optimal symptom management improves quality of life and adherence to treatment. Symptoms result from cancer or antineoplastic therapies and many patients only reveal symptoms when directly questioned. As a result, all patients should have a systematic review of symptoms at each visit. A simple and validated symptom screening instrument for cancer patients is the Edmonton Symptom Assessment System (ESAS). It examines nine of the most common cancer-related symptoms (pain, tiredness, drowsiness, nausea, lack of appetite, shortness of breath, depression, anxiety, and overall sense of well-being). Appropriate symptom management includes a thorough symptom history, physical examination, and a stepwise plan for management over time with frequent reassessments. For complete symptom management algorithms, refer to the National Cancer Care Network Guidelines® for Supportive Care.

Pain

Overview

- Pain may be nociceptive (somatic or visceral and related to tissue injury) or neuropathic (caused by damage to nerves, spinal cord, or brain). Treatment options vary depending on the type of pain. Pain severity and goals of pain relief will guide the intervention. The ability of the patient to tolerate the route of administration must be considered (e.g. level of oral intake).

Assessment

CLINICAL PEARLS

Pain assessment:

- Intensity: baseline pain score (1–10) and minimum/maximum in past 24 hours.
- Goal pain score (e.g. "If you couldn't become pain free, what level of pain is tolerable to you and allows you to function?").
- Characteristics: location, radiation, quality, severity, frequency, onset, aggravating factors, alleviating factors.
- Functional impairment secondary to pain.
- Response to current therapy (e.g. how much does pain score change after as needed (prn) dose, how long does pain relief last, how many prn doses are required per day?).
- Side effects from current opioids (sedation, nausea, constipation, myoclonus).
- If the patient is cognitively impaired, assess nonverbal signs of pain (grimacing, moaning, furrowed brow, agitation).

- Assessment depends on whether the patient has the cognitive capacity to self-report pain scores and provide a pain history.

Management

- After detailed review of pain, further assessment and treatment are determined by source, type, and severity of pain.
- Initiating an opioid: in an opioid-naïve patient with moderate to severe pain and normal renal function, start with 5–15 mg morphine orally (reassess in 60 minutes) or 2–4 mg morphine IV (reassess in 15 minutes).
- Opioid titration: long-acting opioids are indicated when pain is present for more than 50% of the day or if the patient is regularly using at least 4 prn opioid doses per day.

- Stimulant bowel regimen must be initiated with any opioid therapy (e.g. senna 17.2 mg/day). Docusate is a stool softener and is not an effective bowel regimen for opioid-induced constipation.
- Not all pain is opioid responsive. When appropriate titrations cannot achieve pain control, adjuvants should be considered (Figure 48.2).

Nausea and vomiting

Overview

Nausea and vomiting are some of the most distressing symptoms that patients with cancer experience, affecting 40–70% of patients with advanced malignancy. The symptoms are related to the central or peripheral disease burden and/or antineoplastic therapies. Multiple receptors and neurotransmitters have been implicated at the chemoreceptor trigger zone and the vomiting center, including neurokinin, opioid, cannabinoid, dopamine, serotonin, and histamine receptors.

Assessment

> **CLINICAL PEARLS**
> Assessment of nausea/vomiting:
> - Intensity score: mild, moderate, or severe.
> - Characteristics: frequency, appearance of emesis (bilious, bloody, feculent), onset (association with medication, day 1 of chemotherapy or day 5), aggravating factors (unpleasant odors), relieving factors (cool liquids, lying down), contributing factors (radiation exposure, bowel obstruction, constipation).
> - Impairment in function (ability to eat/drink, weight loss, albumin).
> - Response to previous therapy.

- Begin by identifying the cause of the nausea and vomiting, rate the symptom burden, and assess for change over time with various interventions.

Management

- The cause and severity of the nausea and vomiting dictates management in the inpatient or outpatient setting. Consider medication that targets one or more of the receptors implicated in the nausea/vomiting cascade. The National Comprehensive Cancer Network released updated guidelines in 2016 that combined management of both acute and delayed emesis into a single algorithm. Major treatment categories:
  - Dopamine antagonists (e.g. prochlorperazine, olanzapine*, haloperidol, metoclopramide)
  - Antihistamines (e.g. diphenylhydramine, promethazine)
  - Anticholinergics (e.g. scopolamine)
  - 5-HT$_3$ antagonists (odansetron – can cause constipation, palonosetron* which has a longer half-life)
  - Neurokinin/substance P receptor antagonists* (aprepitant, fosaprepitant)
  - Corticosteroids* (dexamethasone)
  - Benzodiazepines (for anticipatory nausea).
  *Indicates agents used for delayed emesis.
- Initiation of an antiemetic: start with a dopamine antagonist as prn either orally, IV, or per rectum (e.g. prochlorperazine 10 mg orally every 6 hours prn). If nausea persists, make regimen standing. If nausea or vomiting persists despite standing regimen, add a second agent to the existing regimen from a different class of drug (e.g. ondansetron 8 mg orally every 8 hours standing).

- The route of administration must be carefully considered based on the patient's ability to tolerate oral intake. Particularly in the outpatient setting, where parental agents are difficult if not impossible to administer in a timely manner, options for a patient who is intolerant of oral medications include: oral disintegrating ondansetron, granisetron or scopolamine patch, or per rectal administration in non-neutropenic patients. However, if these attempts fail, inpatient administration may be required.
- Nonpharmaceutical interventions (acupuncture or acupressure, small meals, avoiding aggravating agents including odors).

Fatigue
Overview
- Cancer-associated fatigue is a distressing, persistent, subjective sense of physical, emotional, and/or cognitive tiredness or exhaustion related to cancer or cancer treatment that is not proportional to recent activity and interferes with usual functioning.
- Fatigue is detected in 75–80% of patients receiving chemotherapy or radiation therapy or in patients with advanced cancer.

Assessment

> **CLINICAL PEARLS**
> Assessment of primary cancer-related fatigue:
> - Cancer disease status.
> - Fatigue/weakness intensity score (mild, moderate, or severe).
> - Level of drowsiness (falling asleep during normal activities).
> - Characteristics: onset (e.g. is it worse during treatment?), duration, timing (e.g. when in the day is it worse?), sleep history (hours asleep, time in bed, time awake), associated symptoms (poor nutrition, emotional distress).
> - Level of functional activity in waking hours (e.g. percentage of the day spent in bed or in a chair?).
> - Impairment in function both physical and emotional/psychologic.
> - Response to previous or current therapies.

- Differentiate between primary cancer-related fatigue and secondary fatigue (side effects of medication such as opioids, anemia, hypothyroidism, sleep apnea).
- All secondary causes of fatigue should be optimally treated first. If fatigue persists despite appropriate treatment of secondary causes, the patient has a primary cancer-related fatigue and the assessment in the Clinical pearls box should be performed.

Management
Initial management of cancer-related fatigue is lifestyle modifications. Evidence suggests pharmacotherapy is most beneficial in those patients who have severe fatigue or advanced disease, rather than those with mild fatigue.
- **Lifestyle modification:** sleep hygiene, exercise/physical therapy, energy saving for most important activities of the day, moderate caffeine intake.
- **Pharmacotherapy:**
  - Psychostimulant (methylphenidate): methylphenidate has the most evidence supporting its use in cancer-related fatigue. A typical starting dose is 2.5 mg orally twice daily at 8:00 a.m. and 12:00 p.m. The dose can be titrated to alleviation of symptoms; the maximum daily dose is generally 20 mg. Doses higher than this often have more side effects without

additional therapeutic benefit. The main side effect is tachycardia. Use of methylphenidate is contraindicated in patients with a recent myocardial infarction.
- Wakefulness-promoting non-amphetamine psychostimulant (modafinil): there are increasing data on the use of modafinil in treating cancer-related fatigue. Dosage begins at 100 mg/day for 1 week then increases to 200 mg/day.
- Corticosteroids (dexamethasone): despite its widespread use, there is a paucity of robust data on the effects of corticosteroids for use in managing fatigue. A randomized controlled trial found a benefit in using dexamethasone but only followed patients for 14 days.

Anorexia–cachexia
Overview
- Anorexia–cachexia syndrome is a catabolic state where weight loss is only partially explained by decreased nutritional intake and is typically unresponsive to supplemental nutrition.
- It is critically important to counsel patients that anorexia–cachexia in the setting of advanced malignancy is not the same as starvation or weight loss from inadequate access to calories.

Assessment

> **CLINICAL PEARLS**
> Anorexia–cachexia assessment:
> - Anorexia intensity score (mild, moderate, severe).
> - Characteristics: number of meals and portions, onset (chemotherapy or radiation induced), duration, aggravating factors, alleviating factors, associated symptoms (nausea, vomiting, pain).
> - Prealbumin and/or albumin.
> - Weight change over the last 6 months.
> - Functional assessment (e.g. can the patient feed herself?, ADLs).
> - Response to previous or current therapies.
> - Goals for therapy (e.g. is the goal appetite improvement or weight gain?).

Management
- No pharmacotherapy will result in an increase in muscle mass and all have side effects. As a result, before initiating therapy it is important to determine whether it is the patient or the caregiver who is most bothered by anorexia–cachexia and whether the most distressing symptom is loss of appetite or weight loss.
  - **Megestrol acetate (MA):** in patients with cancer, MA is associated with weight gain at high doses (>800 mg/day). Fewer than 25% of patients will have a weight gain of >5%. Appetite improvement and improved quality of life are not dose related. Adverse effects include peripheral edema and thromboembolism, which must be considered before prescribing.
  - **Dronabinol:** in a large multicenter clinical trial comparing dronabinol with MA, MA was found to be superior for weight gain and appetite improvement in cancer patients. However, dronabinol still improved appetite by approximately 50% and is associated with fewer side effects. Up to 10% of patients experience somnolence. It should be administered approximately 1 hour prior to lunch and dinner.
  - **Corticosteroids:** in patients with advanced cancer, corticosteroids have been shown to improve appetite, decrease fatigue, and increase patient satisfaction compared with placebo.

The side effects of corticosteroids are considerable, but the benefit to risk ratio in advanced cancer appears in favor of their use especially in patients with limited life expectancy.

Dyspnea
Overview
- Dyspnea is the subjective sensation of breathlessness and may be associated with objective findings of hypoxia.
- The focus must be on assessing and treating the self-reported symptom rather than diagnostic tests such as pulse oximetry value.
- In the absence of underlying cardiac or pulmonary pathology, dyspnea is most often associated with advanced disease or the end of life for patients with cancer.
- Dypsnea can be debilitating physically and psychosocially as it can be associated with anxiety and feelings of impending doom.

Assessment

> **CLINICAL PEARLS**
> Assessment of dyspnea:
> - Dyspnea intensity score (mild, moderate, severe).
> - Past dyspnea experience (asthma, COPD, pulmonary fibrosis).
> - Characteristics: description of dyspnea, frequency, aggravating factors (smells, exercise, anxiety), alleviating factors (open window).
> - Impairment in function both physical and emotional/psychologic.
> - Response to previous or current therapies.

- It is important to identify and treat/optimize the underlying physical cause of the dyspnea whenever possible.

Management
Pharmacologic and nonpharmacologic treatment approaches can be attempted after treating or optimizing the underlying cause of dyspnea. Opioids are the mainstay of treatment.
- **Pharmacologic:**
  - Opioids: the principles of initiation and titration are similar for pain and dyspnea, except starting doses are lower for dyspnea (typically start at 50% of the standard starting dose for pain)
  - Anxiolytics: initiated as an adjuvant to opioids if anxiety is contributing to dyspnea. Evidence does not support the use of anxiolytics to manage dyspnea without the concurrent use of an opioid.
- **Nonpharmacologic:** breath control, modifying environmental factors (being near a window with natural light, limiting noxious odors, directing fan and circulating air to face), and psychosocial support to limit emotional exacerbation of symptoms.

Reading list

Bakitas MA, Tosteson TD, Li Z, et al. Early versus delayed initiation of concurrent palliative oncology care: patient outcomes in the ENABLE III randomized controlled trial. J Clin Oncol 2015;33:1438–1445.

Barbera L, Seow H, Howell D, et al. Symptom burden and performance status in a population-based cohort of ambulatory cancer patients. Cancer 2010;116:5767–5776.

Chang VT, Hwang SS, Feuerman M. Validation of the Edmonton Symptom Assessment Scale. Cancer 2000;88:2164–2171.

Davis MP, Temel JS, Balboni T, et al. A review of the trials which examine early integration of outpatient and home palliative care for patients with serious illnesses. Ann Palliat Med 2015;4:99–121.

Glare P, Virik K, Jones M, et al. A systematic review of physicians' survival predictions in terminally ill cancer patients. BMJ 2003;327:195–198.

Goodman DC, Esty AR, et al. Trends and Variation in End-of-Life Care for Medicare Beneficiaries with Severe Chronic Illness: The Dartmouth Atlas Project Practice. Dartmouth, Center for Health Policy Research: 2011.

Kelley AS, Morrison RS. Palliative care for the seriously ill. N Engl J Med 2015;373:747–755.

May P, Garrido MM, Cassel JB, et al. Prospective cohort study of hospital palliative care teams for inpatients with advanced cancer: earlier consultation is associated with larger cost-saving effect. J Clin Oncol 2015;33:2745–2752.

Nekolaichuk C, Watanabe S, Beaumont C. The Edmonton Symptom Assessment System: a 15-year retrospective review of validation studies (1991–2006). Palliat Med 2008;22:111–122.

Seow H, Barbera L, Sutradhar R, et al. Trajectory of performance status and symptom scores for patients with cancer during the last six months of life. J Clin Oncol 2011;29:1151–1158.

Temel JS, Greer JA, Muzikansky A, et al. Early palliative care for patients with metastatic non-small-cell lung cancer. N Engl J Med 2010;363:733–742.

Weissman DE, Meier DE. Identifying patients in need of a palliative care assessment in the hospital setting: a consensus report from the Center to Advance Palliative Care. J Palliat Med 2011;14:17–23.

Suggested websites
General palliative care
American Academy of Hospice and Palliative Medicine: http://aahpm.org/
Center to Advance Palliative Care: https://www.capc.org/

Communication and shared decision making
VitalTalk: Evidence-based communication trainings for clinicians and institutions: https://www.vitaltalk.org/

Prognosis
Prognosis calculator: http://eprognosis.ucsf.edu/

Advance care planning
http://theconversationproject.org/
https://agingwithdignity.org/
https://prepareforyourcare.org/
https://www.acpdecisions.org/patients/

Advance directives: New York State
http://www.caringinfo.org/files/public/ad/New_York.pdf
https://www.health.ny.gov/professionals/patients/health_care_proxy/
https://www.health.ny.gov/publications/1503.pdf

Guidelines
National society guidelines

Title	Source	Date and weblink
Guidelines for cancer related pain, antiemesis, fatigue, distress, and palliative care	National Cancer Care Network Guidelines for Supportive Care	2019 http://www.nccn.org/professionals/physician_gls/f_guidelines.asp#supportive

Images

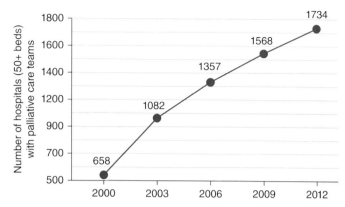

Figure 48.1 Prevalence of US hospital palliative care teams: 2000–2012. (Source: Center to Advance Palliative Care. National Palliative Care Registry 2012 Annual Survey Summary. Accessed 27 November 2015 at https://registry.capc.org/cms/Reports.aspx.)

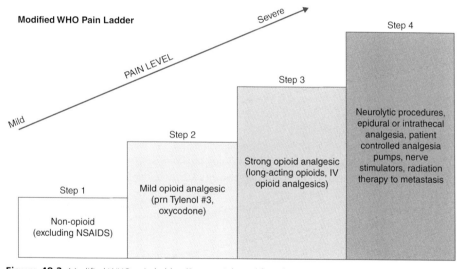

Figure 48.2 Modified WHO pain ladder. (Source: Adapted from http://www.who.int/cancer/palliative/painladder/en/.)

Additional material for this chapter can be found online at:
www.wiley.com/go/oh/mountsinaioncology

This includes a case study, ICD codes, and multiple choice questions.

CHAPTER 49

Nutrition and Symptom Management

Paula Occiano, Melissa Nagelberg, and Raquela Adelsberg
Icahn School of Medicine at Mount Sinai, New York, NY, USA

> **OVERALL BOTTOM LINE**
> - Nutritional management for patients receiving oncologic treatment should focus on maintaining adequate intake of calories and protein, and minimizing nutrition-related side effects of treatment. Weight maintenance and preservation of lean body mass is essential for maintaining patients' strength and energy. Optimal nutrition status assists in preventing nutrient deficiencies, malnutrition, and weight loss as well as decreasing risk for infection.
> - Preventing and managing nutrition-related symptoms can assist in improving treatment outcomes and quality of life.

Nausea and vomiting
- Include easy to tolerate foods such as low fat, bland foods (e.g. chicken noodle soup, toast, crackers, rice or pasta, plain chicken or fish).
- Cold foods may be better tolerated.
- Eat smaller frequent meals or snacks spread throughout the day. Do not go for too long without eating as an empty stomach may trigger nausea.
- Avoid any foods with odors (such as hot meals or eggs), high fat foods, strong spices, high fat dairy products, and creamy soups.
- Try ginger tea, ginger ale, or ginger-flavored hard candies.
- Maintain fluid intake as able via frequent, small sips in between meals.
- Medications: consider antiemetics or prokinetic agents such as ondansetron, reglan, compazine, or erythromycin.
- It is important to verify if antiemetics are being provided in a timely manner; consider standing doses prior to meals to aid in alleviation of nausea and vomiting in order to optimize intake.

Diarrhea
- Consume less insoluble fiber and include foods that are easy to tolerate such as plain white toast, pasta, white rice, and broths.
- Increase fluid intake (water, diluted juice, broth) to 30 mL/kg/day. Try products like G2, coconut water, or Pedialyte for fluid and electrolyte repletion.
- Avoid raw fruits and vegetables, dairy products including milk and cheese, foods that are spicy, acidic, or high in fat, and beverages that are caffeinated, contain sorbitol, or are high in sugar.
- Gradually increase soluble fiber intake (e.g. apple sauce, oatmeal, or potatoes without the skin).
- If chemotherapy-induced, consider L-glutamine 10 g three times daily.

- Medications: consider antidiarrheal medication such as loperamide (if *Clostridium difficile* negative); IV fluid administration; replete electrolytes as needed; discontinue stool softeners or laxative medications.

Constipation

- Gradually increase fiber intake (raw fruits and vegetables, whole grains). Increasing fiber intake too quickly can cause abdominal discomfort.
- Avoid gas forming foods and beverages such as carbonated drinks, cruciferous vegetables, and gas forming protein sources such as beans.
- Increase fluid intake.
- Increase physical activity if possible.
- Place a warm compress or washcloth over the abdomen and gently massage in a clockwise motion (up the right side, cross over, and down the left side). Repeat as needed.
- Medications: consider the addition of stool softeners or laxatives.

Fatigue

- Educate patients on the need for adequate fluid and food intake for energy.
- Promote nutrient dense foods (those high in protein and/or fat as tolerated – nutritional supplements, nuts, seeds, avocado, cheese, oils, yogurt, meat, chicken, fish, eggs).
- Advise patients to keep fluids and snack foods at the bedside for easy access.
- Encourage patients to eat their largest meal at the time of day when they are most awake, with frequent snacks throughout the day.
- Encourage patients to ambulate and consider consulting physical therapy. Movement can help stimulate appetite and increase PO intake.
- Consider use of a multivitamin if oral intake is poor and there are no medical contraindications.
- Encourage family, friends, caregivers and/or nursing staff to encourage intake and help set up meals at mealtimes.
- If fatigue is caused by depression, consider a psychologic consultation and use of antidepressant medications if appropriate.

Anorexia (lack of appetite) and early satiety

- Consider small frequent meals every 2–3 hours.
- Maximize intake and take advantage of times when the appetite is greater.
- Encourage intake of calorically dense as well as protein dense foods (whole-fat dairy products, nut butter, oils, animal proteins).
- Avoid or limit intake of beverages (especially low calorie) prior to or during meals.
- Relaxation techniques and creating pleasant environments for mealtimes can help to increase intake.
- Calorically dense oral nutrition supplements (e.g. Ensure, Enu, Boost) can be used to increase calorie intake. Consider intake in between meals and never prior to meals.
- Keep favorite foods readily available.
- Medications: consider appetite stimulants such as megestrol acetate, corticosteroid agents, dronabinol, remeron if appetite remains low despite alleviation of other nutrition-related symptoms (i.e. mucositis, nausea, and vomiting).

Weight loss

- Encourage patients to consume small, frequent meals of nutrient dense foods (those high in protein and/or fat as tolerated – nutritional supplements, nuts, seeds, avocado, cheese, oils, yogurt, meat, chicken, fish, eggs).

- Provide easy-to-make, nutrient-dense smoothie recipes.
- Provide calorie and protein goals for patients to meet in order to prevent further weight loss.
- Assess for causes of weight loss other than decreased intake (e.g. fever, high tumor burden, diarrhea, emesis); resolve any underlying causes first.
- Advise patients to avoid skipping meals (patients should try to "eat by the clock").
- Assess for signs of malnutrition (protruding ribs/clavicle bones, hollow orbital region, muscle wasting in arms/legs, etc.).
- Consider use of appetite stimulants and/or antidepressant medications if medically appropriate.
- Trend weekly weights.

Steroid induced weight gain
- Provide appropriate calorie goals for weight loss.
- Encourage patients to track oral intake in a food diary.
- Provide education on ways to decrease calorie intake:
  - Limit high calorie foods
  - Limit empty calories (fruit juice, desserts, candy).
- Encourage physical activity, if able – 30–60 minutes of moderate intensity activity daily.
- Encourage an increase in vegetables; whole grains, beans/legumes, and fruits (limit fruits to 2/day; no fruit juice).
- Ensure adequate fluid intake.

Steroid induced hyperglycemia
- When uncontrolled hyperglycemia is present, consider referring to endocrinology. Assess need for medication.
- Limit intake of foods high in sugar (fruit juice, desserts, candy, excess fruit intake).
- Limit 45–75 g carbohydrate (3–5 servings) per meal, depending on severity of hypergycemia.
- Educate patients on choosing fiber-rich carbohydrates (whole grain breads, beans/legumes, green leafy vegetables).
- Encourage adequate amounts of lean protein intake (chicken, fish, turkey, low fat dairy, eggs) which can help patients feel fuller for a longer period of time.
- Promote physical activity, if able; 30–60 minutes of moderate intensity activity daily.

Dysgeusia and hypogeusia
- Rinse mouth with a baking soda and salt solution before and during meals (1 quart water, 1 teaspoon baking soda, and 1 teaspoon salt. Shake well before using). Rinse and spit, do not swallow the solution.
- If a metallic taste is present, use plastic utensils and glass cups.
- Use a straw for liquids to bypass the taste buds, if there is no risk for aspiration.
- Cook foods with seasonings and sauces for a stronger flavor (e.g. teriyaki and BBQ sauces or onion, garlic, and chili powders). *Avoid this if mucositis or mouth sores are present.*
- If the patient has had poor oral intake for a prolonged period of time, consider 220 mg/day zinc sulfate for 2 weeks only (can cause copper deficiency with prolonged use).
- Practice good dental hygiene.
- Use natural sweeteners to combat salty or bitter taste and lemon juice or salt for heightened sweet taste.
- Check to see if dysgeusia and hypogeusia are being caused by fungal growth.

Xerostomia
- Drink plenty of low sugar fluids and stay well hydrated (30 mL/kg/day), unless fluid restriction is necessary.

- Practice good dental hygiene and use a soft bristle toothbrush.
- Rinse mouth with a baking soda and salt solution throughout the day (1 quart water, 1 teaspoon baking soda, and 1 teaspoon salt. Shake well before using). Rinse and spit, do not swallow the solution.
- Try moistening mouth sprays (e.g. Biotene®, Oasis®, Orajel®).
- Try saliva substitutes, if caused by damage to salivary glands.
- Moisten foods with broth, sauces, and gravies.
- Avoid products containing alcohol, caffeine, and tobacco.
- Try using a humidifier. Be sure to keep it clean to avoid bacterial or fungal growth.
- Eat fruits that contain enzymes like papaya and pineapple. Use in smoothies or shakes with crushed ice.

Mucositis
- Consider pain medication and magic mouthwash.
- Consider a calcium phosphate mouth rinse (e.g. Caphosol® or SalivaMax®). Works better if given prophylactically.
- Depending on the grade, follow a soft, pureed, or liquid diet.
- Eat cool or room temperature foods.
- Avoid acidic and spicy foods.
- Practice good dental hygiene and use a soft bristle toothbrush.
- Avoid products with alcohol and tobacco.
- Try sucking on ice to soothe pain.
- Use high calorie, high protein supplemental drinks and shakes to maintain nutritional status as needed.

Odynophagia
- Consider pain medication and magic mouthwash.
- Follow a bland soft, pureed, or liquid diet.
- Moisten foods with broth, sauces, and gravies or blenderize for better tolerance.
- Eat cool or room temperature foods.
- Avoid acidic, salty, and spicy foods.
- Avoid products containing alcohol, caffeine, and tobacco.
- Use high calorie, high protein supplemental drinks and shakes to maintain nutritional status as needed.

Dysphagia
- Refer to speech therapy for evaluation of swallow function and risk of aspiration.
- Depending on grade and if oral feeding is tolerated, follow a soft, mechanical soft, or pureed diet with thin and/or thick liquids per speech therapy evaluation.
- Use a blender to chop or liquefy solids for better tolerance.
- Use high calorie, high protein supplemental drinks and shakes to maintain nutritional status as needed.
- Consider alternative nutrition support, if risk of aspiration:
  - If the gut is functioning, there are no signs of obstruction, and expected need is >5 days, consider feeding tube with enteral nutrition
  - If sign of obstruction, gastrointestinal malabsorption, and expected need is >5 days, consider total parenteral nutrition (TPN)
  - Refer to a registered dietitian for assessment of enteral or parenteral needs and recommendations.

Malnutrition and cancer cachexia

- Follow a high calorie, high protein diet if no renal dysfunction is present.
- Symptom management (see recommendations for specific symptom(s) affecting oral intake).
- Small frequent nutrient dense meals or snacks spread throughout the day.
- Use calorie and protein dense powders, gels, or liquids to add to foods and beverages to increase the item's energy content (e.g. Benecalorie®, Beneprotein®, ProMod Liquid Protein®).
- Use high calorie, high protein supplemental drinks and shakes (e.g. Boost Plus®, Boost Compact®, Boost VHC®, Enu®, Ensure Complete®).
- Consider a daily multivitamin plus minerals that meets close to 100% of the recommended dietary allowance.
- Consider an appetite stimulant, if poor appetite is present with no other symptoms.
- If persistent poor oral intake (<75% of estimated nutrient needs), weight loss, and poor performance status, consider alternative nutrition support:
  - If the gut is functioning, there are no signs of obstruction, and expected need is >5 days, consider feeding tube with enteral nutrition
  - If sign of obstruction, gastrointestinal malabsorption, and expected need is >5 days, consider TPN
  - Refer to registered dietitian for assessment of enteral or parenteral needs and recommendations.

Some foods and supplements can interact with chemotherapeutic agents: CYP3A4 inducers include St. John's wort, phenobarbital; CYP3A4 inhibitors include grapefruit juice, ketoconazole, and erythromycin (see Table 49.1).

Table 49.1 Chemotherapeutic agent specific nutritional considerations and/or interactions.

Drug	Interaction
Axitinib Inlyta*	Avoid CYP3A4 inducers and inhibitors which can alter drug activity
Bexarotene Targretin*	Grapefruit juice can increase concentration and toxicities Limit vitamin A intake to ≤1500 IU/day to avoid possible additive toxicity with drug
Bortezomib Velcade*	Avoid green tea extract and high dose vitamin C supplements CYP3A4 inhibitors or inducers can alter drug activity
Capecitabine Xeloda*	Vitamin B6 (dose of 50–100 mg two to three times a day) can help prevent/reduce the incidence and severity of hand-foot syndrome
Dasatinib Sprycel*	Avoid CYP3A4 inducers and inhibitors which can alter drug activity
Erlotinib Tarceva*	Avoid CYP3A4 inducers and inhibitors which can alter drug activity
Everilimus Afinitor*	Avoid CYP3A4 inducers and inhibitors which can alter drug activity
Exemestane Aromasin*	Avoid CYP3A4 inducers which can decrease drug activity
Fluorouracil 5-FU or Adrucil*, IV	For IV bolus infusions, provide cryotherapy 10–15 minutes before and after IV bolus infusion to reduce incidence of oral mucositis Vitamin B6 (dose of 50–100 mg two to three times a day) can help prevent/reduce the incidence and severity of hand-foot syndrome
Imatinib mesylate Gleevec*	Avoid CYP3A4 inducers and inhibitors which can alter drug activity

Table 49.1 (*Continued*)

Drug	Interaction
Lapatinib Tykerb*	Avoid CYP3A4 inhibitors which can increase drug activity
Methotrexate Folex* or Rheumatrex*	Avoid folic acid and its derivatives during methotrexate drug therapy Avoid alcohol as it can increase hepatotoxicity
Deferasiox Exjade*	Drug contains lactose; recommend lactase enzyme supplement with dosing
Nilotinib Tasigna*	Avoid CYP3A4 inhibitors which can increase drug activity Drug contains lactose; recommend lactase enzyme supplement with dosing
Oxaliplatin Eloxatin *IV	Vitamin B6 (dose of 50–100 mg two to three times a day) can help prevent/reduce the incidence and severity of hand-foot syndrome
Pemetrexed Alimta *IV	To prevent anemia, provide the following dietary supplementation before and after drug therapy • Folic acid (350–100 µg) PO beginning 1 week prior to first treatment continuing daily throughout treatment and post treatment • Vitamin B12 (1000 µg) IM injections given every three cycles, beginning 1 week prior to first treatment and continuing throughout treatment
Procarbazine	Foods containing tyramine should be avoided while taking this drug and for 2 weeks after (aged and strong cheeses, anchovies, avocados, bananas, beer, beef and chicken livers, bologna, brewer's yeast, caffeine, caviar, distilled spirits, dried fruits [raisins and prunes], fava beans, figs, meat extracts, meats such as sausage, miso soup, pepperoni, raspberries, red wine, salami, sauerkraut, sherry, and soy sauce)
Regorafenib Stivarga*	High fat meals can alter the absorption of this drug Take with a low fat meal providing <8 g fat
Sorafenib Nexavar*	Avoid CYP3A4 inducers which can decrease drug activity
Sunitinib Sutent*	Avoid CYP3A4 inducers and inhibitors which can alter drug activity
Tamoxifen Nolvadex*	Avoid CYP3A4 inducers and inhibitors which can alter drug activity
Vinblastine Velban*	Avoid CYP3A4 inducers and inhibitors which can alter drug activity
Vincristine Oncovin*	Avoid CYP3A4 inducers and inhibitors which can alter drug activity
Zoledronic acid Zometa*	Patients should take an oral supplement of 500 mg calcium and 400 IU vitamin D daily
Cyclophosphamide Cytoxan*	Aggressive hydration recommended (3 L/day of fluid)
Cisplatin Platinol*	Encourage adequate hydration to prevent nephrotoxicity

* Trade name.

(Source: Adapted with permission from the Oncology Nutrition Dietetic Practice Group of the Academy of Nutrition and Dietetics: Grant B. Appendix 8: Drug, nutrient, food, and dietary supplement interactions with cancer medications. In: Oncology Nutrition for Clinical Practice. Leser M, Ledesma N, Bergerson S, et al., eds. Chicago, IL: Oncology Nutrition Dietetic Practice Group; 2013: 267–270.)

Additional material for this chapter can be found online at:
www.wiley.com/go/oh/mountsinaioncology

This includes advice for patients, a case study, ICD codes, and
multiple choice questions.

CHAPTER 50

Cancer Survivorship

Lindsay Haines and Charles L. Shapiro
Icahn School of Medicine at Mount Sinai, New York, NY, USA

OVERALL BOTTOM LINE
- Components of survivorship care: surveillance for recurrent and new cancers; addressing long-term and late effects; health promotion and disease prevention; psychosocial care; and communication and care coordination among a multidisciplinary team.
- Special consideration is needed for adult survivors of pediatric cancers, the growing population of geriatric cancer survivors, and caregivers for individuals with cancer.
- The individual needs of cancer survivors vary over time.
- Depending on local practice patterns, a shared care model among the oncologist and primary care or mid-level provider provides the best care for cancer survivors as it maintains continuity and maximizes routine health maintenance.

Background
Definition
- Cancer survivorship focuses on the health and well-being of individuals beginning at diagnosis, throughout active treatment, and continues until the end of life. Functionally, however, it begins after the completion of active treatment.

Incidence and prevalence
- The cancer survivor population will grow from nearly 15 million currently to at least 20 million by 2025.
- About 60% of cancer survivors are over the age of 65 with projections that this percentage will grow over time.
- Figures 50.1 and 50.2 illustrate the most common cancers among survivors.

Economic impact
- Cancer survivors have higher annual medical costs, more productivity losses, higher excess economic burden, and lower employment rates than those without a cancer history.
- There is an anticipated overall shortage of care providers for cancer survivors. Additionally, few physicians and ancillary staff have adequate geriatric expertise to care for the growing number of geriatric cancer survivors.

Etiology
- For most cancers, the precise molecular events (i.e. mutations, amplifications, and pathway alterations) and individual host factors that lead to the development of cancer are unknown.

Mount Sinai Expert Guides: Oncology, First Edition. Edited by William K. Oh and Ajai Chari.
© 2019 John Wiley & Sons Ltd. Published 2019 by John Wiley & Sons Ltd.
Companion Website: www.wiley.com/go/oh/mountsinaioncology

Predictive/risk factors

- Among the strongest risk factors for developing cancer include smoking, excessive alcohol intake, obesity, inherited genetic mutations, and prior cancer therapy.
- Smoking increases the risks of lung, head and neck, as well as bladder cancers.
- Excessive alcohol intake has been linked to hepatocellular carcinomas, head and neck cancers, breast cancers, and both upper and lower gastrointestinal malignancies.
- There are a variety of genetically inherited germline mutations that predispose individuals to cancer, including *BRCA1* and *BRCA2* gene mutations increasing the risks of breast and ovarian cancers, DNA mismatch repair mutations causing hereditary nonpolyposis colorectal cancer (Lynch syndrome), and *APC* gene mutations leading to familial adenomatous polyposis (FAP) and increasing the risk of colorectal cancer. There are many other inherited cancer syndromes that can predispose those with these mutations to cancers at multiple sites.
- Cancer treatment can put individuals at greater risk of developing new primary cancers. For example, mantle irradiation used in Hodgkin lymphoma elevates the risk of breast cancer, while alkylating agents and topoisomerase II inhibitors slightly increase the risk of leukemia.

Prevention

Screening (Table 50.1)

- Like those without a history of cancer, screening and surveillance remain important parts of healthcare maintenance for cancer survivors. There are two types of screening for survivors: cancer recurrence screening and age or gender based screening as recommended to the general population.

Table 50.1 Screening for recurrent, secondary, and metastatic cancers.

Site	Test	Recommendation
Breast cancer	Physical examination	Every 3–6 months for 3 years; every 6–12 months for years 4–5 and annually after 5 years
	Mammogram	About 6 months after completion of radiation post lumpectomy and annually thereafter. After unilateral mastectomy, the contralateral breast annually
	Metastatic/secondary cancer Surveillance: CT scans, bone scan, or PET/CT and tumor markers	None indicated in asymptomatic women. Persistent or new symptoms prompts imaging as clinically indicated
Colorectal cancer	Carcinoembryonic antigen (CEA)	Every 3–6 months for the first 5 years
	Colonoscopy	1 year after initial surgery and every 5 years thereafter if the previous tests are normal
	Metastatic/secondary cancer Surveillance: CT scans	Annually for 3 years but increased frequency for those at high risk
Prostate cancer	Prostate-specific antigen (PSA)	PSA measurements every 6–12 months for the first 5 years and then annually
	Digital rectal examination (DRE)	Annual DRE
	Metastatic/secondary cancer Surveillance: cystoscopy, colonoscopy as clinically indicated for those who have undergone radiation and are symptomatic	None indicated in asymptomatic men. Persistent or new symptoms prompts imaging as clinically indicated

- Recurrence screening allows for early detection of local or metastatic recurrences and prompts initiation of appropriate treatment. In some cases, these screenings can even help identify early stage new primary cancers.
- Routine age and sex appropriate screening for new primary cancers should follow recommendations for the general population.
- There are several germline genetically inherited mutations that increase the risk of cancer for those carriers and warrant additional or alternative screening to monitor for new primary cancers. For example, breast MRI screening rather than standard mammography is recommended for carriers of the *BRCA* mutation.

Primary prevention
- Low dose radiation chest CTs are recommended to monitor for lung cancer in current smokers or ex-smokers who have quit within the last 15 years between the ages of 55 and 80 with at least a 30 pack-year smoking history.
- Known *BRCA* mutation carriers may opt for prophylactic salpingoopherectomy and bilateral mastectomy to prevent the development of ovarian and breast cancer.
- In women who are at high risk of developing breast cancers (e.g. *BRCA* carriers, lobular cancer *in situ*, atypical ductal hyperplasia) tamoxifen, raloxifene, or the aromatase inhibitors reduce their risk.
- While no standardized screening or primary prevention guidelines exist for individuals with FAP, most recommend frequent colorectal cancer screening and total colectomy if and/or when multiple large adenomas or adenomas with more aggressive features are identified.

Secondary prevention
- Tobacco, obesity, and excessive alcohol intake can increase the risk of several cancers. Cancer survivors should be aware of the increased risk of new primary or recurrent cancers related to these modifiable risk factors. Depending on local availability, these patients should be referred to programs and therapies to help with healthy lifestyle changes.

Diagnosis
- Cancer survivors can present with a variety of symptoms ranging from chemotherapy-induced peripheral neuropathy to shortness of breath and ankle edema concerning for anthracycline-induced congestive heart failure. At times the relationship between treatment exposure and symptom onset is not clear, especially with the increasing prevalence of comorbid conditions in an aging population.
- Long-term side effects are complications that appear during and persist after treatment ends. Late effects are complications that present after treatment ends. These effects often overlap as seen in anthracycline and/or trastuzumab related cardiac dysfunction which can develop during or after treatment. Similarly, estrogen or androgen therapy-related bone loss during active treatment might increase the risk of bone fractures or osteoporosis years after treatment completion.
- Common long-term effects include fatigue, pain, peripheral neuropathy, cardiac dysfunction, vasomotor and menopausal symptoms, cognitive problems, bone loss, infertility, sexual dysfunction, insomnia, depression, and anxiety.
- It is important to remember that before the development of primary cancer, patients may have had comorbid conditions, functional limitations, cognitive problems, social isolation, and poor nutrition that can increase the risk of long-term and late effects.

Treatment
Treatment rationale
- Treatment is tailored to individual health problems. In many cases, the treatment for specific diseases are the same regardless of cancer history.
- By 2019, the American College of Surgeons' Commission on Cancer (CoC) as one of the metrics of hospital accreditation will require that all individuals treated for curative intent will be given a cancer treatment summary and individualized survivorship care plan after treatment completion. Included in the treatment summary is a record of the specific treatments received and the most common long-term and late effects to be expected. This treatment summary and care plan is designed to ensure that healthcare providers and cancer survivors are aware of potential late and long-term effects and cancer-specific screening recommendations. Some form of distress screening should also be performed as another CoC requirement for accreditation.
- Cancer survivors are at continued risk for the adverse health conditions that may have predisposed them in the first place to their primary cancer including continued smoking, alcohol, and obesity. Lifestyle modifications have positive effects on survivors' quality of life, and in some cases can reduce the risk of recurrence and mortality.
- Many cancer survivors face increased psychosocial stressors including anxiety, depression, fear of recurrence, reduced social support, and financial problems brought about by the costs of care and lost wages. The Institute of Medicine found that many of these issues remain unaddressed and untreated because of the lack of processes available to identify these needs and resources to link survivors to appropriate care and services. Appropriate referrals should be made to psychosocial and financial support programs.

Models of delivering survivorship care
See Table 50.2.

Special populations
Childhood, adolescent and young adult cancer survivors
- While only 5% of survivors are under the age of 40, there is a growing population of adult survivors of childhood cancer. Childhood cancers have high overall 5-year survival rates, and in 2010 most of them were over the age of 20.
- These survivors have significant rates of premature morbidity and mortality because of second malignant neoplasms and long-term/late effects. The majority will develop a chronic comorbid illness years after treatment completion, and over 40% will develop a severe, disabling, or life-threatening condition from a chronic illness.
- Despite the available guidelines, most in this population do not have appropriate risk-based care and lack knowledge regarding their cancer and treatment-associated health risks. As many have transitioned from pediatric to adult care, they are often followed up by nonspecialists who may lack the training to provide the necessary surveillance in this population.
- There are comprehensive and risk-stratified guidelines for follow-up care for this population.

Older adult cancer survivors
- Cancer survivorship care in this population is focused on "active life expectancy" and helping patients reintegrate into society, work, and familial obligations following completion of cancer treatment.
- The goals of treatment in older adults differ, with some placing more value on quality of life rather than survival time.

Table 50.2 Cancer survivorship care models.

Care model	Overview	Challenges
Oncology Specialist Care	Survivors continue to see their primary oncologist after treatment has ended	This model allows for continuity of care; however, the focus is on illness rather than health promotion. Often, oncologists lack the time or skill set to manage other comorbid illnesses and deliver less routine, noncancer related care
Multidisciplinary Survivorship Clinic	Survivors see multiple providers with expertise in screening and management of long-term/late effects. Survivors who have complex medical problems and require more support may benefit most	This model is often resource and time intensive and is not the most efficient or cost-effective model to serve the majority of survivors
Disease/Treatment Specific Management	Survivors see a provider(s) who specializes in a specific type of long-term or late effect (e.g. seeing a neurologist for cancer-related peripheral neuropathy)	This model alone lacks focus on the significant psychosocial stressors that many cancer survivors face and is impractical. However, depending on the specific problem, this model can help supplement other models
Consultative Survivorship Clinic	Survivors are referred to a survivorship consultant who can recommend a post-treatment care plan and follow-up	This model does not establish long-term follow-up with a provider who is trained to assess survivorship issues
Integrated Survivorship Clinic	This model allows for a survivorship specialist to be a part of the clinical team while the patient is in active treatment and can therefore easily transition to survivorship care while still in the oncology setting	This model only allows patients to receive focused survivorship related care after treatment is over and may not adequately address other comorbid conditions. Additionally, it may be more difficult to transition patients back to their primary care physicians
Community Generalist Model	This model gives the responsibility of cancer survivorship to the primary care physician. The focus of care is on wellness rather than disease surveillance and promotes reintegration into primary care	Primary care physicians may have limited knowledge about long-term and late effects of cancer, treatments, and evolving guideline recommendations
Shared Care of Survivor	Survivors see both their primary care physician and an oncologist who work together to manage survivorship issues. This is useful for those with a high risk of recurrence and complicated cancer-related issues who benefit from continued close surveillance by a specialist	This model can often lead to over or underutilization of resources if the provider roles are not clearly delineated

(Source: Adapted from Providing High Quality Survivorship Care in Practice: An ASCO Guide. American Society of Clinical Oncology, 2014.)

- As advances in cancer treatment continue, increased emphasis will need to extend beyond quantitative outcomes like survival to assess qualitative measures like quality of life in the older adult patient.

Caregivers of cancer survivors
- Across all disease types, many caregivers have clinically significant symptoms of depression or anxiety. Additionally, depression rates and perceived burden increase for this population as the functional status of the care receiver declines.
- Providing support to informal caregivers in addition to the survivor is an integral component of survivorship care.

Reading list
American Cancer Society. Cancer Treatment and Survivorship Facts and Figures 2014–2015. ACS, 2014.

Children's Oncology Group: Long-term follow-up guidelines for survivors of childhood, adolescent and young adult cancers, 2013: http://www.surviorshipguidelines.org/pdf/LTFGuideline_40.pdf (accessed 12 March 2019).

DeSantis CE, Lin CC, Mariotto AB, et al. Cancer treatment and survivorship statistics, 2014. CA Cancer J Clin 2014;64:252–271.

Elston Lafata J, Simpkins J, Schultz L, et al. Routine surveillance care after cancer treatment with curative intent. Med Care 2005;43(6):592–599.

Girgis A, Lambert S, Johnson C, et al. Physical, psychosocial, relationship, and economic burden of caring for people with cancer: a review. J Oncol Pract 2013;9:197–202.

Hewitt, M, Greenfield, S, Stovall, E, et al. From Cancer Patient to Cancer Survivor: Lost in Transition. National Academies Press, Washington DC, 2006.

Keating NL, Nørredam M, Landrum MB, et al. Physical and mental health status of older long-term cancer survivors. J Am Geriatr Soc 2005;53:2145–2152.

Mullen F. Seasons of survival: reflections of a physician with cancer. N Engl J Med 1985;313:270–273.

Oeffinger KC, Mertens AC, Sklar CA, et al. Chronic health conditions in adult survivors of childhood cancer. N Engl J Med 2006;355:1572–1582.

Parr C, Kent EE, Mariotto AB, et al. Cancer survivors: a booming population. Cancer Epidemiol Biomarkers Prev 2011;20(10):1996–2005.

Ward E, DeSantis C, Robbins A, et al. Childhood and adolescent cancer statistics, 2014. CA Cancer J Clin 2014;64:83–103.

Suggested website
ASCO Cancer Survivorship Compendium: http://www.asco.org/practice-research/asco-cancer-survivorship-compendium

Guidelines

Title	Source	Date and weblink
Breast cancer follow-up management after primary treatment	American Society of Clinical Oncology (ASCO)	2013 http://jco.ascopubs.org/content/31/7/961.full
Follow-up care, surveillance protocol and secondary prevention measures for survivors of colorectal cancer	ASCO	2013 http://jco.ascopubs.org/content/31/35/4465
Prostate cancer survivorship care guidelines	ASCO, ACS	2015 http://jco.ascopubs.org/content/early/2015/02/03/JCO.2014.60.2557.full.pdf+html

(*Continued*)

Title	Source	Date and weblink
Prevention and management of chemotherapy-induced peripheral neuropathy in survivors of adult cancers	ASCO	2014 http://www.ncbi.nlm.nih.gov/ pubmed/24733808
Screening, assessment, and management of fatigue in adult survivors of cancer	ASCO	2014 http://jco.ascopubs.org/content/ 32/17/1840.abstract
Screening, assessment, and care of anxiety and depressive symptoms in adults with cancer	ASCO	2014 http://jco.ascopubs.org/content/ 32/15/1605
ASCO Clinical Expert Statement on Cancer Survivorship Care Planning	ASCO	2014 https://ascopubs.org/doi/full/ 10.1200/JOP.2014.001321
Fertility preservation for patients with cancer	ASCO	2013 http://jco.ascopubs.org/content/ 31/19/2500
ASCO statement on achieving high quality cancer survivorship care	ASCO	2013 http://jco.ascopubs.org/content/ 31/5/631.short
Survivorship: screening for cancer and treatment effects version 2	National Comprehensive Cancer Center Network (NCCN)	2014 http://www.jnccn.org/content/ 12/11/1526.short
Survivorship: nutrition and weight management version 2	NCCN	2014 http://www.jnccn.org/content/ 12/10/1396.abstract
Survivorship: healthy lifestyles version 2	NCCN	2014 http://www.jnccn.org/content/ 12/9/1222.abstract
Survivorship: cognitive function version 1	NCCN	2014 http://www.jnccn.org/content/ 12/7/976.abstract
Survivorship: sleep disorders version 1	NCCN	2014 http://www.jnccn.org/content/ 12/5/630.abstract
Survivorship: sexual dysfunction male and female version 1	NCCN	2014 http://www.ncbi.nlm.nih.gov/pmc/ articles/PMC4465261/
Survivorship: pain version 1	NCCN	2014 http://www.jnccn.org/content/ 12/4/488.abstract

Images

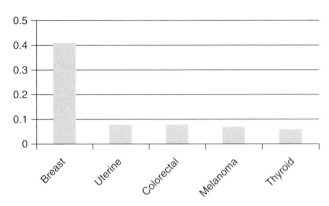

Figure 50.1 Most common cancer types in female survivors. (Data from American Cancer Society. Cancer Treatment and Survivorship Facts and Figures 2014–2015. Atlanta: American Cancer Society; 2014.)

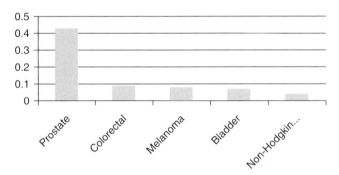

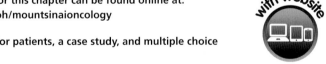

Figure 50.2 Most common cancer types in male survivors. (Data from American Cancer Society. Cancer Treatment and Survivorship Facts and Figures 2014–2015. Atlanta: American Cancer Society; 2014.)

Additional material for this chapter can be found online at:
www.wiley.com/go/oh/mountsinaioncology

This includes advice for patients, a case study, and multiple choice questions.

CHAPTER 51

Pediatric Cancer: Solid Tumors and Lymphoma

Surabhi Batra[1] and Birte Wistinghausen[2]
[1] Icahn School of Medicine at Mount Sinai, New York, NY, USA
[2] Children's National Health System, The George Washington University, Washington, DC, USA

OVERALL BOTTOM LINE
- Childhood cancer is rare, but the leading cause of death in children <15 years of age.
- Malignant solid tumors account for almost 50% (>4000 new diagnoses a year in the USA), and lymphomas for ~20% of pediatric cancers.
- The treatment requires a multidisciplinary approach.
- Cure rates overall exceed 75%.
- A major focus of research is tailoring therapy to reduce short- and long-term toxicities and improve outcome.

Background
Definition of disease
Cancer arises from a monoclonal uncontrolled cell proliferation caused by somatic somations conveying a survival and growth advantage. This chapter focuses on the most common childhood solid tumors and lymphoma.

Disease classification
Pediatric solid tumors are classified by cell and/or organ of origin.
- Sarcoma: arising from bone and soft tissues:
  - Rhabdomyosarcoma (RMS)
  - Nonrhabdomyosarcoma soft tissue sarcomas (synovial sarcomas and others)
  - Osteosarcoma
  - Ewing sarcoma (unknown cell of origin, postulated to be of neuroectodermal origin; EWS).
- Hepatoblastoma (HB).
- Wilms tumor (WT, nephroblastoma).
- Neuroblastoma.
- Retinoblastoma.

  Pediatric lymphomas are classified by Hodgkin disease (HD) and non-Hodgkin lymphoma (NHL) and further classified by immunophenotype into:
- Lymphoblastic lymphoma (40% of NHL in young children decreasing with age).
- Burkitt lymphoma (40% of NHL in young children decreasing with age).
- Diffuse large B-cell lymphoma (increasing with age, most common type in adolescence).
- Anaplastic large cell lymphoma (most prevalent in adolescence and young adults, ~5%).
- Low grade NHL such as mycosis fungoides and follicular lymphomas (up to 17% of NHL in adolescence) are rare in childhood but have been reported to have more favorable prognoses.

Mount Sinai Expert Guides: Oncology, First Edition. Edited by William K. Oh and Ajai Chari.
© 2019 John Wiley & Sons Ltd. Published 2019 by John Wiley & Sons Ltd.
Companion Website: www.wiley.com/go/oh/mountsinaioncology

Incidence/prevalence

- Cancer in children is rare. The incidence of childhood solid tumors is 7.4 in 100 000 per year and childhood lymphoma 2.4 in 100 000 per year. The distribution varies with age in HD, bone tumors, carcinomas, and melanomas becoming more prevalent in adolescence.

Etiology

- Most pediatric cancers are not linked to specific risk factors or exposures. There are rare familial syndromes.

Pathology/pathogenesis

Pediatric solid tumors and NHL are usually high grade and often summarized as "blue round cell tumors." Immunohistochemistry is usually needed to determine the type of tumor. Distinctive translocations are found in many tumor types.

Prevention
Screening

- Routine screening is not recommended.
- Some rare familial conditions warrant screening.

Primary prevention

- There are no primary prevention strategies.

Secondary prevention

- Survivors of childhood cancer are followed for the first 5 years for signs of recurrence and lifelong for long-term toxicities.

Diagnosis (Algorithm 51.1)

Algorithm 51.1 Diagnosis of pediatric tumors

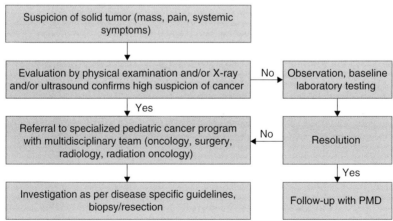

- Most children present with large palpable masses and/or localized pain but vague symptoms might be present for weeks to months.
- Acute presentations can be caused by bleeding into the tumor.
- Final diagnosis requires imaging and pathology.

Differential diagnosis

Differential diagnosis	Features
Infection	History of exposure/travel/other symptoms of infection
Benign tumor	Final diagnosis made on pathology

Typical presentation

Type of tumor	Typical presentation
Bone tumors and soft tissue sarcomas	Swelling or mass +/– pain Acute pain with pathologic fracture Functional deficits
Abdominal tumors including: • Hepatoblastoma • Wilms tumor • Neuroblastoma • Rhabdomyosarcoma • Lymphomas	Abdominal mass Hypertension, hematuria, anemia in Wilms tumor Chronic diarrhea, hypertension, vague systemic symptoms in neuroblastoma Bladder/urinary obstruction in rhabdomyosarcoma arising in the genitourinary tract
Orbital tumors: • Retinoblastoma • Orbital rhabdomyosarcoma	Loss of red reflex (retinoblastoma) • Dilated pupil Amblyopia Proptosis
Lymphoma	Lymphadenopathy Respiratory compromise or superior vena cava syndrome with mediastinal masses (Figure 51.1)

Clinical diagnosis
History
- Systemic symptoms:
  - Weight loss/gain
  - Fever
  - Anorexia
  - Fatigue
  - Pain
  - Localized growing mass.
- Chest tumors:
  - Respiratory symptoms.
- Orbital tumors:
  - Changes in vision.
- Abdominal tumors:
  - Diarrhea/constipation
  - Changes in urination, hematuria.
- Family history of cancer or other genetic syndromes.

Physical examination
Pediatric patients with suspected cancers require a comprehensive physical examination because they are not reliable historians. Special attention should be given to the following:
- Pallor and tachycardia from anemia.

- Lymphadenopathy, especially regional.
- A comprehensive neurologic examination:
  - Pupillar responses, vision, red reflex
  - Opsoclonus-myoclonus (random eye and motor movements) in neuroblastoma.
- Chest examination and auscultation.
- Gentle examination of abdominal masses because of risk of hemorrhage.
- Skin for signs of bruises, petechiae.
- Genitourinary examination for Tanner stage, testicular masses.

Useful clinical decision rules and calculators

Exposure to ionizing radiation should be limited as much as possible.
- Plain X-rays are useful in bone tumors as first line imaging to rule out pathologic fractures (Figure 51.2).
- Ultrasound is the preferred first line imaging modality for soft tissue masses and abdominal tumors.

Disease severity classification

Pediatric solid tumors are staged with disease-specific staging systems including extent of disease and resectibility of disease. Risk classification (risk of relapse) also includes age, location, and histologic features depending on cancer type.

The most important disease specific stages are:
- International Neuroblastoma Staging System:
  - Stage 4S: only in patients <365 days, exceedingly favorable prognosis.
- RMS stages and groups:
  - Modified TNM staging to account for favorable/unfavorable locations
  - Grouping according to amount of postoperative disease.
- National Wilms Tumor Study Staging:
  - Stage V: bilateral WT (5–7% of patients; Figure 51.3).
- Ann-Arbor staging for HD.
- Murphy Staging for NHL.
- Response Evaluation Criteria In Solid Tumors (RECIST) criteria for response evaluation by imaging.

Laboratory diagnosis
List of diagnostic tests
- Complete blood count.
- Comprehensive metabolic function with uric acid.
- Coagulation studies including fibrinogen and D-dimer.
- Urinalysis.
- Tumor markers as needed:
  - Alpha-fetoprotein: HB, germ cell tumor (GCT)
  - Beta-human chorionic gonadotropin (bHCG): GCT
  - Homovanillic acid (HVA) and vanillylmandelic acid (VMA) in spot urine: neuroblastoma.
  - Lactate dehydrogenase (LDH): lymphomas.
- Pathology:
  - Biopsy/resection and pathology is needed for all tumors except for stage IV neuroblastoma with elevated urine VMA and HVA and neuroblasts in bone marrow biopsy
  - Fresh tissue for cytogenetic analysis and fluorescence *in situ* hybridization is highly recommended.

- Staging:
  - Bilateral bone marrow aspiration and biopsies for RMS, EWS, neuroblastoma, NHL, and HD (Figure 51.4 bone marrow infiltration with neuroblasts)
  - Lumbar puncture for NHL and parameningeal RMS
  - Regional lymph node sampling: RMS, WT.

Lists of imaging techniques
- Ultrasound with Doppler to assess vessel patency/invasion (HB, WT).
- CT of the chest to rule out lung metastasis (solid tumors).
- CT/MRI with contrast of primary site
  - Bone tumor: MRI of the entire bone
  - Brain and head-and-neck primary: MRI required
  - Abdominal tumors: MRI preferred.
- Positron emission tomography (PET) if available.
- Bone scan (RMS, osteosarcoma, EWS) or as guided by symptoms.
- CT of the chest, abdomen, and pelvis (HD, NHL).
- Methyl-iodine benzylguanine (MIBG) scan neuroblastoma.

Potential pitfalls/common errors made regarding diagnosis of disease
- Pediatric cancers are rare and patients usually present with nonspecific symptoms, especially in preverbal children. Subtle symptoms often precede diagnosis for weeks to months.
- Because children are vague historians, and refer pain and/or symptoms, a comprehensive physical examination is necessary.

Treatment
Treatment rationale
Solid tumors:
- Pediatric cancers are mostly high grade tumors sensitive to chemotherapy.
- Cure requires two components to treatment:
  - Local control
  - Control of micro- and/or macrometastatic disease.
- Local control:
  - Debilitating surgery should be avoided because of the chemotherapy and/or radiosensitivity of most tumors
  - Local control is achieved with combinations of surgery, chemotherapy, and/or radiotherapy. Guidelines are tumor specific.
- Control of micro- and/or macrometastatic disease:
  - Chemotherapy is needed to treat microscopic local and distant disease
  - Macrometastatic disease must be eliminated as outlined for local control.

Lymphomas:
- Most NHL are cured with chemotherapy alone.
- Most high grade NHL can disseminate to the central nervous system requiring repeated lumbar punctures with intrathecal chemotherapy because of the blood–brain barrier.
- HD is treated with chemotherapy +/– radiation.

When to hospitalize
- Fever and neutropenia.
- Complications of chemotherapy and some chemotherapy regimens.
- Neurologic symptoms.
- Postoperative management.

Managing the hospitalized patient

- Management of pediatric cancer patients requires multidisciplinary care in specialized centers.
- Important aspects of managing hospitalized patients include the following:
  - Intravenous antibiotic coverage in febrile neutropenic patients
  - Monitoring fluid balance
  - Maintaining nutrition
  - Management of pain and/or nausea/emesis
  - Knowledge of chemotherapy-specific complications
  - Psychosocial support.

Table of treatment (Algorithms 51.2 and 51.3)

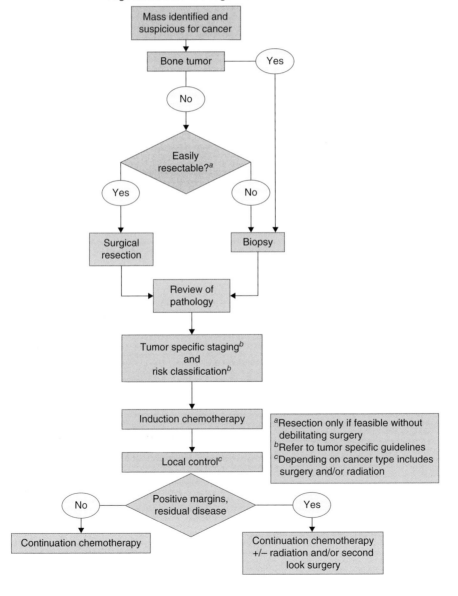

Algorithm 51.2 Management of solid tumors

Algorithm 51.3 Management of lymphoma

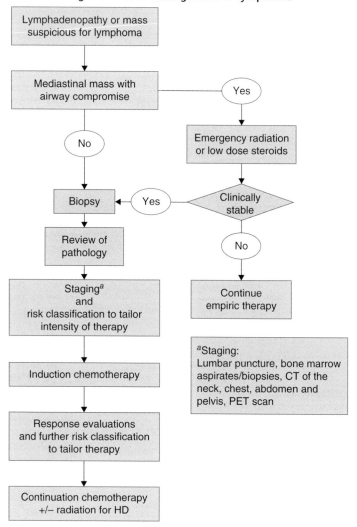

^aStaging:
Lumbar puncture, bone marrow aspirates/biopsies, CT of the neck, chest, abdomen and pelvis, PET scan

Tumor	Comments
Conservative	
Neonatal and stage IVs neuroblastoma	Spontaneous remission is common. Observation is the treatment of choice unless organ dysfunction is present
Chemotherapy	
Rhabdomyosarcoma	All stages require chemotherapy (vincristine, dactinomycin, cyclophosphamide) Neoadjuvant chemotherapy is indicated if upfront resection is not feasible

(Continued)

(*Continued*)

Tumor	Comments
Neuroblastoma	All stages outside infancy require chemotherapy; intensity of therapy depends on stage, histology and n-myc status Neoadjuvant chemotherapy is indicated if upfront resection is not feasible High risk neuroblastoma is treated with a combination of chemotherapy, radiotherapy, surgery, high dose chemotherapy with hematopoietic stem cell transplant (HSCT), cis-retinoic acid and biotherapy with anti-GD2-Ab
Wilms tumor	All stages except stage I with weight <500 g and age <2 years require chemotherapy (vincristine, dactinomycin +/– doxorubicin, additional drugs for advanced stages) Neoadjuvant therapy only for stage V in the USA, guidelines by the International Society of Pediatric Oncology recommend neoadjuvant therapy for all stages
Hepatoblastoma	All stages except for stage I with fetal pathology require chemotherapy (cisplatin, 5-fluorouracil, vincristine, and doxorubin) Neoadjuvant chemotherapy is indicated if upfront resection is not feasible
Osteosarcoma	All stages require chemotherapy (cisplatin, doxorubicin, and high dose methotrexate) Neoadjuvant chemotherapy is the standard of care
Ewing sarcoma	All stages require chemotherapy (vincristine, doxorubicin, cyclophosphamide, ifosfamide, and etoposide) Neoadjuvant chemotherapy is the standard of care Interval compression (14-day cycles instead of 21-day cycles) has been shown to improve outcome
Retinoblastoma	Some advanced stages require chemotherapy Administration options include systemic, intravitriolic, or intra-arterial
Non-Hodgkin lymphoma	Chemotherapy regimens are specific for subtype Lymphoblastic lymphoma is treated on acute lymphoblastic leukemia (ALL) regimen Burkitt lymphoma is cured with very intensive chemotherapy lasting 12–16 weeks Diffuse large B-cell lymphoma in children is treated with Burkitt regimens and has a better prognosis than in adults Anaplastic large cell lymphoma (ALCL) has been treated with several chemotherapy regimens
Surgery	
Rhabdomyosarcoma Neuroblastoma Hepatoblastoma	Upfront resection *only* recommended if negative margins can be easily obtained Otherwise delayed resection of all residual disease after chemotherapy and/or radiotherapy Liver transplant is indicated for unresectable, residual hepatoblastoma after chemotherapy

(Continued)

Tumor	Comments
Wilms tumor	Upfront resection is the standard of care in the USA except of bilateral Wilms tumor
Osteosarcoma	Delayed resection at week 12 of therapy Surgical control of all measurable disease is needed for cure
Ewing sarcoma	Delayed local control at week 12 Surgery preferred but radiation is equally efficacious
Radiation	
Rhabdomyosarcoma Wilms tumor Neuroblastoma	Radiation is indicated if there is residual or locoregional spread of disease
Ewing sarcoma	Ewing sarcoma is a radiosensitive tumor and radiation can be used for local control instead of surgery
Hodgkin disease	Radiation therapy can be avoided in most patients with a good early response but is used in patients who are low responders to chemotherapy
Biologic	
Lymphoma	There are several monoclonal antibodies targeting antigens expressed by some lymphomas that have been incorporated into some treatment protocols Rituximab against CD20 for Burkitt lymphoma and diffuse large B-cell lymphoma Brentuximab vedotin against CD30 in HD and ALCL and crizotinib, a TKI targeted alk in ALCL, are in clinical trials
Complementary	
All pediatric cancers	Intensive psychosocial support of the entire family Intensive supportive care to manage nausea/emesis, pain, nutrition Consider neuropsychologic testing

Prevention/management of complications

- Adrenal suppression:
  - Stress dose steroids if appropriate.
- Management of complications of chemotherapy requires the guidance of an experienced oncologist.
- Fever and neutropenia:
  - Broad spectrum antibiotic coverage.

CLINICAL PEARLS
- For most solid tumors, local control plus control of micrometastatic disease are key to cure and prevention of recurrence.
- Metastatic disease and/or multifocal disease confer a worse prognosis.

Special populations
Immunodeficiency and Down syndrome
• Patients with immunodeficiency and Down syndrome are at higher risk for infections and must be monitored closely during therapy.

Inherited defects of DNA repair
• Patients with Fanconi anemia and other DNA repair defects have an increased sensitivity to chemotherapy. Close monitoring and dose reductions are necessary.

Prognosis

BOTTOM LINE/CLINICAL PEARLS
• Overall, the prognosis of children with cancer now exceeds 75%.
• There is significant physical and psychosocial burden of therapy.
• Patients require lifelong monitoring for potential late effects of therapy.

Natural history of untreated disease
• Cancer is a lethal disease if untreated with few exceptions.
• Spontaneous regression is seen in some infantile neuroblastoma.

Prognosis for treated patients
• The prognosis of children with cancer exceeds 75% but cure rates for patients with metastasis continue to be poor.

Follow-up tests and monitoring
• See section on secondary prevention.

Reading list
Adamson P. Children's Oncology Group's 2013 five year blueprint for research. Pediatr Blood Cancer 2013;60:955–1068.
Pizzo PA, Poplack DG. Principles and Practice of Pediatric Oncology, 7th edition. Wolters Kluwer.
Ravindranath Y. Evolution of modern treatment of childhood acute leukemia and cancer: adventures and battles in the 1970s and 1980s. Pediatr Clin North Am 2015;62:1–10.

Suggested websites
Children's Oncology Group: https://www.childrensoncologygroup.org/
National Cancer Institute: https://www.cancer.gov/
National Comprehensive Cancer Network: https://www.nccn.org/

Guidelines
National society guidelines

Title	Source	Date and weblink
COG Supportive Care Guidelines	Children's Oncology Group (COG): Supportive care endorsed guidelines	2015 https://www.childrensoncologygroup.org/index.php/cog-supportive-care-guidelines
Guidelines for Pediatric Cancer Centers	American Academy of Pediatrics	2004 http://pediatrics.aappublications.org/content/pediatrics/113/6/1833.full.pdf
Long-term follow-up guidelines	Children's Oncology Group (COG): Long-term follow up guidelines	2013 http://www.survivorshipguidelines.org/pdf/LTFU Guidelines_40.pdf

Evidence

Type of evidence	Title and comment	Date and weblink
Clinical studies	Cooperative Group Clinical Studies by the Children's Oncology Group **Comment:** Multiple trials defining current standard of care for most childhood cancers	2019 PubMed
Clinical studies by smaller cooperative group such as TACL, PBTC, PBMTC	**Comment:** Trials defining new therapies mostly in the relapse setting	2019 PubMed

Images

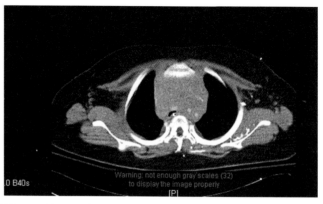

Figure 51.1 CT image of large mediastinal mass with tracheal compression. Pathology showed T-cell lymphoma.

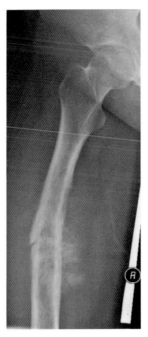

Figure 51.2 X-ray of right femur with osteosarcoma. Please note neoplastic bone formation in the soft tissue (sunburst appearance) and pathologic fracture.

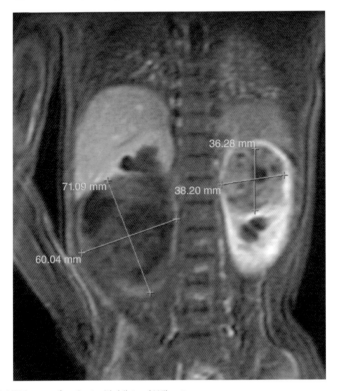

Figure 51.3 MRI image of patient with bilateral Wilms tumor.

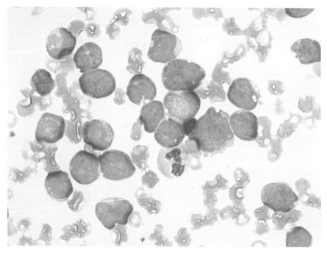

Figure 51.4 Bone marrow aspirate showing numerous large undifferentiated blasts with few trapped hematopoietic cells. Immunostaining (not shown) confirmed neuroblastoma. See website for color version.

Additional material for this chapter can be found online at:
www.wiley.com/go/oh/mountsinaioncology

This includes advice for patients, a case study, ICD codes, and multiple choice questions. The following image is available in color: Figure 51.4.

CHAPTER 52

Pediatric Cancer: Brain Tumors

Surabhi Batra[1] and Birte Wistinghausen[2]
[1] Icahn School of Medicine at Mount Sinai, New York, NY, USA
[2] Children's National Health System, The George Washington University, Washington, DC, USA

OVERALL BOTTOM LINE
- Brain tumors are the second most common malignancy in children and overall account for ~20% of childhood cancers.
- About 4350 children up to the age of 19 are diagnosed with a brain tumor each year in the USA.
- Management of pediatric brain tumors requires a multidisciplinary team of neurosurgeons, neurologists, neuro-oncologists, neuropsychologists, and rehabilitation specialists.
- A major focus of research is tailoring therapy to reduce short- and long-term toxicities.

Background
Definition of disease
A mass arising in the brain in children 0–21 years of age.

Disease classification
The most common pediatric brain tumors:
- Gliomas:
  - Low grade:
    - Pilocytic astrocytomas (PA)
    - Optic pathway tumors (OPT).
  - High grade:
    - Anaplastic astrocytoma
    - Glioblastoma (GBM)
    - Diffuse intrinsic pontine gliomas (DIPG; Figure 52.1).
- Primitive neuroectodermal tumors (PNET):
  - Medulloblastoma (MB)
  - Supratentorial PNET.
- Ependymoma (Figure 52.2).
- Germ cell tumors (GCT; Figure 52.3).

Incidence/prevalence
- The incidence of brain tumors in children aged between 0 and 19 is 3.1 in 100 000 per year.
- MB (20% of childhood brain tumors) has a bimodial peak at age 3–4 and 8–9.
- Gliomas account for the majority of pediatric brain tumors, most commonly PA.
- DIPG peaks at age 6–7, GBM and anaplastic astrocytoma at age 9–10.

Mount Sinai Expert Guides: Oncology, First Edition. Edited by William K. Oh and Ajai Chari.
© 2019 John Wiley & Sons Ltd. Published 2019 by John Wiley & Sons Ltd.
Companion Website: www.wiley.com/go/oh/mountsinaioncology

- Ependymoma is most common in the preschool age child and accounts for 10% of childhood brain tumors.
- GCT account for 3–5% of pediatric brain tumors.

Etiology

- The cause is unknown in most brain tumors.
- Neurofibromatosis type I is associated with OPT.
- Turcot and Gorlin syndromes can give rise to MB.
- The risk of high grade gliomas is increased in kindreds with Li–Fraumeni syndrome.

Pathology/pathogenesis

- PNETs are small round blue cell tumors requiring immunostaining for diagnosis and have to be distinguished from atypical teratoid rhabdoid tumors, a rare embryonal tumor of infancy with a very poor prognosis.
- Gliomas are graded according to World Health Organization (WHO) criteria I–IV.
- Ependymomas arise from the ependymal lining of the ventricles and can be differentiated into WHO grade II or anaplastic (WHO grade III).
- GCT are divided into pure germinomas (undifferentiated) and mixed GCT with embryonal and yolk sac components.

Prevention
Screening

- Routine screening is not recommended.
- Some rare familial conditions warrant screening, (e.g. serial fundoscopies for patients with neurofibromatosis type I because of risk of OPT).

Primary prevention

- There are no primary prevention strategies.

Secondary prevention

- Survivors of childhood brain tumors are followed for 5 years for signs of recurrence and lifelong for long-term toxicities and/or morbidities.

Diagnosis (Algorithm 52.1)

- Symptoms of increased intracranial pressure (ICP) include headaches and vomiting in school aged children, enlarging head circumference, unexplained vomiting, and loss of developmental milestones in younger children.
- Other presenting symptoms include cranial nerve palsies, ataxia, seizures, changes in vision.
- A thorough neurologic examination is necessary in all children with a suspicion of a brain tumor.
- Final diagnosis requires imaging and/or pathology.

Differential diagnosis

Differential diagnosis	Features
Meningoencephalitis	History of exposure or travel Symptoms of infection such as fever, elevated white blood cell count
Metabolic disease	Hepatosplenomegaly, elevated liver enzymes, elevated ammonia
Seizure disorders	No focal neurologic deficits or signs of increased ICP

Algorithm 52.1 Diagnosis of pediatric brain tumors

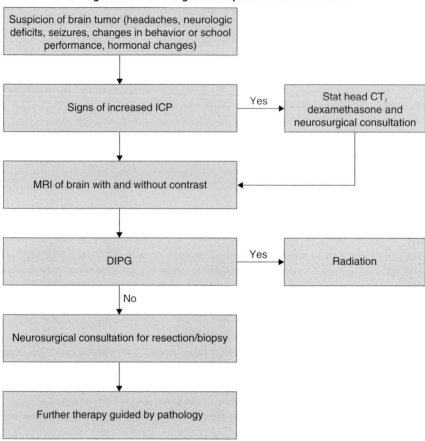

Typical presentation

Location	Typical presentation
Any	Elevated ICP: • Morning headache, vomiting in older children • Enlarging head circumference, loss of milestones, vomiting in young children
Posterior fossa tumors: • MB • Cerebellar PA • Ependymoma • DIPG	More common in preschooler aged children Cranial nerve deficits Ataxia Vision changes
Supratentorial tumors: • Gliomas • GCT • PNET • Ependymoma	Suprasellar (GCT): • Polydypsia, polyuria, • Hormonal changes • Vision changes

(Continued)

Location	Typical presentation
	Hypothalamus, optic chiasm (PA): • Obesity • Slowing of personality • Vision changes Temporal lobe: • Seizures • Behavior changes Frontal lobe: • Behavioral/personality changes Parietal lobe: • Unilateral motor or sensory deficits

Clinical diagnosis
History
- Systemic symptoms:
  - Weight loss/gain
  - Anorexia
  - Fatigue
  - Nausea/vomiting, mostly in the morning.
- Neurologic symptoms:
  - Headache
  - Changes in personality and/or school performance
  - Increased clumsiness
  - Seizures
  - Localized deficits
  - Vision changes.
- Family history of cancer or other genetic syndromes.

Physical examination
Pediatric patients with a suspected brain tumor require a comprehensive physical examination. Special attention should be given to:
- Dysmorphic features
- Skin examination (e.g. café-au-lait spots)
- A comprehensive neurologic examination of:
  - Cranial nerves
  - Vision, including visual fields and fundoscopy
  - Deep tendon reflexes and muscle strength
  - Sensation
  - Signs of ataxia.
- Genitourinary examination for Tanner stage.

Useful clinical decision rules and calculators
- Noncontrast computed tomography (CT) of the head is the fastest way to rule out increased ICP and/or herniation.
- Increased ICP is a medical emergency and requires emergency neurosurgical consultation. Dexamethasone can reduce edema from the tumor and improve signs of increased ICP.

Disease severity classification
- Classifications use histologic grading using WHO criteria.
- PNET, GCT, and ependymoma can disseminate along the neuroaxis and classification includes dissemination of disease.
- Four molecular subtypes of MB have been recognized that correlate with outcome.

Laboratory diagnosis
List of diagnostic tests
- Tumor markers in suprasellar or pineal tumors:
  - Alpha-fetoprotein and beta-human chorionic gonadotropin (bHCG) in serum and cerebrospinal fluid (CSF) to rule out GCT.
- Pathology:
  - Biopsy/resection and pathology is needed for all tumors except for DIPG (distinctive MRI appearance).
- Staging:
  - Lumbar puncture for PNET, GCT, and ependymoma.

Lists of imaging techniques
- MRI of the brain with and without contrast.
- MRI of the spine with and without contrast in ependymoma, PNET, and GCT.

Potential pitfalls/common errors made regarding diagnosis of disease
- Pediatric brain tumors are rare and patients usually present with nonspecific symptoms, especially in preverbal children. Subtle symptoms can precede diagnosis for weeks to months.
- Failure to thrive and loss of developmental milestones as well as unexplained vomiting can be an early sign of brain tumors in preverbal children.

Treatment (Algorithm 52.2)
Treatment rationale
- Except for DIPG and GCTs, the primary treatment is resection when feasible.
- Most pediatric brain tumors are radiosensitive. Radiation alone is used in DIPG, ependymomas, and pure germinomas.
- Combination chemotherapy and radiotherapy is used in MB and PNET.
- High grade gliomas are treated with postoperative radiation and temozolamide.
- Low grade gliomas are cured with complete resection. Unresectable progressive tumors can be treated with carboplatin and vincristine or radiation.
- Radiation is being avoided in children <3 years of age because of neurocognitive sequelae. High dose chemotherapy and autologous transplant have been used in this age group.

When to hospitalize
- Fever and neutropenia.
- Complications of chemotherapy.
- Neurologic symptoms.
- Postoperative management.

Managing the hospitalized patient
- Management of pediatric brain tumor patients requires multidisciplinary care in specialized centers.

Algorithm 52.2 Management of common pediatric brain tumors

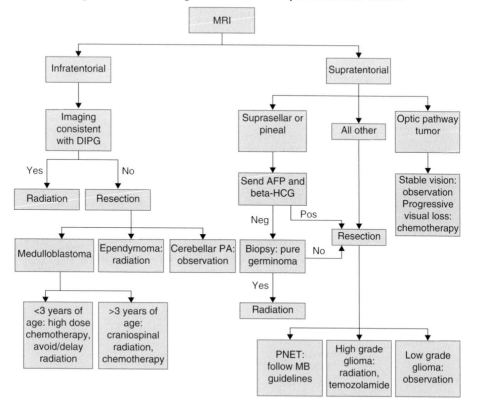

- Important aspects of managing hospitalized patients:
  - Monitoring of neurologic status
  - Multidisciplinary team management with oncology, neurology, neurosurgery, psychologists, and rehabilitation specialists
  - Intravenous antibiotic coverage in febrile neutropenic patients
  - Monitoring fluid balance
  - Maintaining nutrition
  - Management of pain and/or nausea/emesis
  - Knowledge of chemotherapy-specific complications
  - Psychosocial support.

Table of treatment

Tumors	Comments
Surgery	
Upfront resection	Standard of care for all brain tumors except for diffuse brainstem gliomas and GCT
Biopsy	Unresectable tumors Suspicion of GCT or CNS lymphoma
Delayed resection	Indicated for GCT with residual after chemotherapy and/or radiotherapy

(Continued)

(*Continued*)

Tumors	Comments
Chemotherapy	
DIPG Ependymoma	Chemotherapy has no proven efficacy Refer for clinical trial
PA	For unresectable tumors or progressive disease: vincristine, carboplatin
MB PNET Atypical teratoid/ rhabdoid tumor	Combination chemotherapy–radiotherapy for children >3 years of age High dose chemotherapy with autologous hematopoietic stem cell transplant for children <3 years of age
Radiation	
Radiation is avoided in children <3 years of age because of the long-term neurocognitive sequelae; guidelines are for children >3 years of age	
DIPG	Radiation is standard of care, even in younger children
Ependymomas	Radiation indicated in infratentorial and/or anaplastic ependymoma, or for residual disease
MB Atypical teratoid/ rhabdoid tumor PNET	Craniospinal radiation with local boost followed by chemotherapy Radiation doses have been safely reduced by addition of multiagent chemotherapy
Gliomas including PA	Radiation for high grade gliomas Residual/progressive disease in low grade tumors can be treated with radiation
GCT	Radiation of primary site and intraventricular volume Radiation is often combined with chemotherapy in mixed GCTs
Complementary	
All pediatric brain tumors	Intensive psychosocial support of the entire family Neuropsychologic testing Intensive supportive care to manage nausea/emesis, pain, nutrition

Prevention/management of complications

- Cerebellar mutism/posterior fossa syndrome:
  - ~25% of MB after resection
  - Inability to speak and agitation/irritability
  - No known medical intervention
  - Intensive rehabilitation.
- Adrenal suppression:
  - Stress dose steroids if appropriate.
- Complications of chemotherapeutic agents:
  - Hemorrhagic cystitis with alkylator agents
    - Hydration
    - Mesna.
  - Mucositis
    - Pain control
    - Nutritional support.

- Renal tubular dysfunction with cisplatin
  - Hydration
  - Mannitol diuresis.
- Fever and neutropenia:
  - Timely initiation of Gram negative coverage including *Pseudomonas*.

CLINICAL PEARLS
- CNS radiation is avoided in children <3 years because of neurocognitive sequelae.
- Dexamethasone reduces edema surrounding the tumor and often provides symptomatic relief.

Special populations
Inherited defects of DNA repair
- Patients with Fanconi anemia, neurofibromatosis, and other DNA repair defects have an increased sensitivity to radiation and chemotherapy so radiation should be avoided. During chemotherapy, close monitoring, and dose reductions may be necessary.

Prognosis

BOTTOM LINE/CLINICAL PEARLS
- There are a significant physical and psychosocial burdens of therapy and long-term morbidities requiring prolonged rehabilitation.
- Patients require lifelong monitoring for potential late effects of therapy.

Natural history of untreated disease
Brain tumors are lethal if untreated, with few exceptions. OPT in patients with neurofibromatosis I are indolent.

Prognosis for treated patients
Overall, the survival of children with brain tumors exceeds 75%.

Follow-up tests and monitoring
See section on Secondary prevention.

Reading list
Chintagumpala M, Gajjar A. Brain tumors. Pediatr Clin North Am 2015;62(1):167–178.
Gajjar A, Packer RJ, Foreman NK, et al. Children's Oncology Group's 2013 blueprint for research: central nervous system tumors. Pediatr Blood Cancer 2013;60(6):1022–1026.
Pizzo PA, Poplack DG. Principles and Practice of Pediatric Oncology, 7th edition. Wolters Kluwer, 2015, pp. 628–699.

Suggested websites
National Cancer Institute: www.cancer.gov
Children's Oncology Group: www.childrensoncologygroup.org
National Comprehensive Cancer Network (NCCN): www.nccn.org

Guidelines
National society guidelines

Title	Source and comment	Date and weblink
COG Supportive Care Guidelines	Children's Oncology Group (COG) **Comment:** Supportive care endorsed guidelines	2015 https://www.childrensoncologygroup.org/ index.php/cog-supportive-care-guidelines
Guidelines for Pediatric Cancer Centers	American Academy of Pediatrics	2004 http://pediatrics.aappublications.org/content/ pediatrics/113/6/1833.full.pdf
Long-term follow-up guidelines	Children's Oncology Group (COG) **Comment:** Long-term follow-up guidelines	2013 http://www.survivorshipguidelines.org/pdf/ LTFUGuidelines_40.pdf

Evidence

Type of evidence	Title and comment	Date and weblink
Cooperative Group Clinical Studies by the Children's Oncology Group	Multiple trials defining current standard of care for most childhood cancers	PubMed
Clinical studies by smaller cooperative group such as PBTC, St. Jude	Trials defining new therapies mostly in the relapse setting	PubMed

Images

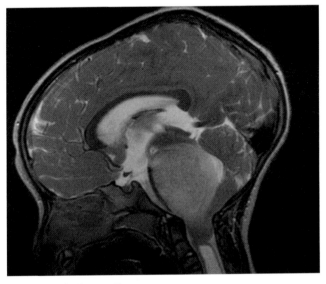

Figure 52.1 Diffuse intrinsic brainstem glioma.

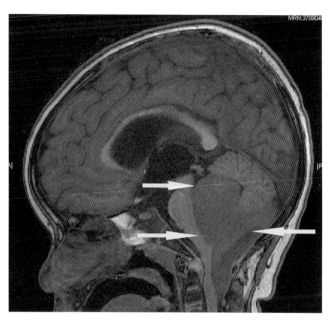

Figure 52.2 Posterior fossa ependymoma compressing the brainstem and cerebellum and causing hydrocephalus.

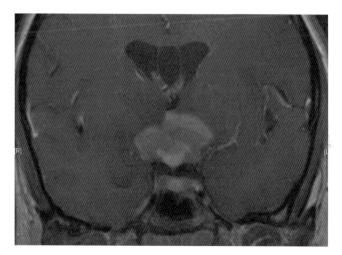

Figure 52.3 Large enhancing suprasellar mass consistent with CNS germinoma.

Additional material for this chapter can be found online at:
www.wiley.com/go/oh/mountsinaioncology

This includes advice for patients, a case study, ICD codes, and
multiple choice questions.

Index

Note: Page numbers in *italic* refer to figures. Page numbers in **bold** refer to tables, boxes or algorithms.

ABCDs (mnemonic), skin lesions, 207
abdominal diameter, esophageal cancer, 140
abdominal tumors, children, 545
abdominoperineal resection, anal cancer, 153, 160, **161**
Abelson murine leukemia gene, 272
abiraterone, prostate cancer, 27, 29
ABL1 gene, 272
abscesses
  brain, 243, 367
  renal, 46
absolute neutrophil count
  IPSS-R, **291**
  neutropenic fever, 428, 429
  recovery, 387
ABVD (adriamycin-bleomycin-vinblastine-dacarbazine), 358, 359, 362
  pregnancy, 360
achalasia, 143
acquired Fanconi syndrome, **299**
acral erythema (palmar-plantar erythrodysesthesia), 52, 414
acral lentiginous melanoma, 204
acromegaly, **257**
AC-T (regimen), breast cancer, **14**
ACTHomas, **257**
active surveillance, prostate cancer, 30
acute demyelinating encephalomyelitis, 367
acute kidney injury, tumor lysis syndrome, 426–427
acute lymphoblastic leukemia, 310, 319–331
  allogeneic stem cell transplantation, 386
  diagnosis, 320–323
  evidence, 329
  guidelines, 329
  prognosis, 328
  severity classification, 322–323
  treatment, 324–328
acute myeloid leukemia (AML), 308–318
  acute lymphoblastic leukemia *vs*, 320
  allogeneic stem cell transplantation, 313, 385, 392–399
  diagnosis, 309–311, 393–394

  evidence, 316–317, 398
  guidelines, 316, 398
  myelodysplastic syndromes *vs*, 290, 310
  prognosis, 316, 397
  severity classification, 311
  treatment, 311–315, 394–397
acute promyelocytic leukemia, 308
  bleeding, 315
  promyelocytes, *318*
  severity classification, 311
  treatment, 311, **314**
acyclovir
  acute myeloid leukemia, **313**
  allogeneic stem cell transplantation, **395**
  herpes simplex virus, 407, 429
adaptive planning, radiotherapy, 457
adenocarcinomas
  bladder, 40
  colorectal, 118, *130*
  esophagus, 140
  gastric, 131
  lung, 66, 67, 73
    mesothelioma *vs*, 81
adenomas
  colorectal, 119, 120
  hepatic, 91
  renal, 46
  thyroid, 223
adnexal tumors, ophthalmologic, 473
adrenal glands, imaging, **451**
adriamycin-bleomycin-vinblastine-dacarbazine (ABVD), 358, 359, 362
  pregnancy, 360
AETHERA trial, 355
afatinib, lung cancer, **76**
aflatoxin B1, 90
African Americans
  cardiotoxicity treatment, 493
  colorectal cancer screening, 121
age
  acute lymphoblastic leukemia, 319
  CRASH score, 517

Mount Sinai Expert Guides: Oncology, First Edition. Edited by William K. Oh and Ajai Chari.
© 2019 John Wiley & Sons Ltd. Published 2019 by John Wiley & Sons Ltd.
Companion Website: www.wiley.com/go/oh/mountsinaioncology

endometrial cancer, 182, 189
  meningiomas, 241
Agent Orange, 56, 333
AGO-AVAR (regimen), ovarian cancer, **174**
AIDS *see* HIV
airway compromise, acute lymphoblastic leukemia,
    327
AKT inhibitors, ovarian cancer, 175
AL amyloidosis *see* amyloidosis
albumin, Hodgkin lymphoma, 357
alcohol
  cancer risk, 536
  colorectal cancer risk, 119
  head and neck cancer, 230
aldosterone receptor antagonists, 493
alectinib, lung cancer, 74, **76**
ALK gene, non-small cell lung carcinoma, 73
alkaline phosphatase, 466
ALK/ROS inhibitors, lung cancer, **76**
alkylating agents, acute myeloid leukemia from,
    309
allogeneic stem cell transplantation, 385–391
  acute myeloid leukemia, 313, 385, 392–399
  antibiotics, **395**, 405
  chronic lymphocytic leukemia, 402
  cytomegalovirus infection, 406
  for follicular lymphoma, 402
  infections, 404–411
    phases, *411*
  for lymphoproliferative disorders, 400, 401
  mantle cell lymphoma, 402
  myelodysplastic syndromes, 294, 296, 386,
    392–399
  non-malignant conditions in which used,
    386
  primary myelofibrosis, 284
  procedures, 386–387
  relapse after, 391
  T-cell lymphoma, 403
allopurinol, tumor lysis syndrome, 426–427,
    428
all-trans-retinoic acid (ATRA)
  acute promyelocytic leukemia, **314**, 317
  teratogenicity, 315
alpha fetoprotein (AFP)
  liver cancer, 91, 94, 95
  pediatrics, 546
  testicular cancer, 59, 60, **61**
alpha particles, 459
alprazolam, **504**
alveolar hemorrhage, diffuse, 389
ambeciclib, breast cancer, 12
amenorrhea, endometrial cancer, 185
American College of Surgeons, Commission on
    Cancer, survivorship care, 538
American Joint Commission on Cancer Staging for
    Esophageal Cancer, 7th edition, 144

American Joint Committee on Cancer, staging
  anal cancer, 158
  gallbladder carcinoma and cholangiocarcinomas,
    106
  lung cancer, 70, **71**
  melanoma, 208, 209
American Psychosocial Oncology Society helpline,
    510
amitriptyline, **505**
amniotic fluid embolism, 440
amputation, 219, 467, **469**
amyloidosis, **299**, 302, 379
  autologous stem cell transplantation for, 379–384
    follow-up, 382–383
    maintenance therapy, 382
    timing, 381
  prognosis, 306
  treatment, 303
anagrelide, essential thrombocythemia, 283
anal canal, anatomy, *165*
anal cancer, 153–165
  diagnosis, 156–158
  evidence, 163–164
  guidelines, 163
  prognosis, 162
  screening, 156
  treatment, 159–162
anal intraepithelial neoplasia, 154, 155
anal margin, 154
anal verge, 154, *165*
anaplastic astrocytomas, 244, 246, 249
  incidence, 556
anaplastic large cell lymphoma, 543
anaplastic oligodendrogliomas, 244, 246, 250
anaplastic thyroid carcinoma, 221
anastomotic leak, esophagectomy, 148
anastrozole, breast cancer, 20
ANC recovery, 387
androgen deprivation therapy, 25, 27
androgen receptor, prostate cancer, 24
anemia
  aplastic, 290, 294, 320
  autoimmune hemolytic, 320
  esophageal cancer, 146, 147
  gastric cancer, 132, 133
  heart failure, 492
  iron deficiency, 123
  pemetrexed causing, **533**
angiomyolipoma
  hepatic, 92
  renal, 46
angiotensin-converting enzyme inhibitors, 493, 496
Ann Arbor staging system, 346, **357**
  graft versus host disease, 416
anorexia, nutritional management, 529
anorexia–cachexia syndrome, 524–525, *see also*
    cachexia; weight loss

anthracyclines
  acute myeloid leukemia, 316
  breast cancer, 10
  cardiotoxicity, 218, 488, 489, *499, 500*
    dexrazoxane for, 489, 495, *499*
    doxorubicin, 10, 488, *499, 500*
    histopathology, *500*
    precaution, 218, 358
    risk factors, 488
    trastuzumab compared, 15
    trastuzumab potentiating, 11
    treatment algorithm, **493**
  myelodysplastic syndromes, 294
antibiotics
  acute myeloid leukemia, **313**
  allogeneic stem cell transplantation, **395**, 405
  autologous stem cell transplantation, 381, 405
  myelodysplastic syndromes, 293, 294
  neutropenic fever, 430
anticoagulants, **442**, 443, 495, *see also* heparin; low
      molecular weight heparin;
      thromboprophylaxis
antidepressants, **505**
antiemetics, 522, 528
antiepileptics, **247**
anti-estrogens, breast cancer, **4**, 9, 15
  metastases, 11
anti-factor Xa monitoring, 443
antiseizure prophylaxis, **395**
antithrombotic drugs, 495
anus *see entries beginning* anal...
anxiety, **502**, **503**
  drugs for, **504**
  dyspnea, 525
anxiety disorders, 502
  management guidelines, 541
APC mutations, 127
apheresis, 380
aplastic anemia, 290, 294, 320
APML4 regimen, **314**
APML17 regimen, **314**
appendix, carcinoids, 258–259
appetite stimulants, 529
apple core filling defect, esophageal, *151*
Ara-C
  acute myeloid leukemia, 313
  acute promyelocytic leukemia, **314**
  myelodysplastic syndromes, 294
  side effects, **326**
armodafinil, **505**
aromatase inhibitors
  breast cancer, 9, 10
    follow-up, 17
  ovarian cancer, 175
arrhythmias *see* QT prolongation
arsenic trioxide (ATO), acute promyelocytic leukemia,
      314, 317

arteriovenous malformations, colorectal, 122
asbestos, 79, 80, 81
ascending cholangitis, 116
ascites, 122
ASCO 2013 trial, ovarian cancer, 172
ASPEN trial, phase III, 50
Aspergillus infection
  prevention, 429
  stem cell transplantation, 388, 409
aspiration, esophageal cancer, 146
aspirin
  colorectal cancer prophylaxis, 121
  esophageal cancer and, 142
  essential thrombocythemia, 282
  polycythemia vera, 281
  on venous thromboembolism risk, 444
ASSURE trial, phase III, 46
astrocytomas, 244, 245, 248
  anaplastic, 244, 246, 249
    incidence, 556
  histopathology, *252*
  magnetic resonance imaging, *252*
  prognosis, 249
atezolizumab
  bladder cancer, 38, **39**
  breast cancer, 21
  lung cancer, **76**
  non-small cell lung carcinoma, 74, 75
  small cell lung carcinoma, 72
ATO (arsenic trioxide), acute promyelocytic leukemia,
      314, 317
atovaquone
  allogeneic stem cell transplantation, **395**
  Pneumocystis pneumonia prevention, 429
ATRA *see* all-trans-retinoic acid
atrial fibrillation, 495
ATRX, loss of expression, gliomas, 245
atypical hemangioma, hepatic, 92
atypical teratoid rhabdoid tumors, 557
  radiotherapy, **562**
Auerbach's plexus, gastric cancer, 133
AURELIA Trial, ovarian cancer, 175
autoimmune hemolytic anemia, 320
autoimmune toxicity, 212
autologous stem cell transplantation (ASCT)
  antibiotics, 381, 405
  complications, 382
  Hodgkin lymphoma, 358
  infections, 404–411
  for lymphoproliferative disorders, 400–403
  maintenance therapy, 382
  for plasma cell disorders, 379–384
    evidence, 384
    guidelines, 383–384
    multiple myeloma, 303
  primary CNS lymphoma, **369**, **370**, 371, 373
  procedures, 380–383

single *vs* double, 381
timing, 381
axitinib
  nutrition and, **532**
  renal cell carcinoma, **51**
  side effects, 52
azacitidine
  acute myeloid leukemia, 313, 317
  acute promyelocytic leukemia, **314**
  myelodysplastic syndromes, 293, 296
azoles, 409

B symptoms, 334
bacillus Calmette–Guérin, intravesical, 34, 37, **38**,
    41
bacterial infections, *see also Clostridium difficile*
    infection; *Helicobacter pylori*; *Pneumocystis*
    pneumonia
  neutropenic fever, 429
  stem cell transplantation, 405–406
baking soda and salt solution, 530, 531
BAP1 gene, mesothelioma, 80
Barcelona Clinic Liver Cancer staging, 93
bare metal stenting, coronary, 494, 495
barium swallow, 144
Barrett's metaplasia, 140, 141
basal cell carcinoma, skin, 208
basal like (triple negative) breast cancer, **4**, 11
  metastases, 12
B-cell acute lymphoblastic leukemia, 319, *330*, *331*
  lymphoid progenitor markers, 320
B-cell lymphoma, 343, *see also* diffuse large B-cell
    lymphoma
  germinal center B-cell lymphoma, 352
  primary mediastinal, 355
B-cell receptor immunoglobulin, 333
B-cell receptor signaling, lymphomas, 343
Bcl-2, uveal melanoma, 474
BCNU *see* carmustine
BCR immunoglobulin, 333
BCR-ABL fusions, 271, *see also ABL1* gene
BEACOPP (regimen), Hodgkin lymphoma, 359, 362
beam shaping, linacs, 455, 456
bendamustine, plasma cell disorders, **304**
benign necrotizing lymphadenitis, 345
benzodiazepines, **504**, **508**
BEP (regimen), testicular cancer, **61**, 62, 64
beta particles, 459
(1–3)-β-D-glucan, 409
β2-microglobulin, 347
beta-blockers, 493
beta-human chorionic gonadotropin, 546
bevacizumab, **125**, 126
  gliomas, **247**
  lung cancer, **76**
  mesothelioma, 83, 85, 87
  monitoring, 248

non-small cell lung carcinoma, 74
ovarian cancer, 173, **174**, 175
renal cell carcinoma, **51**
side effects, 52
bexarotene, nutrition and, **532**
bicarbonate, tumor lysis syndrome, **428**
biliary tract carcinoma *see* cholangiocarcinomas
binimetinib, melanoma, 211
biopsy, *see also* fine needle aspiration biopsy
  bone marrow. *see* biopsy *under* bone marrow
  for cardiotoxicity, *500*
  colorectal cancer, 123
  graft versus host disease, 416
  lymph nodes, 347, 349, *see also* sentinel node
    biopsy
  melanoma, 207, 209
  orthopedic tumors, 467
  primary CNS lymphoma, 368
  prostate, risks, 27
  sarcomas, 216
biphenotypic acute leukemia, 310
Birt–Hogg–Dubé syndrome, 44
bisphosphonates
  for hypercalcemia, 424–425
  plasma cell disorders, **304**
bladder cancer, 32–42
  diagnosis, 34–36
  follow-up, 41
  guidelines, 41
  imaging, **451**
  prognosis, 40–41
  from renal transitional cell carcinomas, 50
  treatment, 36–40
bladder dysfunction, 199
bladder outlet obstruction, prostate cancer, 28
blast crisis, chronic myelogenous leukemia, 281
blast phase, chronic myelogenous leukemia, 274
blasts, myeloid, *317*
bleeding/hemorrhage
  acute promyelocytic leukemia, 315
  anal cancer, 157
  on anticoagulants, 443
  bevacizumab, 52
  diffuse alveolar, 389
  endometrial cancer, 185
  esophageal cancer, 143
  neuroendocrine tumors, 265
  prostate cancer, 28
  sarcomas, 216
  upper gastrointestinal
    esophageal cancer, 146
    occult, 122
bleomycin
  side effects, 62, 63, 358, 360
  testicular cancer, 64
blue round cell tumors, 544, 557
Bolero-2 trial, 11

bone marrow
  biopsy
    acute lymphoblastic leukemia, 323
    essential thrombocythemia, **275**
    Hodgkin lymphoma, 357
    myelodysplastic syndromes, 295
    neuroblastoma, *555*
    plasma cell disorders, 302
    polycythemia vera, **275**
  fibrosis, causes, 278
  older people, 515
  stem cell collection, 387
  suppression, chemotherapy, 199
  transplantation, *see also* stem cell transplantation
    acute lymphoblastic leukemia, 324, **326**,
      327
bone scan, 467
  prostate cancer, 27, **28**
bone tumors, 463–471
  diagnosis, 465–467
  guidelines, 470–471
  metastases, 463, *see also* pathologic fractures
    breast cancer, 14–15, 464
    prostate cancer, 27, 464
  presentation, 545
  treatment, 467–470
borderline ovarian tumors, 166
bortezomib
  autologous stem cell transplantation, 382
  nutrition and, **532**
  plasma cell disorders, **304**
bosutinib, chronic myelogenous leukemia,
  280
bowel regimens, stimulant, 522
brachytherapy, 458–459, *see also* plaque
    brachytherapy
  cervical cancer, **198**
  endometrial cancer, **188**, 191
  prostate cancer, 29
bradycardia, drugs causing, **491**
BRAF mutations
  cholangiocarcinomas, 102
  colorectal cancer, 123–124, 127
  melanoma, 204, 205, 209, 211
    inhibition, 211, 212
  thyroid cancer, 222
brain abscess, 243, 367
brain metastases, 244, *251*, 367
  breast cancer, 15
    treatment, **247**
  diagnosis, 243
  esophageal cancer, 144
  incidence, 241
  melanoma, 210, 212, **247**, *251*
  MRI, 245
  testicular cancer, 62
  treatment, **246**, **247**, 248

brain tumors, 241–254, *see also* brain metastases;
    central nervous system
  children, 248, 556–565
    presentation, 558–559
  diagnosis, 243–245, 557–560
  evidence, 250–251, 564
  guidelines, 250, 564
  prognosis, 248–249
  treatment, 245–248, 560–563
BRCAn genes
  breast cancer, 3, 5
    prophylactic surgery, 6, 537
  ovarian cancer, 167, 168, 175, *180*, 537
  prostate cancer, 24
breakthrough fever, autologous stem cell
    transplantation, 381
breast, benign changes, 7
breast cancer, 3–22, *see also* hereditary
    breast–ovarian cancer syndrome
  acute myeloid leukemia from chemotherapy,
    309
  allogeneic stem cell transplantation, 390
  bone metastases, 464
  brain metastases, 15
    treatment, **247**
  diagnostic tests, 8–9
  elderly people, 20
  evidence, 19–21
  follow-up, 16–17
  guidelines, 18–19
  history-taking, 7
  imaging, 8–9, **452**, *see also* mammography
  physical examination, 7
  prevention of recurrence, 537
  screening, 6, 360, 516, **536**, *see also*
    mammography
  secondary to Hodgkin lymphoma, 360
  subtypes, 3, **4**
  survivorship guidelines, 540
  treatment, 9–16, 19–21
Breast Cancer Index, 8
breast conserving therapy (BCS), 9, 20
  pregnancy, 16
Bremsstrahlung, 454
brentuximab, 355, 358, 361, **551**
Breslow thickness, 208, **210**, 212
brigatinib, lung cancer, 75, **76**
bronchoscopy, 68
Bruton's tyrosine kinase inhibitor *see* ibrutinib
Burkitt lymphoma, 543
  primary CNS lymphoma, 368
  translocations, 343
  treatment, 351, **550**
busulfan, in myeloablative regimens, **395**

C (regimen), breast cancer, **14**
CA 19-9, biliary tract carcinoma, 105

CA-125
    endometrial cancer, 186
    ovarian cancer, 171, 174
    risk of ovarian cancer algorithm (ROCA), 169
cabazitaxel, prostate cancer, 27, 29
cabozantinib
    clear cell renal cell carcinoma, 50
    liver cancer, 89, **96**, 99
    renal cell carcinoma, **51**
    side effects, 52, 96
    thyroid cancer, 225, 228
cachexia, 532, *see also* anorexia–cachexia syndrome
CAF (regimen), breast cancer, **14**
calcineurin inhibitors, **395**
    GVHD prevention, 413
calcitonin, 425
calcitriol secretion, **424**
calcium gluconate, tumor lysis syndrome, **428**
calcium levels, 424
    tumor lysis syndrome, **427**
calcium phosphate mouthwash, 531
calcium supplement, zoledronic acid with, **533**
CALGB 8811 (regimen), acute lymphoblastic
        leukemia, **326**
CALGB Prognostic Index, mesothelioma, 82
CALYPSO (regimen), ovarian cancer, **174**
canalicular fibrosis, docetaxel, 479
Cancer and Aging Research Group, chemotherapy
        toxicity prediction, 40, 516–517
Cancer and Leukemia Group B Prognostic Index,
        mesothelioma, 82
cancer antigen 19-9, biliary tract carcinoma, 105
cancer treatment summaries, 538
cancer-associated retinopathy, 479
Candida, 409
cannabidiol (CBD), **247**
capecitabine
    anal cancer, 153, 159, **160**
    breast cancer, **12**, **13**
        brain metastases, **247**
    nutrition and, **532**
    pancreas cancer, 113
    side effects, **125**
Capizzi methotrexate, acute lymphoblastic leukemia,
        329
carbohydrates, hyperglycemia, 530
carboplatin
    bladder cancer, **39**
    breast cancer, 11
    head and neck cancer, 235, **237**
    lung cancer, **75**
    mesothelioma, 83
    ovarian cancer, 172, 173, **174**, **176**
    testicular cancer, 64
        secondary prevention, 58
carcinoembryonic antigen (CEA), colorectal cancer,
        123

carcinoid crisis, 264, 265
    octreotide for, **265**
carcinoid syndrome, 256, **257**, **258**, 261
carcinoid tumors, 255, 256, *see also* neuroendocrine
        tumors
    appendix, 258–259
    colorectal, 122, 259
    small bowel, 259, 260
    stomach, 258, 259
    tumor markers, 262
carcinoma *in situ*
    bladder, 35
    breast, 3, 7, 10, 20
cardiotoxicity, 360, 486–500
    anthracyclines. *see* cardiotoxicity *under*
            anthracyclines
    diagnosis, 489–493
    follow-up, 496
    guidelines, 497
    prevention, 488–489
    prognosis, 496
    risk scores (CRS), 488, 490
    trastuzumab, 10, 15, 489
        treatment algorithm, **494**
    treatment, 493–496
cardiovascular disease, 487, *see also* cardiotoxicity
    allogeneic stem cell transplantation, 389
caregivers of cancer survivors, 540
carfilzomib, plasma cell disorders, **304**
carmustine (BCNU)
    brain tumors, **247**
    plasma cell disorders, **304**
Castleman disease, 345
catheter-related venous thromboembolism, 438, **442**
cauda equina syndrome, 432
CCNU (lomustine), brain tumors, **247**
CD4 counts, anal cancer treatment, 162
CD34 levels, stem cell mobilization, 380
CEF (regimen), breast cancer, **14**
central nervous system, *see also* brain metastases;
            brain tumors; primary central nervous system
            lymphoma
    acute lymphoblastic leukemia, **326**
    non-Hodgkin lymphomas, 344
cerebellar mutism, 562
cerebrospinal fluid, primary CNS lymphoma, 366,
        368
ceritinib, lung cancer, 74, 75, **76**
cervical cancer, 194–203
    diagnosis, 195–197
    endometrial cancer *vs*, 184
    evidence, 201
    follow-up, 200
    geographic distribution, *202*
    guidelines, 201
    imaging, **452**
    prognosis, 200

cervical cancer (*Continued*)
  screening, 195, 516
  treatment, 197–199
cervical cytology, endometrial cancer, 184, 185
cervical lymph nodes, occult primary, 236
cetuximab
  head and neck cancer, 235–236
    combination chemotherapy, 237
    radiotherapy, **237**
    RAS and *BRAF* mutations and, 124
charged particle EBRT, 457–458
CHECKMATE trials, 74
chemoembolization, liver cancer, 96, 99
chemoprevention, breast cancer, 6
chemo-radiation, gastric cancer, **136**
chemotherapy
  bone marrow suppression, 199
  childhood tumors requiring, **549–550**
    brain tumors, **562**
  DNA repair defects, 552, 563
  gastric cancer from, 132
  hypersensitivity, 177
  long-term side effects, 537
  nephrotoxicity, 199
  ocular complications, 477–479
  toxicity prediction, 516–517
Chemotherapy Risk Assessment Scale for High age
    (CRASH) score, 517
children, 543–565
  acute myeloid leukemia, 315
  brain tumors, 248, 556–565
    presentation, 558–559
  cancer survivors, 538
  colorectal cancer, 126
  diagnosis of neoplasms, 544–547
  evidence, 553
  guidelines, 553
  orthopedic tumors, 469
  radiotherapy, 460
  sarcomas, 214, 216, 218–219
    types, 543
  staging of solid tumors, 546, 547
  thyroid cancer, 226–227
  treatment, 547–552
chlorpromazine, **508**
cholangiocarcinomas, 101–110
  diagnosis, 103–106
  imaging, **451**
  intrahepatic, 91, 109
    IDH1/2 mutations, 102
  prognosis, 108–109
  staging, *110*
  treatment, 106–108
cholangitis, 104, 116, *see also* primary sclerosing
    cholangitis
cholecystitis, 104
cholelithiasis, 102, 104

choriocarcinomas, 57, 62
chorioretinal biopsy, 368
choroidal hemangioma, 476
choroidal melanoma *see* uveal melanoma
choroidal nevus, 475
choroidal osteoma, 476
chromoendoscopy, 141
chromogranin A, 114
  neuroendocrine tumor prognosis, 266
chromophobe RCC, 45
chromosomes 1p/19q deletion, gliomas, 245
chronic eosinophilic leukemia (CEL), diagnosis, 277
chronic lymphocytic inflammation with pontine
    perivascular enhancement responsive to
    steroids (CLIPPERS), 367
chronic lymphocytic leukemia, 332–341
  diagnosis, 334–337
  guidelines, 340–341
  prognosis, 339–340, 352
  stem cell transplantation, 337, 339, 402
  treatment, 337–339
    eligibility for, 336
chronic myelogenous leukemia (CML), 271, 272
  accelerated phase, **275**
  diagnosis, 274
  guidelines, 287
  prognosis, 286
  risk scores, 278
  treatment, 280–281
    allogeneic stem cell transplantation, 386
    pregnancy, 284
chronic neutrophilic leukemia (CNL)
  diagnosis, 276, **277**
  treatment, 284
ciprofloxacin, neutropenic fever prevention, 429
cirrhosis
  cancer screening, 91
  liver cancer, 93
cisplatin
  anal cancer, 162
    metastases, 160, 164
  cervical cancer, 198
  head and neck cancer, 235, 236, **237**
  lung cancer, **75**
  mesothelioma, 83
  nutrition and, **533**
  ovarian cancer, 172, 173
  side effects, 63
  testicular cancer, 64
cisplatin-based combination chemotherapy, *see also*
    platinum-based chemotherapy
  bladder cancer, 37, 38, **39**, **42**
  renal cell carcinoma, 53
citalopram, **504**, **505**
cKIT mutation, melanoma, 212
classic Hodgkin lymphoma (cHL), 354, 355, **356**
clear cell renal cell carcinoma, treatment, 50

Clinical Practice Guidelines in Oncology for Distress
    Management (NCCN), 501, *510–513*
clinical tumor lysis syndrome, 427
CLIPPERS (chronic lymphocytic inflammation with
    pontine perivascular enhancement responsive
    to steroids), 367
clofarabine, myelodysplastic syndromes, 294
clonality, non-Hodgkin lymphomas, 342
clonazepam, **504**
Clostridium difficile infection
    acute myeloid leukemia after, **313**
    graft versus host disease *vs*, 414
    stem cell transplantation, 405
CLOT trial, 441, 445
cobalt- 60, 454, 455
cobimetinib, melanoma, 211
coffee, colorectal cancer and, 121
cognitive-behavioral therapy, 509
cold agglutinin disease, 301
colectomy, prophylactic, 121
colloid nodule, thyroid, 223
colon
    carcinoid tumors, 122, 259
    diverticular disease, 122
colonography, computed tomography, 449
colonoscopy, 120, 121, 124, 128
colorectal cancer, 118–130
    diagnosis, 121–124
    evidence, 129
    5-year survival rates, 127, *129*
    follow-up, 127–128
    guidelines, 128
    imaging, **451**
    prevention, 120–121, 537
    prognosis, 127–128
    screening, 120–121, 516, **536**
    staging, 122–123
    survivorship guidelines, 540
    treatment, 124–127
Commission on Cancer, American College of
    Surgeons, survivorship care, 538
community generalist model, cancer survivors, **539**
complementary therapies, 509
complete hematologic response (CHR), chronic
    myelogenous leukemia, 280
complete molecular response (CMR), chronic
    myelogenous leukemia, 280
Comprehensive Geriatric Assessment, 40, 514
computed tomography, 447–448, *see also* positron
    emission tomography/CT
    colonography, 449
    colorectal cancer, 124
    cone beam CT, 456
    dynamic contrast-enhanced CT, liver cancer, 94
    low dose, 449, 516, 537
    lung cancer, 68, *453*
    mesothelioma, *87*

pneumonia, *432*
prostate cancer, 27
renal cancer, 49
spinal cord compression, 433, *434*
thyroid cancer, 224
conditioning
    allogeneic stem cell transplantation, 387
    autologous stem cell transplantation, 381
    enteritis from, 414
    myeloablative regimens, 387, **395**
        for lymphoproliferative disorders, 400
condoms, anal cancer prevention, 156
condylomas, 157, 158
    ranpirnase on, 156
cone beam computed tomography, 456
congenital hypertrophy of the retinal pigmented
    epithelium, 475
congenital immunodeficiencies, primary CNS
    lymphoma, 365
conjunctivitis, 5-fluorouracil, 479
CONKO-001 trial, 113
consensus molecular subtypes, colorectal cancer,
    119
constipation, 529
consultative survivorship clinics, **539**
conventional T cells (from donors), 412, 413
copy number gene variations, thyroid cancer, 222
cord blood, 387
    graft failure, 389
CORRECT trial, 129
corticosteroids *see* steroids
co-trimoxazole (trimethoprim-sulfamethoxazole),
    406, 429
    allogeneic stem cell transplantation, **395**
Cowden syndrome, endometrial cancer risk, 182
cranial irradiation
    acute lymphoblastic leukemia, **326**
    small cell lung carcinoma, 71, 72
cranial nerve palsies, from chemotherapy, **478–479**
crizotinib, lung cancer, 75, **76**
Crohn disease, neuroendocrine tumors *vs*, 260
crude oil, acute myeloid leukemia from, 309
cryoglobulinemia, 301
cryotherapy, prostate cancer, 28
cryptorchidism, 56, 57
cryptorchidism, 56, 57
CSF3R mutations, 272, **277**
CTLA-4 inhibitors, 211
    autoimmune toxicity, 212
Cushing syndrome, ectopic, **257**
cyclin D2 gene, 57
cyclin-dependent kinase inhibitors, breast cancer,
    12, 21
cyclobutane pyrimidine dimers, 205
cyclophosphamide
    breast cancer, 11
    GVHD prevention, 413
    in myeloablative regimens, **395**

cyclophosphamide (*Continued*)
    nutrition and, **533**
    plasma cell disorders, **304**
    side effects, **326**
        dry eye, 479
        stem cell mobilization, 380
cyclosporine, **396**, 413
CYP3A4 inducers and inhibitors, 532, **533**
cystectomy, 37, **39**, 40
cystic disease of kidney, 44
cystoscopy, 34, 35
cysts, renal, 46
cytarabine *see* Ara-C
cytogenetic markers, acute lymphoblastic leukemia,
        323
cytokine therapy, clear cell renal cell carcinoma,
        50
cytology
    anal, 156
    cervical, endometrial cancer, 184, 185
cytomegalovirus infection, 406–407
cytopenias, *see also* neutropenia; thrombocytopenia
    causes, 278
    chronic lymphocytic leukemia, 335
    lymphopenia, Hodgkin lymphoma, 357
    myelodysplastic syndromes, 290–291
cytoreduction
    essential thrombocythemia, 282
    ovarian cancer, 169, **176**
    polycythemia vera, 282
cytoreductive nephrectomy, 50, **51**
cytosine arabinoside, keratitis, 479
cytoxan, **395**

dabrafenib, melanoma, 211
dacomitinib, lung cancer, 75, **76**
dalteparin, 441, **442**, 445
daratumumab, plasma cell disorders, **304**
dasatinib
    chronic myelogenous leukemia, 280
    nutrition and, **532**
daunorubicin (DNR)
    acute myeloid leukemia, 313
        pregnancy, 315
    acute promyelocytic leukemia, **314**
    side effects, **326**
DC (regimen), breast cancer, **14**
ᴅ-dimer, 437, 495
Deauville criteria, PET/CT, **358**
debulking, ovarian cancer, 169, **176**
decitabine
    acute myeloid leukemia, 313
    acute promyelocytic leukemia, **314**
    myelodysplastic syndromes, 293
decortication, pleurectomy with, 84
deep venous thrombosis, 437, **438**, 441, *see also*
        venous thromboembolism

deferasiox, nutrition and, **533**
defibrillators, intracardiac, 494
defibrotide, 388, 396
dehydration, 116, 146
delirium, 504, 508–509
    causes, **507**
    drugs for, **508**
    management, **507**
    NCCN guidelines, *513*
denosumab
    bone metastases, 14–15
    for hypercalcemia, 425
    hypercalcemia prevention, 423
    plasma cell disorders, **304**
    prostate cancer, 29
dental complications, head and neck cancer,
        237
dentate line, anal canal, *165*
depressive disorders, 502–503
    caregivers of cancer survivors, 540
    management guidelines, 541
    NCCN guidelines, *512*
dermatopathologic lymphadenopathy, 345
dermoscopy, 206
desipramine, **505**
desmoid tumor, 214
desquamation, anal cancer treatment, 161
desvenlafaxine, **505**
dexamethasone, **14**
    acute lymphoblastic leukemia, 329
    for differentiation syndrome, 315
    on fatigue, 524
    plasma cell disorders, **304**
    side effects, **326**
    spinal cord compression, 28, 433
dexmedetomidine, **508**
dexrazoxane, 488, 489, 495, *499*
dextroamphetamine, **505**
diabetes mellitus
    allogeneic stem cell transplantation, 390
    endometrial cancer risk, 182
    fluorodeoxyglucose, 449
dialysis
    autologous stem cell transplantation and, 383
    for hypercalcemia, 425
    tumor lysis syndrome, 427
diarrhea, 116
    anal cancer treatment, 161
    graft versus host disease, 414, **415**
    nutritional management, 528–529
diazepam, **504**
diethylstilbestrol, *in utero* exposure, 56
difference between involved and uninvolved light
        chain (dFLC), 383
differentiation syndrome, **314**, 315
diffuse alveolar hemorrhage, 389
diffuse astrocytomas, 244, 245, 249

diffuse intrinsic pontine gliomas (DIPG), *564*
  incidence, 556
  radiotherapy, **562**
diffuse large B-cell lymphoma, 543
  bone, 465
  primary CNS lymphoma, 364, 368
  prognosis, 352
  stem cell transplantation, 401
  treatment, **550**
diffuse type gastric cancer, 131
diffusing capacity for carbon monoxide, 360
digital rectal examination
  anal cancer, 156, 158
  colorectal cancer, 122
  neutropenic fever and, 430
DIPSS-Plus (dynamic international prognostic scoring
     system), 279
direct fluorescent antibody, 408
Disease Risk Index, 393, **394**
disease/treatment specific management (care
     model), cancer survivors, **539**
disseminated intravascular coagulation, 444
distress, 501–502
Distress Thermometer (NCCN), *511*
diverticular disease, colon, 122
diverticulum, esophagus, 143
DNA mutation panels, 290, 295
DNA repair defects, chemotherapy, 552, 563
docetaxel (D)
  breast cancer, 11, **12**, **13**
  canalicular fibrosis, 479
  lung cancer, **75**
  prostate cancer, 27, 29
docusate, 522
donor cell procurement, 387
donor conventional T cells (Tcons), 412, 413
donor selection
  cytomegalovirus infection, 406
  ethnicity, 397
  stem cell transplantation, 386
Down syndrome, acute lymphoblastic leukemia,
     328
doxorubicin, *see also* anthracyclines; liposomal
     doxorubicin
  breast cancer, 10
  cardiotoxicity, 10, 488, *499*, *500*
  ovarian cancer, **174**, **175**
  plasma cell disorders, **304**
  sarcomas, 220
dronabinol, 524
drug reactions
  phenytoin, 345, 355
  serum sickness, 345
dry eye, cyclophosphamide, 479
dry mouth, 237, 530–531
DTaP (tetanus, diphtheria, acellular pertussis), 410
dual antiplatelet therapy, 495

ductal carcinoma *in situ* (DCIS)
  breast, 3, 7, 20
    radiotherapy, 10
duloxetine, **505**
duodenum
  imaging, **451**
  neuroendocrine tumors, 258
durvalumab, lung cancer, 75, **76**
dynamic contrast-enhanced CT, liver cancer, 94
dynamic international prognostic scoring system
     (DIPSS-Plus), 279
dysgeusia, 530
dysphagia, 143, 144, 146, 148, 531
dysplastic nevi, 208
dyspnea, 525

Early Breast Cancer Trialists' Collaborative Group, 19
early satiety, 529
early stage NSCLC, management, 72–73
Eastern Asia, gastric cancer, 131
Eastern Cooperative Oncology Group, performance
     status, 70
Eastern Europe, gastric cancer, 131
echocardiography, 489, 492, 493, 496, *498*
ectopic Cushing syndrome, **257**
ectopic parathyroid hormone secretion, **424**
Edmonton Symptom Assessment Scheme, 521
ejection fraction (left ventricular), 486, 493
elderly people *see* geriatric oncology
electricity, glioblastoma treatment, **247**
electrocardiography (EKG), 492
electrocautery, anal intraepithelial neoplasia, 154
electrons, radiotherapy, 455
electrophoresis, urine, 302
elotuzumab, plasma cell disorders, **304**
eloxatin, nutrition and, **533**
embolectomy, **442**
embryonal carcinoma, 57, 62
emergencies, 423–434, *see also* hypercalcemia;
     spinal cord compression
  bleeding on anticoagulants, 443
  neutropenic fever, 428–432
  psychiatric, **506**
  raised intracranial pressure, 559
  tumor lysis syndrome, 319, 327, 425–428
EMILA trial, 21
empyema, mesothelioma *vs*, 81
enchondroma, 215
encorafenib, melanoma, 211
endocrine disorders, allogeneic SCT, 390
endometrial cancer, 181–193
  diagnosis, 183–187
  evidence, 191–192
  guidelines, 190, 191
  imaging, **452**
  prognosis, 189–190
  treatment, **183**, 187–189

endometrial hyperplasia, 184, 187
endometrial sampling, 185, 187
endometrioid carcinoma, 181–193
endometriosis, ovarian cancer risk, 167
endoscopic resection, esophageal cancer, 146, 149
endoscopic ultrasound (EUS), gastric cancer, 134, **135**
endoscopy, gastric cancer, 132, **135**, *138*
engraftment, stem cells, 387
engraftment syndrome, 414
Enneking staging system, **466**, **467**
enoxaparin, **442**
 bleeding, 443
 renal insufficiency, 443
enteral nutrition, 146–147
enteritis, from conditioning, 414
enucleation, eye, 481
enzalutamide, prostate cancer, 27, 29
EORTC Prognostic Index, mesothelioma, 82
eosinophilia, causes, 278
ependymomas, 244, **246**, *564*
 dissemination, 560
 grading, 557
 incidence, 557
 radiotherapy, **562**
epidermal growth factor receptor genes
 gliomas, 245
 non-small cell lung carcinoma, 73
epidermal growth factor receptor inhibitors, *see also* cetuximab
 lung cancer, **76**
epidermal growth factor receptor tyrosine kinase inhibitors, brain metastases, **247**
epidermal growth factor receptor tyrosine kinases, 102
epidermoid anal cancer, trial, 163–164
epididymitis, 58
epigenetics
 prostate cancer, 24
 thyroid cancer, 222
epiphora, docetaxel, 479
epirubicin, breast cancer, **13**
epithelial ovarian cancer *see* ovarian cancer
epithelioid cell melanoma, uveal, 476
Epstein–Barr virus
 head and neck cancer, 231
 Hodgkin lymphoma, 354
 post-transplant lymphoproliferative disorders, 343–344
ERG gene, prostate cancer, 24
eribulin, breast cancer, **13**
erionite, 80
erlotinib
 biliary tract carcinoma, 108
 lung cancer, **76**
 nutrition and, **532**
ERSPC trial, 31

erythema, anal cancer treatment, 161
erythrocytosis
 causes, 277
 diagnosis, **274**
erythroderma, GVHD, **415**
erythrodysesthesia, palmar-plantar, 52, 414
erythropoiesis stimulating agents, myelodysplastic syndromes, 293
escitalopram, **504**, **505**
esophageal cancer, 139–152
 diagnosis, 142–145
 evidence, 149
 guidelines, 149
 imaging, **451**
 prevalence, *150*
 prognosis, 148–149
 screening, 141
 treatment, 145–148
esophageal extrinsic compression, 143
esophagectomy, 146, 147–148, 149, *151*
esophagitis, 76, 143
ESPAC-3 (European Study Group for Pancreatic Cancer periampullary trial), 107
ESPAC-4 trial, 113
essential thrombocythemia (ET), 271, 272
 diagnosis, 274, **275**
 guidelines, 287
 perioperative management, 285
 pre PMF *vs*, 280
 thrombotic risk, 278
 treatment, 282–283
 pregnancy, 284
estrogen, endometrial cancer, 182, 183
estrogen levels, breast cancer, 5
estrogen receptors (ER)
 breast cancer, 5, 10
 pathways, *22*
ethnicity
 biliary tract carcinoma, 102
 breast cancer, 4, 16
 donor selection, 397
 endometrial cancer, 182
 melanoma, 205
 neuroendocrine tumors, 259
 prostate cancer, 24
 testicular cancer, 56
etoposide
 lung cancer, **75**
 ovarian cancer, **175**
 plasma cell disorders, **304**
 testicular cancer, 64
etoposide/cisplatin, extensive SCLC, 72
European Organisation for Research and Treatment of Cancer Prognostic Index, mesothelioma, 82
European Study Group for Pancreatic Cancer periampullary trial, 107

European Treatment and Outcome Study risk score, CML, 278
Evans syndrome, 320
everolimus
  breast cancer, 21
    metastases, 11
  nutrition and, **532**
  renal cell carcinoma, **51**
  side effects, 52–53
Ewing sarcoma, 219
  chemotherapy, 217, **550**
  radiotherapy, 469, **551**
  surgery, **551**
examination under anaesthesia, head and neck cancer, 233, 236
exemestane
  breast cancer, 11, 21
  nutrition and, **532**
extensive SCLC, management, 72
external beam radiotherapy, 454–458
extrapleural pneumonectomy, 84, 87
extrinsic compression, esophagus, 143
eye, 473–485
  lymphomas. *see* ocular lymphoma
eye wall resection, 481

facial flushing, 261, 263
familial adenomatous polyposis (FAP), 127
familial pancreatic carcinoma, 112
familial retinoblastoma, 475, 483
familial syndromes *see* inherited disorders
family history
  neuroendocrine tumors, 261
  on ovarian cancer risk, 167
Fanconi syndrome (acquired), **299**
fat embolism, 440
fatigue, 523–524, 529
  management guidelines, 541
febrile neutropenia
  sarcomas, 217, 218
  stem cell transplantation, 405
fecal occult blood *see* stool tests
feeding tubes, head and neck cancer treatment, 237
ferritin, criterion for iron chelation, 294
fever, *see also* breakthrough fever; neutropenic fever
  BRAF inhibitors, 212
  carcinoid tumors, 265
  Hodgkin lymphoma, 356
FGFR2 fusions, gallbladder carcinoma, 102
fibroids, 184
fibromatosis, 214
fibrosis, carcinoid tumors, 265
fiducials, 456
field cancerization, 238
FIGO *see* Joint International Federation of Gynecology and Obstetrics

filgrastim, allogeneic SCT, **395**
fine needle aspiration biopsy
  lung cancer, 71
  lymph nodes, 236, 349
  mesothelioma and, 80
  thyroid cancer, 221, 226
fistula
  esophageal cancer, 146, **147**
  ureterovaginal, 199
  vesicovaginal, 199
5-fluorouracil *see* fluorouracil
5-HT$_3$ antagonists, 522
fixation, pathologic fractures, 15
FLAG (regimen), myelodysplastic syndromes, 294
flow cytometry, chronic lymphocytic leukemia, 337
FLT3 inhibitor (midostaurin), acute myeloid leukemia, 313
fluconazole, neutropenic fever prevention, 429
fludarabine
  in myeloablative regimens, **395**
  side effects, 396
fluid intake, 528, 530
fluid therapy *see* hydration
fluorescence *in situ* hybridization, lung cancer, 70
fluorodeoxyglucose, 449
  lung cancer, 71
fluoroquinolones, 405, 429, 431
fluorouracil (5-fluorouracil)
  anal cancer, 159, 160, **160**, 162, 164
  anal intraepithelial neoplasia, 154
  biliary tract carcinoma, 107
  bladder cancer, **39**
  breast cancer, **13**
  colorectal cancer, 127, 129
  conjunctivitis, 479
  in FOLFOX 6, 160
  nutrition and, **532**
  side effects, **125**
fluoxetine, **504**, **505**
flushing, facial, 261, 263
focal nodular hyperplasia, hepatic, 91
FOLFIRINOX (regimen), **116**
FOLFOX 6, anal cancer metastases, 160
folic acid, pemetrexed with, **533**
follicular lymphoma
  prognosis, 352
  stem cell transplantation, 402
follicular thyroid carcinoma, 221, 227
folliculin, 44
fondaparinux, 441, **442**, 444
food supplements, 532
foscarnet, 407
fractures *see* pathologic fractures
frailty index, 383
free light chain analysis (FLC), 303
free PSA, 27
frontal lobe, tumor presentation, 559

frozen section, endometrial hyperplasia, 187
Fuhrman scale, renal cancer, 48
fulvestrant, breast cancer, 12, 21
fungal infections
  neutropenic fever, 429, 430
  prevention, **313**, 430
  stem cell transplantation, 388, 408–409
furosemide, for hypercalcemia, 424

gadolinium
  MRI of spinal cord compression, 433
  renal failure, 383
galactomannan, 409
gallbladder carcinoma, 101–110
  diagnosis, 103–106
  prognosis, 109
gallium nitrate, 425
gallium-68 scan, neuroendocrine tumors,
    263
gallstones, 102, 104
Gamma Knife®, 457
gamma rays, iodine- 131, 459
gammopathies
  heavy chain disease, **299**
  light chain disease, **299**
  MGUS, **298**, 300
  polyclonal, 301
ganciclovir, 407
gastric cancer, 131–138
  guidelines, 138
  imaging, **451**
  prognosis, 137
  screening, 132
  treatment, 135–137
gastric MALT lymphoma
  follow-up, 352
  Helicobacter pylori, 344
gastric outlet obstruction, 136
gastrinomas, **257**, 261
  tumor markers, 262
gastroduodenal artery, pancreas cancer, 115
gastroesophageal reflux disease (GERD), esophageal
    cancer, 140
gastrointestinal stromal tumor, 133, 214
  chemotherapy, 217
  imatinib, 216, 220
gastrointestinal tract
  graft versus host disease, **415**
  neuroendocrine tumors, 256
gastroscopy, gastric cancer, 132, **135**, *138*
gastrostomy, esophageal cancer and, 147
gefinitib, lung cancer, **76**
gemcitabine
  biliary tract carcinoma, 107, 108
  bladder cancer, **39**, **42**
  breast cancer, **12**
  lung cancer, **75**

mesothelioma, 83, 84
  ovarian cancer, **174**, **175**
  pancreas cancer, 113
GEMOX (regimen), biliary tract carcinoma, 108
gemtuzumab ozogamicin
  acute myeloid leukemia, 313
  acute promyelocytic leukemia, **314**
gender, biliary tract carcinoma, 102
genetically inspired prognostic scoring system
    (GIPSS), 279
genomic markers, acute lymphoblastic leukemia,
    323
genomic study
  breast cancer, 19
  lung cancer, 70, 71
geriatric oncology, 514–518
  allogeneic stem cell transplantation, 385
  bladder cancer, 40
  breast cancer, 16
  cancer survivors, 538–540, *see also* survivorship
  dysphagia, 148
  frailty index, 383
  glioblastomas, 251
  mitomycin, 160, 161
  radiotherapy, 460
  screening assessment, 517
  warfarin, 443
germ cell tumors (GCT)
  brain, 557, 560, *565*
    treatment, **562**
  markers, 546
  testicular, 56, 63
    imaging, **451**
    nonseminomatous, 62
    staging, 59
germinal center B-cell lymphoma, 352
GIPSS (genetically inspired prognostic scoring
    system), 279
Gleason scores, 26
glioblastomas (GBM), 241, 242, 245, 246, *253*
  incidence, 556
  prognosis, 249, 251
  treatment, **247**
gliomas, 556
  diagnosis, 243, 244
  diffuse intrinsic pontine (DIPG), *564*
    incidence, 556
    radiotherapy, **562**
  genetic disorders, 245
  magnetic resonance imaging, 245
  MGMT promoter methylation, 245, 248, 250
  pathology, 242
  prognosis, 248
  treatment, **246**, **247**, 248, 560, **562**
gliomatosis cerebri, 245, 246
global longitudinal strain (GLS), echocardiography,
    489, 492, 493, *498*

glomerular disease of kidney, 34
glucagonomas, **257**, 261
   tumor markers, 262
(1–3)-β-ᴅ-glucan, 409
glucocorticoids *see* steroids
glucose 6-phosphate deficiency, rasburicase and,
    427
L-glutamine, 528
goal pain score, 521
GOG 252 trial, ovarian cancer, 173
Göteborg trial, 31
graft failure, allogeneic SCT, 389
graft versus host disease
   acute, 388, 412–419
   bacterial infections, 406
   chronic, 388–389
   diagnosis, 413–416
   grading, 415
   guidelines, 419
   prevention, 413
   prognosis, 418
   risk factors, 413
   staging, **415**
   treatment, 416–418
Gram-negative bacterial infections
   neutropenic fever, 429
   stem cell transplantation, 405
Gram-positive bacterial infections
   neutropenic fever, 429
   stem cell transplantation, 405
granulocyte colony-stimulating factor
   myelodysplastic syndromes, 293
   stem cell mobilization, 380, 387
GRFomas, **257**

HAART, Hodgkin lymphoma, 361
Haemophilus influenza vaccine, 410
haloperidol, **508**
hamartin, 44
haploidentical transplants, 386
Hasford score, CML, 278
head and neck cancer, 230–240
   diagnosis, 231–233
   follow-up, 238
   guidelines, 239
   prevention, 231
   prognosis, 238
   treatment, 233–238
headaches, brain tumors, 244
healthcare value, 520
heart failure, 487–488, *see also* cardiotoxicity
   anemia, 492
   drugs causing, **490–491**
   pregnancy, 496
heated chemotherapy, *see also* hyperthermic
    intraperitoneal chemotherapy
   mesothelioma, 84

heavy chain disease, **299**
heavy charged particle beam EBRT, 458
Helicobacter pylori
   gastric cancer, 132
   gastric MALT lymphoma, 344
hemangioma
   atypical, 92
   choroidal, 476
hematocrit, polycythemia vera, **275**
hematopoietic stem cell transplantation *see*
    allogeneic stem cell transplantation;
    autologous stem cell transplantation; stem
    cell transplantation; transplantation *under*
    bone marrow
hematuria, 33, 34, 36, 39, 40, 48
hemodialysis *see* dialysis
hemoglobin levels
   Hodgkin lymphoma, 357
   polycythemia vera, **275**
hemolytic anemia, autoimmune, 320
hemolytic–uremic syndrome, mitomycin, 161
hemorrhage *see* bleeding/hemorrhage
hemorrhagic cystitis, 562
hemorrhoids, 158
heparin
   hepatic veno-occlusive disease, 388
   unfractionated, 441
heparin-induced thrombocytopenia, 444
hepatic veno-occlusive disease (VOD), 388, 414
hepatitis A, vaccination, 410
hepatitis B, 90, 91
   allogeneic stem cell transplantation, 389–390
   liver cancer, 91, 93
   vaccination, 410
hepatitis C
   allogeneic stem cell transplantation, 389–390
   liver cancer, 91, 93, 95
   renal cancer, 45
hepatoblastoma, 97
   treatment, **550**
hepatocellular carcinoma, 89–100, *see also* mixed
    hepatocellular cholangiocarcinomas
   biliary tract carcinoma *vs*, 104
   diagnosis, 91–95
   evidence, 98–99
   guidelines, 98
   imaging, **451**
   prognosis, 97
   rupture, 95
   screening, 90–91
   treatment, **94**, 95–97
HER2 enriched breast cancer, **4**
HER2 gene
   breast cancer, 5, 10, 11, 19
    chemotherapy, **13**, 15
   gastric cancer, **136**
HER2/NEU tyrosine kinases, 102

herbicides, 333
  Agent Orange, 56, 333
hereditary breast–ovarian cancer syndrome, ovarian
    cancer risk assessment, 168
hereditary leiomyomatosis and renal cell carcinoma,
    44
hereditary nonpolyposis colorectal carcinoma
    syndrome *see* Lynch syndrome
hereditary papillary renal carcinoma, 44
hereditary paraganglioma/pheochromocytoma,
    44
herpes simplex virus infection
  cervix, 196
  prevention, 429
  stem cell transplantation, 407
herpes virus (modified; T-VEC), 211
HiDAC (regimen), acute promyelocytic leukemia,
    314
high dose rate implants, brachytherapy, 459
high grade squamous intraepithelial lesions, anus,
    154
high-dose methotrexate (HD-MTX)
  drugs delaying clearance, 370
  primary CNS lymphoma, 368, **369**, 370
HIPEC (hyperthermic intraperitoneal chemotherapy),
    83, *see also* heated chemotherapy
histone deacetylase inhibitors (panobinostat),
    plasma cell disorders, **304**
HIV
  acute myeloid leukemia, 309
  anal cancer, 153, 154, 156, 161–162
  cervical cancer, 195, 196, 199
  Hodgkin lymphoma, **356**, 361
  lymphadenopathy, 345
  non-Hodgkin lymphomas, 351
  primary CNS lymphoma, 364, 365, **366**,
    367
    prognosis, 372
    treatment, **370**, 371
  testicular cancer, 57
HLA matching, 394, 413
hoarseness, 69, 144
Hodgkin lymphoma, 354–363
  diagnosis, 355–358
  evidence, 362
  follow-up, 361
  guidelines, 362
  prognosis, 357, 361
  radiotherapy, **551**
  stem cell transplantation, 401
  treatment, 358–361
hospice care, criteria for eligibility, 520–521
HOXB13 gene, prostate cancer, 24
human chorionic gonadotropin (HCG)
  endometrial cancer, 186
  testicular cancer, 59, 60, **61**
human leukocyte antigen typing, AML, 311

human papillomavirus (HPV)
  anal cancer, 153, 154, 155
  cervical cancer, 194, 195
  oropharyngeal cancer, 230, 231, 233, 236,
    238
  testing, 233
  vaccination, 155–156
humoral hypercalcemia, **424**
Hurthle thyroid carcinoma, 221, 227
hydralazine, 493
hydration
  chemotherapy, **533**
  hypercalcemia, 424
  tumor lysis syndrome, 426
hydrocele, 58
hydrocortisone, for hypercalcemia, 425
hydroxyurea
  essential thrombocythemia, 282
  polycythemia vera, 282
  primary myelofibrosis, 284
  sperm banking, 284
hypercalcemia
  malignancy-associated, 423–425
  multiple myeloma, management, 305
hyper-CVAD/methotrexate-cytarabine, ALL, **326**
hyperglycemia, steroids, 530
hyperkalemia, tumor lysis syndrome, 426, **428**
hyperleukocytosis, *see also* leukocytosis
  acute lymphoblastic leukemia, 327
  acute myeloid leukemia, 311
hypermetabolic areas, colorectal cancer metastases,
    130
hyperparathyroidism, **257**
hyperphosphatemia, tumor lysis syndrome, **428**
hypersensitivity, chemotherapy, 177
hypertension
  bevacizumab, 52
  drugs causing, **491**
  management, 495
  renal cancer, 45
  VEGF TKIs, 52
hyperthermic intraperitoneal chemotherapy, 83,
    see also heated chemotherapy
hypertrophic osteoarthropathy, 70
hyperuricemia, tumor lysis syndrome, **428**
hyperviscosity syndrome, retinopathy, 479
hypocalcemia, 225
  tumor lysis syndrome, 426, **428**
hypocellular MDS, 294
hypogeusia, 530
hypoglycemia, neuroendocrine tumors, 256, 261
hypomethylating agents
  acute myeloid leukemia, **314**, 315
  myelodysplastic syndromes, 293
hyponatremia, brain tumors, 248
hypopharyngeal cancer, presentation, 232
hypophosphatemia, 424

hypospadias, 57
hypotension, drugs causing, **491**
hypothalamus, tumor presentation, 559
hypothyroidism
  allogeneic stem cell transplantation, 390
  Hodgkin lymphoma, 360
hypoxia-inducible factors, VHL, 44
hysterectomy, **188**
hysteroscopy, 184

ibrutinib
  chronic lymphocytic leukemia, 338, 339
  non-Hodgkin lymphomas, **350**, 351
ibupropion, **505**
ICON-4 (regimen), ovarian cancer, **174**
idarubicin (IDA)
  acute myeloid leukemia, 313, 317
  acute promyelocytic leukemia, **314**
idelalisib
  chronic lymphocytic leukemia, 338, 339
  non-Hodgkin lymphomas, **350**
IDH1/2 mutations
  gallbladder carcinoma, 102
  gliomas, 245
idiopathic thrombocytopenic purpura, 320
ifosfamide
  ovarian cancer, **175**
  sarcomas, 220
  testicular cancer, 64
IGF1-R, gallbladder carcinoma, 102
ileal conduit urinary diversion, 37
imaging, 447–453, *see also specific modalities*
  breast cancer, 8–9, **452**, *see also* mammography
  children, 547
  guidelines, 452
  radiotherapy guidance, 456
  for staging, 449
imatinib
  acute lymphoblastic leukemia, 329
  chronic myelogenous leukemia, 280
  gastrointestinal stromal tumor, 216, 220
  nutrition and, **532**
imiquimod, anal intraepithelial neoplasia,
    154
immune checkpoint inhibitors, *see also* PD-L1
    inhibitor
  bladder cancer, 38, **39**
  non-small cell lung carcinoma, 74
immunodeficiency, allogeneic stem cell
    transplantation, 388
immunofixation (SIFE; UIFE), 302, 303, 382
immunoglobulin
  cytomegalovirus infection, 407
  graft versus host disease, 416
  stem cell transplantation, 410
immunomodulatory drugs *see* lenalidomide;
    pomalidomide; thalidomide

immunosuppression
  allogeneic stem cell transplantation, **395**
  cervical cancer, 196
  lymphomas, 343
  methotrexate, **396**
  primary CNS lymphoma, 364, 365
immunotherapy, *see also specific drugs*
  melanoma, 211
  non-small cell lung carcinoma, 74–75
  ovarian cancer, 175–176
  pneumonitis from, 76
infarction, renal, 46
infections, *see also Clostridium difficile* infection;
      fungal infections; *Helicobacter pylori*;
      Pneumocystis pneumonia; viral infections
  bone tumors *vs*, 465
  chronic lymphocytic leukemia, 333, 335
  graft versus host disease, 416
  mycobacterial, non-Hodgkin lymphomas *vs*, 345
  neutropenic fever, 429
  non-Hodgkin lymphomas *vs*, 344, 345, 346
  stem cell transplantation, 388, 396–397, 404–411
  stool tests, 416
infectious mononucleosis, 355
inferior vena cava filter, **442–443**
infertility, *see also* sperm banking
  allogeneic stem cell transplantation, 390
  Hodgkin lymphoma treatment, 360
  ovarian cancer risk, 167
inflammatory bowel disease
  colorectal cancer risk, 119, 120, 121
  neuroendocrine tumors *vs*, 260, 261
influenza
  chronic lymphocytic leukemia and, 333
  stem cell transplantation, 408
  vaccination, 410
infusion reactions, 339, 351
inguinal hernia, 58
inherited disorders
  colorectal cancer, 120, 126–127
  sarcomas, 215
inositol polyphosphate multikinase mutation, 261
insulin, tumor lysis syndrome, **428**
insulinomas, 256, **257**, 261
  tumor markers, 262
integrated survivorship clinics, **539**
intensity modulated radiotherapy, 455–456
  image-guided, 456
  prostate cancer, 29
interferon
  essential thrombocythemia, 283
  melanoma, 211
  polycythemia vera, 282
interim PET, Hodgkin lymphoma treatment, 358,
      361, 362
interleukin 2, melanoma, 211
International Bone Marrow Transplant Registry, 385

International Germ Cell Consensus Classification, 59
International Intraocular Retinoblastoma
        Classification, 477
International Metastatic Database Consortium
        model, renal cell carcinoma, 54
International Multicenter InterAACT study, anal
        cancer, 160
International Neuroblastoma Staging System, 546
International Prognostic Index Score (CLL IPI),
        chronic lymphocytic leukemia, 336
International Prognostic Score, advanced stage
        Hodgkin lymphoma, 357
International Prognostic Scoring System, Revised
        (IPSS-R), 290, 291, **292**, 295, 302
International Union Against Cancer, anal cancer
        staging, 158
interval compression, Ewing sarcoma treatment,
        550
interventional radiology, sarcomas, 217
intestinal type gastric cancer, 131, 132
intracranial hemorrhage, ALL, 327
intracranial pressure, raised, 558, 559
intracranial tumors *see* brain tumors
intraepithelial neoplasia, anus, 154, 155
intralesional resection, bone tumors, 469
intraocular tumors, 473–485
    lymphomas. *see* ocular lymphoma
intraoperative radiotherapy, 459
intraperitoneal chemotherapy
    hyperthermic, 83, *see also* heated chemotherapy
    ovarian cancer, 172, 173, 177
intrathecal chemotherapy
    primary leptomeningeal lymphomatosis, 371
    side effects, **326**
intrauterine devices, ovarian cancer risk, 167
intravesical bacillus Calmette–Guérin, 34, 37, **38**, 41
intravesical chemotherapy, 34, 37, **38**
invasive epithelial ovarian cancer *see* ovarian cancer
inverse planning, intensity modulated radiotherapy,
        456
ipilimumab
    melanoma, 211
    mesothelioma, 84
IPSS-R (International Prognostic Scoring System,
        Revised), 290, 291, **292**, 295, 302
irinotecan
    lung cancer, **76**
    side effects, **125**
Irish node, gastric cancer, 133
iron chelation, myelodysplastic syndromes, 294
iron deficiency anemia, 123
iron overload, allogeneic SCT, 390
irritable bowel syndrome, neuroendocrine tumors *vs*,
        260, 261
ischemia (cardiac)
    drugs causing, **491**
    management, 494

ischemic brain injury, ALL, 327
Ivor Lewis esophagectomy, **147**, *151*
ixabepilone, breast cancer, **13**
ixazomib, plasma cell disorders, **304**

JAK2V16F mutation, diagnosis, **274**
Japanese Trial, ovarian cancer, 172
jaundice
    biliary tract carcinoma, 108
    graft versus host disease, 414
    from octreotide therapy, 265
Joint International Federation of Gynecology and
        Obstetrics (FIGO)
    endometrial cancer staging, **186**, **190**
    ovarian cancer staging, **171**
juvenile idiopathic arthritis, 321

Katherine Trial, 11
keratitis, from chemotherapy, 479
KEYNOTE 010 trial, 74
Khorona risk score, 437, 439
Ki-67, breast cancer, **4**, 10
kidney function, *see also* renal failure; renal tubular
        dysfunction
    cervical cancer, 197
    older people, 515
Kikuchi disease, 345
Kimura disease, 345
KIT inhibitors, melanoma, 212
Klatskin tumor, 101
KRAS mutations, 102

laboratory tumor lysis syndrome, 427
lactate dehydrogenase (LDH)
    melanoma, 208
    testicular cancer, 59, 60, **61**
lanreotide, 264, **265**
laparoscopy, gastric cancer, 134, **135**
laparotomy, ovarian cancer, 169
lapatinib
    breast cancer, **13**
    nutrition and, **533**
large granular lymphocytic leukemia, 290
laryngeal cancer
    lymph node metastases, 233
    presentation, 232
laryngitis, CLL and, 333
late effects, chemotherapy, 537
leaves, beam shaping, 455, 456
left ventricular ejection fraction, 486,
        493
lenalidomide
    myelodysplastic syndromes, 293, 296
    plasma cell disorders, **304**
    primary myelofibrosis, 284
    thromboprophylaxis, 437
lentigo maligna, 204

lenvatinib
 liver cancer, 89, **96**, 99
 side effects, 96
 thyroid cancer, 225, 228
leptomeningeal carcinomatosis, 245, **247**
leptomeningeal lymphomatosis, **370**, 371
letermovir, 407
letrozole
 breast cancer, 10, 12
 ovarian cancer, 175
leucovorin, **125**
 colorectal cancer, 127, 129
 in FOLFOX 6, 160
leukapheresis, 311
leukemia, *see also specific types*
 ophthalmologic complications, 479
 secondary to Hodgkin lymphoma, 360
leukocoria, 475
leukocytosis
 acute lymphoblastic leukemia, 327
 acute myeloid leukemia, 311
 cancer-related thrombosis, 439
 causes, 277, 280
 diagnosis, **273**
 Hodgkin lymphoma, 357
leukoencephalopathy, methotrexate-induced, *375*
leukoerythroblastosis, 276
levetiracetam, **395**
levofloxacin
 acute myeloid leukemia, **313**
 allogeneic stem cell transplantation, **395**
 neutropenic fever prevention, 429
L-glutamine, 528
Li–Fraumeni syndrome, 242, 557
light chain analysis (FLC), 303, 383
light chain disease, **299**
limited SCLC, management, 71
linear accelerators, 454
lipomas, 215
liposomal doxorubicin
 breast cancer, **13**
 mesothelioma, 84
liver biopsy, GVHD, 416
liver cancer, 89–100, *see also* hepatocellular
  carcinoma
 anal cancer metastases, 160
 diagnosis, 91–95
 evidence, 98–99
 guidelines, 98
 imaging, 449, **451**
 prognosis, 97
 treatment, **94**, 95–97
 uveal melanoma metastases, 477, 481
liver disease
 allogeneic stem cell transplantation, 389–390
 nonalcoholic fatty liver disease, 90, 97
 signs, 93

liver function
 graft versus host disease, 416
 older people, 515
Liver Imaging Reporting and Data System, 95
liver screen, 93
liver transplantation, **95**, 96, 99
lobectomy, 72–73
lobular carcinoma *in situ* (LCIS), breast, 3, 7
locally advanced SCLC, management, 73
lomustine (CCNU), brain tumors, **247**
longitudinal strain *see* global longitudinal strain
long-term side effects, chemotherapy, 537
lorazepam, **504**, **508**
lorlatinib, lung cancer, 75, **76**
low dose computed tomography, 449, 516, 537
low dose rate implants, brachytherapy, 459
low molecular weight heparin, 437, 441, **442**, 495,
  see also specific drugs
 bleeding, 443
 guidelines, 445
 renal insufficiency, 443
lumbar puncture, primary CNS lymphoma, 366, 368
luminal A breast cancer, **4**, 10
luminal B breast cancer, **4**, 10
luminal HER2 breast cancer, **4**
lumpectomy (breast conserving therapy), 9, 20
 pregnancy, 16
lung, *see also* pneumonia; pneumonitis; pulmonary
  embolism; pulmonary function tests
 bleomycin toxicity, 360
 carcinoid tumors, 258
 extrapleural resection, 84, 87
 graft versus host disease, 389
 transplantation-related injury, 389
lung cancer, 66–78
 computed tomography, 68, *453*
 diagnosis, 68–71
 guidelines, 77–78
 imaging, **450**
 mesothelioma *vs*, 81
 prevention, 68
 prognosis, 77
 sarcoma metastases, 216
 screening, 68, 516
 secondary to Hodgkin lymphoma, 360
 treatment, 71–77
lymph nodes
 biopsy, 347, 349, *see also* sentinel node biopsy
 chronic lymphocytic leukemia, 336
 colorectal cancer, 122, 123
 edema from enlargement, 438
 fine needle aspiration biopsy, 236, 349
 gastric cancer, 133
 head and neck cancer, 233
 melanoma, 208, 209, 211
 non-Hodgkin lymphomas, 344–345, 346, 349
 occult primary, 236

lymph nodes (*Continued*)
   retroperitoneal, dissection, 62, 64
   thyroid cancer and, 225
lymphedema, DVT *vs*, 438
lymphoblastic lymphoma, 543, **550**
lymphoblasts, 320
lymphocytosis
   chronic lymphocytic leukemia, 332
   malignant causes, 335
   monoclonal B-lymphocytosis, 332, 333
   reactive, 320
lymphomas, *see also specific types*
   acute lymphoblastic leukemia *vs*, 321
   B-cell receptor signaling, 343
   biologic agents, **551**
   bone, 465
   brain, 245
   children
      presentation, 545
      treatment, 547, **549**
      types, 543
   eye complications, 479, *see also* ocular lymphoma
   imaging, **452**
   immunosuppression, 343
   mesothelioma *vs*, 81
   neuroendocrine tumors *vs*, 260
   stomach, 133
lymphopenia, Hodgkin lymphoma, 357
lymphoproliferative disorders, *see also*
      post-transplant lymphoproliferative disorders
   ophthalmologic complications, 479
   stem cell transplantation for, 400–403
Lynch syndrome (HNPCC), 121, 126–127
   endometrial cancer, 182
   ovarian cancer risk, 168, *180*
   prophylactic colectomy, 121

M protein, 383
MA-17 trial, breast cancer, 10
maculopapular rashes, GVHD, **415**, *419*
magnetic resonance imaging, 448
   brain tumors, 243, 244, 245
      astrocytomas, *252*
      glioblastomas, *253*
      melanoma metastases, *251*
      meningiomas, *254*
   breast, 6
   cardiac, 492
   children, 547
   hepatocellular carcinoma, **92**
   primary CNS lymphoma, 365–366, 368, *374*
   renal cancer, 48
   spinal cord compression, 433, *434*
magnetic resonance spectroscopy, brain tumors,
   245
major molecular response (MMR), chronic
   myelogenous leukemia, 280

malignant spinal cord compression *see* spinal cord
   compression
malnutrition, 532
   esophageal cancer, 146
   head and neck cancer treatment, 237
MALT lymphoma *see* gastric MALT lymphoma
mammalian target of rapamycin inhibitors, breast
   cancer, 11
mammography, 6, 7, 360, 449, 516
   after breast cancer treatment, 16, **536**
   allogeneic stem cell transplantation, 390
Mammoprint, 8
mantle cell lymphoma, stem cell transplantation,
   402
margins, melanoma resection, 210
MARIANNE trial, 21
markers *see* tumor markers
masses
   mediastinal
      acute lymphoblastic leukemia, 327, *330*
      imaging, **450**
   ovarian cancer *vs*, 170
   renal, 46, 48
   testicular, 59
mastectomy, 9, *see also* breast conserving therapy
   prophylactic, 6
McDonald regimen, gastric cancer, **136**
McKeown esophagectomy, **147**
measles, mumps and rubella vaccine, SCT and, 391,
   410
mediastinum
   acute lymphoblastic leukemia, 327, *330*
   B-cell lymphoma, 355
   imaging, **450**
medullary thyroid carcinoma, 221, 227
   follow-up, 227
medulloblastomas (MB)
   incidence, 556
   radiotherapy, **562**
   syndromes causing, 557
megakaryocytes, primary myelofibrosis, **276**
megestrol acetate, 524
MEK inhibition, melanoma, 211
melanocytoma, optic nerve, 476
melanoma, 204–213
   brain metastases, 210, 212, **247**, *251*
   diagnosis, 207–210
   guidelines, 213
   prognosis, 213
   screening, 206
   treatment, 210–212
   uveal. *see* uveal melanoma
melanoma-associated retinopathy, 479
melphalan
   autologous stem cell transplantation, 381, 383
   multiple myeloma, 303, **304**
   reduced intensity myeloablative regimens, **395**

meningiomas
  diagnosis, 243, 244, 245
  incidence, 241
  magnetic resonance imaging, 245, *254*
  pathogenesis, 242
  prognosis, 249
  treatment, 245, **246**, 248
meningoencephalitis, 557
menopause
  endometrial cancer risk, 182
  ovarian cancer risk and, 167
mercaptopurine, side effects, **326**
mesothelioma, 79–88
  diagnosis, 80–82
  evidence, 87
  guidelines, 86
  prognosis, 85–86
  staging, *87*
  treatment, 82–85
MET oncogene, 44, 45
metachronous cancer, neuroendocrine tumors, 261
metastases, *see also under* bone tumors
  acute lymphoblastic leukemia *vs*, 321
  anal cancer, 160
    cisplatin, 160, 164
  bladder cancer, 35, 38, **39**, 40, *42*
  to brain. *see* brain metastases
  breast cancer, 8, 11–12, 14–15
  colorectal cancer, 122, 124
    hypermetabolic areas, *130*
  to eye, 473, 476, 479
  gastric cancer, treatment, **136**, 137
  head and neck cancer, 236–237
  to heart, *499*
  hepatocellular carcinoma *vs*, 92
  to kidney, 46
  non-Hodgkin lymphomas *vs*, 345
  non-small cell lung carcinoma, 73–74
  plasma cell disorders *vs*, 301
  prostate cancer, 30
  renal cell carcinoma, 50
  sarcomas
    to lung, 216
    mortality, 215
  testicular cancer, 63
  transitional cell carcinomas, 51
  upper respiratory cancer, 233
  uveal melanoma, 477, 481
  venous compression, 438
methotrexate
  acute lymphoblastic leukemia, 329
  immunosuppression, **396**
  keratitis, 479
  nutrition and, **533**
  primary CNS lymphoma, 368, **369**, **370**
  serosal fluid collections, **370**
  side effects, **326**

methotrexate (M)F (regimen), breast cancer, **14**
methotrexate-induced leukoencephalopathy, *375*
methylphenidate, **505**, 523–524
methylprednisolone, GVHD, 416, **417**
MGMT promoter methylation, gliomas, 245, 248, 250
microangiopathy, transplant-associated thrombotic, 396
microlithiasis, testicular, 57
microsatellite instability (MSI), colorectal cancer, 123
midazolam, **508**
midostaurin, acute myeloid leukemia, 313
MIPSS70 + v2.0 (mutation-enhanced international prognostic scoring system plus karyotype, version 2.0), 279
Mirels criteria, orthopedic tumors, **468**
mirtazapine, **505**
mithramycin, 425
mitomycin
  anal cancer, 153, 159–160, 162, 164
  biliary tract carcinoma, 107
  bladder cancer, **39**
  elderly people, 161
  side effects, 161
mitoxantrone, prostate cancer, 29
mixed hepatocellular cholangiocarcinomas, 101
modafinil, **505**, 524
Monalessa trial, 12
Monarch trial, 12
monoclonal B-lymphocytosis (MBL), 332, 333
monoclonal gammopathy of undetermined significance (MGUS), **298**, 300, **301**
mood disorders, *see also* depressive disorders
  NCCN guidelines, *512*
morphine, 521
MOSAIC trial, 129
mouthwashes, 531
MSI (microsatellite instability), colorectal cancer, 123
mTOR inhibitor
  clear cell renal cell carcinoma, 50
  side effects, 52–53
mucosa-associated lymphoid tissue lymphoma *see* gastric MALT lymphoma
mucositis, 237, 388, 531
  vancomycin for, 430
multidisciplinary survivorship clinics, **539**
multiple gated acquisition scan, nuclear medicine, 492
multiple myeloma, 298–307, 379, 465
  allogeneic stem cell transplantation, 386
  autologous stem cell transplantation 379–384
    follow-up, 382
    maintenance therapy, 382
    timing, 381
  computed tomography, 447

multiple myeloma (*Continued*)
  imaging, **452**
  non-secretory, 303
  ophthalmologic complications, 479
  presentation, 302
  prognosis, 305–306
  risk factors, **300**
  treatment, 303–305
  venous thromboembolism, 444
multiple sclerosis, 367
  tumefactive, 243, 245
muscularis propria
  bladder cancer invading, 32, 35, 37–38
  TURBT specimens, 40
mutation panels (DNA mutation panels), 290, 295
mutation-enhanced international prognostic scoring
      system plus karyotype, version 2.0
      (MIPSS70 + v2.0), 279
mutism, cerebellar, 562
MVAC (regimen), bladder cancer, **39**, **42**
mycobacterial infections, non-Hodgkin lymphomas
      vs, 345
mycophenolate, **396**
  colitis, 396
myeloablative regimens, 387, **395**, *see also*
      conditioning
  for lymphoproliferative disorders, 400
myelodysplastic syndromes (MDS), 288–297
  acute lymphoblastic leukemia *vs*, 321
  acute myeloid leukemia *vs*, 290, 310
  acute myeloid leukemia with changes related,
      308, 309
  allogeneic stem cell transplantation, 294, 296,
      386, 392–399
  classification, 288–289
  diagnosis, 290–292, 393–394
  evidence, 296, 398
  guidelines, 295–296, 398
  neuropathy, 305
  neutropenia, 293, 305
  prognosis, 295, 397
  risk stratification, 393
  treatment, 292–294, 394–397
myelofibrosis *see* primary myelofibrosis
myeloid blasts, *317*
myeloperoxidase, 492
myeloproliferative neoplasms (MPNs), 271–287
  acute myeloid leukemia from, 308, 309
  BCR-ABL –, risk prediction, 278–279, 285
  diagnosis, 272–280
  guidelines, 287
  overlap syndromes, 290
  perioperative management, 285
  prognosis, 285–286
  treatment, 280–285
myelosuppression, ABVD (regimen), 359
myocardium *see* cardiotoxicity; ischemia (cardiac)

nabothian cysts, 196
nab-paclitaxel
  breast cancer, 21
  lung cancer, **75**
nab-T, breast cancer, **12**
nadroparin, 445
nanoparticle albumin bound (nab-T), breast cancer,
      12
nasal congestion, 233
nasopharyngeal cancer
  lymph node metastases, 233
  presentation, 232
National Comprehensive Cancer Network, 18
  Clinical Practice Guidelines in Oncology for
      Distress Management, 501, *510–513*
National Institute for Health and Clinical Excellence,
      on renal cancer, 43–44
National Wilms Tumor Study Staging, 546
nausea, 522–523
  graft versus host disease, 414
  nutritional management, 528
NCCN *see* National Comprehensive Cancer Network
necitumumab, non-small cell lung carcinoma, 74
necrolytic migratory erythema, 261
neobladder, 37
nephrectomy
  cytoreductive, 50, **51**
  radical, 49, **51**
nephrotoxicity, chemotherapy, 199
nephroureterectomy, transitional cell carcinomas, **51**
neuroblastoma
  acute lymphoblastic leukemia *vs*, 321
  bone marrow aspirate, *555*
  markers, 546
  opsoclonus-myoclonus, 546
  regression, 552
  staging, 546
  treatment, **549**, **550**
neuroendocrine tumors, 255–267
  diagnosis, 259–263
  guidelines, 262, 267
  pancreas, 111, 113, 114, 256, 258, 260
  prognosis, 265
  stomach, 133
  treatment, 263–266
neurofibromatoses, 242, 557
neuropathy, 116
  management guidelines, 541
  myelodysplastic syndromes, 305
  oxaliplatin, 126
  plasma cell disorders, **299**
neurotoxicity, delayed, 370
neutropenia, 428, *see also* febrile neutropenia
  ABVD (regimen), 359
  myelodysplastic syndromes, 293, 305
neutropenic enterocolitis, 414
neutropenic fever, 428–432

neutropenic sepsis, 116
nevi, 206, 208
  choroidal, 475
niacin deficiency, 256
nicotinic-acetylcholine receptor genes, lung cancer,
      67
nilotinib
  chronic myelogenous leukemia, 280
  nutrition and, **533**
nitrates, 493
nitroso compounds, gastric cancer, 132
nivolumab
  clear cell renal cell carcinoma, 50
  Hodgkin lymphoma, 358
  liver cancer, 89, **96**
  lung cancer, **76**
  melanoma, 211
  mesothelioma, 84
  non-small cell lung carcinoma, 74, 77
  renal cell carcinoma, **51**
NK/T-cell lymphoma, 343
nodular lymphocyte predominant Hodgkin
      lymphoma (NLPHL)
  diagnosis, **356**
  pathology, 355
  prognosis, 361
nodular melanoma, 204
nodular regenerative hyperplasia, hepatic, 92
nonalcoholic fatty liver disease, 90, 97
non-Hodgkin lymphomas, 342–353
  children, 543
    treatment, 547, **550**
  diagnosis, 344–349
  follow-up, 352
  guidelines, 353
  plasma cell disorders vs, 301
  prognosis, 346–347, 351–352
  secondary to Hodgkin lymphoma, 360
  treatment, 349–351
    children, 547, **550**
nonpulmonary visceral metastasis, testicular cancer,
      63
nonseminomatous germ cell tumors, 56, 62, 63
non-small cell lung carcinoma, 66, 68
  management, 72–75
  prognosis, 77
nonsteroidal anti-inflammatory drugs
  colorectal cancer prophylaxis, 121
  esophageal cancer and, 142
  renal cancer, 45
nortriptyline, **505**
novel oral anticoagulants, **442**
NRAS mutations, melanoma, 204
NSCLC-NOS (non-small cell lung carcinoma), 66
nuclear medicine, 448, see also positron emission
      tomography
  bone tumors, 27, **28**, 467

multiple gated acquisition scan, 492
  somatostatin receptor scintigraphy, 260, 262
nucleic acids, tumor lysis syndrome, 426
nulliparity, endometrial cancer risk, 182
nutritional management, 528–534, see also
      malnutrition
  esophageal cancer, 146–147
  gastric cancer, 136

obesity, see also abdominal diameter
  colorectal cancer risk, 119
  endometrial cancer, 182
  gastric cancer, 132
  pancreas cancer, 112
  renal cancer, 44, 45
  sarcopenic, 515
obinutuzumab, infusion reaction, 339
occult primary, cervical lymph nodes, 236
occult upper gastrointestinal bleeding, 122, see also
      stool tests
occupational exposure
  asbestos, 79, 80, 81
  bladder cancer rate, 33
  sinonasal tract tumors, 231
  uveal melanoma, 474
OCEANS (regimen), ovarian cancer, **174**
OctreoScan see somatostatin receptor scintigraphy
octreotide, 264, **265**
ocular lymphoma, 367, 368
  treatment, **369**, **370**
ocular slit lamp examination, primary CNS
      lymphoma, **366**, 368
odynophagia, 143, 531
olanzapine, 502, **508**
olaparib, ovarian cancer, 173, 175
older people see geriatric oncology
oligodendrogliomas, 242, 244, 246, 254
  prognosis, 249, 250
omacetaxine, chronic myelogenous leukemia, 281
oncocytomas, kidney, 45
oncology specialist care, cancer survivors, **539**
Oncotype DX® (RT-PCR assay), 8, 10, 16
ondansetron, 522
(1–3)-β-D-glucan, 409
ophthalmology, 473–485, see also ocular lymphoma
  primary CNS lymphoma, **366**
opioids, 521, 525
opsoclonus-myoclonus, 546
optic nerve, melanocytoma, 476
oral cavity cancer
  lymph node metastases, 233
  presentation, 232
  treatment, 234
oral contraceptives, endometrial cancer and, 183
oral ulcers, mTOR inhibitors, 53
orbital tumors, children, 545
orchiectomy, 60

orchiopexy, 58
oropharyngeal cancer
  human papillomavirus, 230, 231, 233, 236, 238
  presentation, 232
  treatment, 236
orthopedic fixation, pathologic fractures, 15
orthopedic oncology *see* bone tumors; soft tissue
    tumors
osimertinib, lung cancer, 74, **76**
osteolysis, **424**
osteoma, choroidal, 476
osteomyelitis, 321
osteosarcomas, 219, *471*, *554*, *see also* bone tumors
  chemotherapy, 217, **550**
  radiotherapy and, 216
  surgery, **551**
otitis, chronic lymphocytic leukemia and, 333
Ottawa prognostic score, 437, 439
OUTBACK trial, 201
ovarian cancer, 166–180
  BRCAn genes, 167, 168, 175, *180*, 537
  diagnosis, 169–172
  differential diagnosis, 170
  guidelines, 179
  imaging, **452**
  prognosis, 178
  screening, 169
  treatment, 172–178
overlap syndromes, myelodysplastic syndromes, 290
oxaliplatin
  colorectal cancer, 126
  in FOLFOX 6, 160
  nutrition and, **533**
  side effects, **125**, 126

p16 (tumor suppressor)
  loss in head and neck cancer, 231
  loss in melanoma, 205
P53 tumor suppressor gene, head and neck cancer,
    231
pacemakers, 494
paclitaxel
  breast cancer, 11, **12**, 20
  lung cancer, **75**
  ovarian cancer, 172, 173, **174**, **176**
pain
  anal cancer, **161**
  management, 521–522, *527*
  radiotherapy for, 15
    mesothelioma, 84
  WHO ladder, *527*
palbociclib, breast cancer, 12, 21
PALETTE trial, 220
palivizumab, 408
palliative care, 519–527
  guidelines, 526
  prevalence of teams (USA), *527*

palliative radiotherapy
  mesothelioma, 84
  sarcomas, 217
palliative surgery, sarcomas, 217
palmar-plantar erythrodysesthesia, 52, 414
Paloma III trial, 12
palonosetron, 522
PAM50 (RT-PCR test), 8
pamidronic acid
  for hypercalcemia, 424
  hypercalcemia prevention, 423
  plasma cell disorders, **304**
pancreas, neuroendocrine tumors, 111, 113, 114,
    256, 258, 260
pancreas cancer, 111–117
  diagnosis, 113–115
  guidelines, 117
  imaging, **451**
  prognosis, 117
  treatment, 115–117
pancreastatin, neuroendocrine tumor prognosis, 266
pancreatitis, pancreas cancer, 112
panitumumab, *RAS* and *BRAF* mutations and, 124
panobinostat, plasma cell disorders, **304**
Papanicolaou smears
  anal cancer, 154
  cervical cancer, 195
papillary renal carcinoma, hereditary, 44
papillary thyroid carcinoma, 221, 222, 225, 227
  children, 227
papillary tumors, bladder, 35
paranasal sinuses, cancer, presentation, 232
paraneoplastic syndromes
  lung cancer, 68
  ocular, 479
parathyroid hormone secretion, ectopic, **424**
parenteral nutrition, 147
parietal lobe, tumor presentation, 559
PARMA trial, 401
paroxetine, **505**
paroxysmal nocturnal hemoglobinuria (PNH), 290
partial mastectomy, 9, 20
  pregnancy, 16
partial nephrectomy, **51**
particle beam radiotherapy, 457–458
pathologic fractures
  breast cancer, 15
  prevention, 305
  sarcoma metastases, 217
patient education, 509–510
patient selection, allogeneic SCT, 386–387
pazopanib
  ovarian cancer, 173
  renal cell carcinoma, **51**
  sarcomas, 220
  side effects, 52
PCA3 gene, 27

PCarbo-AC (regimen), breast cancer, **14**
PCV (pneumococcal conjugate vaccine), 410
PCV regimen, **247**, 250
PD-1 checkpoint inhibitors
 non-small cell lung carcinoma, 74
 ovarian cancer, 176
 side effects, 53
PD-L1, melanoma, 205
PD-L1 inhibitor, breast cancer, 21
pectinate line, anal canal, *165*
pediatric regimens in adults, acute lymphoblastic
  leukemia, 329
peg-asparaginase, side effects, **326**
pegylated interferon α
 essential thrombocythemia, 283
 polycythemia vera, 282
pegylated liposomal doxorubicin, breast cancer, **13**
Pel–Ebstein fever, 356
pellagra, 256
pelvis, computed tomography, prostate cancer, 27
pembrolizumab
 bladder cancer, 38, **39**, **42**
 liver cancer, 89
 lung cancer, 74, 75, **76**, 77
 melanoma, 211
 mesothelioma, 84
 ovarian cancer, 176
pemetrexed
 lung cancer, 73, 74, **75**
 mesothelioma, 83, 84, 85, 87
 nutrition and, **533**
percutaneous coronary intervention, 494
perforation, esophageal cancer, 147
perianal skin, squamous cell carcinomas, 153, 158
pericardial effusion, 70, *499*
 drugs causing, **492**
 management, 495
pericarditis
 drugs causing, **492**
 management, 495
perihilar cholangiocarcinomas, 101
peripheral blood stem cells, 387
 graft failure, 389
peripheral nerve sheath tumors, *472*
peripheral neuropathy *see* neuropathy
peritoneum
 chemotherapy
  hyperthermic, 83
  ovarian cancer, 172, 173, 177
 gastric cancer, 134
permanent implants, brachytherapy, 458
pernicious anemia, gastric cancer, 132
pertussis, vaccines, 410
pertuzumab, breast cancer, 11, **13**
Peter's criteria, cervical cancer, 197
phenytoin, drug reaction, 345, 355
pheochromocytomas, **257**

PHI (test for prostate cancer), 27
Philadelphia chromosome, 271
 acute lymphoblastic leukemia, imatinib, 329
phlebotomy, polycythemia vera, 281
phlegmasia cerulea dolens, 437, 441
phobias, **503**
phosphatidylinositol-3 kinase inhibitors *see* idelalisib
phosphorus levels, tumor lysis syndrome, **427**
photocoagulation, uveal melanoma, 481
PI3K/AKT inhibition, ovarian cancer, 175
PIK3CA mutations, 102
pilocytic astrocytomas, 244, 245, 249
pineal gland, primitive neuroectodermal tumor, 477
plaque brachytherapy, uveal melanoma, 475, 481,
  482
plasma cell disorders, 298–307, *see also* multiple
  myeloma *and specific disorders*
 autologous stem cell transplantation for, 379–384
  evidence, 384
  guidelines, 383–384
  multiple myeloma, 303
 diagnosis, 301–303
 guidelines, 306
 prognosis, 305–306
 treatment, 303–305
plasma cell leukemia, **299**
plasma cells, malignant, *307*
plasmacytomas, **299**, 303
plasmapheresis, 305
platelet recovery, 387
platelet transfusion, acute myeloid leukemia, **314**
platinum-based chemotherapy, *see also*
   cisplatin-based combination chemotherapy
 non-small cell lung carcinoma, 73
 side effects, 177
platinum-free interval, ovarian cancer, 174
PLCO trial, 31
plerixafor, stem cell mobilization, 380, 381
pleural tumors
 imaging, **451**
 mesothelioma, 79–81
pleurectomy with decortication, 84
pneumococcal conjugate, 410
Pneumocystis pneumonia
 prophylaxis, **247**, 248, **395**, 405–406, 429
 stem cell transplantation, 388, **395**, 405–406
pneumonectomy, extrapleural, 84, 87
pneumonia, *see also Pneumocystis* pneumonia
 aspiration, esophageal cancer, 146
 computed tomography, *432*
 viral infections, 408
pneumonitis
 allogeneic stem cell transplantation, 389
 from immunotherapy, 76
 mTOR inhibitors, 52–53
 radiation, 85
 sirolimus, 396

POEMS (syndrome), **299**
polio vaccine, 410
poly (ADP-ribose) polymerase inhibitors, ovarian
    cancer, 173, 174, 175
polyclonal gammopathies, 301
polycystic ovarian syndrome
    endometrial cancer risk, 182
    ovarian cancer risk, 167
polycythemia vera (PV), 271, 272
    diagnosis, 274, **275**
    guidelines, 287
    masked, 280
    perioperative management, 285
    prognosis, 286
    thrombotic risk, 278
    treatment, 281–282
        pregnancy, 284
polymerase chain reaction (PCR)
    Oncotype DX®, 8, 10, 16
    PAM50, 8
    respiratory viral infections, 408
polyps, see also papillary tumors
    cervix, 196
    colorectal, 119
    endometrial, 184
    familial adenomatous polyposis, 127
polystyrene sulfonate, tumor lysis syndrome, **428**
pomalidomide
    plasma cell disorders, **304**
    primary myelofibrosis, 284
ponatinib, chronic myelogenous leukemia, 280
portal vein, pancreas cancer, 115
posaconazole
    acute myeloid leukemia, **313**
    allogeneic stem cell transplantation, **395**
    neutropenic fever prevention, 429
positron emission tomography
    endometrial cancer recurrence, 190
    lung cancer, 71
    neuroendocrine tumors, 263
positron emission tomography/CT, 449
    anal cancer, 158
    chronic lymphocytic leukemia, 335
    esophageal cancer, 144
    head and neck cancer, 233
    Hodgkin lymphoma, **358**
    mesothelioma, 82
    non-Hodgkin lymphomas, 349
    orthopedic tumors, 467
    testicular cancer, 63
posterior fossa syndrome, 562
posterior fossa tumors, 565
    presentation, 558
postmenopausal bleeding, endometrial cancer, 185
post-remission therapy, acute myeloid leukemia,
    313
post-thrombotic syndrome, 438

post-transplant lymphoproliferative disorders, 390
    Epstein–Barr virus, 343–344
    plasma cell disorders vs, 301
    primary CNS lymphoma, 365, 371
potassium levels, tumor lysis syndrome, **427**
PPoma, 262
prednisone
    for hypercalcemia, 425
    side effects, **326**
pregnancy
    acute myeloid leukemia, 315
    anticoagulants, 443
    breast cancer treatment, 15–16
    cardiotoxicity and, 496
    cervical cancer, 199
    colorectal cancer, 126
    esophageal cancer, 148
    gliomas, 248
    Hodgkin lymphoma, ABVD, 360
    ibrutinib and idelalisib, 339
    myeloproliferative neoplasms, 284–285
    radiotherapy, 460
    thyroid cancer, 226
    uveal melanoma, 482
primary central nervous system lymphoma, 364–375
    children, 547
    diagnosis, 365–368
    evidence, 373
    guidelines, 372–373
    pathology, 374
    prognosis, 371–372
    stem cell transplantation, 401–402
    treatment, 368–371
primary leptomeningeal lymphomatosis, treatment,
    370, 371
primary mediastinal B-cell lymphoma, 355
primary myelofibrosis (PMF), 271, 272
    diagnosis, 276
    essential thrombocythemia vs, 280
    guidelines, 287
    prognosis, 278, 286
    treatment, 283–284
primary sclerosing cholangitis (PSC), 102, 103, 104
primitive neuroectodermal tumors (PNET), 556
    dissemination, 560
    pathology, 557
    pineal gland, 477
    treatment, **562**
Prinzmetal angina, **125**, 161
procarbazine
    brain tumors, **247**
    nutrition and, **533**
prochlorperazine, 522
progesterone receptors (PR)
    breast cancer, 10
        pathways, 22
progestins, endometrial cancer and, 183, **188**

programmed death ligand 1, melanoma, 205
progression-free survival (PFS), primary CNS
  lymphoma, 372
promyelocytes, acute promyelocytic leukemia, *318*
propofol, **508**
prostate cancer, *23–31*
  bone metastases, 464
  diagnosis, 25–27
  evidence, 31
  guidelines, 31
  imaging, **451**
  radiotherapy, 29, *461*
  risk assessments, **28**
  screening, 25, 26, 27, 30, 31, 515–516, **536**
  survivorship guidelines, 540
  treatment, 27–30
prostate cancer gene 3, 27
prostatectomy (radical), 28, 30
  side effects, 29
prostate-specific antigen (PSA), **25**, 26, 27, 30, 516
proteasome inhibitors, plasma cell disorders, **304**
PROTECHT (trial), 445
proteinuria, 218
  bevacizumab, 52
proton beam therapy, 457–458
  prostate cancer, 29
  uveal melanoma, 481
pseudoachalasia, 133
pseudohypopyon, *484*
pseudoprogression, brain tumors, 243
psychological dimensions, 501–513
  cancer survivors, 538
psychological symptoms, testicular cancer, 62
psychostimulants, **505**, 523–524
psychotherapies, 509–510
PTEN mutation, gliomas, 245
PTHrPomas, **257**
pulmonary embolism, 439, 440, 441
pulmonary function tests, 144, *see also* bleomycin
  allogeneic stem cell transplantation, 389
pulsus paradoxus, 70

QT prolongation
  drugs causing, **491**
  management, 495
  monitoring, 492
QUASAR trial, 129
quetiapine, **508**

rabbit ATG, **396**
radiation
  acute myeloid leukemia from, 309
  myelodysplastic syndromes from, 289
radiation pneumonitis, 85
radical cystectomy, 37, **39**, 40
radical nephrectomy, 49, **51**
radical pleurectomy, 84

radical prostatectomy, 28, 30
  side effects, 29
radioactive iodine (RAI)
  ablation, 225, 226
  follow-up scanning, 227
  uptake, 224
radiofrequency ablation, liver cancer, side effects, 96
radiopaque markers, 456
radiopharmaceuticals
  diagnostic, 448, *see also* nuclear medicine
  therapeutic, 458–459
radiotherapy, 454–462, *see also* whole brain
      radiotherapy
  acute lymphoblastic leukemia, **326**
  bladder cancer, 37–38, **39**
  breast cancer, 10, 19
    bone metastases, 15
    brain metastases, 15
  breast cancer risk from, 5
  cardiotoxicity follow-up, 496
  childhood tumors requiring, **551**
    brain tumors, **562**
  complications, 460
  Ewing sarcoma, 469, **551**
  for gastric cancer, **136**
  gastric cancer from, 132
  guidelines, 461
  for mesothelioma, 84
  mesothelioma from, 80
  non-small cell lung carcinoma, 72–73
  prostate cancer, 29, *461*
  retinopathy, 481, 482
  sarcomas, 216, 217
  small cell lung carcinoma, 71
  for spinal cord compression, 433
  total body irradiation, 387, 390, **395**
  whole brain, primary CNS lymphoma, **369**, **370**,
      371, 373, 401
radium-223, prostate cancer, 27, 29
Rai Stage Classification, chronic lymphocytic
      leukemia, **336**
ramucirumab
  liver cancer, 89, **96**, 99
  non-small cell lung carcinoma, 74
  side effects, 96
ranpirnase, 156
RAS mutations
  colorectal cancer, 123–124, 127
  thyroid cancer, 222
rasburicase, 427, **428**
Rb mutation, brain tumors, 242
RB1 gene, 474
R-CHOP, non-Hodgkin lymphomas, 351
reactive lymphocytosis, 320
reactive oxygen species, melanoma, 205
RECIST (Response Evaluation Criteria In Solid
      Tumors), 450

rectum
carcinoid tumors, 259
squamous cell carcinomas, 153
recurrence, *see also* relapse therapy; second primary
tumors
colorectal cancer, 127
head and neck cancer, 236
ovarian cancer, 174–175, **177**
screening for, 537
recurrence score, Oncotype DX®, 8
recurrent laryngeal nerve injury, 225
recurrent venous thromboembolism, 444
treatment, **442**, **443**
red cell mass, polycythemia vera, **275**
red flag symptoms, brain tumors, 244
red meat, colorectal cancer risk, 119
reduced intensity regimens, myeloablative, 387,
395, 397, 400
Reed–Sternberg cells, 355
Reese–Ellsworth classification, 477
REG3α (GVHD biomarker), 416
regorafenib
colorectal cancer, **125**, 129
liver cancer, 89, **96**, 99
nutrition and, **533**
side effects, 96
relapse therapy, **327**, 328, *see also* recurrence, acute
lymphoblastic leukemia
renal cancer, 43–55
diagnosis, 46–49
evidence, 55
guidelines, 55
imaging, **451**
screening, 45–46
treatment, 49–54
renal cell carcinoma
chemotherapy, 50–51, 53
hereditary leiomyomatosis and, 44
metastases, 50
prognosis, 54
sporadic, 45
renal clearance, for plerixafor dosing, 381
renal failure, *see also* acute kidney injury; renal
tubular dysfunction
anticoagulants, 443
prevention, 305, 383
renal medullary carcinoma, 54
renal transplant
EBV nucleic acid testing, 343–344
primary CNS lymphoma, 365
renal tubular dysfunction, 563
respiratory viral infections, stem cell transplantation,
408
Response Evaluation Criteria In Solid Tumors
(RECIST), 450
retinal pigmented epithelium, congenital
hypertrophy, 475

retinoblastoma, 473, 474
diagnosis, 475–479
follow-up, 483
guidelines, 483–484
presentation, 545
prognosis, 482–483
pseudohypopyon, *484*
treatment, 479–482, **550**
retinopathy, 479
radiotherapy, 481, 482
retroperitoneal lymph node dissection, 62, 64
rhabdomyosarcoma, 219
chemotherapy, 217, **549**
genitourinary, 545
orbital, 545
surgery, **550**
ribavirin, 408
ribociclib, breast cancer, 12
Richter transformation, 340
risk of ovarian cancer algorithm (ROCA), 169
risperidone, **508**
ritonavir, Hodgkin lymphoma, 361
rituximab
infusion reaction, 339, 351
lymphomas, **551**
non-Hodgkin lymphomas, 350
primary CNS lymphoma, 368
R-MPV (regimen), primary CNS lymphoma, **369**,
370, 373
ROS gene, non-small cell lung carcinoma, 73
Rosai–Dorfman syndrome, 345
RTOG 1016 (trial), 236
rucaparib, ovarian cancer, 175
ruxolitinib
polycythemia vera, 282
primary myelofibrosis, 283–284

sadness, 502
saline
for hypercalcemia, 424
tumor lysis syndrome, 426
salivary gland dysfunction, 237
salpingo-oophorectomy, prophylactic, 6, 169
salt, gastric cancer, 132
sarcoidosis, 344
brain, 367
sarcomas, 214–220, 463–470, *see also* Ewing
sarcoma; osteosarcomas; rhabdomyosarcoma
children, 214, 216, 218–219
types, 543
diagnosis, 215–216
evidence, 220
guidelines, 220
prevention, 215
renal, 46
treatment, 216–219
uterine, 184

sarcopenia, 515
Schistosoma haematobium, 33
scleromyxedema, 301
screening
    anal cytology, 156
    breast cancer, 6, 360, 516, **536**, *see also*
        mammography
    cancer survivors, 536–537
    cervical cancer, 195, 516
    colorectal cancer, 120–121, 516, **536**
    Epstein–Barr virus, 343–344
    esophageal cancer, 141
    gastric cancer, 132
    hepatocellular carcinoma, 90–91
    imaging, 449
    lung cancer, 68, 516
    melanoma, 206
    older people, 515–516
    ovarian cancer, 169
    prostate cancer, 25, 26, 27, 30, 31, 515–516,
        536
    renal cancer, 45–46
second primary tumors, 536
    head and neck cancer, 238
    proton beam therapy and, 457
    retinoblastoma, 481–482
secondary malignancies
    allogeneic stem cell transplantation, 390
    Hodgkin lymphoma, 360
Sedlis criteria, cervical cancer, 197
seizures, prophylaxis, **395**
selective serotonin reuptake inhibitors, 265, **504**,
    505
self-examination, breast, 6
seminomas, 56, 57, 61
senna, 522
sentinel node biopsy
    breast cancer, 9
    melanoma, 210–211, 212
serotonin, 256
serous carcinoma, ovary, 166
sertraline, **505**
serum free light chain analysis (FLC), 303
serum sickness, drug reactions, 345
17p deletion, CLL, prognosis, 352
sex cord stromal tumors, 56
shared care of survivors, **539**
siblings, allogeneic SCT, 386
sickle cell disease, 54
sigmoidoscopy, 120, 124
silver sulfadiazine cream, anal cancer treatment,
    161
simian virus 40 large-tumor antigen, 80
simulations, radiotherapy, 455
sinus histiocytosis with massive lymphadenopathy,
    345
sinusitis, CLL and, 333

sinusoidal obstruction syndrome (VOD), 388, 414
sipuleucel-T, prostate cancer, 27, 29
sirolimus, **396**
    pneumonitis, 396
Sister Mary Joseph node, gastric cancer, 133
skeletal-related events (SRE), breast cancer, 14–15
skin
    acute myeloid leukemia, 310
    allogeneic stem cell transplantation, 390
    graft versus host disease
        biopsy, 416
        rashes, 414, **415**, *419*
    melanoma, 206, 207, 208
    non-Hodgkin lymphomas, 345
    squamous cell carcinomas, 153, 158, 208, 212
slit lamp examination *see* ocular slit lamp
        examination
small bowel carcinoids, 258, 259, 260, 261
small bowel malignant tumors, imaging, **451**
small cell carcinomas
    bladder, 40
    lung (SCLC), 71–72
small lymphocytic lymphoma, 332
    stem cell transplantation, 402
smoking, 536
    acute myeloid leukemia, 309
    bladder cancer, 32, 33
    cervical cancer, 195
    colorectal cancer risk, 119
    esophageal cancer, 140
    head and neck cancer, 230, 231, 238
    lung cancer, 67, 68
    ovarian cancer risk, 167
    pancreas cancer, 112, 113
    prostate cancer, 24, 29
    renal cancer, 44, 45
smoldering multiple myeloma, **298**, 300, **301**
soft tissue tumors (orthopedic), 463–470
    diagnosis, 465–467
    guidelines, 470–471
    treatment, 467–470
Sokal score, CML, 278
soluble fiber, 528
somatostatin analogs, 264, **265**, 266
somatostatin receptor scintigraphy (SSRS), 260, 262
somatostatinomas, **257**
somatuline (lanreotide), 264, **265**
sorafenib
    FLT3 positive patients, 394
    liver cancer, 89, **96**, 98
    nutrition and, **533**
    renal cell carcinoma, **51**
    side effects, 52, 96
    thyroid cancer, 225, 228
sore throat, 233
sperm banking, 284, **314**, 360
spermatocele, 58

spinal cord compression, 432–434
  prostate cancer, 28
  sarcomas, 217
spindle-A cell melanoma, uveal, 476
spine, surgery, plasma cell disorders, **305**
spironolactone, 493
splanchnic venous thrombosis, 435
splenectomy, primary myelofibrosis, 284
splenomegaly
  causes, 278
  non-Hodgkin lymphomas, 346
squamous cell carcinomas
  anus, 154, 155, 158
  bladder, 40
  esophagus, 140
  head and neck, 230–240
  lung, 67
  rectum, 153
  skin, 153, 158, 208, 212
ST2 (GVHD biomarker), 416
stage migration strategy, liver cancer, **94**, 97
stem cell mobilization, 380–381
  granulocyte colony-stimulating factor, 380,
    387
Stem Cell Transplant Comorbidity Index, 393
Stem Cell Transplant Outcomes Database, 385
stem cell transplantation, *see also* allogeneic stem
    cell transplantation; autologous stem cell
    transplantation; transplantation *under* bone
    marrow
  chronic lymphocytic leukemia, 337, 339, 402
  costs, 289
  EBV nucleic acid testing, 344
  infections, 388, 396–397, 404–411
stents, coronary, 494, 495
stereotactic radiosurgery, 456–457
stereotyped chronic lymphocytic leukemia, 333
steroids
  acute lymphoblastic leukemia, 319, 323
  anorexia–cachexia syndrome, 524–525
  brain tumors, 248
  on fatigue, 524
  graft versus host disease, 388, 416, **417**
  for hypercalcemia, 425
  hyperglycemia, 530
  plasma cell disorders, **304**
  primary CNS lymphoma, 368, **370**
  spinal cord compression, 433
  weight gain, 530
stimulant bowel regimens, 522
stomach
  cancer. *see* gastric cancer
  carcinoid tumors, 258, 259
stool tests
  colorectal cancer, 120, 516
  infections, 416
strain rate imaging *see* global longitudinal strain

strictures
  esophagus, 143
  ureter, 199
stroke, acute lymphoblastic leukemia, 327
subsegmental pulmonary embolism, 439
suicide risk, 503–504, **506**
sun protection measures, 206
sunitinib
  nutrition and, **533**
  renal cell carcinoma, 50, **51**
  side effects, 52
superficial spreading melanoma, 204
superior mesenteric vessels, pancreas cancer, 115
superior sulcus tumor, 69
superior vena cava obstruction, 69
  acute lymphoblastic leukemia, 327
supraclavicular adenopathy, colorectal cancer, 122
suprasellar tumors, *565*
  presentation, 558
supratentorial tumors, presentation, 558
surgery, *see also specific resections*
  childhood tumors requiring, **550–551**
  myeloproliferative neoplasms, 285
  oropharyngeal cancer, 236
  orthopedic tumors, 217, **469**
  spine, plasma cell disorders, **305**
surgical staging, endometrial cancer, 188
surprise question, 520
survivorship, 535–542
  cancer types in cancer survivors, *542*
  care plans, 538
  guidelines, 540–541
symptom management, palliative care, 521–525
systemic lupus erythematosus, 345

T1 tumors, bladder, 35
TACE (transarterial chemoembolization), 96, 99
tacrolimus, GVHD prevention, 413
tacrolimus CIV, **395**
Takotsubo cardiomyopathy, **125**, 161
talc pleurodesis, 83
tamoxifen
  breast cancer, 9, 10, 19
  endometrial cancer risk, 182
  nutrition and, **533**
  ovarian cancer, **175**
tandem transplant (ASCT), 381
TAS-102 (drug), **125**
taxanes, side effects, 177
TBC (regimen), primary CNS lymphoma, **370**, 373
T-cell acute lymphoblastic leukemia, 319
  lymphoid progenitor markers, 320
  management, **325**
T-cell depletion, 413
T-cell lymphoma
  primary CNS lymphoma, 368
  stem cell transplantation, 402–403

TDM-1 (trastuzumab emtansine), breast cancer, 11, **13**, 21
temozolomide, brain tumors, **246**, **247**, 248, 250, 251
TEMPI syndrome, **299**
temporal lobe, tumor presentation, 559
temporary implants, brachytherapy, 459
temsirolimus
  renal cell carcinoma, 50, **51**
  side effects, 52–53
teratogenicity, 284, 315
teratoid rhabdoid tumors (atypical), 557
  radiotherapy, **562**
teratomas, 62
TERT gene
  lung cancer, 67
  promoter mutation, gliomas, 245
testicular cancer, 56–65
  diagnosis, 59–60
  evidence, 64
  guidelines, 64
  imaging, **451**
  prognosis, 63
  treatment, 60–63
testicular radiation, ALL, **326**
testosterone, target level, prostate cancer metastases, 30
tetanus, diphtheria, acellular pertussis (vaccine), 410
tetrahydrocannabinol (THC), **247**
TH (regimen), breast cancer, **13**
TH3RESA (trial), 21
thalidomide
  plasma cell disorders, **304**
  primary myelofibrosis, 284
  thromboprophylaxis for, 437
therapeutics-related cardiac dysfunction, 486
13q deletion, chronic lymphocytic leukemia, 352
thoracentesis, 83
Thorotrast, 80
THP (regimen), breast cancer, **13**
three-dimensional conformal radiotherapy, 455
  image-guided, 456
  prostate cancer, *461*
three-hole esophagectomy, **147**
thrombectomy, **442**
thrombocytopenia
  heparin-induced, 444
  VTE treatment, **442**
thrombocytosis
  cancer-related thrombosis, 439
  causes, 277
  cervical cancer, 196
  diagnosis, **273**
thrombolysis, **440**
thromboprophylaxis, 437, *see also* anticoagulants

thrombosis, 435–446
  bevacizumab, 52
  causes, 277, 280
  drugs causing, **492**
  evidence, 445
  guidelines, 445
  management, 495
thrombotic microangiopathy, transplant-associated, 396
thymomas
  chronic lymphocytic leukemia *vs*, 335
  imaging, **450**
  mesothelioma *vs*, 81
thymus, carcinoid tumors, 258
thyroid adenoma, 223
thyroid cancer, 221–229
  diagnosis, 223–225
  evidence, 228
  guidelines, 228
  prevention, 222
  prognosis, 227
  treatment, 225–227
thyroid hormone replacement, **225**
thyroid stimulating hormone, 223, 225, 238
thyroidectomy, 225, **226**
tinzaparin, **442**
tissue markers, liver cancer, 91
TMPRSS2 gene, prostate cancer, 24
TNM staging
  colorectal cancer, **123**
  gastric cancer, **134**
topoisomerase inhibitors, 488, *499*
  acute myeloid leukemia from, 309
topotecan
  extensive SCLC, 72
  ovarian cancer, **175**
torsade de pointes, drugs causing, **491–492**
total abdominal hysterectomy/bilateral salpingo-oophorectomy, 169
total body irradiation, 387, 390, **395**
toxocariasis, ocular, 476
toxoplasmosis, 243, 367, 368
TP53 gene, ovarian cancer risk, *180*
tracheoesophageal fistula, 146, **147**
trametinib, melanoma, 211
transarterial chemoembolization, liver cancer, 96, 99
transfusions
  acute myeloid leukemia, **314**
  criteria, **395**
trans-hiatal esophagectomy, **147**
transitional cell carcinomas, *see also* urothelial cancer
  kidney, 43, **47**, 48, 50
  metastases, 51
  nephroureterectomy, **51**
transitional zone, anal canal, *165*
translocations, B-cell lymphoma, 343

transoral robotic surgery, oropharyngeal cancer, 236
transplant-associated thrombotic microangiopathy, 396
transpupillary thermal therapy, 481
transurethral resection of bladder tumor (TURBT), 34, 35
trastuzumab, *see also* TDM-1
  breast cancer, 5, 11, **13**, 20
  cardiotoxicity, 10, 15, 489
    treatment algorithm, **494**
  gastric cancer, **136**
treatment planning (radiotherapy), 455
  adaptive planning, 457
treatment response, imaging, 449–450
treatment specific management, cancer survivors, **539**
treatment summaries, 538
tricyclic antidepressants, **505**
trifluridine-tipiracil, side effects, **125**
trilateral retinoblastoma, 477
trimethoprim-sulfamethoxazole (Bactrim; co-trimoxazole), 406, 429
  allogeneic stem cell transplantation, **395**
triple negative breast cancer (TNBC), **4**, 11
  metastases, 12
troponin I, 492
tryptophan, 256
TTFields, glioblastoma treatment, **247**, 250
tuberculomas, cerebral, 367
tuberin, 44
tuberous sclerosis, 242
tuberous sclerosis complex, 44
tumefactive multiple sclerosis, 243, 245
tumor lysis syndrome (TLS), 319, 327, 425–428
tumor markers
  biliary tract carcinoma, 105
  brain tumors, 560
  breast cancer, 8
  children, 546
  colorectal cancer, 123
  liver cancer, 91
  neuroendocrine tumors, **259**, 260, 262, 266
  testicular cancer, 58, 59, 60, **61**
tumor necrosis, carcinoid tumors, 265
tumor suppressor genes, biliary tract carcinoma and, 103
tumor thrombus, 438, 440
tumor-treating fields *see* TTFields
Turcot syndrome, 242
T-VEC (modified herpes virus), 211
twins, acute lymphoblastic leukemia, 320
typhlitis, 414
tyramine, foods with, **533**
tyrosine kinase inhibitors, *see also* ibrutinib
  brain metastases, **247**
  chronic myelogenous leukemia, 280–281
    resistance, **275**

metastatic non-small cell lung carcinoma, 73
  side effects, 225, 226
  thyroid cancer, 226
  VEGF tyrosine kinase inhibitors, side effects, 52

ulcers
  cervix, 196
  melanoma staging, 209
  oral, mTOR inhibitors, 53
ultrasound, 447
  breast, 6
  endometrial cancer, 187
  gastric cancer, 134, **135**
  liver screening, 449
  thyroid cancer, 222, 224
ultraviolet radiation, melanoma, 205
umbilical cord units, cord blood, 387
understaging, esophageal cancer, 145
unsealed source radiotherapy, 459
upper endoscopy, gastric cancer, 132, **135**, *138*
upper extremity thromboembolism, 437
upper gastrointestinal bleeding
  esophageal cancer, 146
  occult, 122, *see also* stool tests
upper respiratory tract infections
  chronic lymphocytic leukemia and, 333
  stem cell transplantation, 408
urachus, cancer from, 40
ureterectomy, **52**
ureteric obstruction
  bladder cancer, 39
  prostate cancer, 28
ureteroscopy, renal cancer, 48
ureterovaginal fistula, 199
ureters, stricture, 199
uric acid, tumor lysis syndrome, 426, **427**, **428**
urinary diversion, 37
urinary tract tumors, imaging, **451**
urothelial cancer, 32, 33, *see also* transitional cell carcinomas
ursodiol, hepatic veno-occlusive disease, 388
US Preventive Services Task Force, ovarian cancer testing, 168
uterus, *see also* cervical cancer; endometrial cancer
  imaging, **452**
  sarcomas, 184
uveal melanoma, 473, 474
  diagnosis, 475–479
  follow-up, 483
  guidelines, 483–484
  immunohistochemistry, *484*
  prevention, 475
  treatment, 479–482

vaccination
  human papillomavirus (HPV), 155–156
  for plasma cell disorders, **304**

pneumococcal conjugate, 410
  stem cell transplantation, 390–391, 410
valacyclovir, 407
valganciclovir, 407
vancomycin, 430
vandetanib, thyroid cancer, 225, 228
varicella, vaccination, 410
varicocele, 58
Varivax, 410
VEGF monoclonal antibodies, side effects, 52
VEGF pathway inhibitors
  clear cell renal cell carcinoma, 50
  proteinuria, 218
VEGF tyrosine kinase inhibitors (VEGF TKIs), *see also*
      tyrosine kinase inhibitors
  side effects, 52
vemurafenib, melanoma, 211, **247**
venlafaxine, **505**
veno-occlusive disease (VOD), hepatic, 388, 414
venous thromboembolism, 435–436, 438–439, 444
  drugs causing, **492**
  evidence, 445
  guidelines, 445
  management, 495
  treatment, **442–443**
vesicovaginal fistula, 199
VHL (gene), 44
vinblastine, nutrition and, **533**
vincristine
  nutrition and, **533**
  R-CHOP and, 351
  side effects, **326**
vinorelbine
  breast cancer, **12**
  lung cancer, **76**
  mesothelioma, 84
  ovarian cancer, **175**
VIPomas, **257**
viral infections, *see also* Epstein–Barr virus; herpes
      simplex virus infection; human papillomavirus
  graft versus host disease *vs*, 414
  stem cell transplantation, 406–408
Virchow node, gastric cancer, 133
Virchow's triad, 436
viscosity (serum), 302

VitalTalk, 526
vitamin B6, **532**, **533**
vitamin B12, pemetrexed with, **533**
vitamin D
  colorectal cancer and, 121
  zoledronic acid with, **533**
vitamin K, 443
vitamin K antagonists, **442**, 443
vitrectomy, 368
vomiting, 522–523
  graft versus host disease, 414
  nutritional management, 528
von Hippel–Lindau (VHL), 44
voriconazole, 409, 429

waist *see* abdominal diameter
wakefulness-promoting psychostimulant, 524
Waldenström macroglobulinemia, **299**, 303
warfarin, 443
  bleeding, 443
Watchman device, 495
weight gain, steroids, 530
weight loss
  chronic lymphocytic leukemia, 334, 335
  Hodgkin lymphoma, 356
  nutritional management, 529–530
whole brain radiotherapy (WBRT), primary CNS
      lymphoma, **369**, **370**, 371, 373, 401
Wilms tumor, 53, *554*
  staging, 546
  treatment, **550**, **551**

xerostomia, 237, 530–531
X-rays
  bone tumors, 467, 546
  radiotherapy, 455

yolk sac tumors, 57, 62

zinc sulfate, 530
zoledronic acid, 14–15, 29
  for hypercalcemia, 425
  nutrition and, **533**
  plasma cell disorders, **304**
Zollinger–Ellison syndrome, 256, **257**, 261